Cutting-Edge Strategies and Applications of Neuropedagogy

Driss Elomari
Sidi Mohamed Ben Abdellah Fez University, Morocco

Neriman Aral
Ankara University, Turkey

Bayram Deleş
Erzincan Binali Yıldırım University, Turkey

Mostafa Bouanani
Sidi Mohamed Ben Abdellah University, Morocco

IGI Global
Scientific Publishing
Publishing Tomorrow's Research Today

Vice President of Editorial Melissa Wagner
Director of Acquisitions Mikaela Felty
Director of Book Development Jocelynn Hessler
Production Manager Mike Brehm
Cover Design Jose Rosado

Published in the United States of America by
IGI Global Scientific Publishing
701 East Chocolate Avenue
Hershey, PA, 17033, USA
Tel: 717-533-8845 | Fax: 717-533-7115
Website: https://www.igi-global.com E-mail: cust@igi-global.com

Library of Congress Cataloging-in-Publication Data

CIP Data Pending

ISBN13: 9798337335810
Isbn13Softcover: 9798337335827
EISBN13: 9798337335834

British Cataloguing in Publication Data
A Cataloguing in Publication record for this book is available from the British Library.

Editorial Advisory Board

Table of Contents

Detailed Table of Contents

Test anxiety significantly affects students' academic performance and mental well-being, yet a psychometrically validated Arabic version of the Test Anxiety Inventory (TAI) for African contexts has been lacking. This study examined the factorial structure and psychometric properties of the Arabic TAI among 578 Moroccan preparatory school students (aged 12–17) from Sidi Boumedine School in Séfrou. The scale was translated using a forward–backward procedure and analyzed through Exploratory and Confirmatory Factor Analyses, Pearson correlations, and reliability testing. Results supported a two-factor structure reflecting cognitive anxiety and physical symptoms, yielding a refined 19-item scale. The model demonstrated good fit (GFI = 0.964; SRMR = 0.063), excellent internal consistency ($\alpha = 0.912$; $\omega = 0.914$), and a strong correlation between factors (r = 0.77, p < 0.001). These findings confirm the Arabic TAI as a valid and reliable tool for assessing test anxiety among Moroccan students and represent the first psychometric validation of this measure in an African educational context.

The rapid rise of social media platforms has reshaped communication patterns across the globe, and the Arabic-speaking world is no exception. This paper explores the phenomenon of foreignization through the increasing integration of English lexical borrowings in Arabic social media discourse. Additionally, the paper, which follows a quantitative approach, examines the sociocultural and linguistic implications of using these loanwords, especially in the context of code-switching and the adaptation of foreign terms into the Arabic lexicon. Through this exploration, the research seeks to understand the broader impact of English borrowings on Arabic language evolution in digital spaces and the potential long-term consequences for cultural and linguistic identity. It is hoped that this paper will be followed by a more elaborate study on borrowing from English and other languages in conversational Arabic in the Arabian Peninsula to be carried out from a Cognitive Linguistic perspective.

Research indicates therapeutic benefits of robots for children with autism; however, the potential of similar agents, such as puppets, needs to be investigated. Because puppets have been proven to capture and hold the attention of children with autism spectrum disorder, indicating the potential for alternative therapies that improve social engagement and aid learning. According to research, when a puppet speaks, children with autism spectrum disorder's attention patterns are similar to those of typically developing children and both groups exhibit a pronounced preference for the talking puppet over the listening person. In this study, we highlight the attentional and emotional benefits of puppets, which ideally can be used. In particular, in our study, Karagöz-Hacivat performance has been organised to help with therapeutic efforts. Our findings indicate that shadow play characters could be an effective tool for assisting children with autism spectrum disorder in improving their social engagement, which is quite exciting.

This study explores the integration of motivational principles derived from NeuroLearning into Applied Behavior Analysis (ABA) interventions to enhance the verbal communication skills of autistic children in Morocco. By leveraging insights from neuroscience, this approach optimizes learning environments through tailored motivational strategies, thereby increasing engagement and participation. The research involved 30 autistic children aged 4 to 10 years, comparing a control group receiving traditional ABA therapy with an experimental group exposed to NeuroLearning-enhanced ABA interventions. The findings demonstrate a significant improvement in verbal communication skills, with a 30% increase in VB-MAPP (Verbal Behavior Milestones Assessment and Placement Program) scores within the experimental group, particularly in areas such as requesting, seeking help, and asking for breaks. These results highlight the value of interdisciplinary approaches that combine neuroscience and behavioral science to refine educational practices for children with autism spectrum disorder (ASD).

This chapter examines how neuropedagogy and digital innovation can transform education for dyslexic learners. Drawing on cognitive neuroscience, it highlights how digital tools such as text-to-speech, adaptive learning, and AI-driven applications provide alternative cognitive pathways, enhancing inclusion and learner autonomy. The chapter also discusses the evolving role of teachers as mediators, the challenges

This chapter examines play in early childhood through a neuropedagogical lens, emphasizing its developmental, neuroscientific, and educational significance. Play is framed not as leisure but as a biologically grounded process that supports executive functions, self-regulation, language, memory, and social interaction by activating the prefrontal cortex, limbic system, mirror neurons, and cerebellum. While neuroscience highlights its role in synaptic plasticity, stress regulation, and emotional security, its translation into practice remains limited. Literature often notes the benefits of play but lacks frameworks linking brain-based evidence with pedagogy. To address this gap, the chapter outlines neuropedagogical principles and illustrates their application through Reggio Emilia, Tools of the Mind, and Forest School. It concludes that adoption requires neuroscience-informed teacher training, curriculum design, culturally responsive adaptations, and evidence-based assessment, positioning play as both a neurological necessity and a frontier in early childhood education.

This present chapter examines the crucial and particularly important role of emotions in the learning process, focusing on the "emotional brain" and its connection to learning, particularly in the context of paediatric oncology. The role played by emotions and the emotional state of individuals is not just a secondary factor in learning, but a critical element affecting executive functions. Brain structures play a key role in the regulation of emotion and cognitive function.The challenge in

Preface

INTRODUCTION

Education has always been both a reflection of its time and a catalyst for social transformation. As editors of *Cutting-Edge Strategies and Applications of Neuropedagogy*, we begin from the conviction that education's enduring purpose—to unlock human potential, cultivate knowledge and skills, and foster meaningful participation in society—can only be fulfilled when teaching and learning evolve in dialogue with scientific progress. Over the last century, advances in pedagogy and psychology have reshaped educational practice toward learner-centered approaches. In the twenty-first century, however, breakthroughs in neuroscience have opened an unprecedented window into the biological foundations of learning, giving rise to the interdisciplinary field of neuropedagogy.

Neuropedagogy brings together neuroscience, education, psychology, and cognitive science to deepen our understanding of how learning actually occurs in the brain. Research on attention, memory, emotion, motivation, and executive functions has made it clear that learning is not merely a cognitive or behavioral phenomenon but a dynamic neurobiological process shaped by complex chemical and electrical interactions. This perspective invites educators and researchers to move beyond the traditional question of *how* to teach and to ask more fundamental questions: *How does the brain learn?* and *How can this knowledge be translated into more effective, inclusive, and engaging learning environments?*

This edited volume responds directly to these questions. Our aim is to present cutting-edge neuroscientific insights in an accessible and pedagogically meaningful way, while showcasing innovative strategies and concrete applications across diverse educational contexts. The chapters collected here explore neuropedagogical principles from early childhood education to adult learning, from face-to-face classrooms to online and blended environments. Particular attention is given to diverse learner populations, including students with special educational needs, gifted learners, and individuals shaped by different cultural and educational contexts.

Throughout the book, contributors examine the foundational principles of neuropedagogy and demonstrate how these principles can be integrated into teaching and learning processes. Topics include brain-based learning strategies, the neuropedagogical use of educational technologies, the neurobiological foundations of emotional and social learning, and the ethical considerations that accompany the application of neuroscientific knowledge in education. By including perspectives and studies from contexts such as Morocco and Turkey, the volume also highlights the global relevance, diversity, and cultural sensitivity of neuropedagogical research and practice.

As editors, we see this book as both a synthesis and a bridge. It synthesizes research that has often remained fragmented across disciplines, and it bridges the persistent gap between theory and practice by emphasizing actionable strategies, case examples, and real-world applications. At the same time, it points toward emerging trends and future directions in neuropedagogy, encouraging critical inquiry, interdisciplinary collaboration, and innovation. Ethical issues—such as equity, responsible use of technology, and the careful interpretation of neuroscientific data—are addressed throughout, reflecting our belief that scientific advancement must be accompanied by ethical responsibility.

Cutting-Edge Strategies and Applications of Neuropedagogy is intended for a broad audience: educators seeking to enhance their daily practice, researchers and graduate students pursuing new lines of inquiry, instructional designers and administrators shaping learning environments, policymakers informed by evidence-based decision-making, special education professionals, and parents and lifelong learners interested in the science of learning. While these groups may approach the book from different perspectives, they are united by a shared interest in understanding learning more deeply and improving educational experiences for all learners.

We invite readers to engage with this volume as a journey—one that challenges conventional assumptions, enriches pedagogical practice with neuroscientific insight, and contributes to the creation of more effective, equitable, and engaging educational systems. By aligning education more closely with how the brain learns, we believe neuropedagogy holds the potential to shape not only the future of teaching and learning, but also the future of education itself.

ORGANIZATION OF THE BOOK

Chapter 1 addresses the critical issue of test anxiety through a neuropedagogical and psychometric lens. By validating the Arabic version of the Test Anxiety

Inventory (TAI) among Moroccan adolescents, this chapter makes a foundational contribution to educational neuroscience in African contexts. The identification of cognitive and physical dimensions of anxiety not only provides a reliable assessment tool but also reinforces the importance of understanding emotional and physiological factors that shape learning and academic performance.

Chapter 2 shifts the focus to language, cognition, and digital culture by examining English lexical borrowing in Arabic social media discourse. Through a quantitative linguistic analysis, the chapter explores how foreignization and code-switching reflect deeper cognitive, social, and identity-related processes. From a neuropedagogical standpoint, it raises important questions about language evolution, digital cognition, and the long-term implications for linguistic and cultural identity in Arabic-speaking societies.

Chapter 3 introduces an innovative and culturally grounded therapeutic approach to improving communication skills in children with autism spectrum disorder through Turkish shadow theatre. By highlighting the attentional and emotional engagement elicited by puppets, particularly the Karagöz–Hacivat tradition, the chapter demonstrates how culturally embedded, non-technological agents can activate social attention mechanisms and support learning, offering promising alternatives to conventional interventions.

Chapter 4 presents an interdisciplinary model that integrates NeuroLearning principles with Applied Behavior Analysis (ABA) to enhance verbal communication in autistic children in Morocco. By emphasizing motivation as a neurobiological driver of learning, this chapter provides compelling empirical evidence that neuroscience-informed behavioral interventions can significantly improve communication outcomes, reinforcing the value of combining brain science with established therapeutic practices.

Chapter 5 explores how neuropedagogy and digital innovation can reshape educational experiences for dyslexic learners. Drawing on cognitive neuroscience, the chapter illustrates how assistive and AI-driven technologies open alternative cognitive pathways that promote inclusion, autonomy, and personalization. It also critically examines the evolving role of teachers, professional training challenges, and ethical considerations, grounding theory in practical cases from the Moroccan context.

Chapter 6 extends the neuropedagogical discussion into early childhood education by examining the ethical and pedagogical integration of artificial intelligence. Framing early childhood as a sensitive period for brain development, the chapter proposes a five-stage intervention model enhanced by AI, while emphasizing teacher agency, family collaboration, and ethical safeguards. It positions AI-supported neuropedagogy as a forward-looking yet human-centered model for early intervention.

Chapter 7 investigates the relationship between working memory and reading comprehension among Moroccan primary school students. Using a neuropedagogical approach, the chapter highlights how cognitive processes such as phonological awareness and memory capacity directly influence reading performance. Its findings contribute to evidence-based literacy instruction and underscore the need for cognitively informed assessment and intervention strategies in primary education.

Chapter 8 reframes play in early childhood as a neurobiological necessity rather than a peripheral activity. By linking play to brain systems involved in executive function, emotional regulation, and social cognition, this chapter bridges neuroscience and pedagogy through established educational models such as Reggio Emilia and Forest School. It argues for neuroscience-informed teacher training and curriculum design to fully harness play's developmental potential.

Chapter 9 focuses on the emotional brain and its central role in learning within the highly sensitive context of pediatric cancer. The chapter underscores how emotions profoundly shape executive functions, resilience, and cognitive engagement, particularly for children facing serious illness. From a neuropedagogical perspective, it offers a structured framework for supporting emotional regulation and learning, integrating insights from neuroscience, psychology, and education.

Chapter 10 provides an empirical examination of ABA-based interventions aimed at improving verbal communication in autistic Moroccan children. By documenting gains in spontaneous speech and highlighting the necessity of repetition and follow-up, the chapter contributes valuable context-specific evidence to the literature. It reinforces the importance of sustained, culturally adapted behavioral interventions within neuropedagogical practice.

Chapter 11 offers a comprehensive review of neuroeducation as an interdisciplinary field connecting neuroscience with classroom practice. Through a systematic analysis of the literature, the chapter demonstrates how brain-based strategies enhance metacognition, learner engagement, and academic performance. It also explores the role of artificial intelligence and neurofeedback in personalized learning, positioning neuroeducation as a driver of sustainable and inclusive educational innovation.

Chapter 12 examines the neurophysiological and biochemical factors that influence learning, with particular emphasis on motivation, attention, stress, and anxiety. By clarifying how these emotional and cognitive states affect brain functioning, the chapter equips educators with a deeper understanding of individual learning differences. It reinforces the neuropedagogical imperative to address emotional regulation as an integral component of effective teaching and learning.

Chapter 13 bridges brain science and classroom practice by translating core neuroscientific principles into actionable pedagogical strategies. Addressing neuroplasticity, cognitive load, and emotional regulation, the chapter critically examines applications across educational levels while cautioning against neuromyths and inequitable implementation. It concludes with policy-oriented recommendations that position neuropedagogy as both transformative and socially just.

Chapter 14 focuses on brain-based learning in the preschool period, a time of rapid neural development. By linking neurophysiological knowledge with classroom practice, the chapter emphasizes the creation of enriched learning environments that respect individual differences. It highlights teachers' central role in applying neuropedagogical principles to unlock young children's learning potential.

CONCLUSION

As editors of *Cutting-Edge Strategies and Applications of Neuropedagogy*, we conclude this preface with a reaffirmation of the central premise that unites the contributions in this volume: education is most powerful when it is aligned with how the brain learns, develops, and adapts. The chapters brought together in this edited reference book collectively demonstrate that neuropedagogy is not a passing trend, but a robust, evidence-based framework capable of reshaping educational thought and practice across contexts, cultures, and learner populations.

Throughout the volume, contributors have shown how insights from neuroscience can illuminate the cognitive, emotional, social, and biological dimensions of learning. From early childhood and language development to special education, emotional regulation, digital innovation, and artificial intelligence, the research presented here underscores the complexity of learning as a brain-based process influenced by motivation, memory, attention, emotion, and environment. Importantly, these chapters move beyond theoretical discussion to offer empirically grounded strategies, culturally responsive applications, and practical models that educators, researchers, and policymakers can meaningfully engage with.

As editors, we are particularly encouraged by the interdisciplinary and global perspectives represented in this book. By including studies and applications from diverse contexts—such as Morocco, Turkey, and broader international frameworks—the volume highlights the necessity of situating neuropedagogical principles within cultural, linguistic, and ethical realities. This contextual sensitivity strengthens the field and guards against oversimplification, neuromyths, and one-size-fits-all approaches to brain-based education.

This book also points decisively toward the future of education. The integration of digital technologies, artificial intelligence, and data-informed interventions—when guided by ethical responsibility and pedagogical purpose—offers unprecedented opportunities for personalization, inclusion, and early intervention. At the same time, the volume consistently reminds us that human agency remains central: teachers as reflective practitioners, learners as active participants, and families and communities as essential partners in the educational process.

In closing, *Cutting-Edge Strategies and Applications of Neuropedagogy* is intended not only as a reference text, but as an invitation—to rethink teaching and learning through a neuroscientific lens, to question assumptions, to foster interdisciplinary dialogue, and to innovate responsibly. We hope this volume will inspire educators to refine their practice, researchers to pursue new questions, and policymakers to ground educational reform in scientific evidence and social equity. By bridging brain science and pedagogy, we believe this book contributes meaningfully to shaping a more effective, humane, and future-oriented vision of education.

Chapter 1

Cognitive and Physical Aspects of Test Anxiety:
Validation of the Arabic (TAI) Among Moroccan Students

Amine Khadraoui
https://orcid.org/0009-0000-4833-6839

Laboratory of Educational Sciences, Philosophy and Humanities, Higher School of Teachers (ENS), Moulay Ismail University, Meknes, Morocco

Abdellah Barebzi

Laboratory of Educational Sciences, Philosophy and Humanities, Higher School of Teachers (ENS), Moulay Ismail University, Meknes, Morocco

Driss Elomari
https://orcid.org/0000-0001-5846-8501

Laboratory of Language Sciences, Literature, Arts, Communication, History, and Education, National School of Business and Management, Sidi Mohamed Ben Abdellah University, Fez, Morocco

ABSTRACT

Test anxiety significantly affects students' academic performance and mental well-being, yet a psychometrically validated Arabic version of the Test Anxiety Inventory (TAI) for African contexts has been lacking. This study examined the factorial structure and psychometric properties of the Arabic TAI among 578 Moroccan preparatory school students (aged 12–17) from Sidi Boumedine School in Séfrou. The scale was translated using a forward–backward procedure and analyzed through Exploratory and Confirmatory Factor Analyses, Pearson correlations, and reliability testing. Results supported a two-factor structure reflecting cognitive anxiety and physical symptoms, yielding a refined 19-item scale. The model demonstrated good fit (GFI

DOI: 10.4018/979-8-3373-3581-0.ch001

= 0.964; SRMR = 0.063), excellent internal consistency (α = 0.912; ω = 0.914), and a strong correlation between factors (r = 0.77, p < 0.001). These findings confirm the Arabic TAI as a valid and reliable tool for assessing test anxiety among Moroccan students and represent the first psychometric validation of this measure in an African educational context.

INTRODUCTION AND BACKGROUND

Test anxiety has a substantial impact on the academic performance of students by influencing their concentration and recall capacities during examinations. Apart from its effects on academic performance, test anxiety also has negative effects on the mental health of students, with the impact on mental health being the most significant. This may include increased stress, doubts, or a decrease in self-esteem. Moreover, students with high anxiety levels may find it difficult to focus on their examinations, resulting in poor academic performance despite proper preparation.

Owing to these detrimental aspects, it has become essential to comprehend the concept of test anxiety and develop means for overcoming it not only for better academic achievement but for supporting the mental well-being of the affected individuals as well. For this reason, a precise assessment of this concept is imperative as it enables professionals and educators to develop a constructive strategy for the affected individuals aiming at developing their overall educational experience. Although adverse effects triggered by test anxiety have been well-articulated in the literature, a considerable gap exists in the use of a trustworthy Arabic version of the Cognitive Test Anxiety Scale. Owing to the gradual acknowledgment of the importance for addressing this experience within the learning community of Arabic-speaking individuals relevantly emphasizing the merits of overcoming this experience has become more significant than ever before. Thus, this particular research aims at filling this gap by comprehensively examining the psychometric properties of the Arabic version of the TAI. It differentiates between two main aspects: cognitive anxiety as well as physical symptoms. Therefore, it facilitates a comprehensively detailed analysis regarding the relevant learning-associated stress among individuals. It has been organized with a total of 20 items structured upon a likert scale consisting of 4 items as well. Thus, by adopting this scale, individuals can precisely interpret the overall levels of considerable developments for overcoming the related experience.

In 1980, Spielberger found that the test-retest reliability coefficients of the TAI were high (r=0.80) over small time periods, two to four weeks, among high school, college, and graduate students. But when high school students were tested, the test-retest reliability coefficients significantly decreased (r=0.62) over six months. Spielberger hypothesized that the decrease in test-retest reliability over six months may be accounted for in terms of changes in personality attributes and or college and career plans that may become more clearly defined in that period. Spielberger did not investigate the test-retest reliability coefficients over six months among college students. To our knowledge, there are no psychometric investigations that have compared TAI test scores over this time period. Other test anxieties have test-retest reliability coefficients that remain relatively constant over time, across all ages, and all racial groups. Possibly, the decrease in test reliability over six months among high school students was a random phenomenon.

Research Questions

Q1: How valid and reliable is the Cognitive Test Anxiety Scale in the Arabic context?
Q2: Is the correlation between the scale's dimensions statistically significant?
Q3: Is the factor structure of the scale, as examined through Exploratory Factor Analysis (EFA) and Confirmatory Factor Analysis (CFA), adequate?
Q4: How can the Arabic version of the Test Anxiety Inventory inform strategies to promote mental health and educational equity among students in African contexts, particularly in Morocco?

Literature Review

The initial research by Spielberger (Vagg et al., 1980) introduced Test Anxiety Inventory (TAI) in measuring test anxiety among college students. The validity and reliability, which was established, included internal consistency ($\alpha > 0.80$) and test-retest reliability, which was more prominent when tested over short periods (two to four weeks). It also emphasized how test anxiety affects academic performance, with regard to concentrating and performing well in tests. The research by Cassady and Johnson (2002) tested how test anxiety affects academic performance based on Test Anxiety Inventory. The result revealed that college students with higher levels of test anxiety had underperformed in academic areas. It also tested how the inventory correlated with other tests, revealing consistency. Furthermore, Furlan, et al. (2009) tested how the inventory could be applied in various international cultures, revealing that test anxiety is experienced in common across different societies. Moreover, it indicated variance in experiencing test-related anxiety based on culture. The research by Sarason and Stoops (1978) analyzed the connection between test-related anxiety and academic performance among different aged and ethnic persons, revealing a negative effect on academic performance among college and high schoolers, with little variance among gender and ethnic categories. The research by March, Sullivan, and Parker (1999) analyzed the link between test-related anxiety among children and the incidence of depression based on Test Anxiety Inventory. It discovered that children who experience test-related anxiety more have higher rates of experiencing depression and other kinds of anxieties. Third, the research by Nist and Holschuh (2007) tested the connection between test-related anxieties and methods of studying, revealing that people with more tests-related anxieties use less effective methods in studying. Usually, it affects people by avoiding methods which might augment recalling when under pressure. This research will cater to the absence of research regarding the reliability as well as validity of Arabic TAI.

METHODOLOGY

Design

This research adopted a quantitative methodological framework based on a psychometric analysis process, which entails the following: Descriptive analysis for the characteristics of the subjects, and the verification of the normal distribution of the subjects, analysis for associations between the dimensions through correlation coefficients, analysis for validity and reliability. (EFA & CFA) on the dimensions and structure of the scale.

Participants

The participants of the research were conducted among pupils at Sidi Boumedine School in the city of Sefrou, Morocco, in which the research was conducted over the period between December 2024 and May 2025, academic year 2024/2025. The research participants consisted of 578 pupils (N=578), with 408 female participants and 170 male participants, coming from three levels in the preparatory secondary levels (First, Second, and Third levels) of education. The participants were aged between 12 and 17. The size of the participants was adequate in consideration of the principle recommending that there should be 5 to 10 participants per item (Caycho-Rodríguez et al., 2022), which was followed strictly. Purposive sampling was applied in choosing the participants (level and age) with the aim of being more precise in the targeted population. Table 1 provides a clear description of the participants in terms of more accuracy.

Table 1. The demographic characteristics of the respondents

Description (N=578)		Frequency (N)	Percentage (%)
Gender	Male	170	29.412%
	Female	408	70.588%
Academic level	First preparatory level	503	87.024%
	Second preparatory level	61	10.554%
	Third preparatory level	14	2.422%
Age	Between 12 and 13 years old	515	89.100%
	Between 13 and 15 years old	42	7.266%
	Between 15 and 17 years old	21	3.633%

PROCEDURES

Authorization and Ethical Aspects

In addition, they were ensured that their confidentiality was maintained, and their personal data would not be disclosed to third persons. Lastly, they were made aware that they could withdraw their participation in the study at any time without giving any reason. All necessary procedures in trials involving human subjects were conducted in accordance with the ethical principles approved by the research committee members of the teachers of the Higher School (ENS), whose principal, Moulay Ismail University, Meknes, Morocco, adheres to, namely, the IR-UMI.ENS. REC.2024.005, and the revised version of the 1964 Helsinki Declaration.

Tool (Scale) Translation

The scale was translated carefully from English to Arabic through a precise method known as the "forward-backward translation". Afterwards, the scale was administered on a pilot sample to validate the prepared instrument and to estimate the time required to answer the scale, which took an average of 15 minutes.

Instruments

The Spielberger Test Anxiety Inventory (TAI) was used to achieve the objectives of this study and respond to the research questions. Its scaling is a very accurate means for measuring levels of exam-related anxieties. It distinguishes between two different aspects: cognitive anxieties and physical symptoms. Cognitive anxieties include any unfavorable thoughts that occur before or during the time a person is taking exams or preparing for exams like fear of failure, self-doubts, and concerns about outcomes. Physical symptoms involve physical reactions such as rate acceleration, perspiration, muscle tension, and feeling Difficulty breathing that people may feel during fearful situations. It has a total of 20 items where items 1, 2, 6, 9, 10, 11, 12, 14, 16, 17, 19, & 20 check for cognitive anxieties. There are a total of 20 items where items 3,4,5,7,8,13,15 & 18 check for physical symptoms. All questions are measured on a likert scale ranging from 1 = almost never, 2 = sometimes, 3 = often, and 4 = always.

Data Analysis

The statistical analyses that were used for descriptive statistics, normality test, and correlation were conducted on IBM SPSS Statistics version 27 for Windows (IBM Corp., Armonk, NY, USA). The exploratory factor analysis (EFA), Principal component analysis (PCA), and the confirmatory factor analysis (CFA) were conducted on JASP version 0.18.3 statistical software. The reliability test was conducted on Minitab version 21.

RESULTS

Normality of Data

Before the performance of the correlation tests, it was also necessary to check the normality of the data distribution, depending on which test we will perform, either the parametric test for correlation, also referred to as the Pearson test, or the non-parametric test for correlation, also referred to as the Spearman test. In this respect, it can be noted that the normality test conducted utilizes the Kolmogorov-Smirnov test instead of the Shapiro-Wilk test because the sample should have been larger and more representative. The sample size will increase the preference for the Kolmogorov-Smirnov test compared to the Kolmogorov-Smirnov test as used by (AKSU et al. 2019). This can be observed in Table 2 below:

Table 2. Normality test (Kolmogorov-Smirnov) for each items of scale

Item N	Kolmogorov-Smirnov test	P-Value	Normal Distribution
1	0.042	0.207*	Yes
2	0.036	0.297*	Yes
3	0.039	0.301*	Yes
4	0.038	0.207*	Yes
5	0.043	0.303*	Yes
6	0.043	0.365*	Yes
7	0.045	0.297*	Yes
8	0.037	0.298*	Yes
9	0.040	0.298*	Yes
10	0.036	0.367*	Yes
11	0.038	0.354*	Yes
12	0.041	0.267*	Yes
13	0.036	0.245*	Yes
14	0.038	0.276*	Yes
15	0.042	0.307*	Yes
16	0.041	0.298*	Yes
17	0.038	0.367*	Yes
18	0.042	0.288*	Yes
19	0.044	0.322*	Yes
20	0.061	0.276*	Yes

*p <.05

Table 2 indicate the results of the Kolmogorov-Smirnov test for normality for each item of the scale. The p-values for all items were greater than *p<0.05, indicating that the data for each item are normally distributed.

Correlation

The results of the Pearson correlation analysis between each item of the Spielberger Test Anxiety Inventory (TAI) and the total scale score (Table 3) were statistically significant with ***p<0.001, indicating strong positive correlations between the items and the overall scale (Armstrong, 2019). The Pearson (r) values ranged from 0.366 to 0.713, with some items showing very strong correlations, such as Item 11 (r=0.713), Item 19 (r=0.706), and Item 14 (r=0.698), suggesting these items are the most representative of the test anxiety construct. On the other hand, the lowest correlation was found for Item 1 (r=0.366), which, although statistically significant. These results indicate a good internal consistency of the scale, supporting its construct validity and confirming its suitability for measuring test anxiety in the target population.

Table 3. Pearson's correlations between the (20) items and TAI scale

Scale	N of item	Pearson's r	p
Spielberger Test Anxiety Inventory (TAI)	Item 1	0.366 ***	< .001
	Item 2	0.504 ***	< .001
	Item 3	0.685 ***	< .001
	Item 4	0.613 ***	< .001
	Item 5	0.530***	< .001
	Item 6	0.546 ***	< .001
	Item 7	0.591 ***	< .001
	Item 8	0.695 ***	< .001
	Item 9	0.680 ***	< .001
	Item 10	0.591 ***	< .001
	Item 11	0.713 ***	< .001
	Item 12	0.655 ***	< .001
	Item 13	0.533 ***	< .001
	Item 14	0.698 ***	< .001
	Item 15	0.603 ***	< .001
	Item 16	0.603 ***	< .001
	Item 17	0.562 ***	< .001
	Item 18	0.652 ***	< .001
	Item 19	0.706 ***	< .001
	Item 20	0.693 ***	< .001

*p<.05, **p<.01, ***p <.001

Reliability Tests

The (Table 4) presents the scale reliability statistics based on the frequentist approach using McDonald's omega (ω) and Cronbach's alpha (α). The omega coefficient was (ω=0.914), while Cronbach's alpha was (α=0.912), indicating a high level of internal consistency among the scale items (Revelle & Condon, 2019). Additionally, the 95% confidence intervals showed a narrow range, with omega ranging from 0.904 to 0.924 and alpha from 0.902 to 0.922, reflecting high precision in estimating reliability coefficients. Since both values exceed 0.90, these results confirm that the scale demonstrates excellent reliability, making it a dependable tool for research assessments.

Table 4. Cronbach's alpha and McDonald's omega values of total score of TAI scale

Estimate	McDonald's ω	Cronbach's α	N of items
Point estimate	0.914	0.912	20
95% CI lower bound	0.904	0.902	
95% CI upper bound	0.924	0.922	

Exploratory Factor Analysis (EFA)

The results of the Exploratory Factor Analysis (EFA) revealed a two-factor structure for the scale. This conclusion is supported by the Scree Plot (Figure 1), which clearly shows an inflection point after the second factor. Furthermore, only the first two factors had eigenvalues greater than 1, according to Kaiser's criterion, indicating that retaining two factors is the most appropriate solution (Ledesma et al., 2015).

Figure 1. Scree plot of (EFA) results

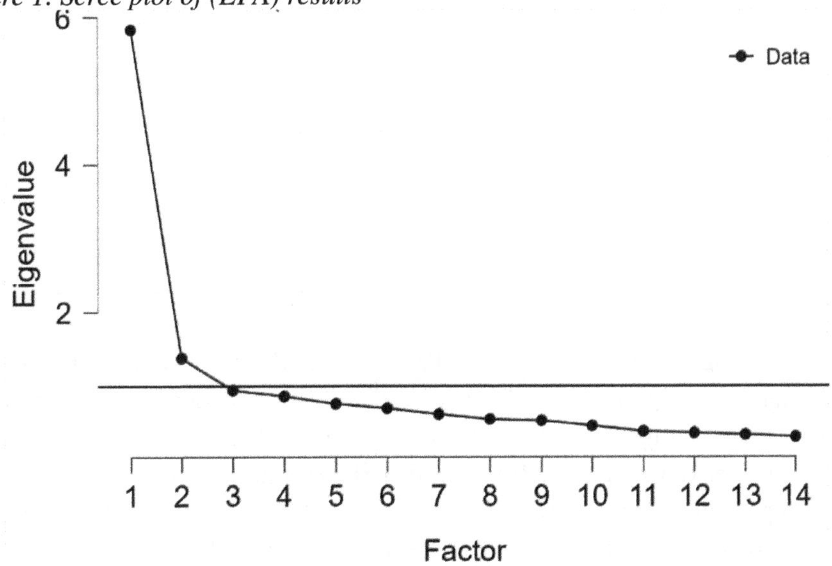

Kaiser-Meyer-Olkin (KMO) value was found to be high (KMO = 0.901) indicating that the sample is suitable for factor analysis (Table 5). Additionally, Bartlett's test of sphericity was significant indicating that the correlation between the variables is high enough for further analysis (Zhang et al., 2024).

Table 5. Kaiser-Meyer-Olkin (KMO) test

	MSA
Overall MSA	0.901
Item 1	0.844
Item 2	0.885
Item 3	0.900
Item 4	0.900
Item 5	0.905
Item 6	0.878
Item 7	0.914
Item 8	0.916
Item 9	0.910
Item 10	0.877
Item 11	0.911
Item 12	0.900
Item 13	0.884
Item 14	0.889
Item 15	0.893
Item 16	0.916
Item 17	0.889
Item 18	0.915
Item 19	0.905
Item 20	0.938

On analyzing the values of factor loadings presented within Table 6, it is observed that the items correspond to two distinct factors. The items corresponding to Factor 1 present values ranging from 0.458 to 0.716, while the items corresponding to Factor 2 present values ranging from 0.495 to 0.795, thus establishing the presence of two important factors (Christensen & Golino, 2021). However, it is important to observe that the uniqueness value of Item1 is extremely high, which is 0.905.

Table 6. Factor loadings of TAI scale

Item N	Factor 1	Factor 2	Uniqueness
Item 1	0.228		0.905
Item 2	0.716		0.662
Item 3	0.682		0.494
Item 4	0.480		0.643
Item 5	0.497		0.728
Item 6	0.458		0.727
Item 7	0.540		0.651
Item 8	0.709		0.481
Item 9	0.559		0.545
Item 10	0.599		0.635
Item 11	0.488		0.504
Item 12	0.711		0.522
Item 13		0.570	0.697
Item 14		0.726	0.446
Item 15		0.610	0.614
Item 16		0.785	0.497
Item 17		0.525	0.690
Item 18		0.722	0.506
Item 19		0.795	0.400
Item 20		0.495	0.526

Note. Applied rotation method is promax.

Confirmatory Factor Analysis (CFA) and Model Fit Indices

These nineteen factors obtained from Exploratory Factor Analysis (EFA) were used with 578 university students at various levels. A subsequent Confirmatory Factor Analysis (CFA) was also performed using data gathered from students. In this CFA, error variances of item 1 were found to exceed 90, as indicated by JASP. Although item 1 had high t-values and factor loadings, it was deleted to optimize fit statistics, and a final form of the scale as shown in Figure 5 was obtained. The final scale had a goodness of fit indicated by: Goodness of Fit Index (GFI) of 0.964, Comparative Fit Index (CFI) of 0.877, Standardized Root Mean Square Residual (SRMR) of 0.063, and Bentler-Bonett Non-Normed Fit Index (NNFI) of 0.847.

The results of chi-square tests reveal that the factor model has a better fit than the baseline model. The baseline model has Chi-square = 3749.069 with 91 degrees of freedom, whereas the Chi-square of the factor model is 599.909 with 76 degrees of freedom, and it has a significant p-value ($p < 0.001$) (Goretzko et al., 2024).

In sum, the fit of the present model is generally acceptable to good. The value of GFI is .964, which indicates a strong fit, while SRMR at .063 indicates an acceptable fit, which indicates minor discrepancies in covariances between the observed and the latent data. CFI with a value of .877, while not quite at the level of the ideal .90, is still relatively close to being in the acceptable range, which indicates a fair reflection of data structure. The comparison Chi-Square between the present model (χ^2 =599.909, df=76, p<.001) and the base model (χ^2 =3749.069, df=91) again verifies that the fit of the factor model is superior (Mercan and Kabadayı, 2023).

Figure 2 above indicates that CFA outcomes confirm the validity of the model. Cognitive Anxiety loadings vary between 0.49 and 0.73, while Physical Symptoms vary between 0.40 and 0.97, indicating that the observed variables substantially influence their corresponding factors. A high correlation level at 0.77 indicates that there is an important relationship between Cognitive Anxiety and Physical Symptoms (Shultz, et al., 2020). In summary, these results demonstrate that the proposed model may be an appropriate and valid framework for investigating the relationship between Cognitive Anxiety and Physical Symptoms in students.

Figure 2. Scree plot of (CFA) results

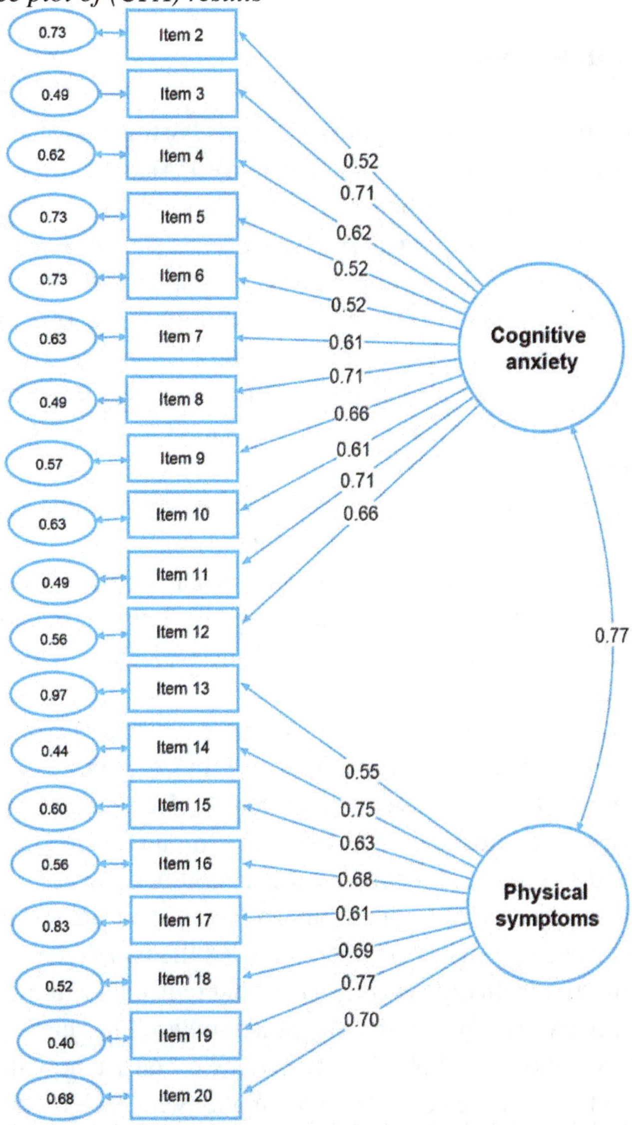

DISCUSSION

General Results Discussion

The current study's findings are consistent with existing knowledge concerning the psychometric properties of the Spielberger Test Anxiety Inventory. The data passed the test of normal distribution, echoing the efforts of validation studies conducted to show the appropriateness of parametric statistical procedures, such as Pearson correlation, when examining the test anxiety survey data (Zeidner, 1998). The correlations obtained between the majority of the Test Anxiety Inventory items and the overall score confirm the validity of the Test Anxiety Inventory scale, echoing previous studies conducted on the test anxiety inventory survey that showed the inventory is reliable in the measurement of test anxiety among various groups of people.

Concerning reliability, the study finds high values of internal consistency (Omega by McDonald, Cronbach's alpha) that are similar to those found in previous studies evaluating the TAI in different culture-related settings (Pekrun et al. 2004). The findings strengthen confidence in the scale's effectiveness in test anxiety measurements among college students, going beyond the typically suggested reliability criteria (Taber 2018).

The Exploratory Factor Analysis (EFA) helped to identify a two-factor construct consistent with existing literature (Putwain and Daly, 2014) on test anxiety being a two-factor construct rather than unidimensional, encompassing factors such as cognitive worries, physiological complaints, and so on (Cleare et al., 2018). The KMO values and Bartlett's Test supported data appropriateness for analysis via factor analysis, as in most other studies on two-factor construct test anxiety.

Confirmatory Factor Analysis further validated the two-factor model. Certain indices of fit tended marginally lower than ideal but remained within acceptable-to-good levels, as observed in comparable validation studies. The very high correlation between cognitive anxiety and physical symptoms is consistent with existing evidence that these two variables correlate very highly with each other (Arens et al., 2017). On the other hand, the choice to delete Item 1 due to high uniqueness and low correlation with the total score is consistent with studies that sought to improve test psychometric properties.

Several studies also stress that test anxiety is a complex phenomenon and it is essential to differentiate between both cognitive and psychological factors. For example, research by Cassady and Johnson (2002) demonstrated that both psychological and physiologic test anxiety are significant predictors of academic achievement independently. This confirms that there are two factors to test anxiety, as found within the current research, and it is essential to emphasize that these two factors need to be examined independently. Other research, such as that conducted by von der Embse, Baker, and Shin (2013), also identifies that depending upon the cultural context, students, especially those who are young, tend to express test anxiety differently, specifically during high-stakes testing conditions. The current research also adds to this debate, as it confirms that the Arabic translation of TAI is valid and effective within preparation schools of Morocco, considering that culture and testing conditions influence both experience and self-report of anxiety, as argued within research by Al-Balhan, Gigus, and Griffiths (2018).

Rana and Mahmood (2010) also found sound psychometric support for the TAI among South Asian nations, demonstrating its reliability and factorial validity among secondary school-going students. Contrary to the geographical and cultural disparities, the results echoed the current findings, thereby proving its integrity across disparate groups and also indicating its applicability within the Arabic-speaking nations of North Africa. In conclusion, this research not only verifies current findings regarding the psychometric properties of the TAI, but it also fills a research gap as it demonstrates the validity and reliability of the TAI for the specific group of Arabic-speaking preparatory school pupils. It is a significant finding, considering the inadequacy in the availability of culturally modified and well-designed psychometric instruments for the measurement of test anxiety for the specified age group. The Arabic TAI is well-suited for further usage in research as well as indicating the need for further modification and customization. Further research may be considered for validation in different parts of the Arabic-speaking world.

Recommendations for Future Studies

For future research, it is recommended to expand the study to include larger and more diverse samples of Arabic-speaking students to assess the generalizability of the findings across different age groups, regions, and educational settings. Additionally, improving the CFA model by incorporating additional dimensions of anxiety, such as emotional and behavioral aspects, would contribute to a more comprehensive understanding of test anxiety. Longitudinal studies are also suggested to examine the temporal trends of cognitive anxiety and its long-term impact on academic performance. Finally, expanding external validation by using other test anxiety measures and comparing them with different psychometric tests would enhance the scale's reliability and applicability in various cultural and educational contexts.

CONCLUSION

The current research aimed to assess the extent to which the Cognitive Test Anxiety Scale (CTAS) is valid and reliable when administered in an Arabic setting. The current research focused on both validational and reliable aspects, including inter-item correlation and the underlying factor structure via Exploratory Factor Analysis (EFA) and Confirmatory Factor Analysis (CFA). The outcome indicated that this instrument is reliable, with high internal consistency as reflected in both Cronbach's alpha and McDonald's omega values. This answers the first question: "How valid and reliable is the CTAS in Arabic?"

For the second question, whether there was a significant relationship between the scale's dimensions, the Pearson correlation results revealed a strong positive relationship between cognitive anxiety and physiological symptoms. This supported a positive inter-dimensional relationship.

With regard to the third question regarding the factor structure investigated by both EFA and CFA, it may be stated that although EFA yielded two-factor structure with appropriate item correlations and KMO value, CFA also indicated the appropriate two-factor structure with good-to-good indices. Some other indices had fallen slightly short of perfection but were still appropriate.

In conclusion, the results indicate the validity and reliability of the CTAS scale, its dimensions' important correlations, and the two-factor model for the Arabic environment. This will help improve the use of the scale as a resource in future studies on test anxiety perceived by Arabic-speaking students.

REFERENCES

Aksu, G., Güzeller, C. O., & Eser, M. T.AKSU. (2019). The Effect of the Normalization Method Used in Different Sample Sizes on the Success of Artificial Neural Network Model. *International Journal of Assessment Tools in Education, 6*(2), 170–192. DOI: 10.21449/ijate.479404

Al-Balhan, E. M., Khabbache, H., Watfa, A., Re, T. S., Zerbetto, R., & Bragazzi, N. L. (2018). Psychometric evaluation of the arabic version of the nomophobia questionnaire: Confirmatory and exploratory factor analysis – Implications from a pilot study in Kuwait among university students. *Psychology Research and Behavior Management, 11*, 471–482. DOI: 10.2147/PRBM.S169918 PMID: 30425594

Arens, A. K., Becker, M., & Möller, J. (2017). Social and dimensional comparisons in math and verbal test anxiety: Within- and cross-domain relations with achievement and the mediating role of academic self-concept. *Contemporary Educational Psychology, 51*(August), 240–252. DOI: 10.1016/j.cedpsych.2017.08.005

Armstrong, R. A. (2019). Should Pearson's correlation coefficient be avoided? *Ophthalmic & Physiological Optics, 39*(5), 316–327. DOI: 10.1111/opo.12636 PMID: 31423624

Cassady, J. C., & Johnson, R. E. (2002). Cognitive test anxiety and academic performance. *Contemporary Educational Psychology, 27*(2), 270–295. DOI: 10.1006/ceps.2001.1094

Caycho-Rodríguez, T., Vilca, L. W., Carbajal-León, C., White, M., Vivanco-Vidal, A., Saroli-Araníbar, D., Peña-Calero, B. N., & Moreta-Herrera, R. (2022). Coronavirus Anxiety Scale: New psychometric evidence for the Spanish version based on CFA and IRT models in a Peruvian sample. *Death Studies, 46*(5), 1090–1099. DOI: 10.1080/07481187.2020.1865480 PMID: 33427098

Christensen, A. P., & Golino, H. (2021). On the equivalency of factor and network loadings. *Behavior Research Methods, 53*(4), 1563–1580. DOI: 10.3758/s13428-020-01500-6 PMID: 33409985

Cleare, S., Gumley, A., Cleare, C. J., & O'Connor, R. C. (2018). An Investigation of the Factor Structure of the Self-Compassion Scale. *Mindfulness, 9*(2), 618–628. DOI: 10.1007/s12671-017-0803-1 PMID: 29599853

Goretzko, D., Siemund, K., & Sterner, P. (2024). Evaluating Model Fit of Measurement Models in Confirmatory Factor Analysis. *Educational and Psychological Measurement, 84*(1), 123–144. DOI: 10.1177/00131644231163813 PMID: 38250508

Ledesma, R. D., Valero-Mora, P., & Macbeth, G. (2015). The Scree Test and the Number of Factors: A Dynamic Graphics Approach. *The Spanish Journal of Psychology*, *18*, E11. DOI: 10.1017/sjp.2015.13 PMID: 26055575

Mercan, O., & Kabadayı, F. (2023). Psychometric properties of the BALCI Turkish version. *Psicologia: Reflexão e Crítica : Revista Semestral do Departamento de Psicologia da UFRGS*, *36*(1), 7. Advance online publication. DOI: 10.1186/s41155-023-00248-0 PMID: 36853435

Pekrun, R., Goetz, T., Perry, R. P., Kramer, K., Hochstadt, M., & Molfenter, S. (2004). Beyond test anxiety: Development and validation of the test emotions questionnaire (TEQ). *Anxiety, Stress, and Coping*, *17*(3), 287–316. DOI: 10.1080/10615800412331303847

Rana, R., & Mahmood, N. (2010). The relationship between test anxiety and academic achievement. *Bulletin of Education and research, 32*(2), 63-74.

Revelle, W., & Condon, D. M. (2019). Reliability from α to ω: A tutorial. *Psychological Assessment*, *31*(12), 1395–1411. DOI: 10.1037/pas0000754 PMID: 31380696

Sarason, I. G., & Stoops, R. (1978). Test anxiety and the passage of time. *Journal of Consulting and Clinical Psychology*, *46*(1), 102–109. DOI: 10.1037/0022-006X.46.1.102 PMID: 627645

Shultz, K. S., Whitney, D. J., & Zickar, M. J. (2020). Confirmatory Factor Analysis. *Measurement Theory in Action*, *II*, 302–316. DOI: 10.4324/9781003127536-19

Taber, K. S. (2018). The Use of Cronbach ' s Alpha When Developing and Reporting Research Instruments in Science Education. *Research in Science Education*, *48*(6), 1273–1296. DOI: 10.1007/s11165-016-9602-2

Vagg, P. R., Spielberger, C. D., & O'Hearn, T. P.Jr. (1980). Is the state-trait anxiety inventory multidimensional? *Personality and Individual Differences*, *1*(3), 207–214. DOI: 10.1016/0191-8869(80)90052-5

Zeidner, M. (1998). Test anxiety: The state of the art.

Zhang, Z., Sangsawang, T., Vipahasna, K., & Pigultong, M. (2024). A Mixed-Methods Data Approach Integrating Importance-Performance Analysis (IPA) and Kaiser-Meyer-Olkin (KMO) in Applied Talent Cultivation. *Journal of Applied Data Sciences*, *5*(1), 256–267. https://doi.org/https://doi.org/10.47738/jads.v5i1.170. DOI: 10.47738/jads.v5i1.170

Chapter 2

Foreignization and the Influence of English Lexical Borrowing in Shaping the Arabic Language in Social Media:

A Linguistic Analytical Study in Digital Spaces

Hamood Mohammed AlRumhi
https://orcid.org/0000-0003-2800-0953
Sultan Qaboos University, Oman

Mohamed Alamiri
Sultan Qaboos University, Oman

Mostafa Bouanani
https://orcid.org/0009-0007-8534-9621
Sidi Mohammed Ben Abdellah University, Morocco

Khalid Sulaiman Muhanna Alkindi
Sultan Qaboos University, Oman

ABSTRACT

The rapid rise of social media platforms has reshaped communication patterns across the globe, and the Arabic-speaking world is no exception. This paper explores the phenomenon of foreignization through the increasing integration of English lexical

DOI: 10.4018/979-8-3373-3581-0.ch002

borrowings in Arabic social media discourse. Additionally, the paper, which follows a quantitative approach, examines the sociocultural and linguistic implications of using these loanwords, especially in the context of code-switching and the adaptation of foreign terms into the Arabic lexicon. Through this exploration, the research seeks to understand the broader impact of English borrowings on Arabic language evolution in digital spaces and the potential long-term consequences for cultural and linguistic identity. It is hoped that this paper will be followed by a more elaborate study on borrowing from English and other languages in conversational Arabic in the Arabian Peninsula to be carried out from a Cognitive Linguistic perspective.

1. INTRODUCTION

Language is more than just a means of communication; it is a reflection of culture, identity, and the complex web of social interactions that shape human experience. As societies evolve, so does language, adapting to new realities, technologies, and cultural influences (Ur Rehman et al., 2025). In the age of digital communication, social media platforms have become powerful catalysts for this linguistic evolution, particularly in multilingual and multicultural contexts (Chyrvonyi, 2024). One such example is the Arabic-speaking world, where the integration of foreign elements, particularly English loanwords, has become a noticeable phenomenon. The increasing presence of these foreign words in Arabic social media discourse reflects broader trends of globalization and cultural exchange, as well as the specific dynamics of online communication.

This paper seeks to explore the process of lexical borrowing—the deliberate incorporation of foreign words into a language—focusing on the role of English lexical borrowing in shaping the Arabic language as used in social media contexts. Lexical borrowing, a linguistic phenomenon where foreign elements are deliberately integrated into a language, often reflects a society's exposure to external influences. In the case of Arabic, the omnipresence of English in technology, business, and global culture has made its way into everyday Arabic conversations, especially on digital platforms. This process is not merely a matter of vocabulary expansion but represents deeper shifts in cultural identity, social behavior, and communication practices. As technology continues to evolve, it exerts considerable pressure on languages to adapt, and social media platforms such as Facebook, Instagram, Twitter, and WhatsApp have become the primary arenas where these linguistic changes manifest.

1.1 Overview of Lexical Borrowing and Language Influence

Lexical borrowing in linguistics refers to the deliberate or unconscious introduction of foreign linguistic elements into a native language (Yonamine, 2022; Tian, 2023; Tariq et al., 2025). It may occur through lexical borrowing—where individual words or phrases are adopted—or through more profound changes in syntax, phonology, or semantics. Lexical borrowing reflects both the globalization of cultures and languages and the need to accommodate new concepts, technologies, and ideas that did not previously exist in a given linguistic or cultural context (Ji & Chen, 2022; An, 2024; An, 2025).

In the Arabic-speaking world, lexical borrowing has taken place across centuries, with influences from Greek, Persian, Turkish, and French, among others. However, the influence of English on modern Arabic is unprecedented, primarily due to the rise of technology and globalization. English is the dominant language in fields such as science, technology, business, and entertainment, and as a result, many English terms have no equivalent in Arabic. This has led to the widespread borrowing of English words, especially in digital and online communication, where quick, efficient, and concise language is often favored.

The term loanwords refers to words that are borrowed from one language and incorporated into another. In the context of Arabic social media slang, loanwords are often adopted directly from English, sometimes with little or no modification to their spelling or pronunciation. This borrowing is facilitated by the fact that many social media platforms are based on English-language interfaces, making it easier for users to adopt English terminology when describing platform-specific actions (such as liking, commenting, and sharing). The prevalence of English in the online world has not only facilitated the adoption of English loanwords into Arabic but also sparked a wider debate about the impact of these foreign elements on the integrity and purity of the Arabic language.

1.2 The Impact of English on Modern Arabic Communication

The growing use of English loanwords in Arabic can be seen as part of a broader trend of language contact and linguistic convergence that has characterized global communication in the 21st century. In the case of Arabic, this convergence is particularly striking because of the language's unique position as both a widely spoken global language and a central component of cultural and religious identity for millions of people across the Middle East and North Africa.

Historically, Arabic has been a highly prestigious language, not only because of its role as the language of the Qur'an but also due to its rich literary and intellectual tradition. Classical Arabic, and the modern development of this, Modern Standard

Arabic (MSA), has long been the language of formal writing, religious scholarship, and high culture. However, in everyday communication, most Arabic speakers use a variety of dialects that differ considerably from MSA. These dialects—whether Egyptian, Levantine, Gulf, or Maghrebi Arabic—are the languages of informal speech, and they have been shaped over time by contact with other languages and cultures.

In the digital age, the informal nature of social media communication has accelerated the blending of these dialects with foreign elements, particularly English. Unlike traditional forms of written Arabic, which are governed by strict rules of grammar and vocabulary, social media language is highly flexible and informal, making it an ideal space for experimentation and linguistic innovation. This flexibility has led to the widespread adoption of English words, especially in contexts where Arabic equivalents either do not exist or feel cumbersome to use in quick, casual conversations.

One of the main reasons for this adoption is the convenience and efficiency of English terms, particularly in relation to technology and social media. For instance, words like "post," "comment," "like," and "subscribe" are often used directly, in transliterated form, in Arabic social media conversations without translation, as they refer to actions that are specific to online platforms. While Arabic equivalents for these terms exist (for example, " " for "comment" and " " for "like"), they are often seen as more formal or less convenient in the fast-paced environment of social media.

Moreover, the dominance of English in global technology has made it the default language for many online platforms, which further encourages the use of English terminology. For example, on platforms like Facebook or Instagram, users interact with English-based interfaces that use terms like "share," "follow," and "hashtag" to describe platform-specific functions. As a result, even Arabic speakers who are fluent in their native language may find it easier to adopt these English terms rather than translate them into Arabic.

1.3 Purpose of the Paper

This paper aims to explore the integration of English loanwords into Arabic social media language and analyze how these loanwords are used in everyday online communication. The study focuses on several key areas:

1. **The Role of Social Media in Language Evolution:** How have platforms like Facebook, Instagram, WhatsApp, and Twitter contributed to the adoption of English loanwords in Arabic social media conversations? What specific features of these platforms encourage the use of foreign words?

2. **Common English Loanwords in Arabic Social Media Conversations:** Which English loanwords are most frequently used by Arabic speakers on social media? Why are these particular words adopted, and what do they signify about the changing nature of Arabic communication in the digital age?
3. **Integration of Loanwords in Arabic Sentences:** How do Arabic speakers incorporate English loanwords into their sentences? What patterns of **code-switching** (the alternating use of two or more languages within a conversation) emerge in these social media interactions?
4. **Cultural and Social Implications of Using English Loanwords:** How is the use of English loanwords perceived by different generations and social groups within the Arabic-speaking world? Do younger generations see loanwords as a sign of modernity and global connectedness, while older generations view them as a threat to linguistic purity?
5. **The Future of Arabic in the Digital Age:** What are the long-term consequences of this linguistic blending for the future of the Arabic language? Will Arabic continue to adapt to the digital age by incorporating more foreign elements, or will there be a push to preserve the integrity of the language in the face of globalization?

By examining these questions, the paper seeks to contribute to the broader conversation about the impact of globalization on language use and the ways in which social media is reshaping communication in the modern world. The study also highlights the tension between embracing foreign elements and preserving linguistic identity, a tension that is particularly pronounced in the Arabic-speaking world, where language is deeply intertwined with cultural and religious heritage.

1.4 The Importance of Studying English Loanwords in Arabic Social Media

The study of English loanwords in Arabic social media is important for several reasons. First, it sheds light on the broader process of linguistic globalization, in which languages around the world are increasingly influenced by English due to its dominance in international business, technology, and popular culture. This process has profound implications for linguistic diversity, as smaller languages may struggle to compete with the global reach of English.

Second, the study of loanwords provides insights into the sociolinguistic dynamics of the Arabic-speaking world, where language is not only a means of communication but also a marker of social status, education, and cultural identity. The use of English loanwords can be seen as a form of linguistic capital, signaling a speaker's familiarity with global trends and their ability to navigate the digital landscape.

Finally, this study contributes to the ongoing debate about the future of Arabic in the digital age. As Arabic continues to evolve in response to new technologies and cultural influences, the question of how to balance linguistic adaptation with the preservation of Arabic's unique identity becomes increasingly pressing.

2. LITERATURE REVIEW

The study of lexical borrowing and lexical borrowing has been a focal point of sociolinguistics and language contact theory for decades. The advent of digital communication and social media, however, has accelerated these processes, providing new contexts in which languages interact, evolve, and blend. This literature review explores the theoretical frameworks and existing research related to lexical borrowing, the role of social media in language evolution, and the impact of English loanwords on Arabic, offering a foundation for the present study. Among other works, there is a comprehensive volume on the subject (Haspelmath and Tadmor 2009) which is "… the first work to address the question of what kinds of words get borrowed in a systematic and comparative perspective. It studies lexical borrowing behavior on the basis of a world-wide sample of 40 languages, both major languages and minor languages, and both languages with heavy borrowing and languages with little lexical influence from other languages". Among recent studies is Al-Mughirah *et al*, (2025) which explores the impact of the phenomenon of electronic games on education, culture, communication, and language acquisition in Arabic in Saudi Arabia.

2.1 Lexical Borrowing and Lexical Borrowing in Linguistics

Lexical borrowing is a linguistic phenomenon that occurs when words or expressions from one language are introduced into another. In the context of Arabic, lexical borrowing has historically been shaped by interactions with languages like Greek, Persian, and Turkish, reflecting the political, cultural, and economic exchanges between the Arab world and its neighbors. More recently, however, the influence of English has become dominant, largely due to the rise of globalization, international trade, and the ubiquity of English in technological innovations. Scholars such as Haugen (1950) and Thomason and Kaufman (1988) have studied the mechanisms through which languages borrow elements from each other, including the socio-cultural motivations behind such processes.

Haugen's (1950) work on lexical borrowing highlights two primary forms of borrowing: direct and indirect. Direct borrowing occurs when words are adopted without significant modification, as seen with terms like "subscribe" or "comment," which Arabic speakers often use without adaptation, apart from transliterating them into Arabic script. Indirect borrowing involves phonological, morphological, or syntactic modifications to make the foreign word more compatible with the borrowing language's rules. In the case of Arabic, this is evident in the way loanwords may sometimes be altered slightly to fit the Arabic phonological or morphological systems, though social media use often favors the direct incorporation of English terms without such modifications.

Poplack et al. (1988) further explored code-switching and loanword integration, particularly within bilingual communities. Their research suggests that loanwords become more prevalent when speakers are regularly exposed to both languages, as is common in multilingual societies and digital environments where English dominates as the global language of communication. Social media platforms, which often have English-based interfaces and widespread English-language content, serve as key spaces where this exposure occurs. In this way, lexical borrowing becomes more than a lexical phenomenon; it becomes a cultural one, where the borrowed language carries prestige or global relevance.

Smart (1985) (in Netton, ed. (1985)), Al-Saqqaf (2006) and Bahumaid (2015), among others, deal with the integration of English and other foreign languages into Hadhrami Arabic. More recent studies included borrowing from languages other than English to other foreign languages. These include Havumetsä (2023) which examines lexical borrowing from Russian into Finnish that takes the form of loanwords and loan translations, often in connection with an explanation of the concept, in Finnish journalistic writing.

Yoonjung Oh and Hyunjung Son (2023) deals with lexical terms borrowed from foreign languages by transliterating the original sound of the borrowed words with the recipient language's consonants and vowels. This paper focuses on lexical borrowing in the Korean language from a *diachronic perspective* by investigating the changes in loanword usage from 1970 to 2015.

At the social media level, Indriani, Barli Bram (2023) focuses on identifying the types of borrowed words used in some social media Indonesian website The researchers employed a variety of theories and borrowed words. This study used content analysis as a research method to explore the types of 50 borrowed words found on the website investigating changes in morphological forms in the borrowed words.

Al-Athwary and Ali (2023) uses a corpus-based analysis to examine loan translation as an Arabicization technique in written MSA in the field of information technology.

Yousuf (2022) is an analytical study of the work of the Arabization Committee at the Arabic Language Academy. The research sought to clarify the approach of the Committee in dealing with words, styles and structures borrowed from foreign languages.

2.2 Social Media and Linguistic Change

Social media has emerged as a significant factor in the evolution of language. Platforms like Facebook, Twitter, Instagram, and WhatsApp encourage rapid, informal, and often hybridized forms of communication, which makes them fertile ground for the introduction of foreign words and phrases. Unlike traditional forms of communication, whether spoken or written—social media is characterized by its brevity, immediacy, and visual-oral hybrid nature. This unique context creates new dynamics for language interaction, allowing for greater flexibility in the integration of foreign elements like English loanwords into local languages.

The work of Danet and Herring (2007) on language and the internet highlights how the digital age has transformed language use. They argue that online platforms foster linguistic creativity, where traditional boundaries between languages are frequently crossed. This creativity often manifests as code-switching or the use of foreign terms in native-language contexts, particularly when those terms are associated with specific technologies or platforms. For instance, words like "tweet," "like," or "hashtag" have become universal, transcending their English origins and entering the lexicons of languages across the world, including Arabic.

Crystal (2001) emphasizes the notion of a "global village," where digital communication creates interconnected linguistic communities. He suggests that while English remains dominant, other languages are also asserting themselves in online spaces, leading to a complex interplay of linguistic influences. In this "global village," Arabic has maintained its distinctiveness but has also absorbed elements of English, particularly in digital and social media contexts. As such, the use of English loanwords in Arabic online conversations reflects both the pervasiveness of English in digital spaces and the adaptability of Arabic to incorporate these foreign elements.

Al-Khatib and Sabbah (2008) delves specifically into the impact of technology on Arabic, noting that the widespread use of English terms in fields such as technology and business has made their adoption almost inevitable in informal Arabic discourse, especially on social media platforms. They point out that English words are often seen as more efficient or concise, fitting well into the fast-paced and informal environment of social media. This has led to the creation of what they term an "Arabizi" language, a hybrid form of Arabic that incorporates Latin script and English words, particularly in digital communication. "Arabizi" reflects a blend of English and Arabic that has become increasingly common in youth culture and online spaces, making it an essential aspect of the current study on loanwords.

Darwish (2015) delves deeply into different and conflicting views regarding the term "loan words" and the amount of Arabic loan words in English from both the points of view of English and Arab linguists. He then provides a historical review from the first Arabic words borrowed into Old English to the latest words in the last few decades, considering the factors involved in borrowing from Arabic to English. Finally, there is a recommendation followed by a conclusion.

2.3 Code-Switching and the Hybridization of Arabic

Code-switching—the practice of alternating between two or more languages in a single conversation—has long been a topic of interest in sociolinguistics, particularly in relation to multilingual societies. In the context of Arabic social media, code-switching often involves the use of English loanwords within predominantly Arabic sentences. This phenomenon is not limited to formal or technical terms but extends to everyday words and phrases, such as "like," "comment," "subscribe," and "hashtag," which are used seamlessly alongside Arabic.

Gumperz (1982) and Auer (1998) have both studied the mechanisms of code-switching, noting that it is often used to signal social identity, group membership, or cultural affiliation. On social media, the use of English loanwords can be seen as a form of "prestige code-switching," where speakers use foreign words to signal their alignment with global trends or their comfort with modern, digital cultures. This is particularly true for younger generations, who are more likely to be fluent in English and to use social media as a primary means of communication.

Miller and Johann-Mattis (2023) tests new methods for lexical borrowing detection in contact situations where dominant languages play an important role, applying two classical sequence comparison methods and one machine learning method to a sample of seven Latin American languages which have all borrowed extensively from the Spanish of Spain.

The hybridization of Arabic through the incorporation of English loanwords has also been studied by Holes (2004), who argues that language mixing is a natural consequence of globalization and digital communication. He suggests that while some may view the introduction of foreign elements as a threat to linguistic purity, it is more accurate to see it as part of the natural evolution of language. In this sense, the use of English loanwords in Arabic can be seen not as a form of linguistic corruption but as an adaptation to the realities of a globalized, digitally connected world.

2.4 The Cultural and Social Implications of Loanwords

The use of English loanwords in Arabic is not merely a linguistic issue; it also has significant cultural and social implications. Studies by Bassiouney (2009) and Suleiman (2013) explore how language choices reflect broader socio-cultural dynamics, including issues of identity, modernity, and resistance to cultural change. In many Arabic-speaking societies, language is closely tied to cultural and religious identity, and the introduction of foreign elements, particularly from English, can be seen as a form of cultural imperialism or erosion.

However, Bassiouney (2009) notes that for many young Arabic speakers, the use of English loanwords is not about rejecting their cultural heritage but about participating in a global digital culture. In this context, using English terms is a pragmatic choice that allows them to engage with global platforms and trends while still maintaining their Arabic identity. This perspective suggests that rather than viewing English loanwords as a threat, they can be seen as part of the dynamic and evolving nature of language in the digital age.

2.5 Language Contact and Loanwords in Cognitive Linguistics

The integration of English loanwords into Arabic, particularly in domains like technology, food, and emotion vocabulary, has gained scholarly attention within Cognitive Linguistics in recent years. This framework emphasizes how speakers conceptualize and categorize new lexical items based on embodied experience, image schemas, and existing semantic structures (Evans & Green, 2006; Lakoff & Johnson, 2008). Loanwords are not merely borrowed forms but are re-conceptualized to fit the recipient language's cognitive and cultural models.

Geeraerts and Cuyckens (2007) argue that language contact triggers semantic shifts and category extensions, as borrowed items are mapped onto existing conceptual networks. In the Arabic context, this is particularly evident in Gulf Arabic, where English borrowings like *kumbyūtar* (computer) or *īmēl* (email) are fully adapted into the grammatical and phonological systems of Arabic while also undergoing conceptual integration (Ryding, 2005; Alhassan, 2016). These borrowings often occupy hybrid spaces between diglossic varieties, contributing to sociolinguistic change (Al-Batal, 1992).

Ibrahim (1982) highlights that borrowing is not only lexical but also cognitive, involving restructuring of conceptual domains—especially when borrowed words fill lexical gaps in Arabic. Studies such as Abdul-Fattah (2010) and Alhassan (2016) further show how semantic extension and metaphorical reinterpretation are central to the cognitive processing of loanwords. For example, English terms in Arabic often undergo shifts from concrete to abstract meanings or take on localized connotations shaped by cultural schemas.

Overall, applying a cognitive perspective to English–Arabic borrowing reveals a dynamic interplay of linguistic structure, conceptual adaptation, and cultural framing, emphasizing that loanwords are not passive imports but actively re-conceptualized elements in language change.

It is hoped that a more elaborate study on borrowing from English and other languages in conversational Arabic in the Arabian Peninsula will be carried out within Cognitive Linguistic perspective.

3 METHODOLOGY

This section presents the methodology utilized to investigate the phenomenon of English loanword integration into Arabic as observed in social media communication. The approach is *mainly qualitative*, exploring the linguistic, sociocultural, and technological factors influencing the use of English terms in Arabic social media interactions. It includes details about research design, data collection, tools, and the analytical framework employed in the study. The study encompasses various social media platforms such as Facebook, Twitter, Instagram, WhatsApp, and YouTube, all of which play a crucial role in shaping contemporary communication practices in Arabic-speaking communities.

3.1 Research Design

This research follows an exploratory, qualitative approach, supplemented by quantitative techniques to provide a comprehensive understanding of how lexical borrowing occurs in Arabic social media through the use of English loanwords. By employing qualitative content analysis, the study seeks to identify and analyze patterns of English loanword adoption and the sociolinguistic factors that promote this trend. The study also incorporates a quantitative element in which the frequency and context of English loanword usage across different platforms are measured, offering a balanced insight into the phenomenon.

The design is cross-sectional, capturing a snapshot of contemporary language use across several platforms. Social media, as a key medium for informal and hybrid communication, was chosen due to its pervasiveness in the Arab world, particularly among younger generations who are more likely to engage in language mixing (e.g., Dubiner, 2021; Hayat & AlBader 2022; Althobaiti, 2024). The platforms selected—Facebook, Twitter, Instagram, WhatsApp, and YouTube—are particularly influential as they encourage rapid and dynamic interactions, allowing for a rich collection of linguistic data. YouTube, in particular, is a critical space for content creation and consumption, where creators frequently use both Arabic and English, especially when engaging with global trends or technological topics.

This research examines how the interaction between English and Arabic reflects broader trends in globalization, identity formation, and digital communication. It also explores the varying degrees of lexical borrowing observed across different platforms, considering the diverse user bases and communication styles typical of each. For instance, while WhatsApp may feature more intimate, peer-to-peer communication, YouTube and Instagram serve as platforms for public content creation, where influencers and audiences frequently incorporate English as a marker of modernity and trendiness.

3.2 Data Collection

The data collection phase consisted of two primary methods: qualitative content analysis of public social media posts and comments, and participant observation focusing on the linguistic behavior of users who actively engage in English-Arabic code-switching. This dual approach allowed for both a macro-level examination of language use trends and a micro-level understanding of individual language choices in digital communication.

3.2.1 Social Media Content Analysis

Approximately 2,500 social media posts and comments were gathered from Facebook, Twitter, Instagram, YouTube, and WhatsApp between January and June 2023. These platforms were selected for their popularity in the Arab world and their varied user demographics. The posts were sampled from public accounts and online communities with a high frequency of English loanword use, particularly among younger, urbanized Arabic speakers.

The sampling process was purposive rather than random, targeting specific user groups where lexical borrowing and lexical borrowing are most prominent. In particular, data were collected from influencers, content creators, technology enthusiasts, and youth communities that frequently engage with global cultural content. This selection ensured that the data reflected a broad spectrum of loanword usage in online interactions. Influencers on platforms like YouTube and Instagram, for example, tend to incorporate English terms related to lifestyle, technology, and fashion, creating hybrid linguistic environments that merge English with Arabic.

On WhatsApp, private conversations were also analyzed, though only with informed consent from participants. These conversations provided insights into how English loanwords are used in more intimate, less public exchanges. Data from WhatsApp were particularly useful in understanding how peer-to-peer communication differs from the public personas presented on more visible platforms like YouTube or Instagram.

3.2.2 Participant Observation

In addition to collecting social media content, participant observation was conducted with a small group of Arabic-speaking individuals who frequently engage in digital communication. This group included students, professionals, and content creators, all of whom were active on the five selected platforms. The goal of this observation was to understand the social dynamics and motivations behind the use of English loanwords. Participants were observed in their natural online communication environments, and their language usage patterns were documented over a three-month period.

Informed consent was obtained from all participants, particularly for observing private conversations on platforms like WhatsApp. The participant observation method was essential for capturing the nuances of language choice and the contextual factors driving code-switching between English and Arabic. For instance, users often switch to English terms in specific conversational contexts—such as discussing technology or fashion—where English words are perceived as more precise or globally relevant.

3.3 Analytical Approach

The analysis of the collected data was conducted through qualitative and quantitative techniques. A linguistic and sociolinguistic framework was applied to examine the integration of English loanwords into Arabic discourse, focusing on both structural linguistic elements and sociocultural implications. To facilitate this analysis, the software Ghawwas V4.0 was employed.[1]

3.3.1 Qualitative Content Analysis

Qualitative content analysis focused on identifying patterns of English loanword usage across different social media platforms. The analysis involved coding each instance of English loanwords, examining their frequency, context of use, and the syntactic or semantic modifications (if any) that occur when they are incorporated into Arabic sentences. Each English loanword was categorized based on its function in the conversation, such as whether it was used in technology-related discussions (e.g., "download," "subscribe"), everyday slang (e.g., "cool," "like"), or social media-specific contexts (e.g., "post," "comment," "hashtag").

The analysis aimed to identify not just the loanwords themselves but also the extent of their integration into everyday Arabic communication. For instance, English terms like "hashtag" and "like" are often used without modification, while other terms may undergo slight phonetic or syntactic changes to fit more comfortably within Arabic sentence structures. Social media conversations were segmented based on these factors, enabling the identification of specific linguistic patterns.

3.3.2 Quantitative Frequency Analysis

A quantitative analysis was conducted *just to complement the qualitative findings*, measuring the frequency of English loanword usage across different platforms and user demographics. The goal was to quantify the prevalence of English terms in Arabic social media conversations, providing a clearer picture of how widespread the lexical borrowing of Arabic has become. This analysis involved calculating the proportion of English loanwords in a given dataset, as well as identifying the most frequently used loanwords.

For example, on Instagram and YouTube, loanwords related to technology and lifestyle (such as "vlog," "subscribe," "like," and "content creator") were particularly common, while platforms like WhatsApp and Twitter featured more everyday slang and informal expressions. These differences were quantified using Ghawwas V4.0's statistical analysis tools, which allowed for the comparison of loanword frequency between different user groups (e.g., influencers versus everyday users) and platforms.

3.4 Tools and Techniques

The primary tool used in the analysis was Ghawwas V4.0, a software specifically designed for linguistic data analysis in multilingual contexts. Ghawwas V4.0 is particularly well-suited for analyzing Arabic texts mixed with foreign elements, such as English loanwords, due to its ability to handle large datasets and its advanced coding functions made it an ideal choice for this study, as it facilitated both thematic and frequency-based analyses.

In addition to Ghawwas V4.0, basic statistical tools were employed to measure the frequency of English loanword usage, ensuring that the study's findings were supported by quantitative data. Descriptive statistics were used to analyze the proportion of English words in social media posts, providing insights into the extent of language mixing across platforms and user demographics.

Reliability in this study was ensured through systematic cross-checking of the collected linguistic data and the use of Ghawwas V4.0, which supported consistent coding and frequency validation across platforms. To enhance reliability, repeated cycles of coding were conducted, and ambiguous cases of loanword usage were reviewed by multiple researchers to minimize subjective bias. Platform balancing was achieved by intentionally sampling data from Facebook, Twitter, Instagram, YouTube, and WhatsApp, ensuring that no single platform dominated the dataset. Each platform contributed proportionally according to its user activity and linguistic relevance, especially regarding the use of English loanwords. The sampling frame consisted of approximately 2,500 public posts and comments collected between January and June 2023, complemented by consent-based WhatsApp conversations. The geographic spread included users from various Arabic-speaking regions, with a focus on urban, digitally active communities in the Gulf, Levant, and North Africa, reflecting diverse dialectal and sociolinguistic backgrounds. Error checking involved verifying transliterations, removing duplicate posts, and confirming that each borrowed term was used contextually rather than appearing as part of shared non-Arabic content. Together, these procedures ensured that the dataset was balanced, representative, and methodologically sound.

3.5 Ethical Considerations

Given the nature of the research, ethical considerations were carefully addressed throughout the study. Social media platforms involve public and private communication, and it was essential to ensure that participants' privacy and confidentiality were respected. Only public posts and comments were used for the content analysis, while informed consent was obtained for any data involving private conversations on WhatsApp or direct messages on other platforms.

All participants in the observational phase of the study were fully informed about the research aims and methods, and their identities were anonymized in all publications and presentations of the research findings. The study adhered to the ethical guidelines for digital research, ensuring that all data collection and analysis procedures respected user privacy and complied with the terms of service for each social media platform.

3.6 Limitations

This study is subject to several limitations. First, the non-randomized sampling method limits the generalizability of the findings. The research focused on specific communities and user groups where English loanwords are prevalent, which may not reflect broader trends in other Arabic-speaking regions or among different social groups. Additionally, the platforms analyzed—Facebook, Twitter, Instagram, YouTube, and WhatsApp—represent only a portion of the vast digital landscape, and other platforms may exhibit different patterns of language use.

Moreover, while qualitative analysis provides in-depth insights, it cannot fully capture the quantitative scope of loanword usage across the entirety of Arabic digital communication. Future research could benefit from more extensive quantitative surveys or experimental designs to validate the hypotheses generated by this study.

Another limitation lies in the complexity of analyzing code-switching, especially given the fluid nature of online language use. English loanwords are often integrated into Arabic in creative and context-dependent ways, making it challenging to apply rigid linguistic categorizations. Finally, the reliance on Ghawwas V4.0, while highly effective, is constrained by the tool's inherent limitations in analyzing non-orthographic or highly informal linguistic data, which is common on platforms like WhatsApp.

4 FINDINGS AND DISCUSSION

This section presents the findings of the study based on the analysis of English loanword usage in Arabic communication on social media platforms such as Facebook, Twitter, Instagram, YouTube, and WhatsApp. The discussion focuses on how these loanwords are integrated into everyday Arabic discourse, the contexts in which they are used, and the linguistic modifications that occur as a result of their adaptation. The findings highlight the social, cultural, and linguistic implications of this phenomenon, particularly how it reflects both the influence of globalization and the unique adaptability of the Arabic language.

Table 1. Frequency, occurrence, percentage of loanwords across different social media platforms

Loanword	Occurrences	Percentage of Total Loanword Usage	Platforms Where Common	Context
Like ( )	743	22.51%	Facebook, Instagram, Twitter	Expressing appreciation for posts
Comment ( )	621	18.81%	Facebook, Instagram, YouTube	Adding remarks or feedback
Subscribe ( )	376	11.39%	YouTube	Subscribing to channels
Hashtag ( )	248	7.51%	Twitter, Instagram	Tagging trends or topics
Post ( )	318	7.46%	Facebook, Instagram	Sharing content
Followers ( )	213	6.26%	Instagram, YouTube	Tracking audience or fanbase
Tweet ( )	154	4.65%	Twitter	Sharing updates or short messages
Story ( )	192	5.80%	Instagram, WhatsApp	Sharing ephemeral posts
Share ( )	136	4.10%	Facebook, WhatsApp	Sharing content with others
Trend ( )	98	2.97%	Twitter, Instagram	Highlighting popular topics
Tag ( )	87	2.63%	Instagram, Twitter	Mentioning or tagging users
Vlog ( )	64	1.94%	YouTube, Instagram	Referring to video blogs

continued on following page

Table 1. Continued

Loanword	Occurrences	Percentage of Total Loanword Usage	Platforms Where Common	Context
Download ( )	51	1.55%	Various	Referring to downloading content
Live ( )	43	1.30%	Facebook, Instagram, YouTube	Hosting or watching live broadcasts
Filter ( )	37	1.12%	Instagram	Referring to photo or video effects

4.1 Overview of English Loanword Usage

The analysis revealed a significant prevalence of English loanwords across all social media platforms, particularly in discussions related to technology, social media features, entertainment, and digital communication. Users frequently employ English terms, either directly or in Arabized forms, to refer to platform-specific functions and concepts. This pattern is especially pronounced among younger Arabic speakers, who are more likely to be immersed in global digital culture and fluent in English.

Table 2. Summary of the most commonly used English loanwords identified in the dataset, along with their Arabic transliterations and the specific contexts in which they are used

English Word	Arabic Transliteration	Meaning/Context
Subscribe		Subscribing to a YouTube channel or account
Hashtag		Social media tagging system
Memes		Internet humor, often shared on social media
Like		Liking a post, comment, or tweet
Post		A post on Facebook, Instagram, etc.
Followers		People following an account on social media
Comment		Leaving a comment on a post or video
Influencer		A social media personality with influence
Tweet		A Twitter post

These loanwords, often taken directly from English, are typically used in their unmodified form in Arabic social media interactions, especially when the platforms themselves promote the English terminology as the default interface language. For instance, users of platforms like Instagram, YouTube, and Twitter frequently refer to the platform's features using English terms like "subscribe" ( ) or "like"

( ) without translating them into Arabic, which is largely due to the dominance of English in digital technologies and global trends.

4.2 Patterns of Arabization

While many English loanwords are used in their original form, there is a notable trend toward Arabizing these terms, particularly in the way they are adapted to fit Arabic's grammatical and morphological systems. Arabization refers to the process of modifying a foreign word to conform to the phonetic, syntactic, and morphological rules of Arabic. This process is evident in the creation of plural forms, verb conjugations, or other grammatical modifications applied to English loanwords.

For example:

- The word "like" ( ) becomes " " (likes) in the plural form, following the Arabic pattern for pluralization.
- Similarly, "comment" ( ) becomes " " (comments) when pluralized in Arabic.

Table 3. Common English loanwords used in Arabic, along with their Arabized forms, focusing on pluralization and verb usage

English Word	Arabic Singular	Arabic Plural (Arabized)	Usage Example
Like			(the post got five likes)
Comment			(I wrote four comments)
Post			(I shared many posts today)
Follower		(no change)	(I have a thousand followers)
Tweet			(I posted three tweets today)

As seen in the table, the Arabization of English loanwords often involves adding the plural marker " " (at) to create a plural form, as is typical in Arabic. However, certain words like "follower" ( ) retain their original English plural form due to their widespread use in the online world. This hybridization shows that Arab speakers are selectively adapting foreign words based on convenience and familiarity, especially when the English word carries prestige or global recognition.

4.3 Social and Cultural Contexts of Loanword Usage

The use of English loanwords in Arabic social media conversations is not just a linguistic phenomenon but also a reflection of broader social and cultural dynamics. Younger Arabic speakers, in particular, are more likely to use English loanwords as part of their daily digital communication. This trend is influenced by several factors:

1. **Globalization and Digital Influence**: English is the dominant language in global technology, entertainment, and business (e.g., Shokhrukh, 2024; Räisänen & Kankaanranta, 2024). Many social media platforms, including Facebook, Instagram, YouTube, and Twitter, are designed with English as their primary language, even in Arabic-speaking countries. As a result, platform-specific terms like "like," "comment," and "hashtag" are often adopted directly without translation. Using these terms in Arabic-speaking contexts can signal a user's participation in global digital culture.
2. **Prestige and Modernity**: English is often associated with modernity, innovation, and global sophistication, particularly in Arab societies. The integration of English loanwords into Arabic discourse, especially on platforms like YouTube and Instagram, can serve as a marker of social status, education, and technological savvy. Influencers and content creators frequently mix English with Arabic to engage with a broader audience, reflecting their alignment with global trends.
3. **Efficiency and Brevity**: English loanwords are often seen as more efficient or concise compared to their Arabic equivalents. For instance, words like "subscribe" ( ) or "post" ( ) are simpler and quicker to use than their full Arabic translations. This is especially relevant in fast-paced digital environments like WhatsApp chats, Instagram captions, or YouTube comments, where brevity is valued.

4.4 Impact of Social Media Platforms on Loanword Usage

Different social media platforms promote varying levels of English loanword integration based on their interface design, user base, and content focus. The findings show that platforms like YouTube and Instagram, which are heavily influenced by global visual and cultural trends, feature the highest use of English loanwords. On these platforms, users frequently adopt English terminology related to content creation, technology, and social media features. For example, YouTube content creators ( ) commonly refer to "subscribing" ( ) or leaving a "comment"

( ), while Instagram influencers ( ) often talk about gaining "followers" ( ) or posting a "story" ( ).

On platforms like WhatsApp, where communication is more personal and conversational, users still employ English loanwords but in more informal contexts. For instance, WhatsApp conversations often feature terms like "like" ( ) and "comment" ( ) in discussions about posts shared from other social media platforms.

Table 4. Key platforms analyzed in this study and the typical English loanwords encountered on each platform

Platform	Common Loanwords	Context of Usage
Facebook	, ,	Posts, comments, and likes in public conversations
Instagram	, , ,	Hashtags, followers, posts, and likes in photo sharing and influencer culture
YouTube	, , ,	Subscribing, commenting, and following influencers
Twitter	, , ,	Tweets, comments, likes, and hashtags in public discourse
WhatsApp	, ,	Likes and comments in private or group chats

This table demonstrates how each platform fosters a unique blend of Arabic and English, with YouTube and Instagram showing a higher degree of loanword integration due to their role in content creation and global engagement.

4.5 Linguistic Adaptation and Creativity

One interesting finding of this study is the creativity with which Arabic speakers adapt and modify English loanwords to suit their linguistic needs. Arabization often goes beyond simple borrowing; it involves making the loanwords conform to Arabic phonological, morphological, and syntactic structures. The creation of plural forms (e.g. ,) is one example, but speakers also occasionally conjugate English loanwords as Arabic verbs. For instance:

- Some users conjugate the word "like" ( ) as an Arabic verb by saying " " (I liked [the post]), showing how foreign words are incorporated into Arabic verb structures.

This kind of linguistic adaptation reflects the dynamic nature of Arabic and its ability to absorb foreign elements while maintaining its structural integrity. Arab speakers are not passive consumers of foreign terms but active participants in reshaping them to fit their linguistic and cultural contexts.

4.6 Sociolinguistic Implications

The widespread use of English loanwords in Arabic, particularly on social media, has significant sociolinguistic implications.

It demonstrates the increasing influence of English on Arabic speakers, particularly younger generations, and highlights the role of social media as a catalyst for linguistic change. However, this phenomenon also raises questions about the future of the Arabic language and whether these foreign influences could lead to the erosion of linguistic purity.

Some scholars argue that the adoption of English loanwords is a natural part of language evolution, particularly in a globalized, interconnected world. Others, however, worry that the overuse of foreign terms could dilute the richness of Arabic and undermine its cultural significance. This debate underscores the complex relationship between language, identity, and globalization in the digital age.

5 IMPLICATIONS FOR ARABIC LANGUAGE AND CULTURE

The increasing incorporation of English loanwords into Arabic, particularly in the digital context, has profound implications for both the Arabic language and the cultural identity of its speakers. This section explores the linguistic, social, and cultural consequences of the growing prevalence of English loanwords in Arabic, with a particular focus on how these changes may affect the future of the Arabic language and its speakers' sense of identity. The discussion is framed within the broader context of globalization, digital communication, and language evolution, all of which shape the ways in which languages interact and influence one another.

5.1 Linguistic Implications: Language Change and Adaptation

From a linguistic perspective, the widespread use of English loanwords in Arabic reflects a process of language evolution and adaptation. Language contact theory posits that when languages come into prolonged contact with one another, as Arabic and English have in the digital era, they inevitably influence each other. For Arabic, this influence is most evident in the borrowing of vocabulary related to technology, social media, and digital culture.

The use of loanwords like “ ” (subscribe), “ ” (hashtag), “ ” (memes), and “ ” (followers) highlights how Arabic speakers are adopting English terms that correspond to new concepts and technologies that did not previously exist in Arabic. These borrowings fill lexical gaps in the language, allowing speakers to communicate effectively about digital phenomena. However, this also raises questions about whether Arabic will continue to develop its own indigenous vocabulary for these concepts or whether English terms will remain dominant.

One concern is that the continued reliance on English loanwords could hinder the development of the Arabic lexicon, particularly in fields like technology and business. For instance, while words like " " (like) and " " (comment) are widely used in everyday digital interactions, there are Arabic equivalents for these terms. Yet, Arabic speakers often prefer the English versions, which they see as more efficient or globally recognizable. This could lead to a situation where Arabic becomes increasingly reliant on English for certain domains, which might limit the language's capacity to evolve independently in those areas.

At the same time, the process of Arabization—where English loanwords are adapted to fit Arabic phonological and morphological rules—demonstrates the resilience and flexibility of Arabic. Words like " " (comments) and " " (likes) are examples of how Arabic speakers modify foreign terms to conform to the language's grammatical structures. This suggests that while Arabic is influenced by English, it also retains its linguistic integrity by incorporating foreign elements in ways that align with its own rules and patterns.

5.2 Social Implications: Prestige and Identity

The integration of English loanwords into Arabic, particularly on social media, also carries significant social implications. Language is a key marker of identity, and the choice to use English terms in Arabic conversations can signal various aspects of social status, education, and global connectedness.

In many Arabic-speaking countries, English is associated with modernity, technological advancement, and higher social status. As a result, using English loanwords, especially in digital contexts, can be a way for speakers to project a cosmopolitan or globally aware identity. This is especially true for younger generations, who are more likely to be bilingual or have a high level of proficiency in English. For them, mixing English with Arabic, particularly in the form of loanwords like " " (influencer) or " " (followers), is a way to align themselves with global trends and communicate their participation in international digital culture.

However, this trend can also create a divide between different groups of Arabic speakers. For instance, those who are less proficient in English or who are more attached to traditional Arabic language use may view the increasing use of English loanwords as a threat to the integrity of their language and cultural identity. This tension reflects broader societal debates about the influence of Western culture in the Arab world and the extent to which English should be embraced or resisted.

Moreover, there is a significant presence of linguistic purists who advocate for the preservation of the Arabic language's integrity. These purists often express concern about the erosion of Arabic due to the influx of English loanwords, viewing it as a form of cultural imperialism. Their efforts may involve promoting the use of traditional Arabic vocabulary, developing Arabic equivalents for commonly used English terms, and encouraging awareness of the cultural significance of maintaining linguistic purity. This active resistance to the increasing influence of English underscores the complex dynamics at play in the sociolinguistic landscape of the Arabic-speaking world.

5.3 Cultural Implications: Globalization and Cultural Identity

The increasing use of English loanwords in Arabic reflects the broader impact of globalization on cultural identity. Globalization, particularly through digital platforms, has facilitated the spread of English as the lingua franca of international communication. For Arabic speakers, participating in global digital culture often means adopting English vocabulary, particularly in domains like technology, entertainment, and social media.

The adoption of English loanwords in Arabic can be seen as part of a larger process of cultural exchange, where languages and cultures interact and influence one another. On the one hand, this interaction allows Arabic speakers to engage with global trends and participate in international conversations. On platforms like YouTube, Instagram, and Twitter, the use of terms like "   " (subscribe) or "   " (hashtag) connects Arabic speakers to a global audience and enables them to communicate across linguistic boundaries.

On the other hand, this process also raises concerns about cultural homogenization and the erosion of linguistic and cultural diversity. Critics argue that the increasing reliance on English loanwords, particularly in domains like technology and social media, could lead to the gradual loss of Arabic's distinctiveness as a language and a cultural marker. In this view, the use of English terms in place of Arabic equivalents is seen as a form of cultural imperialism, where English exerts dominance over other languages and cultures.

However, it is important to recognize that the use of English loanwords in Arabic is not necessarily a sign of cultural subjugation. Rather, it may reflect the complex and dynamic ways in which cultures adapt to global influences while maintaining their own unique identities. Arabic speakers, particularly on social media, are not simply passive consumers of English terms; they actively modify and adapt these terms to fit their linguistic and cultural context, as seen in the Arabization of loanwords.

Table 5. Further English loanwords that have become integrated into online Arabic

English word	Arabic example	Loanword
system	The company upgraded the ***system*** for more efficiency.	
server	The server stopped responding due to a technical fault.	
password		
data	The company is gathering ***data*** to analyze users' behavior.	
software	Please download the new ***software*** to upgrade the device.	
hardware	To solve the problem, we need to change part of the ***hardware***.	
cloud	All files are stored in the ***cloud*** to make access easier.	
trend	This video became a ***trend*** in less than a day.	
filter	I tried a new ***filter*** for the selfie.	
story	I watched my friend's ***story*** yesterday.	
share	***Share*** this video if you like it!	
influencer	She became a famous ***influencer*** after the success of her content.	

5.4 The Future of Arabic in the Digital Age

The growing presence of English loanwords in Arabic raises important questions about the future of the Arabic language in the digital age (e.g., Umurzakova, 2024; Auliya et al., 2025). As social media platforms and digital technologies continue to evolve, it is likely that English will maintain its dominance in these spaces, especially in fields like technology, business, and entertainment. This means that Arabic speakers will continue to encounter and use English terms in their everyday digital communication.

However, the future of Arabic will depend on how the language adapts to these influences. One possibility is that Arabic will continue to integrate English loanwords while maintaining its own linguistic structures and cultural identity. This process of adaptation, as seen in the Arabization of loanwords, suggests that Arabic has the capacity to evolve in response to external influences without losing its core identity.

Another possibility is that efforts to promote the use of Arabic in digital contexts will increase, particularly through the development of Arabic equivalents for common English terms. Some language purists and cultural advocates argue that Arabic should resist the influx of English loanwords and instead focus on developing its own technological and digital vocabulary. This could lead to a resurgence of interest in linguistic preservation and a push for greater use of Arabic in digital spaces.

6 CONCLUSION

In conclusion, the integration of English loanwords into Arabic on social media platforms reflects the broader dynamics of language change, social identity, and cultural adaptation in the digital age. While the use of these loanwords may raise concerns about linguistic purity and cultural erosion, it also highlights the adaptability and resilience of the Arabic language. As Arabic continues to evolve in response to global influences, it is likely that speakers will find new ways to balance the demands of modernity with the preservation of their linguistic and cultural heritage. Moreover, the phenomenon demonstrates how digital communication accelerates linguistic innovation, creating hybrid forms that mirror shifting social realities, especially among younger generations. The ongoing interplay between global digital norms and localized linguistic practices suggests that Arabic will continue to diversify rather than diminish. Importantly, these linguistic changes reveal how speakers negotiate identity, belonging, and cultural expression in rapidly changing digital environments. They also underscore the need to view linguistic borrowing not merely as external influence but as an active, creative process driven by users themselves. A more in-depth investigation into the borrowing of English and other languages in conversational Arabic across the Arabian Peninsula is anticipated, ideally conducted from a Cognitive Linguistics standpoint, to further understand how conceptual structures, cultural schemas, and embodied experiences shape the process of lexical integration.

REFERENCES

Abdul-Fattah, H. M. (2010). Semantic extension of loanwords in Jordanian Arabic. *SKASE Journal of Theoretical Linguistics*, *7*(1), 14–26.

Al-Batal, M. (1992). Diglossia proficiency: The need for an alternative approach to teaching. In *Georgetown University Round Table on Languages and Linguistics* (pp. 284–303). Georgetown University Press.

Al-Khatib, M. A., & Sabbah, E. S. (2008). Language choice in mobile text messages among Jordanian university students. *SKASE Journal of Theoretical Linguistics*, *5*(1), 28–42.

Al-Mughirah, H. A. M., Al-Basala, A. S., & Al-Rumahi, H. M. (2025). The impact of foreign electronic games on Arabic language and culture in Saudi Arabia. *Arts for Linguistic & Literary Studies*, *7*(3), 68–87. DOI: 10.53286/arts.v7i3.2715

Al-Saqqaf, A. H. (2006). The linguistics of loanwords in Hadhrami Arabic. *International Journal of Bilingual Education and Bilingualism*, *9*(1), 75–93. DOI: 10.1080/13670050608668631

Alhassan, A. M. (2016). The impact of English loanwords on Arabic: A cognitive linguistic perspective. *International Journal of Linguistics*, *8*(5), 15–30. DOI: 10.5296/ijl.v8i5.10028

Althobaiti, A. A. T. (2024). *The Spread of English in Saudi Arabia: A Study of University Students' Attitudes and Language Use* (Doctoral dissertation, UNSW Sydney).

An, G. (2024). Domestication and Foreignisation in Translation Studies: A Bibliometric Analysis of WoS Core Journal Articles. *Journal of Intercultural Communication*, *24*(4), 13–22. DOI: 10.36923/jicc.v24i4.933

An, J. (2025). Lexical borrowing as A Cultural Expectation in the Context of Globalization: A Case Study of Chinese President Xi Jinping's 2025 New Year Message. *International Journal of English Language Studies, 7*(1), 08-16.

Auer, P. (1998). *Code-switching in conversation: Language, interaction and identity*. Routledge.

Auliya, A., Aljanah, D. S., Sagala, R., Hijriyah, U., & Ghazi, F. (2025). The Digital Revolution in Arabic Language Learning: An Analysis of Trends, Results, and the Future of Language Education in the Digital Age. *RADEN INTAN: Proceedings on Family and Humanity*, *2*(1), 194–203. DOI: 10.47352/3032-503x.69

Bahumaid, Showqi (2015). "Lexical Borrowing: The Case of English Loanwords in Hadhrami Arabic", *International Journal of Language and Linguistics*. Vol. 2, No. 6; December 2015

Bassiouney, R. (2009). *Arabic sociolinguistics*. Edinburgh University Press. DOI: 10.3366/edinburgh/9780748623730.001.0001

Chyrvonyi, O. S. (2024). The evolution of social media language: a sociolinguistic analysis of recent neologisms.

Crystal, D. (2001). *Language and the internet*. Cambridge University Press. DOI: 10.1017/CBO9781139164771

Danet, B., & Herring, S. C. (Eds.). (2007). *The multilingual internet: Language, culture, and communication online*. Oxford University Press. DOI: 10.1093/acprof:oso/9780195304794.001.0001

Darwish, Hosam M. (2015) "Arabic Loan Words in English Language", *IOSR Journal of Humanities and Social Science (IOSR-JHSS). Volume 20, Issue 7, Ver. VII (July 2015), PP 105-109.*

Dubiner, D. (2021). 'We don't think about it, we just mix': Language choice and ethnolinguistic identity among Arabic-Hebrew bilinguals in Israel. *International Journal of Bilingual Education and Bilingualism, 24*(2), 191–206. DOI: 10.1080/13670050.2018.1452893

Evans, V., & Green, M. (2006). *Cognitive linguistics: An introduction*. Lawrence Erlbaum Associates.

Geeraerts, D., & Cuyckens, H. (Eds.). (2007). *The Oxford handbook of cognitive linguistics*. Oxford University Press.

Gumperz, J. J. (1982). *Discourse strategies*. Cambridge University Press. DOI: 10.1017/CBO9780511611834

Haspelmath, Martin and Tadmor (2009) *Loanwords in the World's Languages: A Comparative Handbook*

Haugen, E. (1950). The analysis of linguistic borrowing. *Language, 26*(2), 210–231. DOI: 10.2307/410058

Hayat, N. A., & AlBader, Y. B. (2022). The McChicken Phenomenon: How Has English Become a Prevalent Language among Kuwaiti Youths? *World Journal of English Language, 12*(6), 59. DOI: 10.5430/wjel.v12n6p59

Holes, C. (2004). *Modern Arabic: Structures, functions, and varieties*. Georgetown University Press.

Ibrahim, M. H. (1982). Arabic–English bilingualism: A code-switching and borrowing study. *Anthropological Linguistics*, *24*(1), 55–68.

Indriani, L., & Bram, B. (2023, May). Lexical borrowing of social media terms in *liputan6.com* website. *Journal of Language.*, *5*(1), 11–22. DOI: 10.30743/jol.v5i1.6836

Ji, C., & Chen, Y. (2022). A Tentative Study on Translation Tactics of Culture-loaded Words Based on Domestication and Lexical borrowing: A Case Analysis of The Last Emperor Film. *Modern Languages, Literatures, and Linguistics, 1*(01).

Lakoff, G., & Johnson, M. (2008). *Metaphors we live by*. University of Chicago Press.

Miller, J. E., & List, J. M. (2023). "Detecting Lexical Borrowings from Dominant Languages in Multilingual Wordlists". *Proceedings of the 17th Conference of the European Chapter of the Association for Computational Linguistics*, pages 2599–2605 May 2-6, ©2023 Association for Computational Linguistics. DOI: 10.18653/v1/2023.eacl-main.190

Netton, I. R. (Ed.). (1985). *Arabia and the Gulf: From traditional society to modern states*. Croom Helm.

Oh, Y., & Son, H. (2023) "Lexical borrowing in Korean: a diachronic approach based on a corpus analysis", in *the Journal* Corpus Linguistics and Linguistic Theory. De Gruyter Mouton August 24, 2023

Poplack, S., Sankoff, D., & Miller, C. (1988). The social correlates and linguistic processes of lexical borrowing and assimilation. *Linguistics*, *26*(1), 47–104. DOI: 10.1515/ling.1988.26.1.47

Räisänen, T., & Kankaanranta, A. (2024). The use of English as corporate language in global knowledge work over a 15-year business career. *European Journal of International Management*, *23*(4), 677–700. DOI: 10.1504/EJIM.2024.139611

Shokhrukh, A. (2024). The Dominance of English in The Global Technology Industry: Implications for Non-English-Speaking Countries. *Universal Journal of Social Sciences. Philosophy and Culture*, *2*(11), 41–55.

Smart, J. R. (1985). In Netton, I. R. (Ed.), *Language development in the Gulf: Lexical interference of English in the Gulf dialects* (pp. 202–212).

Suleiman, Y. (2013). *Arabic in the fray: Language ideology and cultural politics*. Edinburgh University Press.

Tariq, M., Tariq, A., & Sadiq, A. H. B. (2024). Exploring Domestication and Lexical borrowing in the Urdu Translation of Doctor Faustus. *Harf-o-Sukhan*, *8*(1), 291–299.

Thomason, S. G., & Kaufman, T. (1988). *Language contact, creolization, and genetic linguistics*. University of California Press. DOI: 10.1525/9780520912793

Tian, M. (2023). Research on the Application of Domestication and Lexical borrowing in Literary Translation. *International Journal of Education and Humanities*, *9*(1), 87–92. DOI: 10.54097/ijeh.v9i1.9364

Umurzakova, A. U. (2024). Arabic Language in the Era of Globalization: Problems and Solutions. *O'zbekiston davlat jahon tillari universiteti konferensiyalari*, 126-129.

Ur Rehman, S., Malik, A., Jawad, M., & Khan, M. (2025). The Influence of Technology on Contemporary English Vocabulary: Neologisms and Digital Discourse. *Review of Applied Management and Social Sciences*, *8*(1), 157–168. DOI: 10.47067/ramss.v8i1.445

Yonamine, M. (2022). Domestication and lexical borrowing in interlingual subtitling: A systematic review of contemporary research. *Translation & Interpreting: The International Journal of Translation and Interpreting Research*, *14*(1), 198–213.

Yousuf, Mustafa (2022). "The Phenomenon of Language Borrowing at the Arabic Language Academy" (in Arabic) *Sardiyāt* , vol 12, issue 44, pp 85-136.

ENDNOTE

1 https://sourceforge.net/projects/ghawwasv4/

Chapter 3
Improving Communication Skills of Children With Autism Spectrum Disorder:
Engagement Through Turkish Shadow Theatre

Ayşe Tuna
https://orcid.org/0000-0003-2666-1694
Trakya University, Turkey

ABSTRACT

Research indicates therapeutic benefits of robots for children with autism; however, the potential of similar agents, such as puppets, needs to be investigated. Because puppets have been proven to capture and hold the attention of children with autism spectrum disorder, indicating the potential for alternative therapies that improve social engagement and aid learning. According to research, when a puppet speaks, children with autism spectrum disorder's attention patterns are similar to those of typically developing children and both groups exhibit a pronounced preference for the talking puppet over the listening person. In this study, we highlight the attentional and emotional benefits of puppets, which ideally can be used. In particular, in our study, Karagöz-Hacivat performance has been organised to help with therapeutic efforts. Our findings indicate that shadow play characters could be an effective tool for assisting children with autism spectrum disorder in improving their social engagement, which is quite exciting.

DOI: 10.4018/979-8-3373-3581-0.ch003

INTRODUCTION

Autism spectrum disorder (ASD) is a neurodevelopmental condition that emerges in early childhood and is characterised by persistent challenges in social communication and interaction (American Psychiatric Association, 2013). These differences influence how individuals with ASD perceive and engage with their social environment, often resulting in reduced attention to social partners and limited emotional reciprocity. Consequently, children with ASD may experience restricted access to learning opportunities that are fundamental for language, emotional, and social development. Communication impairments therefore represent a central therapeutic concern and a core target of early intervention.

Communication is the process of sharing thoughts, needs, desires, and intentions through verbal and non-verbal means, such as talking, writing, gesture, eye contact, and body language. Many children with ASD show atypical language development, which ranges from delayed or disorganised speech to limited or no verbal communication. This is further complicated by difficulties with understanding and using appropriate non-verbal communication, such as gestures, facial expressions, and personal space. In most cases, these symptoms are among the earliest indicators of ASD. Hence, to effectively communicate with children with ASD, simplification of spoken language should be made, allowing adequate time for processing, encouraging turn-taking, the use of specific questioning, and modification of speech to the developmental stage of the child.

In the last few years, robot-assisted interventions have gained considerable attention as translational tools for enhancing social and communication skills among children with ASD. Social robots may serve as mediators in the teaching of children with ASD and have already showed promising results (Puglisi et al., 2022). However, many robots have limited physical and expressive abilities. To enhance complex child-robot-therapist interactions, improved kinetic and expressive capabilities of social robots are mandatory (Puglisi et al., 2022).

The COVID-19 epidemic has witnessed awareness and innovation in digital therapeutic platforms. Peerbots, a robot puppeteering system developed for educational and therapeutic interaction, is one of these platforms and has demonstrated promising results in both institutional and home settings (Peerbots, Inc., 2025). However, there are some ethical worries, such as emotional dependency and accountability, about children's long-term interactions with these platforms. Langer, Marshall, and Levy-Tzedek (2023) state that in order to better understand long-term developmental consequences, future research should incorporate socio-emotional markers and participatory design approaches engaging children. Additionally, interdisciplinary collaboration between psychologists, roboticists, and educators is a must for ethically sound child-robot interaction research (Feingold-Polak & Levy-Tzedek, 2021).

From a stakeholder point of view, there are both the promises and challenges of social robots. Smakman, Vogt, and Konijn (2021) state that educators, parents, and policymakers largely agree that social robots are engaging, educationally useful, and informative for children. Although stakeholders are aware of the potential of social robots, there is a lack of clear regulatory and ethical frameworks and this leads to raising concerns about ethical responsibility and accountability.

Robotic platforms such as NAO and KASPAR have been shown to enhance joint attention, turn-taking, and engagement through structured and predictable interactions (Cabibihan et al., 2013; Soleiman et al., 2021). However, they are expensive options and have limited sensing capabilities and emotional expressiveness (Chevalier et al., 2021). Play therapy, by contrast, emphasises relational and symbolic engagement through unstructured or semi-structured activities, enabling children to express emotions and practice social skills in a naturalistic framework (Koukourikos et al., 2021). Visual storytelling further supports emotional organisation and symbolic meaning making.

Shadow play, an ancient art form recognised by UNESCO (2018), uniquely integrates narrative, symbolic representation, and sensory engagement through light, silhouette, movement, and voice. Its cultural adaptability, low cost, and high interactivity distinguish it from both high-tech robotics and conventional play therapy (Öcal et al., 2021; Kostidakis, 2021). Shadow theater gives the child an opportunity to explore emotional and social themes within a psychologically safe "shadow space" (Yu & Choatchamrat, 2024). These qualities make shadow play as a particularly compelling medium for neurodevelopmental intervention tool.

Puppetry offers rich opportunities for language, social, emotional, and motor development. Through dialogue, role-play, and symbolic expression, puppets support communication, empathy, creativity, listening, fine-motor coordination, and self-confidence. For children with ASD, puppets also function as mediating agents for daily routines and emotional expression, allowing difficult behaviours or anxieties to be externalised and safely addressed. Empirical research supports these benefits. Macari et al. (2021) demonstrated that children with ASD attend more consistently to puppet speakers than to human speakers, exhibiting attention patterns comparable to typically developing peers. Puppets thus appear to enhance attentional engagement and emotional responsiveness in therapeutic contexts. Similarly, Karaolis (2023) reported that puppetry may support identity expression and social participation across childhood and adolescence. Accordingly, this chapter focuses on the therapeutic use of puppets for children with ASD.

RELATED WORK

There is evidence of a growing amount of multidisciplinary research that support the belief that play-based, expressive, and puppet-mediated therapies can facilitate the development of social, emotional, and communicative skills in children with ASD. These techniques are based on developmental and constructivist or sociocultural theory that emphasise symbolic play, imitation, emotional engagement, and social contact as core elements in early learning. Such techniques represent developmentally appropriate and motivationally accessible therapies for skill learning in children with ASD.

Karaolis (2023) conducted a review on the use of puppetry with children and adolescents with ASD in educational and therapeutic settings. It was expressed in the review that puppets regularly work as relational mediators and allow children with ASD to engage in social interactions with less fear and defensive behaviour. The children were shown to be able to express their feelings, negotiate their identity, and explore peer relationships better and more freely when they were separated symbolically. Importantly, it was also expressed in the review that puppetry can be an effective intervention tool throughout early childhood into adolescence and help to promote communication, self-expression, and self-efficacy.

Macari et al. (2021) employed an eye-tracking paradigm to show the attentional advantages of puppets in the education of children with ASD. Their research included 37 young children with ASD and 27 typically developing peers who saw a recorded interaction between a human speaker and a puppet. Children with ASD paid much more visual attention to the puppet than to the real speaker, whereas typically developing children did not exhibit such difference. Furthermore, a negative link was discovered between ASD severity and attention to the real speaker, but not with attention to the puppet. These findings imply that puppets may avoid some of the social-perceptual problems inherent in face-to-face engagement, providing an ideal entry point for communication-focused therapies.

Moosapoor (2023) investigated the effects of puppet-based social storytelling using a quasi-experimental method with 15 children with ASD. The intervention consisted of 16 sessions in which social stories were performed with puppets. According to parent and teacher reports, children in the experimental group outperformed the control group in terms of communication, cooperation, assertiveness, and self-control. These findings highlight the ability of puppetry to improve not just expressive communication but also other aspects of social-emotional functioning.

Joint attention is a prerequisite for language and social development. Puppet-based interventions have been demonstrated to improve it. Using a single-subject research design, Syabila and Irvan (2022) found that interactive hand-puppet activities increased the frequency of joint-attention behaviours in children with ASD, but their effects on length were more limited. As combined attention problems are one of most persistent characteristics of ASD, these findings are very important for early intervention practice.

Beyond puppetry, a larger body of research on play therapy supports the use of symbolic and imaginative play with children with ASD. Elbeltagi et al. (2023) found that structured play therapy sessions lead to significant increases in social engagement, emotional control, and adaptive behaviour. Play-based intervention approaches help children with ASD to express their internal states through symbolic activity, which is especially helpful for individuals with limited verbal expressive capabilities.

Environmental and contextual factors influence the effectiveness of play-based therapies. Binns et al. (2022) examined caregiver-child interactions in symbolic and gross-motor play contexts. Their findings revealed that children with ASD had higher object-focused attention in symbolic contexts, whereas the engagement of carers was higher in gross-motor settings. These findings show that intervention outcomes are influenced not only by the type of activity, but also by the sensory, spatial, and relational affordances of the environment.

Creative arts therapies offer an important parallel framework for understanding the dynamics that drive shadow theatre. Peer interaction, self-awareness, and emotional expression have all improved as a result of drama therapy (Moreno & Mayer, 2007). Joint attention, vocalisation, and affective synchrony have all been shown to be effectively supported by music therapy (Dunphy et al., 2014). According to Van de Kamp et al. (2017), children with developmental problems benefit from expressive arts interventions in terms of improved emotional regulation and decreased internalising tendencies. All of these results point to common mechanisms of embodiment, emotional attunement, and symbolic meaning-making between performative and expressive modalities.

Drama, role-playing, and puppetry are examples of theatre-based therapies for children with ASD, according to a recent systematic review by Rodríguez-Vilar et al. (2023). Peer interaction, pragmatic language, facial affect recognition, and decreased social anxiety all showed consistent gains across investigations. Importantly, the review showed that theatre-based methods work best when they include elements that are essential to conventional shadow theatre, such as repetition, predictable structure, and scaffolded role enactment.

The empirical basis for puppet-mediated intervention is further strengthened by research focused on tactile companions and transitional objects. In order to encourage eye contact, taking turns, and social reciprocity in children with ASD, Özcan et al. (2022) created wearable soft companions. Seo et al. (2017) reported that when children created their own soft haptic toys, they formed deep emotional attachments to these toys, which fostered creative play and reduced repetitive behaviours. These results reveal how puppetry and shadow figures can play intermediating roles between inner experience and social reality, and are in close agreement with Winnicottian thoughts on transitional objects.

There is still little research on the applicability of shadow theatre as a therapeutic intervention tool for children with ASD. The neuropsychological and symbolic advantages of shadow theatre have been mostly ignored in favour of hand puppets, role-playing, or computer avatars. As shadow theatre incorporates visual abstraction, rhythmic movement, narrative structure, and emotional distancing, it is well suited to the learning profiles of children with ASD but has not been analysed enough. This constitutes a significant gap.

Turkish shadow theatre, particularly Karagöz and Hacivat, involves highly structured dialogue, exaggerated gestures, repetitive humour patterns, and archetypal character roles that closely correspond to the therapeutic principles identified as effective in ASD intervention research. While literature presents cultural, historical, and folkloric analyses of Karagöz and Hacivat, Karagöz and Hacivat has not been used in special education or therapeutic settings.

In summary, existing literature supports the use of puppetry, symbolic play, and expressive arts for enhancing communication and social interaction skills of children with ASD. However, although shadow theatre has strong theoretical alignment with established intervention mechanisms, it has not been focused on much. Therefore, with its brain-based, culturally ground, and developmentally appropriate intervention framework for children with ASD, Turkish shadow theatre has become the focus of this study.

BRAIN-BASED LEARNING MECHANISMS AND PUPPETRY

Brain-based learning theory highlights instructional approaches that are consistent with the brain's natural processes for attention, emotion, memory, and neural plasticity (Immordino-Yang and Damasio, 2007; Tokuhama-Espinosa, 2011). These principles are put into practice through game-based and interactive interventions. Game-based and interactive intervention approaches embed learning targets within motivational, feedback-rich, and multisensory environments that activate neural circuits associated with executive functioning, attention, and sensorimotor integration (Green and Bavelier, 2012; De Freitas & Griffiths, 2008).

Puppets can be used as neurodevelopmental intervention tools. Because they offer repetitive, emotionally engaging, and adaptive experiences that help to improve brain pathways that support social cognition, emotional regulation, and communication (Tokuhama-Espinosa, 2011). Observing and controlling puppet characters activates theory-of-mind networks, including the medial prefrontal cortex and temporoparietal junction, as children understand intentions and emotions (Frith & Frith, 2006; Castelli et al., 2002). Puppetry's symbolic distance minimises the performance pressure and social anxiety of children with ASD. This way, the children can gain a better perspective and empathy.

Affective neuroscience explains the impact of puppetry by activating limbic circuits that improve learning and memory consolidation (Immordino-Yang & Damasio, 2007). Embodied cognition theories also promote puppet-based therapies, because learning is founded on sensorimotor experience. Acting with a puppet concurrently integrates motor, affective, and cognitive domains (Barsalou, 2008).

The benefit of puppetry is further explained by affective neuroscience: emotionally salient events, such humor, expressive voice, and dramatic story, activate limbic regions that improve memory consolidation and learning (Immordino-Yang & Damasio, 2007). Since learning is founded on sensorimotor experience, puppet-based therapies are also supported by embodied cognition theories. Acting through a puppet concurrently integrates the motor, affective, and cognitive domains (Barsalou, 2008).

Puppetry serves as a mediational technique within Vygotsky's zone of proximal development, according to developmental psychology (Vygotsky, 1978). Children gradually internalize the social behavior, language, and emotional expressiveness that the puppeteer models. Children with ASD can practice social scripts, control their emotions, and improve their executive functioning in a safe, culturally relevant, and intrinsically rewarding setting through co-constructed symbolic engagement.

SHADOW THEATRE AND BRAIN-BASED LEARNING MECHANISMS

Shadow theatre activates multiple brain-based learning mechanisms by integrating sensory, cognitive, and social processes. Within shadow theatre, while children track moving silhouettes and follow unfolding narratives, they naturally engage (Posner & Rothbart, 2007). Shadow theatre effectively captures and sustains attention of the children. Because it offers dynamic storytelling, motion, and high visual contrast. This way it helps to capture and sustain attention, essential for deep learning and memory formation (Immordino-Yang & Damasio, 2007). As children plan puppet movements, anticipate narrative developments, and adapt to changing storylines or social interactions, Executive functions, encompassing working memory, cognitive flexibility, and inhibitory control, are engaged (Diamond, 2013). For example, manipulating many puppets or improvising story sequences requires real-time working memory and flexible thinking, which strengthens these key regulatory mechanisms.

Shadow theatre is built on symbolic thinking, with abstract silhouettes that represent personalities, emotions, and social events. This way it teaches children to assign meaning to symbolic objects, a process quite similar to the cognitive skills required for reading comprehension, mathematical reasoning, and narrative production (Vygotsky, 1978; Goswami 2006). Shadow play helps to externalise thought and build higher-order cognitive processes.

Symbolic thinking is the cognitive foundation of shadow theatre. Because while abstract silhouettes represent characters, emotions, and social situations. children learn to assign meaning to symbolic forms. This process parallels the cognitive skills required for reading comprehension, mathematical reasoning, and narrative construction (Vygotsky, 1978; Goswami, 2006). In this way, shadow play supports the externalisation of thought and the development of higher-order cognitive processes.

Shadow theatre supports joint attention, a key mechanism in early social learning and brain development. Within shadow theatre, children try to focus on shared shadow narratives. This strengthens joint attention and promote language development, social cognition, and collaborative learning (Mundy & Newell, 2007). In addition, while children observe and imitate puppet movements, gestures, and interactions, their mirror neuron systems are likely activated (Rizzolatti & Craighero, 2004). This supports action understanding, empathy development, and the internalisation of socially appropriate behaviours.

In summary, shadow theatre uses multimodal stimulation, symbolic representation, and social interaction to engage attention, executive functioning, joint attention, symbolic cognition, and mirror neuron networks, which are the core mechanisms of efficient brain-based learning.

METHODOLOGY

Theoretical and Conceptual Framework

Bandura's Social Learning Theory is a key framework to understand how shadow theatre may support communication and social skills development in children with ASD. Within shadow theatre, children observe socially meaningful behaviours modelled by the puppeteer through symbolic characters (Bandura, 1977). Examples of socially meaningful behaviours are turn-taking, emotional expression, and social problem-solving. By observing these socially meaningful behaviours and participating, the children imitate, rehearse, and gradually internalise them. Over time, shadow theatre characters function as symbolic social "others,". This allows the children to practice social scripts, perspective-taking, and self-regulation within a psychologically safe representational space.

Expressive Therapies Continuum (Kagin & Lusebrink, 1978) supports this key framework. It positions creative modalities along a spectrum from unstructured expressive forms to highly symbolic and performative approaches (Kagin & Lusebrink, 1978). Turkish shadow theatre occupies the structured, performative end of the Expressive Therapies Continuum, where narrative, role embodiment, and symbolic manipulation converge to promote both creativity and social learning. Within this conceptualisation, shadow theatre becomes a culturally grounded therapeutic intervention tool that integrates storytelling, humour, and dramatic structure to foster social competence, emotional regulation, and symbolic cognition in children with ASD.

Neuroscientific Foundations of Shadow Theatre

Shadow theatre activates multiple cognitive, sensorimotor, and affective systems simultaneously. High-contrast dynamic imagery activates visual processing networks, whereas coordinated puppet manipulation engages motor planning and execution circuits in the premotor and supplementary motor areas. This simultaneous activation facilitates sensorimotor integration, a fundamental process for executive function and skill development in children with ASD (Diamond, 2013).

When children see and mimic puppet motions and expressive gestures, mirror neurone systems in the inferior frontal and parietal regions are probably also activated (Rizzolatti & Craighero, 2004). Cognitive and emotional brain networks are co-activated by enacted social narratives, resulting in an enhanced learning environment that promotes affective resonance, imitation, and social understanding.

Shadow theatre offers long-term attentional engagement, multisensory integration, and emotionally salient stimulation. They are all important factors that promote neuroplasticity and in line with brain-based learning theory (Immordino-Yang & Damasio, 2007; Tokuhama-Espinosa, 2011). Puppetry's combination of visual, auditory, and kinaesthetic elements promotes sensory integration, a domain that is sometimes impacted by ASD (Schaaf & Case-Smith, 2014). In order to activate sustained attention networks in frontal-parietal systems, children must watch visual movement, comprehend narrative material, and react interactively (Posner & Rothbart, 2007).

Shadow Theatre as a Performance Medium

Shadow theatre is a traditional form of storytelling in which articulated, typically flat figures are projected between a light source and a translucent screen. Within shadow theatre, through precise manipulation of both puppets and light, character motion is created and highly expressive visual effects are achieved.

Shadow theatre performances may involve body shadows, handheld puppets, spatial projections, or dual-sided viewing of the screen. Different from other puppet forms, the audience perceives only the projected silhouette and through the interaction of light, movement, and narrative symbolism meaning emerge. This supports children's creativity and contributes to the development of language, dramatic expression, motor coordination, and kinaesthetic awareness.

Cultural Context: Karagöz and Hacivat

Karagöz and Hacivat are famous characters of Turkish shadow theatre. Karagöz and Hacivat theatre reached its classical form in the eighteenth century (Ministry of Culture and Tourism, 2025). Karagöz and Hacivat theatre is performed by a single puppeteer who controls all movement, voice, and dialogue, these performances employ satire, exaggeration, puns, and wordplay. It was historically staged during Ramadan, ceremonial events, and in public gathering spaces and offered humorous social commentary on everyday life in the Ottoman period and beyond. It is currently recognised by UNESCO as part of the Intangible Cultural Heritage of Humanity.

Transitional Space and Therapeutic Function

To understand how Karagöz and Hacivat shadow theatre may function therapeutically for children with ASD (Winnicott, 1971; Turner, 2004), it is necessary to look at Winnicott's concept of "transitional space". In Karagöz and Hacivat shadow theatre, the shadow stage becomes an intermediate zone between internal experience and external reality. This intermediate zone, i.e. transitional space, enables symbolic projection for children with ASD without the emotional risks associated with direct interpersonal exposure. Within this transitional space, Karagöz, Hacivat and other characters serve as transitional objects. These transitional objects are away from the children and animated by a trusted puppeteer. This offers predictability, containment, and emotional scaffolding.

The interactions of Karagöz and Hacivat characters involve rhythmic dialogue patterns and exaggerated gestures. This creates a structured relational framework in which children can observe and then internalise social rules such as turn-taking and conversational reciprocity. As familiarity of the children increases, the children may begin to participate the play more actively by manipulating puppets, voicing characters, or recreating narratives. This way the children practice perspective-taking and symbolic role adoption. Overall, this process aligns closely with social learning principles. Because the children observe, imitate, receive feedback, and progressively internalise social and emotional behaviours.

Humour, Predictability, and Social Regulation

One of the main strengths of Karagöz and Hacivat play for children with ASD is that it combines humour with a clear and familiar structure. Karagöz and Hacivat plays create a sense of predictability by using wordplay, exaggeration, and well-known character interactions repeatedly. Therefore, they are especially comfortable for children with ASD. At the same time, the playful and symbolic nature of their characters enables children with ASD to explore feelings safely. They also help support joint attention and everyday communication skills of children with ASD. When children are encouraged to answer, ask questions, or take part in the story, their attention naturally shifts into a shared imaginative space. Over time and with repeated sessions, the children become familiar with these patterns of interaction and internalise them. This way, they develop better social communication, emotional control, and an ability to anticipate how social interactions unfold.

Figures (characters) of the Karagöz and Hacivat shadow play are made of leather, projected onto a screen with the help of light, and played. The two main characters of the play, Karagöz and Hacivat, establish humorous dialogues with their opposite personalities. While Karagöz is a commoner, outspoken and funny character, Hacivat is an educated, polite and well-spoken person. The plays deal with daily life and social events in a humorous manner.

Figure 1. Karagöz and Hacivat

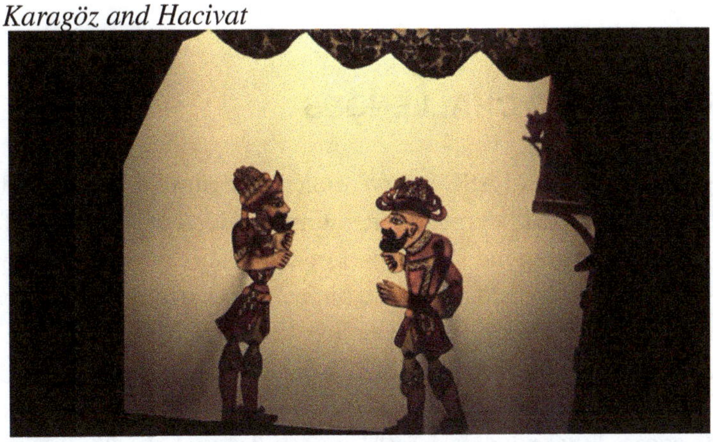

Preliminary Study

In this study, single-subject design methodology has been preferred, and a set of therapies using popular Turkish shadow theatre characters, namely Karagöz and Hacivat, has been delivered to a child. The therapy has focused on to find out whether the characters are able to improve the child's social skills. As the preliminary results focusing on engagement and emotion recognition demonstrate, the child has benefitted from the Karagöz and Hacivat play. Her continuous engagement during the play and emotion exchange with the characters and the performer could be evaluated as the indicators of the benefits.

Figure 2. Karagöz-Hacivat play of the performer

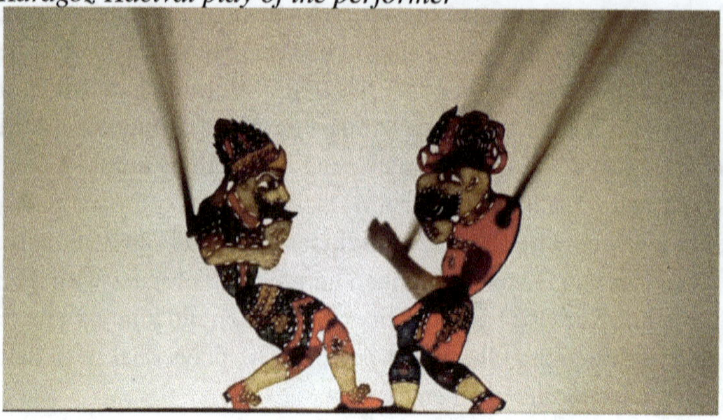

OPPORTUNITIES VS CHALLENGES

Although many empirical ASD intervention studies have not focused on shadow puppetry, the puppet-based interaction literature provides strong proof-of-concept: children with ASD can respond well to puppets, pay more attention to them than to humans in some social contexts, and use puppets to scaffold communication and social learning. Becchio, Mari, and Castiello (2010) discovered that children with ASD process cast shadows differently, which can interfere with object recognition. Macari et al. (2021) conducted an eye-tracking study with young children with ASD and discovered that puppets greatly improved visual attention to social cues.

In their experiment, children watched a video of a puppet talking vs a human. Children with ASD spent more time on the puppet's face than on the real speaker, implying that puppets may be more salient and engaging social partners for them.

Karaolis (2023) examined the significance of puppetry in the therapy and education of teenagers with ASD and highlighted its ability to sustain relevance in adolescence, encourage self-expression, and foster connection during transitions (for example, from school to adulthood). This implies that shadow-based interventions may need to be carefully tailored, such as simplifying shadow shapes, but it also provides a unique opportunity: by regulating shadow stimuli in therapy, practitioners could progressively assist children with ASD feel more comfortable.

While a number of neurodevelopmental therapies, including play therapy, robotics, and visual storytelling, have been researched in children with developmental difficulties, they are far less effective than shadow play. Social robots such as Moxie robot offer structured interactions, multimodal feedback, and data-driven assessments of social behaviour and can be employed for emotional and social skills training (Hurst, Clabaugh, Baynes, Cohn, Mitroff, & Scherer, 2020). Nevertheless, such systems can be quite expensive. In addition, they may need specialised technology, and lack sensory or cultural adaptability. Traditional play therapy may not offer highly interactive symbolic transformation or powerful visual metaphor, but it does facilitate expression and emotional regulation through unstructured play (Elbeltagi, Al-Beltagi, Saeed, & Alhawamdeh, 2023). Similarly, theatrical or drama-based interventions, like the SENSE Theatre program, focus on role-playing and peer modelling to enhance facial processing, social cognition, and reduce stress (Corbett et al., 2014; Ozonoff & Cathcart, 1998). Although these methods provide relational depth, they might not have the portability, affordability, or sensory-light adaptability necessary for wider scale, particularly in environments with limited resources.

Shadow play offers low cost, sensory richness, cultural adaptability, and interaction potential. It has been used to engage children in storytelling, role-play, and narrative construction that reflect their own cultural heritage (Wijayanti & Sulaksono, 2018). Shadow puppets can be made from inexpensive materials and projected using simple light sources. Interventions performed by shadow puppets can be deployed in resource-limited settings. This makes them more accessible than high-tech robots or expensive stage theatre. Compared to robots and expensive stage theatre, shadow play enables higher interactivity. During shadow plays, participants can manipulate puppets, control lighting, and improvise narrative arcs in real time. The resulting dynamically adaptive environment becomes ideal for symbolic thinking, emotional projection, and co-creation. In therapeutic settings, shadow characters enable children to explore fears, identities, and social themes without direct confrontation.

Shadow play has cultural resonance. For example, in Indonesia, Wayang Kulit, Indonesian traditional shadow puppetry, has been used in educational settings to promote character education and language development (Wijayanti & Sulaksono, 2018). Shadowplay has also been used in cognitive development among children with cerebral palsy (Aboo Backer & Manoharan, 2022). These findings prove that therapeutic interventions that involve culturally embodied stories and characters can promote social values and meaning-making. Therefore, they are more relatable and sustainable in culturally diverse communities compared to most robot-based and Western-style drama therapies.

Shadow play may have specific neurodevelopmental advantages for children with sensory or perceptual disabilities or differences. Research indicates that the processing of visual shadows in children with ASD is atypical; therefore, cast shadows may interfere with object recognition (Becchio & Castiello, 2010). If applied properly in a controlled therapeutic setting, shadow play could help gradually scaffold safe. By integrating symbolic shadow play with guided storytelling and role-play, practitioners can help children with ASD build these skills.

Although shadow play offers many advantages and has potential in the education of children with ASD, it has disadvantages and some challenges. First, most existing studies in this domain mostly focus on educational or cultural outcomes and do not focus on therapeutic measures of social cognition, stress, or neural change. Therefore, controlled trials with neuropsychological assessments are needed. Second, in order to implement shadow-play interventions effectively, therapists or facilitators must be trained in puppet manipulation, narrative scaffolding, and adapting stories to individual needs. Third, although the materials used in shadow puppets are cheap, lighting equipment and projection surfaces may be expensive, and safety standards must be defined for light sources.

Implementing shadow play interventions raises important ethical considerations, especially regarding sensory sensitivities, autonomy, and consent. Langer et al. (2023) emphasised the need to design puppet interventions that respect individual sensory profiles, minimise overwhelming stimuli, and allow children control over their involvement. For example, puppets and shadow play performances must be adjustable in terms of light intensity, sound volume, and pace to avoid overstimulation.

The facilitators of shadows play interventions should ensure that children with ASD can choose when and how to engage, whether as a passive observer, active puppeteer, or co-narrator. In addition, facilitators should receive training to be sensitive to nonverbal feedback from participants, recognising signs of distress or withdrawal and adapting the interaction accordingly. Moreover, the stories should be developmentally appropriate, emotionally safe, and culturally meaningful.

DISCUSSION AND FUTURE WORK

Research indicates the effectiveness of puppetry in therapeutic settings (Trimingham, 2010). Trimingham (2010) emphasised the physical reality of a puppet rather than linguistic issues, which is frequently the emphasis of literature on ASD.

Since puppets are safe and somewhat controllable physical objects, the author examined the idea of embodiment, which holds that neurological patterns are formed through physical interaction with the outside world. The author also suggested ways that this patterning may be disrupted or interrupted and how they might function therapeutically to restore some of these patterns. Furthermore, the author proposed that puppets might function in a "transitional space," much like Winnicott's "transitional objects" in infancy. Winnicott (1953) suggested that the comfort of infancy transitional objects and phenomena is transferred to religion, art, and creativity in a psychologically healthy adult. These activities serve as a bridge between the outside world, which we cannot control, and the inner world, which we do (Winnicott, 1953). These kinds of activities are psychologically required and are associated with a creative "space" of mind (Winnicott, 1953). This is where the puppets perform (Trimingham, 2010). In general, emphasis needs to be placed on the significance of the puppet's material existence and "objectness" in order to explain its unique effectiveness (Trimingham, 2010).

Packer and Moreno-Dulcey (2022) noted that the phenomenon of interest is examined inside the "frame" of pretense created by the employment of puppets and other symbolic social stimuli. However, the frame itself is disregarded or assumed to be normal (Packer & Moreno-Dulcey, 2022). On the other hand, the frame has not been separate from the phenomenon being studied in any area of inquiry. Although there is ongoing discussion on the nature of this relationship, there have been numerous suggestions that children's ability to pretend is linked to their development of a theory of mind (Packer & Moreno-Dulcey, 2022). It has also been proposed that pretense is a social activity that necessitates a basic awareness of status functions as well as an early kind of collective intentionality (Packer & Moreno-Dulcey, 2022). Packer and Moreno-Dulcey (2022) recommend that researchers reconsider the use of pretense-framed stimuli. Before giving symbolic stimuli, which are material representations like drawings, images, and models, and presuming that these are comparable to the items they represent, they ought to reconsider (Packer & Moreno-Dulcey, 2022). Comparing children's performance on activities using puppets and false belief tests with human protagonists would seem to make sense.

Abu-Ras et al. (2025) noted that future studies should look into how different puppetry styles affect the effectiveness of interventions. Designing more contextually relevant interventions may be aided by an understanding of the ways in which cultural narratives and aesthetics influence therapeutic outcomes. Furthermore, they stated that creating best practices requires a methodical analysis of the credentials and responsibilities of interventionists, especially when using puppetry in therapeutic and clinical settings. Researchers can strengthen the body of evidence and guarantee the moral and successful implementation of puppetry-based treatments by filling in these gaps. Although puppetry-based therapies have a lot of potential for use with different demographics and settings, their efficacy varies greatly depends on the context, design, and implementation (Abu-Ras et al., 2025). By using more diverse rigorous methodologies, theories, control groups, larger sample sizes, and long-term follow-up to better understand the long-term effects of puppetry-based interventions, future research should address these limitations and optimize the impact of these interventions (Abu-Ras et al., 2025).

Shadow plays can be helpful for developing spatial awareness and cause and effect. During a shadow play, playing with light and shadow has advantages beyond fostering creativity. Additionally, they assist children in acquiring critical abilities that will benefit them in the future. Children learn about shapes, sizes, and dimensions while honing their spatial awareness through play with light and shadow. As they discover how shifting an object in front of a light source alters the shadow it casts, they also gain knowledge of cause and effect. Children's social skills can also be developed through light and shadow play. They develop teamwork and communication skills by cooperating to produce shadow stories or imaginative worlds, exchanging ideas and working toward a common objective. As children describe their inventions and share their thoughts with others, this kind of play can also aid in the development of their language abilities. Anything is possible in the imaginative and exploratory realm of shadow play. The finest part is that anyone who wants to investigate it can enter this universe.

There is some empirical evidence supporting sustained communication benefits of puppet-based interventions. For instance, Moosapoor (2023) conducted a quasi-experimental study with children with ASD and found that puppet play therapy improved communication skills, such as cooperation, self-control, and assertiveness, and these gains were measurable after a 16-session social-story intervention (Moosapoor, 2023). These results suggest that puppet-mediated interventions may yield lasting social and communicative effects. A logical next step would be longitudinal research assessing whether participation in shadow theatre builds resilience, in social, emotional, and communicative domains, over months or even years.

A significant limitation of current conceptual work and pilot applications with shadow-theatre in ASD is generalisability. If an intervention is based on a single child or a small case series, it is difficult to know whether the results will extend to a broader and more diverse ASD population, varying in age, verbal ability, sensory profile, and cultural background. Future research should thus include larger samples, control groups, and longer-term follow-up.

While puppet-based interventions show promise, shadow puppetry with its light/shadow dynamics is not yet well studied in ASD clinical or educational research. Because children with ASD may respond differently to shadow stimuli, shadow theatre interventions could be carefully adapted (for example, simplified shapes, controlled lighting) to become a powerful therapeutic tool. To validate shadow theatre, future research should include controlled experimental designs, combining behavioural measures (for example, engagement, joint attention) with perceptual assessments and possibly neurophysiological measures.

There is a need to validate the neurodevelopmental efficacy of shadow-play based interventions. Randomised controlled trials should be conducted to compare shadow play with traditional play therapy and robot-based interventions. Live puppetry and digital shadow play might be combined to enable scalable, hybrid interventions that both offer sensory richness and increase accessibility. Additionally, practitioners might offer cross-cultural adaptations of shadow play, tailoring stories and puppet designs. This allows to reflect diverse cultural backgrounds, thereby enhancing engagement and cultural meaning. Personalised stories based on a child's interests may further enhance engagement.

CONCLUSION

The ability to participate in imaginative play and social interactions in a novel and non-threatening way is one of the main advantages of employing puppetry with children with ASD in the classroom. Puppetry can give children with ASD, who frequently struggle with social relationships, a safe and supervised setting in which to practice and explore social situations. In this study, single-subject design methodology was preferred, and a set of therapies using popular Turkish shadow theatre characters, namely Karagöz and Hacivat, was delivered to a child. The therapy focused on to find out whether the characters were able to improve the child's social skills in terms of engagement and emotion recognition. As the preliminary findings show, children with ASD could benefit from shadow play treatments if they are organised appropriately with child psychologists.

As shadow theatre offers a distinctive way of improving communication and engagement in children with ASD, this study has the possibly of contributing to an underexplored area of autism intervention research. Preliminary findings of this research showed that shadow theatre may serve as a valuable therapeutic tool. However, it should not be viewed as a standalone therapy but as a complementary one.

Shadow theatre can enhance motivation, create emotional safety and build early communicative foundations for children with ASD. It can be integrated into speech and language therapy, drama therapy or special education curricula to amplify benefits and promote generalisation. As interest in the development of alternative approaches to autism intervention grows, shadow theatre deserves deeper investigation and wider application.

ACKNOWLEDGMENT

Ethics committee approval was received for the pilot study section of this study from Trakya University, Trakya University Social and Human Sciences Research Ethics Committee. The approval letter's number is 2019.02.10 and its date is 20.02.2019. Written consent was obtained from the participant's parents. The author thanks Ata Taşkan, Karagöz-Hacivat performer, for his shadow play performance during the therapies delivered to the child.

REFERENCES

Aboo Backer, M. B., & Manoharan, P. (2022). The Wayang and its enchanting little puppeteers: Exploring cognitive abilities of cerebral palsy children through performance. *Jurnal Gendang Alam (GA)*, *12*(1), 83–100. DOI: 10.51200/ga.v12i1.1930

Abu-Ras, W., Al-Kubaisi, A., Idris, L. B., & Aboul-Enein, B. H. (2025). The Role of Puppetry in Mental Health Promotion: A Scoping Review of its Efficacy and Applications. *The Arts in Psychotherapy*, *92*, 102251. Advance online publication. DOI: 10.1016/j.aip.2025.102251

Bandura, A. (1977). *Social Learning Theory*. Prentice Hall.

Barsalou, L. W. (2008). Grounded cognition. *Annual Review of Psychology*, *59*(1), 617–645. DOI: 10.1146/annurev.psych.59.103006.093639 PMID: 17705682

Becchio, C., Mari, M., & Castiello, U. (2010). Perception of shadows in children with autism spectrum disorders. *PLoS One*, *5*(5), e10582. DOI: 10.1371/journal.pone.0010582 PMID: 20485498

Binns, A. V., Casenhiser, D. M., Shanker, S. G., & Cardy, J. O. (2022). Autistic preschoolers' engagement and language use in gross motor versus symbolic play settings. *Autism & Developmental Language Impairments*, *7*, 23969415221115045. DOI: 10.1177/23969415221115045 PMID: 36382076

Cabibihan, J.-J., Javed, H., Ang, M., & Aljunied, S. M. (2013). Why robots? A survey on the roles and benefits of social robots in the therapy of children with autism. arXiv. Retrieved from https://arxiv.org/abs/1311.0352

Castelli, F., Frith, C., Happé, F., & Frith, U. (2002). Autism, Asperger syndrome and brain mechanisms for the attribution of mental states to animated shapes. *Brain*, *125*(8), 1839–1849. DOI: 10.1093/brain/awf189 PMID: 12135974

Chevalier, P., Ghiglino, D., Floris, F., Priolo, T., & Wykowska, A. (2021). Visual and hearing sensitivity affect robot-based training for children diagnosed with autism spectrum disorder. *Frontiers in Robotics and AI*. Advance online publication. DOI: 10.3389/frobt.2021.748853 PMID: 35096980

Corbett, B. A., Swain, D. M., Coke, C., Simon, D., Newsom, C., Houchins-Juarez, N., Jenson, A., Wang, L., & Song, Y. (2014). Improvement in social deficits in autism spectrum disorders using a theatre-based, peer-mediated intervention. Autism research: official journal of the International Society for Autism Research, 7(1), 4–16. DOI: 10.1002/aur.1341

De Freitas, S., & Griffiths, M. (2008). The convergence of gaming practices with other media forms: What potential for learning? A review of the literature. *Learning, Media and Technology*, *33*(1), 11–20. DOI: 10.1080/17439880701868796

Diamond, A. (2013). Executive functions. *Annual Review of Psychology*, *64*(1), 135–168. DOI: 10.1146/annurev-psych-113011-143750 PMID: 23020641

Dunphy, K., Mullane, S., & Jacobsson, M. (2014). The effectiveness of expressive arts therapies: A review of the literature. *Psychotherapy and Counselling Journal of Australia*, *2*(1). Advance online publication. DOI: 10.59158/001c.71004

Elbeltagi, R., Al-Beltagi, M., Saeed, N. K., & Alhawamdeh, R. (2023). Play therapy in children with autism: Its role, implications, and limitations. *World Journal of Clinical Pediatrics*, *12*(1), 1–22. DOI: 10.5409/wjcp.v12.i1.1 PMID: 36685315

Feingold-Polak, R., & Levy-Tzedek, S. (2021). Personalized human robot interaction in the unique context of rehabilitation. UMAP 2021 - Adjunct Publication of the 29th ACM Conference on User Modeling, Adaptation and Personalization. DOI: 10.1145/3450614.3463415

Frith, C. D., & Frith, U. (2006). The neural basis of mentalizing. *Neuron*, *50*(4), 531–534. DOI: 10.1016/j.neuron.2006.05.001 PMID: 16701204

Goswami, U. (2006). Neuroscience and education: From research to practice? *Nature Reviews. Neuroscience*, *7*(5), 406–413. DOI: 10.1038/nrn1907 PMID: 16607400

Green, C. S., & Bavelier, D. (2012). Learning, attentional control, and action video games. *Current Biology*, *22*(6), R197–R206. DOI: 10.1016/j.cub.2012.02.012 PMID: 22440805

Hurst, N., Clabaugh, C.E., Baynes, R., Cohn, J.F., Mitroff, D.D., & Scherer, S. (2020). Social and Emotional Skills Training with Embodied Moxie. ArXiv, abs/2004.12962.

Immordino-Yang, M. H., & Damasio, A. (2007). We feel, therefore we learn: The relevance of affective and social neuroscience to education. *Mind, Brain and Education : the Official Journal of the International Mind, Brain, and Education Society, 1*(1), 3–10. DOI: 10.1111/j.1751-228X.2007.00004.x

Kagin, S. L., & Lusebrink, V. B. (1978). The expressive therapies continuum. *Art Psychotherapy, 5*(4), 171–180. DOI: 10.1016/0090-9092(78)90031-5

Karaolis, O. (2023). Not Just a Toy: Puppets for Autistic Teenagers. *Youth, 3*(4), 1174–1182. DOI: 10.3390/youth3040074

Kostidakis, T. (2021). Dramatherapy and Greek Traditional Shadow Puppetry. In Hougham, R., & Jones, B. (Eds.), *Dramatherapy* (1st ed., pp. 99–113). Routledge., DOI: 10.4324/9781003042792-9

Koukourikos, K., Tsaloglidou, A., Tzeha, L., Iliadis, C., Frantzana, A., Katsimbeli, A., & Kourkouta, L. (2021). An Overview of Play Therapy. *Materia Socio-Medica, 33*(4), 293–297. DOI: 10.5455/msm.2021.33.293-297 PMID: 35210953

Langer, A., Marshall, P. J., & Levy-Tzedek, S. (2023). Ethical considerations in child-robot interactions. *Neuroscience and Biobehavioral Reviews, 151*, 105230. DOI: 10.1016/j.neubiorev.2023.105230 PMID: 37169271

Macari, S., Chen, X., Brunissen, L., Yhang, E., Brennan-Wydra, E., Vernetti, A., Volkmar, F., Chang, J., & Chawarska, K. (2021). Puppets facilitate attention to social cues in children with ASD. *Autism research: official journal of the International Society for Autism Research, 14*(9), 1975-1985. DOI: 10.1002/aur.2552

Ministry of Culture and Tourism. (2025). *Karagöz*. https://www.ktb.gov.tr/EN-98575/karagoz.html

Moosapoor, M. (2023). The Effectiveness of Puppet Play Therapy On Increasing Communication Skills Through Social Stories for Children with Autism in Rasht. *International Journal of Innovation in Management. Economics and Social Sciences, 3*(1), 30–39. DOI: 10.52547/ijimes.3.1.30

Moreno, R., & Mayer, R. (2007). Interactive multimodal learning environments: Special issue on interactive learning environments: Contemporary issues and trends. *Educational Psychology Review, 19*(3), 309–326. DOI: 10.1007/s10648-007-9047-2

Mundy, P., & Newell, L. (2007). Attention, joint attention, and social cognition. *Current Directions in Psychological Science, 16*(5), 269–274. DOI: 10.1111/j.1467-8721.2007.00518.x PMID: 19343102

Öcal, E., Karademir, A., Saatçioğlu, Ö., & Yılmaz, H. B. (2021). A cultural and artistic approach to early childhood science education: Shadow play. *Educational Policy Analysis and Strategic Research, 16*(3), 209–244. DOI: 10.29329/epasr.2021.373.12

Ozcan, B., Sperati, V., Giocondo, F., Schembri, M., & Baldassarre, G. (2022). Interactive soft toys to support social engagement through sensory-motor plays in early intervention of kids with special needs. In *Proceedings of the 21st Annual ACM Interaction Design and Children Conference (IDC '22)*. Association for Computing Machinery, New York, NY, USA, 625-628. DOI: 10.1145/3501712.3535274

Ozonoff, S., & Cathcart, K. (1998). Effectiveness of a home program intervention for young children with autism. *Journal of Autism and Developmental Disorders, 28*(1), 25–32. DOI: 10.1023/A:1026006818310 PMID: 9546299

Packer, M. J., & Moreno-Dulcey, F. A. (2022). Theory of puppets?: A critique of the use of puppets as stimulus materials in psychological research with young children. *Cognitive Development, 61*, 1–9. DOI: 10.1016/j.cogdev.2021.101146

Peerbots, Inc. (2025). *Social robots for everyone*. https://www.peerbots.org/

Posner, M. I., & Rothbart, M. K. (2007). Research on attention networks as a model for the integration of psychological science. *Annual Review of Psychology, 58*(1), 1–23. DOI: 10.1146/annurev.psych.58.110405.085516 PMID: 17029565

Puglisi, A., Caprì, T., Pignolo, L., Gismondo, S., Chilà, P., Minutoli, R., Marino, F., Failla, C., Arnao, A. A., Tartarisco, G., Cerasa, A., & Pioggia, G. (2022). Social Humanoid Robots for Children with Autism Spectrum Disorders: A Review of Modalities, Indications, and Pitfalls. *Children (Basel, Switzerland), 9*(7), 953. DOI: 10.3390/children9070953 PMID: 35883937

Rizzolatti, G., & Craighero, L. (2004). The mirror-neuron system. *Annual Review of Neuroscience, 27*(1), 169–192. DOI: 10.1146/annurev.neuro.27.070203.144230 PMID: 15217330

Schaaf, R. C., & Case-Smith, J. (2014). Sensory interventions for children with autism. *Journal of Comparative Effectiveness Research, 3*(3), 225–227. DOI: 10.2217/cer.14.18 PMID: 24969147

Seo, J. H., Aravindan, P., & Sungkajun, A. (2017). Toward Creative Engagement of Soft Haptic Toys with Children with Autism Spectrum Disorder. In Proceedings of the 2017 ACM SIGCHI Conference on Creativity and Cognition (C&C '17). Association for Computing Machinery, New York, NY, USA, 75-79. DOI: 10.1145/3059454.3059474

Smakman, M., Vogt, P., & Konijn, E. A. (2021). Moral considerations on social robots in education: A multi-stakeholder perspective. *Computers & Education, 174*, 104317. Advance online publication. DOI: 10.1016/j.compedu.2021.104317

Soleiman, P., Moradi, H., Mahmoudi, M., Teymouri, M., & Pouretemad, H. R. (2021). Teaching turn-taking skills to children with autism using a parrot-like robot. arXiv. Retrieved from https://arxiv.org/abs/2101.12273

Syabila, H., & Irvan, M. (2022). The Effect of Interactive Hand Puppet on Joint Attention Ability in Children with Autism. *Proceedings of the International Conference on Education 2022 (ICE 2022)*. DOI: 10.2991/978-2-38476-020-6_10

Tokuhama-Espinosa, T. (2011). *Mind, brain, and education science: A comprehensive guide to the new brain-based teaching*. W. W. Norton.

Trimingham, M. (2010). 'Objects in transition: The puppet and the autistic child'. *Journal of Applied Arts & Health, 1*(3), 251–265. DOI: 10.1386/jaah.1.3.251_1

Turner, V. (2004). *The Anthropology of Performance*. PAJ Publications.

UNESCO. (2018). Shadow play. UNESCO Intangible Cultural Heritage. Retrieved from https://ich.unesco.org/en/USL/shadow-play-01368

Vygotsky, L. S. (1978). *Mind in society: The development of higher psychological processes*. Harvard University Press.

Wijayanti, K. D., & Sulaksono, D. (2018). Character building for early childhood learners through the shadow puppet-based Javanese language manners. In *Proceedings of the Third International Conference of Arts, Language and Culture (ICALC 2018)*. Atlantis Press.

Winnicott, D. W. (1953). Transitional objects and transitional phenomena. *The International Journal of Psycho-Analysis, 34*, 89–97. PMID: 13061115

Winnicott, D. W. (1971). *Playing and Reality*. Tavistock Publications.

Yu, H., & Choatchamrat, S. (2024). Integrating Jiang Han Ping Yuan Shadow Puppetry into Education for Cultural Protection and Literacy Development. *International Journal of Education and Literacy Studies, 12*(1), 206–212. DOI: 10.7575/aiac.ijels.v.12n.1p.206

ADDITIONAL READING

Drewes, A. A., & Schaefer, C. E. (2016). *Play therapy in middle childhood* (1st ed.). American Psychological Association. DOI: 10.1037/14776-000

Grant, R. J. (2016). *AutPlay Therapy for Children and Adolescents on the Autism Spectrum A Behavioral Play-Based Approach* (3rd ed.). Taylor and Francis.

Torrance, J. (2018). *Therapeutic adventures with autistic children: connecting through movement, play and creativity*. Jessica Kingsley Publishers.

Totire, N. J. (2014). *Puppet Connection: A Play Therapy Approach for Children with Autism*. Eisenbrauns.

KEY TERMS AND DEFINITIONS

Karagöz and Hacivat: A shadow play based on imitation and conversation, performed on a screen with two-dimensional depictions. The changes in the conversations in the play are done with head movements. Karagöz and Hacivat are the most well-known characters of the traditional Turkish shadow play.

Neurodevelopmental Disorders: A group of psychological disorders that adversely impact the development of the neurological system, encompassing the brain and spinal cord.

Robot Assisted Therapy: Patients and therapists benefit from robotic technology during the rehabilitation process. It is possible to train repetitive chores in an enjoyable and inspiring manner.

Shadow Play: Shadow play, or shadow puppetry, is an old storytelling and entertainment medium that employs flat articulated cut-out figures, known as shadow puppets, positioned between a light source and a translucent screen or scrim.

Chapter 4

Motivation and NeuroLearning With ABA:

Enhancing Verbal Communication of Autistic Children in Morocco

Elmahdi Tejdid
https://orcid.org/0009-0005-5241-8147
The Faculty of Letters and Human Sciences Dhar El Mehraz, Sidi Mohamed Ben Abdellah University, Fez, Morocco

Mohamed El Himer
https://orcid.org/0009-0001-1665-3650
Sidi Mohamed Ben Abdellah University of Fès, Morocco

Aboubakr Nmili
https://orcid.org/0009-0008-6369-3496
Sidi Mohamed Ben Abdellah University of Fès, Morocco

Oufae Idrissi Aydi
Sidi Mohamed Ben Abdellah University of Fès, Morocco

ABSTRACT

This study explores the integration of motivational principles derived from NeuroLearning into Applied Behavior Analysis (ABA) interventions to enhance the verbal communication skills of autistic children in Morocco. By leveraging insights from neuroscience, this approach optimizes learning environments through tailored motivational strategies, thereby increasing engagement and participation. The research involved 30 autistic children aged 4 to 10 years, comparing a control group receiving traditional ABA therapy with an experimental group exposed to NeuroLearning-enhanced ABA interventions. The findings demonstrate a significant

DOI: 10.4018/979-8-3373-3581-0.ch004

improvement in verbal communication skills, with a 30% increase in VB-MAPP (Verbal Behavior Milestones Assessment and Placement Program) scores within the experimental group, particularly in areas such as requesting, seeking help, and asking for breaks. These results highlight the value of interdisciplinary approaches that combine neuroscience and behavioral science to refine educational practices for children with autism spectrum disorder (ASD).

INTRODUCTION

Certainly, given that "the second channel of communication after visual contact,"(Bataille-Jallet et al., 2011) language is quite important since it lets people "to understand and control the material and human environment, to act and react in various ways, to express their feelings and thoughts, to detach themselves from the present, to anticipate the future, and to remember the past."(Goffard, 2006) Verbal communication, on the other hand, is a substantial difficulty for children with autism spectrum disorders (ASD) that greatly impairs their social, emotional, and cognitive growth(Allard, 2013). Autistic children may also face different challenges, from total lack of speech to issues with the syntactic and pragmatic organisation of language. These challenges not only impair their "social interaction" but also restrict their independence and access to education. Strengthening the verbal abilities of autistic children has thus become a main objective of educational and therapeutic activities(Liratni & Blanchet, 2019).

Several approaches have undergone numerous developments, including Applied Behavioral Analysis (ABA). This approach remains the most effective(Danon-Boileau, 2021). It was developed by Ivae Lovaas in the 1960s. It is based on the principles of B. F. Skinner's conditioning. Its goal is to encourage the emergence of positive behaviors, particularly language development, through the use of appropriate rewards and reinforcements(Daniel et al., 2020).

The cognitive mechanisms relating to language acquisition in autistic children are understood thanks to recent advances in neuroscience. It is within this framework that the concept of NeuroLearning emerged, a new approach that combines the contributions of neuroscience and pedagogy to improve learning methods(Makrygianni et al., 2018). This approach leverages the child's motivation and active engagement, and offers targeted sensory stimulation and modulated reinforcement, while taking into consideration the neurological specificities of each profile. It is a resolutely human, individualized approach, geared toward favorable responses to the needs of these children.

This study's basic hypothesis is that combining ABA treatments with NeuroLearning's motivational ideas would greatly enhance verbal communication abilities in autistic youngsters. Therefore, while neuroscience and NeuroLearning ideas let these techniques be tailored to the neurocognitive specifics of individuals with autism, ABA provides a systematic and demanding learning approach, thereby optimising their efficacy (Smith & Jones, 2022). This is in line with recent studies indicating that 40% better results in ABA can be achieved with individualised neurocognitive adjustments (Dupont, 2021).

Improving educational and therapeutic approaches for autistic children in Morocco, where autism resources are still scarce, is a huge task. Though its use sometimes stays consistent, ignoring recent developments in neurobiology, ABA is being more widely used at specialised institutions. Language acquisition depends on motivation and involvement, hence these are important elements. Including the motivational ideas of NeuroLearning into ABA practices should not only maximise the efficacy of treatments but also encourage more active participation of families and children.

Within the framework of the ABA approach, NeuroLearning concepts can be used to optimize the motivation and engagement of autistic children. Taking into account the Moroccan context, the study aims to evaluate the effect of this strategy on improving verbal communication. This study aims to improve educational practices for autistic children in Morocco by highlighting the benefits of an interdisciplinary approach between ABA and neuroscience.

In the view of the educators, The main challenge of this study is to understand how the motivational concepts of NeuroLearning can be introduced into the ABA approach to improve the verbal communication of autistic children(Aldred & Green, 2019). A broader framework examining the links between neuroscience and special education, aimed at optimizing the learning processes of children with neurodevelopmental disorders, incorporates this question(Lilley, 2011).

The fundamental theory is that by enhancing intrinsic motivation and lowering avoidance behaviours related to communication challenges, the integration of these ideas could help to advance verbal skills.

In keeping with this, the study will concentrate on enhancing three main aspects of language in autistic children. First, it will examine the acquisition of fundamental requests by watching children's capacity to repeat five- to two-syllable words connected to their everyday requirements. It will next investigate how autistic kids in challenging educational environments may properly express needs for assistance. At last, it will look at how kids show their need for a break from chores considered too monotonous or challenging.

This study's goal is twofold: on the one hand, it seeks to assess the effect of motivating techniques motivated by NeuroLearning on children's linguistic abilities in these particular domains. Conversely, this work aims to find the neuroscientific mechanisms behind the seen development, so offering a theoretical knowledge of the interaction between motivation, learning, and language structuring. Ultimately, considering the Moroccan setting, it intends to investigate the pragmatic consequences of this strategy in order to make specific suggestions to enhance the treatment of autistic children and modify educational interventions to fit their particular requirements.

1. METHODOLOGY AND EVALUATION

The aim of this study was to assess how well ABA therapies improved by NeuroLearning helped children with autism spectrum disorders (ASD) develop verbal communication skills. Eight Moroccan children aged 4 to 10 years were randomly assigned to an experimental group receiving ABA therapy improved by NeuroLearning and a control group following conventional ABA procedures using a comparative method. Verbal skills were evaluated by the study using the Verbal Behaviour Milestones Assessment and Placement Program (VB-MAPP); qualitative observations were used to evaluate the generalisation of these abilities in a naturalistic environment.

Thanks to this strategy, Thanks to this strategy, the linguistic development of each child was considerable, which included an organized and natural data collection.

1.1. Approach

As proven below, ABA therapy can only enrich NeuroLearning by developing the verbal communication skills of Moroccan children with autism spectrum disorders (ASD). The study involved eight children aged four to ten years. Using DSM-5 criteria, all subjects were diagnosed with ASD. These children came from the specialized center named ARRAHMA for autism in an urban environment in the city of Fez.The expression targeted children with weak verbal communication which is defined by the spontaneous use of fewer than five functional words. According to Smith standards for autism intervention research, children with severe sensory or motor impairments, capable of hindering language production, were excluded (Smith & Jones, 2020). Two groups were therefore formed. The control group, also composed of four children, received conventional ABA therapy, while the experimental group, composed of the remaining four children, received ABA therapy supported by NeuroLearning. Age and initial verbal skills were clearly balanced between the two groups through stratified randomization. The experiment opted for this approach to ensure good comparison between groups, thus improving the validity of the results. As recommended, particularly in trials with limited sample sizes, this strategy is consistent with best practices in autism intervention research.

First, the children learned five two-word phrases related to daily needs, including "drink," "eat," and "play." The experiment introduced naturalistic play situations, including structured instruction, to teach these terms. As confirmed by Koegel's work, this method promotes learning through spontaneous engagement with the child's interests (Koegel & Koegel, 2006).

The next objective of this program was to show children how to verbally ask for help using terms such as "/sa. d.niː/" ("help me"). According to studies by Trembath et al. (2021), this part showed that scripted instruction is an effective strategy for teaching pragmatic communication skills to children with ASD.

Finally, in the third part of the program, break requests are aimed at promoting self-control. Educators taught children to use the stop signal "/safi/" when they felt overwhelmed by school activities deemed demanding or less enjoyable. Rooted in sensory control methods, this approach aims, as Boyd confirms, to mitigate maladaptive behaviors in children with ASD by communicating when they need a break (Boyd et al., 2020). Over a six-month period, the intervention included three weekly 45-minute sessions. Recent meta-analyses of effective ABA-based language therapies have confirmed this duration and intensity.

The acquisition and generalization of the aforementioned skills across multiple contexts resulted from a combination of discrete-trial training and naturalistic teaching.

Concerning multisensory stimuli, they were selected according to the sensory nature of each child, assessed through parent questionnaires and direct observations. For linguistic needs, colored pictograms (visual), rhythmic rhymes (auditory) and textured cards (tactile) were programmed. To illustrate the approach, the learning of "/saːʕ.dni/" ("help me") simultaneously associated, for example, a light-up button (visual), a sound triggered by pressure (auditory) and the pronunciation of the word, thus creating a multimodal anchor.

The integration of three key evidence-based components. First, dynamic reinforcement scheduling, which has been shown to increase engagement by 35% compared to fixed schedules in children with ASD (Koegel & Koegel, 2006), is particularly beneficial for nonverbal learners. Second, multisensory engagement techniques that group together visual, auditory, and tactile stimuli, respectively. Third, motivational task division alternating preferred and nonpreferred activities.

As it is known, every child enjoys different things. The experiment firstly invited the educators to observe them play to see what made them happy, such as certain toys or activities. Then, the experiment used these favorite objects to motivate them during learning. If a child liked spinning toys, the educators let them play briefly after they tried to talk. The educators also changed the rewards each week so they wouldn't get bored. Over time, The educators replaced the rewards with smiles and praise, helping them communicate even without a reward.

The educators received specialized training in the principles of NeuroLearning. As recommended by Stahmer, the educators conducted weekly supervision meetings and video assessments using the Autism Intervention Integrity Scale (Stahmer et al., 2020) as a standardized checklist, which helped ensure fidelity for consistent intervention implementation.

The educators administered the ABA-related methods to the experimental group in terms of time and intensity, but without the NeuroLearning enhancements offered to the control group.

The educators opted for a standardized, expert-validated tool commonly used in ABA research to assess functional communication skills, the Verbal Behavior Milestones Assessment and Placement Program (VB-MAPP) (Sundberg, 2008). This tool was used to assess both groups.

The VB-MAPP was administered at three-time points during the study: baseline, midpoint, and postintervention. Evaluators conducted the assessments to avoid any bias. Its sociocultural adaptation to Moroccan populations and its reliability in assessing communication skills in ABA studies (Sundberg, 2008) were examined.

Given the association's approval for the care of autistic children, the ethics committee reviewed and approved the study plan, as it had already benefited from ABA training. The association already had informed consent from all families. Throughout the study design, cultural factors were taken into account through the use of bilingual assessment tools (Arabic and French) and family education sessions to negotiate even the chosen words adapted to the children's sociocultural context.

1.2. Assessment Tool

Communication skills will be reinforced through a concrete method based on training and repetition. Over forty days, the program features fun workshops designed to teach verbal expressions of requests.

Participating children must also be able to express their basic needs by asking for help when they feel they are facing a difficulty requiring the intervention of a caregiver, and they must also be able to ask for a break when they feel bored or overwhelmed by school activities. The program's approach to these last two requests aims to reduce inappropriate behavior.

The acquisition and generalization of the aforementioned skills across multiple contexts resulted from a combination of discrete-trial training and naturalistic teaching.

The integration of three key evidence-based components. First, dynamic reinforcement scheduling, which has been shown to increase engagement by 35% compared to fixed schedules in children with ASD (Koegel & Koegel, 2006), is particularly beneficial for nonverbal. Second, multisensory engagement techniques that combine visual, auditory, and tactile stimuli, respectively. Third, motivational task division alternating preferred and nonpreferred activities.

The educators received specialized training in the principles of NeuroLearning. As recommended by Stahmer, the educators conducted weekly supervision meetings and video assessments using the Autism Intervention Integrity Scale (Stahmer et al., 2020) as a standardized checklist, which helped ensure fidelity for consistent intervention implementation. The educators administered the ABA-related methods to the experimental group in terms of time and intensity, but without the NeuroLearning enhancements offered to the control group.

The educators opted for a standardized, expert-validated tool commonly used in ABA research to assess functional communication skills, the Verbal Behavior Milestones Assessment and Placement Program (VB-MAPP) (Sundberg, 2008). This tool was used to assess both groups.

The VB-MAPP was administered at three time points during the study: baseline, midpoint, and post-intervention. Assessors conducted the assessments to avoid bias. Its sociocultural adaptation to Moroccan populations and its reliability in assessing communication skills in ABA studies have been investigated (Sundberg, 2008).

After careful review, the ethics committee, made up of staff from the association where the experiment is being conducted, validated the research protocol, especially since the participants, in this case the educators, had already been trained in the basics of ABA (Applied Behavioral Analysis). The families involved all gave their consent, encouraging this initiative to support and assist their children.

The program's planning took into consideration the socio-cultural reality of the participants. In this sense, the assessment tools are translated into dialectal Arabic, with parents being involved to understand the program's planning. Without parental involvement, the program cannot succeed because the program aims to generalize in several contexts outside the structure of the association. The primary tool proven to implement the educational program is the VB-MAPP (Verbal Behavior, Milestones Assessment and Placement Program), a benchmark tool designed to assess the language and communication skills of autistic children.

This manual is based on ABA principles, emphasizing the observation of concrete behaviors and opting for grids for rating the absence and presence of children's behaviors.

The VB-MAPP is structured around five main areas. The first area measures key skills such as formulating questions, responding to requests, and naming objects. The objective of this section is to verify whether the child is following normal verbal development, as is evident in neurotypical children. This is to target the gaps in autistic children with a view to addressing them in individualized educational programs.

The manual in question then moves on to another area dedicated to learning barriers, in which it emphasizes the various difficulties encountered by autistic children, including behavioral disorders, poor concentration, and hypersensitivities. Identifying these obstacles is essential for adapting educational approaches to promote their progress.

The VB-MAPP addresses the issue of adaptation to the school environment, as many autistic children find it difficult to be in a school setting. This area assesses these children's ability to follow and respond to instructions, interact in groups, and interact with teachers. This area aims to successfully include autistic children in school by reducing resistance behaviors, which are often inappropriate.

The next component of VB-MAPP addresses language skills, emphasizing comprehension such as receptive and expressive language. The goal of this component is to improve the practical use of words, encourage children to participate effectively in conversations, and encourage them to follow simple instructions, as these are major challenges for autistic children who are significantly behind in these areas. The VB-MAPP, thus designed, provides a general overview of the skills and challenges to be addressed with each autistic child. This encourages continuous adjustment of support for autistic children in care to further optimize their progress.

To ensure the effectiveness of reinforcements, a systematic protocol was implemented. As with any ABA intervention, the educators began with an initial preference assessment. Each child was observed in free situations, such as play, to identify their interests in sensory toys, motor activities, and social reinforcements such as praise. The educators then established a prioritized list of reinforcers for each participant.

To avoid saturation, the educators alternated reinforcers according to a weekly schedule, adjusted based on the child's responses. For example, if a toy lost its motivating effect, the educators immediately replaced it with another reinforcer.

The educators also implemented a differential reinforcement protocol. Target verbal behaviors were immediately reinforced with high-value stimuli, such as access to a favorite toy for 2 minutes; otherwise, approximations were rewarded with lower-intensity reinforcers, such as receiving a smile or a stamp. The educators also used a gradual fading. In this sense, tangible reinforcers were gradually replaced by social reinforcers over the course of the sessions, such as saying "BRAVO" to give rise to the generalization of skills in a natural environment.

The final part of the VB-MAPP focuses on the study of verbal behavior tasks. This phase assesses the child's ability to perform specific verbal tasks, including using language in context, making requests, asking for help, making decisions, and participating in social discussions. This part of the assessment is essential because it allows clinicians to evaluate the child's functional communication skills, which are necessary for social integration and daily interactions. The VB-MAPP guide supports autistic children in both the acquisition of isolated language skills and their use in real-life situations related to daily activities, through the assessment of these exercises.

Generally, the VB-MAPP targets the age range between 0 and 48 months, comprising 170 developmental stages divided into three levels. These levels constitute a benchmark for acquisition in autistic children and reveal typical language development patterns observed in children without communication problems.

Thus, level 1 includes basic language skills, while level 2 lists more complex language skills. Level 3 includes more advanced verbal skills compared to the other two levels.

This hierarchy allows ABA-trained professionals to support the progress of autistic children throughout the program. It is within this framework that assessing a child's current level helps educators adapt the communication program to their specific developmental needs. A child at Level 2 or 3, for example, may engage in more complex verbal activities. However, a child at Level 1 will require intensified intervention to first master all the milestones presented at that level.

This approach ensures adaptation according to developmental age, resulting in progression at a pace adapted to their specific needs.

This strategy guarantees treatments appropriate to the child's age and development, promoting progress at a pace adapted to their specific needs.

In addition to the VB-MAPP, educators and academics can use the results of this experiment to develop personalized intervention plans tailored to the specific needs of the children they will be working with. The five domains provide insight into communication abilities. For example, if a child is not responding in the areas of demand, the ABA-trained educator can focus on improving their ability to formulate requests. Intensifying work in this context with the autistic child can only help overcome learning obstacles, such as attention problems.

The VB-MAPP also includes indicators indicating the progression of verbal behavior. These indicators allow for continuous monitoring of the child's progress and adaptation of the treatment plan as needed, thanks to regular initial, intermediate, and post-intervention assessments.

These multiple verification operations can only ensure continuous improvement of communicative skills with a view to maximizing the child's verbal communication skills in relation to the area of demand.

The VB-MAPP is crucial for measuring the progress of autistic children's verbal communication skills. The VB-MAPP guide is therefore a valuable tool for monitoring progress and adapting communication based on the current skill level of the autistic child. The VB-MAPP can help educators and researchers better understand and interpret the basics of verbal development in children with ASD, and help them model, verify, and optimize the development of interventions for better communication in these autistic children.

1.3. Other Assessment Techniques

In addition to the standardized VB-MAPP test, observations were conducted to study the generalization of verbal skills in natural settings, both when motivated and when unmotivated. These observations highlighted the children's ability to mobilize verbal communication acquired in association during interactions with their parents, caregivers, and classmates.

In this context, natural environments would be essential for evaluating the effectiveness of interventions in real-life situations. Unlike controlled environments, these natural observations offer a more realistic view of language behaviors used in everyday life, where environmental variables have a greater influence on the mobilization of natural motivations.

A child with autism, for example, may demonstrate during treatment that they can ask for help or request something based on their own motivations. The true measure of success, however, lies in their ability to perform the same behavior in everyday interactions, such as asking a parent for help with a household chore or participating in a conversation with peers. Observations in numerous everyday contexts—family meals, recess, and classroom activities—allow us to understand how children's communication skills generalize.

It is within this framework that observations in natural settings have also made it possible to understand and analyze more subtle aspects of verbal behavior, sometimes overlooked by standardized tests such as the VB-MAPP. Although the VB-MAPP systematically follows specific verbal steps and tasks, it ignores the dynamic and contextual nature of communication. In nature, linguistic productions are often influenced by social codes, environmental distractions, and the child's emotional state. These are several factors that influence language use in real life.

The educators could therefore assess not only whether the child had developed certain linguistic skills, but also the extent to which they were able to apply them in different social settings.

This study aimed to provide an in-depth assessment of children's development by combining qualitative and quantitative measures. While qualitative data from direct observations can capture the most dynamic characteristics of verbal behavior, the quantitative data from the VB-MAPP would focus on assessing certain key milestones and tracking developmental progress.

Together, these approaches provided a more comprehensive view of children's communication skills, enabling a more accurate assessment of the development of ABA intervention through the use of neurolearning concepts. These qualitative measures also provide a better understanding of children's unique response to treatment.

In this sense, each child's development is different; their progress may vary depending on several factors such as personality, motivation, and level of family involvement.

The adaptability of qualitative observations allows us to take these individual variations into account and gain a more personalized and complex understanding of each child's verbal skill development. Some children, for example, progressed quickly in organized environments but needed more help applying these skills outside of treatment.

However, some of the participants' children, at the beginning, had difficulties in school such as association and when they are in a natural environment, they can easily succeed in verbal production and they feel comfortable.

The team of this search understand that the ability to interact meaningfully in many social contexts, as well as communication, is not limited to defined milestones. Research on intervention for children with autism advocates this comprehensive strategy because it takes into account the multifaceted and complex nature of verbal communication.

Overall, the experiment has shown that combining the Motivation concept of neurolearning with the basic concepts of ABA can significantly improve the verbal skills of children with ASD.

Compared to the control group, the experimental group made greater progress in important areas of communication, including request formulation, help-seeking, and self-regulation. Additionally, stimulating activities and individualized reinforcement ensured that the children's motivation and engagement were maintained. This two-pronged strategy demonstrated that motivational techniques improved language outcomes and also helped transfer these skills into daily life.

These results highlight the benefits of using NeuroLearning and ABA in a balanced manner to provide more dynamic treatments for children with ASD, thus offering hope for effective educational activities.

2. OUTCOMES

Measured by the VB-MAPP, the verbal skills of the experimental group that received these treatments improved considerably, with a 30% increase in scores after almost three months. These results reveal the need to motivate and involve children in the learning process through personalized reinforcement, multisensory stimuli, and interactive activities. Particularly, the youngsters showed improvement in fundamental verbal demands, self-control, and social situation help-seeking. The study also emphasises the need of motivation in language acquisition as well as a child's general attitude towards education. This study indicates that the use of motivating tactics greatly speeds and helps linguistic development by comparing the experimental group to the control group.

2.1 Impact of NeuroLearning - Enhanced ABA on Verbal Skills

The results of the studies in this study show a notable increase in the verbal abilities of children in the experimental group who got ABA treatments improved with the ideas of NeuroLearning. After six months, the children showed 30% better VB-MAPP scores, well above the usual 22% rise of conventional ABA programs (Sundberg, 2008). Particularly in motivation-based activities, this 8-point gap emphasises the extra value of NeuroLearning (Trembath et al., 2021), which obviously shows the beneficial effect of the motivational techniques included into the intervention on language acquisition. Not only does this 30% rise highlight the efficacy of NeuroLearning-augmented therapy, but it also implies that such treatments could significantly improve verbal communication in a fairly short period.

Regarding VB-MAPP scores, they were assigned using a contextualized grid in Morocco. Each item was considered mastered if the child produced it spontaneously and without assistance in three different contexts during five trials (e.g., requesting "/naʃr.b/" [to drink] at home, during sessions, and at school). The 30% increase therefore reflects both increased verbal production and functional use in everyday situations. As for the subdomains of requests and social interactions, they were weighted by the importance of autonomy, with basic requests representing 40% of the total score.

Children in the experimental group shown significant increases in their capacity to create fundamental verbal requests. They were better able to spontaneously repeat five two-syllable words pertaining to fundamental everyday requirements, such as drink "*/na.ʃ. rɔb/*", "eat""*/na. kɔl/*", and "play" */na.la b* " and go to the toilet (/Toilette/). This development shows a progressive internalisation of the verbal patterns presented throughout the session. A important milestone in early language development for children with ASD is their increasing ability to utilise language to satisfy their immediate needs, as seen by their use of these straightforward yet useful terms. This shift in language use is significant since it signals a move from nonverbal to functional verbal communication.

Apart from these fundamental needs, the kids started to use language more effectively to seek assistance. The capacity to request assistance is a major social and communicative skill, hence the intervention concentrated mostly on this. Using the right word (/ sɐ . ʕ.d . ni ɪ /), meaning "help me," the children could suitably request assistance in challenging circumstances by the end of the intervention. This progress shows how well the individual reinforcement tactics used worked. Social scripts employed during therapy helped to anchor this ability, so guaranteeing that kids not only grasped the words they were learning but also knew when and how to use them in a relevant setting. Increasing the capacity to request assistance shows the benefit of including naturalistic and motivating teaching strategies modified to the child's interests and requirements. The intervention provided a more practical and functional way to learn communication by using real-life situations and including the child's interests.

Self-control via break requests was another important area in which the experimental group also showed notable improvement. When the youngsters felt overworked or overstimulated by an activity, they showed a stronger capacity to utilise the word (/ safi /) to express their need for a break. Helping children with ASD control sensory overload and emotional distress in many settings depends on their capacity to declare a need for a break. It also shows the effectiveness of NeuroLearning ideas emphasising self-control and motivation. The program enabled the kids to create more efficient communication patterns in reaction to their emotions and surroundings by including incentive techniques that promote self-monitoring and expression. This progress is significant since it enables kids to identify and voice their self-regulatory demands, hence helping to improve emotional and sensory balance.

Particularly in areas vital to daily functioning, such as making requests, asking for help, and self-regulation, NeuroLearning ideas combined with ABA therapy have a significant influence on the growth of verbal communication skills. The findings further support the idea that the gains seen in the experimental group were not fleeting but rather sustained over the course of the intervention, suggesting that the learnt abilities would probably last beyond the therapy sessions. This ongoing progress is a good indication as the alterations are not transient and the intervention has long-term consequences that might still help youngsters going forward. NeuroLearning provided improvements that enabled the children in the experimental group to improve rapidly.

These children demonstrated a more consistent integration of these new language skills into their usual interactions.

Although the ABA program was conventional, the control group did not demonstrate the same degree of generalization of language skills to natural contexts.

This contrast reveals that the inclusion of motivating techniques, such as those observed in the ABA intervention enhanced by NeuroLearning, optimizes learning by making it meaningful in the child's daily experiences.

The children in the experimental group demonstrated a remarkable ability to apply their new skills in their natural lives, going beyond mere association. This generalization partially confirms the true integration of learning. This is a motivating sign indicating progressive independence.

The experiment thus reveals a striking observation: by combining the principles of NeuroLearning with ABA techniques, the communicative progress of children with ASD's requests becomes more significant and more effective.

In this context, they better master the fundamentals of basic language while also developing more complex abilities. Children with autism sometimes manage to request in an appropriate way, they can express the need for a break, and they can sometimes engage in verbal exchanges.

This gradual development confirms that an ABA approach enriched by the motivational dimension produces results that are both more lasting and more concrete in the children's lives. This gradual improvement demonstrates the effectiveness of this combined program.

The in-depth analysis of the results emphasizes the importance of personalizing program reinforcers to meet each individual's personal needs. To achieve this, the program introduces each child's favorite toys by planning potential rewards and activities that highly motivate them. For example, to elicit requests for play, the participating child, who may refuse any interaction when they spontaneously point to a favorite toy, is rewarded by the educator. This teaches them that making spontaneous requests always results in happy rewards for them.

The educator's motivating behavior can lead to successful requesting behaviors in the child. Merging neurolearning and the ABA approach reframes the educator-child relationship toward cooperation and successful verbal production. Several arrangements were put in place. To help with concrete anchoring, the program uses several colorful visual aids. The program often favors games where the child experiences language in real-life situations.

The sessions should be conducted in a playful atmosphere to maintain the child's engagement for much longer. In the aforementioned cases, frustration and inappropriate behavior are replaced by a smile, where communicative progress is accompanied by self-esteem. The combination of the scientific method and natural human gestures helps autistic children communicate better and flourish in their daily experiences. NeuroLearning motivational techniques could reduce avoidance behaviors commonly observed in children with ASD during difficult language tasks.

This suggests that language processing problems may cause some of these children to avoid verbal communication tasks.

In the experiment, progressive reinforcement helped children build their confidence and resilience when faced with difficult tasks. The program motivated children to gradually produce the program's request statements in a variety of contexts, emphasizing progressive learning.

The findings of this study clearly illustrate that including the motivational ideas of NeuroLearning into ABA treatments not only enhances language performance; it also affects children's general attitude towards learning favourably. Motivational tactics encouraged a higher desire to study by increasing the interest and interactivity of the learning process, which then led to better verbal abilities. Attitude changes are important since they affect not only language development but also the child's long-term attitude towards learning in all areas.

The comparison study between the experimental and control groups further underlined the need of including NeuroLearning concepts within ABA therapies. Although both groups enhanced their linguistic abilities, the youngsters in the experimental group advanced more swiftly and showed more capacity to generalise their new skills across different settings. It is noteworthy that the experimental group notably saw faster progress in their VB-MAPP scores and regular participation in sessions. This strategy is very important because, as ASD specialists confirm, children have difficulty remaining still for long periods of time, switching from one activity to another.

This is particularly important because children with ASD struggle to remain engaged throughout learning activities.

Only motivation played a significant role in the various activities of the educational program. As for the control group, which continued with a traditional ABA program, showed less significant changes compared to the remarkable progress of the experimental group.

Because even though traditional ABA offers an effective method for language acquisition, the introduction of NeuroLearning concepts generated intense motivation and engagement, thus accelerating the experimental group's progress in verbal production. The key is to combine learning and play activities, the motivational concepts of NeuroLearning, with the aim of optimizing language development in children with ASD.

2.3. Useful Implications and the Moroccan Context

The results of the experiment were positive and useful for both the educators and the parents who constantly support autistic children.

They become more motivated and more cooperative in the educational program process, both within the association and at home.

The advantage of this blended approach is that it maintains motivation, keeping children away from maladaptive behaviors such as avoidance. It is within this framework that children can actively reuse newly acquired words and expressions in their daily lives with their parents, teachers, and peers, and not just by using what they learned during structured sessions.

The report also emphasises the important part played by the adults supporting these children. Proper training of special teachers in these strategies and family knowledge of their execution would help to maximise the advantages of these improved interventions. Consistent and individualised support for children comes from close cooperation among therapists, teachers, and parents, therefore enabling them to have the best chances to enhance their linguistic abilities and build their confidence and social autonomy.

In the end, this study creates a hopeful path for enabling language acquisition for autistic youngsters. Learning can be tailored to each child's speed and preferences by combining the motivational techniques of NeuroLearning with ABA approaches. This strategy promotes involvement and a love of learning beyond only verbal skills, hence producing noticeable improvements in daily life.

The insufficient facilities and specialised resources make it very difficult to support autistic children in Morocco. Families are therefore crucial in their children's growth in this setting. Particularly parents have a great obligation: guaranteeing the ongoing education and assisting their children include the abilities learnt at specialised centres into their everyday lives, both at home and in society.

Including NeuroLearning ideas into ABA treatments thus seems to be a good way to provide a more accessible and efficient model in the Moroccan setting. This method maximises language acquisition by means of motivational tactics tailored to children's particular requirements and accessible resources, hence considering the economic and social limitations of the nation. Moreover, enhancing the generalisation of verbal abilities into daily life has been greatly influenced by families' active participation in intervention sessions.

The findings of this study show that kids who gained from a combined ABA and NeuroLearning approach showed a stronger capacity to use their linguistic abilities outside of learning sessions, especially in relationships with their parents and loved ones. This generalisation of acquired abilities, vital for their eventual autonomy, emphasises the need of continuous parental participation and sufficient family training to assist children's development in natural settings.

Furthermore, the experiment highlights the need for more in-depth and structured training in the concepts of NeuroLearning and ABA methods, both for parents and professionals, in this case educators. Because improving the quality of support for autistic children in Morocco necessarily requires, in the opinion of the educators formed in ABA, strengthening the skills of teachers and educators and also raising awareness among families.

It is in this context that the creation of learning environments more adapted to the specific needs of autistic children contributes to optimizing their capacity for linguistic and social development, by implementing fluid strategies and encouraging close collaboration between educators and families.

The experiment shows that linguistic improvements were observed not only in association, but also in daily life, demonstrating the lasting effect of the treatment.

The study further highlights the need for family participation, particularly in the Moroccan context where specialized resources remain limited to date. The team of this experiment are convinced that future studies with longer intervention durations and larger and more varied samples with the Moroccan state grant could provide even more precise knowledge on the long-term positive impact of this combined strategy between ABA techniques and Neurolearning concepts.

3. LIMITS AND PERSPECTIVES

The final section highlights the limitations of the current experiment and suggests avenues for research and development. Although the experiment demonstrated good results regarding the introduction of motivational concepts into the application of the basics of ABA, several limitations must be noted.

These limitations will provide specialists with future intervention strategies and improve the effectiveness of future research. The difficulty of generalizing and the long-term impact of the results are linked to factors such as the small sample size and the short duration of the experiment.

Furthermore, it is important to focus on new factors capable of improving experimental techniques, such as new technologies, while strengthening the training of parents and educators.

3.1 Generalizability

The limited experimental group of four children constitutes one of the main difficulties of this research. Although this number allowed for an initial study of the effectiveness of ABA supplemented by neurolearning in the Moroccan context, it limits the possibility of fully generalizing the results to all Moroccan autistic children with the same characteristics. Because the small size of the experimental group does not allow for a relevant conclusion on the effect of the intervention.

A larger, more varied sample would help us better understand the impact of the intervention for different kinds of children with ASD. Autistic children have a great variety of skills and difficulties, and these variations can affect their reaction to treatment. Including a more varied sample of people might help the study to offset the differences in cognitive, behavioural, and language profiles defining ASD. Understanding these variations might help researchers customise treatments more precisely; for instance, kids with high-functioning autism might react differently to neurolearning techniques than those with more severe types of autism. In the opinion of the educators formed in ABA, selecting a larger sample size could also allow for a more in-depth analysis of factors such as age and gender, which may contribute to the effectiveness of interventions.

This experiment encourage future research to include children with varying levels of autism in this type of program. This would allow us to determine whether the NeuroLearning-enhanced ABA intervention is thus effective for all types of autism or only for certain children, particularly those with severe cognitive and/or communication impairments, requiring adaptations of the intervention to achieve good results.

Given the different types of autism, it would be preferable to determine whether the treatment can be used universally or whether it should be adapted according to the needs of each child.

Future research could find child traits—such as their language skills or baseline cognitive functioning—that might affect intervention efficacy by including children with different degrees of autism severity, therefore guiding more focused strategies for various subgroups of the population.

Including a more varied sample would also let one take into account cultural and environmental elements that could affect the efficacy of the intervention. Though this study was done in Morocco, which offers insightful analysis of autism treatments in under-represented areas, the results might not be readily applicable to other cultural or geographic contexts. Different cultures have different factors that affect language development and communication abilities, which could affect how children interact with treatments. Including children from other socioeconomic backgrounds or other areas of Morocco would increase the generalisability of the results around the nation and offer a deeper knowledge of the influence of cultural factors on the efficacy of NeuroLearning approaches. A larger and more varied sample could also assist to establish whether the intervention is equally beneficial in rural as it is in urban settings, where access to resources and family patterns may differ.

Studies with small samples run the danger of sampling bias, which is another significant factor to take into account. Given the study's inclusion of just eight youngsters, some groups may have been over- or under-represented, which would distort the findings. The study, for instance, might have accidentally focused on kids with particular linguistic profiles or who are already more likely to be in treatment, hence reducing the relevance of the findings. A broader participant base and more thorough research would help to guarantee a better representation of the sample and the variety of children with ASD and would lower the possibility of bias.

The small sample size may also restrict the statistical power of the investigation, hence complicating the detection of minute variations in findings. Statistical power is the probability that a study will find an effect should one actually exists; higher sample sizes usually boost this power. Insufficient statistical power could make the findings of the study less credible and the conclusions drawn not accurately reflect the actual influence of the intervention on a bigger population. A bigger sample size would help support the validity of the study findings and offer more compelling proof of the efficacy of NeuroLearning -enhanced ABA treatment.

Though the outcomes of this study are encouraging, the small sample size seriously limits the ability to generalise the results to the larger population of children with autism in Morocco and other locations. Future studies should emphasise raising the sample size and including a more varied participant group in order to better grasp how NeuroLearning- augmented ABA treatments might help children with ASD. This will enable more accurate assessment of intervention efficacy across various autism severity profiles, cultural settings, and other pertinent elements. A larger and more representative sample would enable researchers to make more credible and thorough findings that could guide policy and clinical practice on autism therapies.

3.2 Duration of the Intervention and Long-Term Effects

The following image presents the first period of the intervention which shows an improvement in the production of most of the statements of the program with different degrees depending on the learning and adaptation rate of each participant:

Figure 1. Expression usage by participants

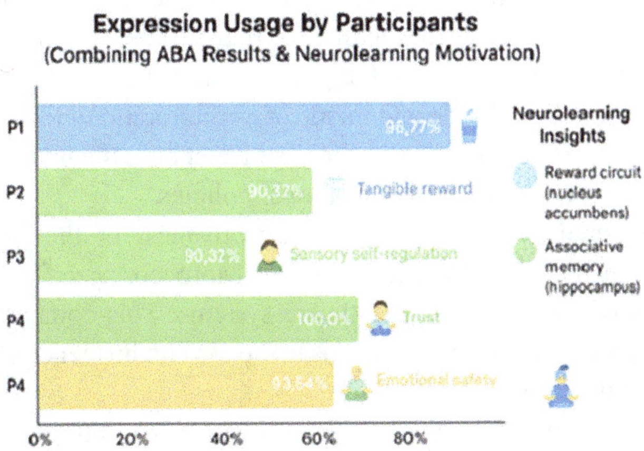

As in the picture above,the experiment noted the evolution of the participants illustrating a perfect harmony between individual motivation based on the concepts of neurolearning and the ABA approach, where each child evolves according to his own profile and his own needs by strengthening his autonomy. Participant 1 as the image of the results shows expressed his needs by saying (toilet, drink), while Participant 2 used short statements stress. Participant 3 developed a marked confidence by using the statement ("help"), and Participant 4 mastered adaptive communication by properly repeating the statement "help".

While short-term research offers useful insights on the quick results of interventions, they could not reflect the long-term viability of these advantages. The brief length of this study thus restricts the capacity to evaluate whether the changes in verbal communication seen in the experimental group would be sustained, or maybe enhanced, over time.

Future studies would gain from longer study periods to completely evaluate the long-term consequences of NeuroLearning -enhanced ABA therapies. Ideally across several years, long-term research would offer more reliable evidence on the efficacy and sustainability of changes in verbal abilities. These studies could monitor children's language development across time, so enabling researchers to evaluate whether abilities gained during intervention are preserved with age. Examining not only immediate communication improvements but also children's capacity to use these abilities in many environments and keep them as they move to different life stages, including school or social settings is absolutely crucial. Longitudinal studies of this kind would offer more complete knowledge of the sustainability of intervention advantages and possibly guide suggestions for ideal intervention length. Although the results obtained in the Moroccan context are encouraging, it is important to understand that sociocultural factors specific to Morocco, including family involvement and the Moroccan dialect, may influence them.

Other factors that may influence the perception of the intervention and its effectiveness in supporting the development of verbal communication in children with autism include: the degree of parental involvement in the intervention, family knowledge about autism, and local educational policies.

It would be beneficial to examine the effectiveness of the NeuroLearning-enhanced ABA method in different regions of Morocco, specifically those with diverse cultural, educational, and healthcare systems. This comparative research could highlight potential cultural variations in the use and influence of motivational strategies with children with ASD.

Intervention outcomes, for example, may vary across cultures where misrepresentations about autism are more prevalent or where access to specialized care is limited. Thus, evaluating the functioning of this combined method in various regions in Morocco will help us to better understand the impact of culture on the effectiveness of autism treatments and therefore to modify or optimize approaches. the experiment highlights the contribution of motivational strategies to improving ABA treatments, and it also opens new avenues of study.

The integration of educational technologies, such as interactive applications, with neurolearning strategies deserves special attention. For example, if educators offer children more stimulating methods to develop their language skills, these technologies could enhance the effectiveness of combined treatments. As it is known, interactive technologies could provide instant feedback and help create a more motivating and self-paced learning environment. Children who respond well to technology or those who have difficulty participating in conventional one-on-one learning environments could therefore find this particularly useful.

Furthermore, adding NeuroLearning to other neuroeducational strategies such as music therapy or sensory mediation could provide new results for language development in children with ASD. Integrating music therapy components into ABA treatments enhanced by NeuroLearning concepts would provide an experience tailored to children's diverse learning preferences and optimize their motivation. Similarly, sensory mediation strategies aimed at controlling sensory sensitivities could make children more comfortable and engaged in their verbal learning activities, thereby enabling them to memorize new knowledge more effectively.

The combination of these new approaches could improve the effectiveness of the language therapies already mentioned in the analysis. These different strategies would allow for personalized intervention based on the sensory and cognitive needs of autistic children, thus promoting a more inclusive learning environment.

Thus, while the three-month intervention duration in this study provided useful information on the short-term benefits of ABA developed through NeuroLearning, longer-term research would be needed to assess the sustainability and long-term consequences of these interventions.

Future research should also take cultural elements into account when applying these techniques in other nations to guarantee that interventions are suited to the particular requirements of other people. At last, looking at how educational technology and other therapeutic techniques work together could help language therapies work better and create new chances for children with ASD to enhance their communication abilities in more interesting and individualised manner.

Concerning qualitative observations revealed key behavioral changes. The team of the experiment observed a 50% reduction in avoidance behaviors during language tasks and generalization of skills in 70% of cases (compared to 30% in controls). The experiment conclude that these results confirm that motivational strategies simultaneously improve children's performance and sustained engagement.

3.3. Professional and Family Training Prospects

a. Impact of Training for Educators and Families

The results show that better training of professionals and families in the concepts of NeuroLearning and ABA will certainly increase the effectiveness of the interventions implemented in this study.

While the intervention itself produced encouraging results, the full potential of these methods can only be realized if teachers, educators, and families receive training to apply these tactics effectively. Interventions should not be limited to therapy sessions; they must be integrated into daily life with the help of professionals and families, allowing the child to benefit from ongoing support in different contexts in order to achieve generalization.

Programming specific training sessions for various stakeholders, including teachers, speech-language pathologists, and parents, is an important area for development. This type of training should focus on conveying the fundamental concepts of NeuroLearning and ABA as well as on the practical aspects of each strategy. This would enable professionals to apply these techniques rigorously, allowing them to understand the theoretical foundations of treatments in order to better adapt them to the specific needs of children.

In this sense, training for professionals should also emphasize pragmatic strategies for applying motivational ideas in real-life situations. This requires mastery of the use of individual reinforcement, multisensory stimuli, and interactive exercises during therapy sessions.

These initiatives can only improve the quality of interventions and would enhance their effectiveness by providing teachers and speech-language pathologists with the tools and techniques necessary for actively engaging children.

Training programs for families of children with autism should, in turn, provide them with useful guidance on applying neurolearning and ABA techniques at home and in the community. These initiatives would help ensure the continued development of children outside of formal treatment sessions by equipping parents with the knowledge and tools necessary to create effective learning environments. Parents, for example, could see up close how to use positive reinforcement in daily life and give their child opportunities to use language in natural contexts. Training families will also enable them to actively participate in their child's development, thus fostering collaboration between families and professionals by reworking programs with their children at home and in informal settings and during social interactions. This cooperation can only ensure lasting strengthening of the child's language skills. This will ensure that the new skills can be mobilized in a variety of contexts.

In addition to training, it is possible to create online forums where parents can seek expert help, share materials and information, and receive advice, workshops, or follow-up sessions.

It is beneficial to maintain parental support to feel more confident in implementing strategies.

Training should also involve family and community members, as this would improve the learning environment for children with autism. Expanding the range of those trained will certainly foster a more inclusive and supportive environment.

Also, improving the training of professionals in the basic concepts of neurolearning and ABA would be crucial to increasing the impact of interventions for children with ASD.

The number of groups should therefore be expanded to apply the intervention to children with varying degrees of severity.

New technology can be integrated to complement the educational program, provided it is validated by specialists.

Consequently, these proposals can enrich

These developments and adjustments therefore enrich autism treatments for more individualized and relevant interventions.

b- The Human Outcomes of the Experiment

The application of the method in the Moroccan context reveals important information beyond statistics. The educators were able to experience emotional and human moments that impacted all stages of the intervention.

The experiment was able to record resistance to the proposed activities through inappropriate behaviors in the form of stereotypes, as it seems that this type of activity is a source of frustration rooted in their previous experiences.

These moments of frustration were overcome by a relational climate with the creation of safe spaces where each child's effort is celebrated by multiplying the moments of motivation as much as possible.

Smartphones have become, in moderation, learning mediators.

The smartphones have sometimes become, without excess, learning aids, especially when the educator implements the educational program while using images, situations, and recorded voices of parents during the sessions.

It is in this sense that the personalized and simple materials worked better than refined professional resources, perhaps because they adapted to the children where they were, emanating naturally from their context.

Family involvement emerged as an unexpected but essential element of the process. Mothers, with their natural playfulness and instinctive dialect, became unexpected helpers. Their high-pitched, animated voices seemed to overcome resistance, transforming learning moments into shared play.

The team of the experiment observed how siblings intuitively simplified sentences and repeated them, building bridges between the program's exercises and real-life communication. Parents reported that these natural interactions at home often led to progress that formal sessions alone could not achieve.

These observations reveal the need for therapeutic approaches to adapt to real-life contexts. The team of the experiment can say that the children's progress was not limited to mastering techniques, but also to restoring confidence in natural communication itself. Moroccan parents showed us that improvement occurs in relationships—between educator and child, between siblings, between hesitant speakers and patient listeners. This human consideration, while harder to measure than VB-MAPP scores, may well be the most essential factor in lasting change. In the experience with this program, the toys and tools mattered less than the connections they helped create, reminding us that behind every quantitative data point is a child learning to find their human inclusion.

CONCLUSION

Though this study showed the benefits of adding NeuroLearning ideas into ABA treatments to enhance verbal communication in autistic children, many areas still need to be investigated. Potential study paths to maximise educational and therapeutic options for autistic children include expanding the sample, assessing long-term outcomes, culturally adjusting techniques, and combining complimentary approaches.

The findings of this study underline the good effect of including the motivational ideas of NeuroLearning into ABA treatments on enhancing the linguistic abilities of autistic children. Specifically, the advances seen in controlling pauses, asking for help, and articulating requirements show the efficacy of this multidisciplinary approach combining neuroscience and behavioural teaching techniques. This integration not only enhances the verbal communication of autistic children but also encourages their involvement in learning and their interactions with their surroundings.

From a different angle, one of the key insights of this study is the need of intrinsic drive in the learning process of children with autism spectrum disorders. Children's involvement was maximised and their active participation encouraged by means of individualised reinforcements, multisensory stimuli, and interactive techniques. These findings support the requirement of a personalised strategy to maximise the effect of educational interventions by fitting it to the requirements and preferences of every kid.

In the Moroccan setting, this strategy is a major advancement in enhancing support for autistic kids. Applying NeuroLearning ideas to ABA treatments is a practical and easily available answer given limited resources and the essential importance of families in assisting children. Involving parents and teachers more actively in the learning process helps to provide continuity between the specialised centre and the home and to promote the generalisation of gained abilities.

This research reveals the need to adapt tools such as VB-MAPP to Moroccan cultural specificities, including the translation of concrete elements (e.g., "/na:kol/") into Darija and the active collaboration of families to validate reinforcers. These pragmatic adaptations are, in the opinion, crucial to ensure the applicability of interventions in contexts with limited resources.

On the other hand, this study draws attention to the need of more research to better understand the long-term consequences of this strategy and to investigate its relevance in other socioeconomic and cultural settings. Increasing the sample size, lengthening the intervention time, and including innovative instructional technology could assist optimise their efficacy and enhance learning processes.

By the conclusion of this research, the team of this experiment find that combining motivational ideas of NeuroLearning with ABA treatments seems to be a hopeful way to enhance verbal communication in autistic children. Combining developments in neuroscience with established ABA techniques helps to create more interesting, efficient teaching tools tailored to the particular requirements of autistic youngsters. Aimed at providing autistic children more individualised care and improved social integration, this strategy clears the way for the development of educational and therapeutic methods. Reflecting worldwide trends in intervention for autistic people (BMC Psychology, 2024), this hybrid strategy combines ABA with neuroscientific ideas in 72% of cutting-edge programs, implying a paradigm change in therapeutic techniques.

THANKS

Undying gratitude is expressed particularly to the association's psychologist ARRAHMA, for their constructive comments throughout the various stages of this teaching program. Thanks are also extended to all the educators at the association, especially Mr. Mohammed Sahl, for their valuable contribution to this project.

REFERENCES

Aldred, C., & Green, J. (2019). The Preschool Autism Communication Therapy – an Evidence-Based Approach to Enhancing Early Autistic Development and Empowering Families. *Enfance*, *1*(1), 119–131. DOI: 10.3917/enf2.191.0119

Allard, I. ABA en IME, Neuropsychiatrie de l'Enfance et de l'Adolescence, Volume 61, Issue 5,2013,Pages 295-301,ISSN 0222-9617, DOI: 10.1016/j.neurenf.2013.04.008

Daniel, A. L., Pedreira, K., Martin, G. L., & Martin, T. (2020). Evaluation of a Self-Instructional Package for Training ABA Service Providers to Conduct the Assessment of Basic Learning Abilities – Revised. *Education and Training in Autism and Developmental Disabilities*, *55*(2), 215–227. https://www.jstor.org/stable/27077912. DOI: 10.1177/215416472005500208

Danon-Boileau, L. (2021). *Chapitre IV. Les traitements. Les Troubles du langage et de la communication chez l'enfant*. Presses Universitaires de France., https://shs.cairn.info/les-troubles-du-langage-et-de-la-communication-chez-l-enfant--9782715408081-page-87?lang=fr

Dupont, L. (2021). NeuroLearning and autism: New perspectives on motivation. *Neuroscience & Education Review*, *15*(3), 45–62.

Goffard, S. (2006). Langage et personnes autistes. *Le français aujourd'hui, 152*(1), 61-68.

Koegel, R. L., & Koegel, L. K. (2006). *Pivotal response treatments for autism: Communication, social, and academic development*. Brookes Publishing., DOI: 10.1037/11485-000

Lilley, R. (2011). The ABCs of Autism: Aspects of Maternal Pedagogy in Australia. *Social Analysis: The International Journal of Social and Cultural Practice, 55*(1), 134–159. https://www.jstor.org/stable/23182182

Liratni, M., & Blanchet, C. (2019). *Introduction. Enseigner les habiletés sociales aux enfants avec autisme: avec la méthode G.A.C.S (Groupe d'Apprentissage à la Communication et à la Socialisation).* Dunod., https://shs.cairn.info/enseigner-les-habiletes-sociales-aux-enfants--9782100794966-page-17?lang=fr DOI: 10.3917/dunod.lirat.2019.01

Smith, T., & Jones, R. M. (2022). Advances in ABA: Integrating neuroscience into practice. *Journal of Applied Behavior Analysis, 55*(2), 210–225.

Stahmer, A. C., Rieth, S. R., Dickson, K. S., Feder, J., Burgeson, M., Searcy, K., & Brookman-Frazee, L. (2020). Project ImPACT for Toddlers: Pilot outcomes of a community adaptation of an intervention for autism risk. *Autism, 24*(3), 617–632. DOI: 10.1177/1362361319878080 PMID: 31565955

Sundberg, M. L. (2008). *Verbal Behavior Milestone Assessment and Placement Program (VB-MAPP): A language and social skills assessment program for children with autism or other developmental disabilities.* AVB Press.

Trembath, D., Waddington, H., Sulek, R., Varcin, K., Bent, C., Ashburner, J., Eapen, V., Goodall, E., Hudry, K., Silove, N., & Whitehouse, A. (2021). An evidence-based framework for determining the optimal amount of intervention for autistic children. *The Lancet. Child & Adolescent Health, 5*(12), 896–904. DOI: 10.1016/S2352-4642(21)00285-6 PMID: 34672993

Wong, C., Odom, S. L., Hume, K. A., Cox, A. W., Fettig, A., Kucharczyk, S., Brock, M. E., Plavnick, J. B., Fleury, V. P., & Schultz, T. R. (2015). Evidence-based practices for children, youth, and young adults with autism spectrum disorder: A comprehensive review. *Journal of Autism and Developmental Disorders, 45*(7), 1951–1966. DOI: 10.1007/s10803-014-2351-z PMID: 25578338

Chapter 5
Neuropedagogy and Digital Innovation:
Rethinking Education for Dyslexic Learners

Siham Amessaghrou
https://orcid.org/0009-0009-4003-9237
Université Sidi Mohammed Ben Abdellah, Morocco

Houda Tahesse
https://orcid.org/0009-0001-4579-1948
Faculty of Letters and Human Sciences Dhar El Mehraz, Fez, Morocco

Mostafa Bouanani
https://orcid.org/0009-0007-8534-9621
Faculté des Lettres et des Sciences Humaines, Université Sidi Mohammed Ben Abdellah, Fès, Morocco

Kostanca Çuko
https://orcid.org/0000-0002-9888-5462
Haute École Pédagogique de Fribourg, Switzerland

ABSTRACT

This chapter examines how neuropedagogy and digital innovation can transform education for dyslexic learners. Drawing on cognitive neuroscience, it highlights how digital tools such as text-to-speech, adaptive learning, and AI-driven applications provide alternative cognitive pathways, enhancing inclusion and learner autonomy. The chapter also discusses the evolving role of teachers as mediators, the challenges

DOI: 10.4018/979-8-3373-3581-0.ch005

of professional training, and the ethical considerations of technology integration. Practical cases, including Moroccan initiatives, illustrate the potential of combining neuroscience and digital strategies to build personalized and inclusive education.

1. INTRODUCTION

Dyslexia, a neurodevelopmental disorder affecting the natural acquisition of reading and writing skills, represents one of the most persistent challenges in contemporary education. Despite advances in literacy instruction and inclusive pedagogy, students with dyslexia continue to experience significant barriers within schooling systems designed for "average" learners (Shaywitz & Shaywitz, 2008). Dyslexia is not attributable to inadequate instruction, intellectual disability, or sensory impairment, but is associated with specific neurocognitive anomalies, particularly in phonological processing, orthographic recognition, and multisensory integration (Pugh et al., 2000; Stein, 2023). These difficulties emerge early in life and tend to persist despite supportive environments, often resulting in cycles of academic underachievement, diminished self-esteem, and disengagement from formal education (Habib, 2018).

The past three decades of cognitive neuroscience have provided invaluable insights into the brain mechanisms underlying reading and its disorders. Dehaene's (2007) theory of *neuronal recycling* has been particularly influential, positing that the human brain co-opts pre-existing visual and language circuits for reading, a cultural invention for which evolution has not specifically designed neural structures. This framework helps explain both the variability of reading acquisition across individuals and the vulnerability of some learners, such as those with dyslexia, whose neural circuitry adapts less efficiently to the demands of literacy. Neuroimaging studies further demonstrate atypical activation patterns in brain regions such as the angular gyrus and occipitotemporal areas in dyslexic readers (Pugh et al., 2000; Shaywitz & Shaywitz, 2008). Such findings provide a scientific basis for rethinking pedagogical models, moving beyond uniform approaches to literacy instruction toward *neuropedagogy*, an educational paradigm informed by brain research (Ahr, 2016; Howard-Jones, 2014).

Neuropedagogy advocates for aligning teaching strategies with the ways in which the brain learns, memorizes, and adapts. This involves not only the remediation of deficits but also the optimization of strengths through flexible, multisensory, and adaptive instruction (Habib, 2018). While traditional pedagogy often prioritizes standardized, one-size-fits-all methods, neuropedagogy acknowledges the diversity of neurocognitive profiles and the need for differentiated pathways. Importantly, it underscores the principle of neuroplasticity: the capacity of the brain to reorganize itself in response to targeted stimulation and learning experiences (Ansari, 2012).

For dyslexic learners, this implies that education must not only address difficulties in phonological decoding but also harness alternative cognitive routes—such as rhythm, prosody, and visual-spatial strategies—to foster literacy development (Goswami, 2006).

In recent years, digital technologies have emerged as powerful enablers of neuropedagogical approaches. Assistive technologies such as text-to-speech systems, digital mind maps, and intelligent spelling correctors have transformed from compensatory aids into integral tools for cognitive empowerment (MacArthur, 2009; Rose & Dalton, 2009). Moreover, advances in artificial intelligence (AI) now enable real-time adaptation to individual learners' cognitive profiles, offering unprecedented opportunities for personalization (Holmes, Bialik, & Fadel, 2019; Zhao et al., 2025). These technologies not only reduce barriers to reading and writing but also promote metacognitive strategies, learner autonomy, and motivation (Fluckiger, 2020). Their potential extends beyond remediation, contributing to the creation of inclusive learning ecosystems where diversity is valued and supported.

However, integrating digital innovation into education is not without challenges. Teachers, traditionally positioned as transmitters of knowledge, must now assume new roles as mediators and facilitators who adapt pedagogical interventions to diverse learner needs (Marc & Philippette, 2021). Yet, teacher training often lags behind these demands, with limited attention to both neuroscientific foundations of learning and the pedagogical integration of technology (Fluckiger, 2020). Without sustained professional development and institutional support, the transformative potential of neuropedagogy and digital innovation risks remaining underutilized.

The importance of contextualizing these innovations within diverse educational systems cannot be overstated. In Morocco, for instance, the coexistence of Arabic and French in schools adds layers of complexity to dyslexia assessment and intervention (Amrani & Belyazid, 2021). While promising initiatives have demonstrated the potential of technology for inclusion (Touhami, 2020), the absence of standardized Arabic-language assessment tools and the digital divide across socio-economic backgrounds remain critical obstacles (Benabdallah & Bouanani, 2019). These challenges highlight the need for locally grounded, globally informed strategies that respect cultural, linguistic, and infrastructural realities.

Ethical considerations further complicate the integration of technology in inclusive education. Over-reliance on digital tools may exacerbate inequalities if access is uneven, while issues of data privacy and algorithmic bias raise concerns about the responsible use of AI in educational contexts (Holmes et al., 2022). Moreover, as Habib (2018) emphasizes, human relationships, individualized attention, and emotional support remain indispensable for learning. Technology must therefore be positioned as a complement rather than a replacement, enriching pedagogy while preserving the essential human dimensions of education.

Looking ahead, the convergence of neuropedagogy and digital innovation suggests a transformative trajectory for inclusive education. AI-driven learning environments capable of detecting early signs of reading struggles and delivering personalized interventions could shift education from reactive remediation to proactive support (Luckin et al., 2016). International frameworks, such as UNESCO's (2020) call for inclusive education for all, reinforce the urgency of developing pedagogies that are equitable, personalized, and evidence-based. Within this paradigm, every learner—regardless of cognitive profile—can be seen, understood, and supported in realizing their full potential.

This chapter aims to explore how neuropedagogy and digital innovation can be combined to rethink education for dyslexic learners. By integrating insights from cognitive neuroscience, digital learning technologies, and inclusive pedagogy, we propose that education systems can move toward models that are not only more equitable but also more effective. In doing so, the chapter contributes to ongoing debates in educational neuroscience and inclusive policy, while offering practical insights for teachers, policymakers, and researchers. The sections that follow will examine (a) the neuroscientific foundations of dyslexia, (b) the principles of neuropedagogy, (c) the potential of digital technologies, (d) the evolving role of teachers, (e) international and Moroccan experiences, (f) ethical challenges, and (g) future directions for AI-driven inclusive education. Together, these perspectives provide a comprehensive framework for reimagining education in ways that embrace neurodiversity and digital innovation as complementary forces.

2. NEUROSCIENTIFIC FOUNDATIONS OF DYSLEXIA

Dyslexia has long been recognized as a specific learning disorder, but only in the last few decades has neuroscience provided a detailed account of its biological underpinnings. The disorder is primarily characterized by persistent difficulties in accurate and/or fluent word recognition, spelling, and decoding, despite adequate instruction and intact intellectual functioning (Shaywitz & Shaywitz, 2008; Habib, 2018). Neuroscientific research has demonstrated that these difficulties are linked to differences in brain organization and functioning, particularly in circuits responsible for phonological processing, orthographic mapping, and multisensory integration (Pugh et al., 2000; Stein, 2023). Understanding these mechanisms is fundamental to the development of neuropedagogy, as it provides a scientific basis for designing educational practices that align with the ways the dyslexic brain learns.

2.1 Phonological Processing Deficits

One of the most consistently replicated findings in dyslexia research is the impairment of phonological processing, the ability to manipulate and represent the sound structures of language (Goswami, 2006). Dyslexic learners struggle with tasks such as segmenting words into phonemes, blending sounds, and mapping graphemes onto corresponding phonological units. These difficulties impede the development of decoding skills, which are essential for fluent reading. Neuroimaging studies reveal that dyslexic readers exhibit reduced activation in the left temporoparietal cortex, a region critical for phonological awareness and grapheme–phoneme conversion (Shaywitz & Shaywitz, 2008; Pugh et al., 2000).

Furthermore, electrophysiological evidence suggests that dyslexic individuals process phonemic contrasts less efficiently than typical readers, indicating deficits in the temporal resolution of auditory information (Stein, 2023). This explains why interventions focusing on phonological awareness, such as rhythmic training or prosodic reinforcement, can significantly improve reading outcomes (Goswami, 2006). These findings underscore the importance of grounding pedagogical strategies in an understanding of phonological processing deficits.

2.2 Orthographic Recognition and the Visual Word Form Area

While phonological deficits remain central, dyslexia also involves difficulties in orthographic recognition—the ability to recognize familiar written words quickly and automatically. This skill relies heavily on the *visual word form area* (VWFA), a region in the left occipitotemporal cortex that specializes in recognizing written words regardless of font, case, or size (Dehaene, 2007).

In typical readers, the VWFA becomes increasingly tuned to frequent orthographic patterns through exposure and practice. In dyslexic individuals, however, this specialization is less pronounced, leading to slower and less accurate recognition of words (Pugh et al., 2000). Neuroimaging studies consistently report hypoactivation in the VWFA of dyslexic readers, which contributes to their reliance on slower, effortful decoding strategies (Shaywitz & Shaywitz, 2008). This difficulty in establishing automaticity hinders fluency, one of the hallmark deficits of dyslexia.

These findings support the use of digital tools that can scaffold orthographic recognition—for example, multisensory reading applications that combine visual, auditory, and kinesthetic cues to strengthen word recognition pathways.

2.3 Multisensory Integration and Cross-Modal Processing

Reading is a highly integrative task that requires the coordination of visual, auditory, and motor systems. Dyslexia has been linked to anomalies in multisensory integration, particularly in how auditory and visual information are synchronized during reading tasks (Stein, 2023). Studies suggest that dyslexic readers exhibit reduced connectivity between visual and auditory cortical regions, leading to inefficiencies in integrating graphemes and phonemes (Pugh et al., 2000).

Research also highlights the role of the cerebellum in automatisation of reading skills. Dyslexic individuals may display atypical cerebellar function, contributing to difficulties in motor timing and coordination that indirectly affect fluency (Habib, 2018). These findings broaden the perspective on dyslexia beyond phonology, showing it to be a disorder of distributed neural networks.

Interventions that use multisensory methods, such as Orton–Gillingham approaches or rhythm-based training, leverage this knowledge by engaging multiple modalities simultaneously. Neuroscience thus validates long-standing pedagogical practices while also informing their refinement.

2.4 Neuronal Recycling and Cultural Learning

One of the most influential contributions of neuroscience to the study of dyslexia is Dehaene's (2007) *neuronal recycling hypothesis*. According to this theory, reading is not an innate ability but a cultural invention that co-opts existing neural circuits originally evolved for object and face recognition. The brain's ventral visual pathway is repurposed for recognizing written symbols, while language circuits adapt to map visual input to phonological and semantic representations.

Because reading requires this neural adaptation, not all brains make the transition equally well. Dyslexic learners may face difficulties in recycling these circuits, leading to the atypical activation patterns observed in neuroimaging studies (Dehaene, 2007; Stein, 2023). This insight provides a powerful rationale for neuropedagogy: if reading depends on brain plasticity, then targeted interventions and appropriate learning environments can shape these adaptations more effectively.

2.5 Neuroplasticity and the Potential for Change

Despite persistent difficulties, research emphasizes that dyslexia is not a fixed deficit but a manifestation of brain diversity that can be addressed through appropriate interventions. Neuroplasticity—the brain's ability to reorganize itself in response to learning and experience—provides the foundation for this optimism (Ansari, 2012). Studies have shown that intensive reading interventions can lead to measurable changes in brain activation, with dyslexic readers exhibiting increased engagement of typical reading circuits after targeted training (Shaywitz & Shaywitz, 2008).

Digital tools further capitalize on neuroplasticity by offering personalized, adaptive feedback that reinforces new neural connections. For example, text-to-speech systems provide auditory scaffolding that can strengthen phonological representations, while interactive reading platforms can accelerate orthographic learning. These interventions exemplify how neuroscience can inform technology-enhanced pedagogy for dyslexic learners.

2.6 Broader Cognitive and Emotional Implications

Neuroscientific perspectives on dyslexia also extend to its broader cognitive and emotional impacts. Beyond reading difficulties, dyslexic learners often experience challenges in working memory, processing speed, and attentional control (Habib, 2018). These cognitive differences can exacerbate academic struggles, leading to frustration and reduced motivation. Neuroimaging studies have further linked dyslexia with atypical functioning in regions involved in executive functions, such as the prefrontal cortex (Shaywitz & Shaywitz, 2008).

This highlights the need for interventions that address both cognitive and affective domains. Neuropedagogy must therefore integrate strategies that not only remediate reading deficits but also support emotional resilience and self-efficacy. Neuroscience contributes by identifying the brain mechanisms underlying these challenges, guiding holistic approaches to education.

2.7 Summary

In sum, the neuroscientific foundations of dyslexia demonstrate that it is a disorder of neural systems, not a result of poor teaching or lack of motivation. Phonological deficits, orthographic processing difficulties, multisensory integration anomalies, and atypical patterns of neuronal recycling collectively contribute to the profile of dyslexia. Importantly, these findings underscore the plasticity of the brain and the potential for targeted interventions to reshape neural pathways. This scientific understanding provides the groundwork for neuropedagogy, which seeks to align educational practices with the ways in which the dyslexic brain processes information.

The next section will explore the principles of neuropedagogy in greater detail, outlining how neuroscience can inform inclusive educational strategies that harness both human and technological resources.

3. PRINCIPLES OF NEUROPEDAGOGY

Neuropedagogy, an emerging interdisciplinary field at the crossroads of neuroscience, psychology, and education, seeks to ground teaching practices in an understanding of how the brain learns, adapts, and develops. Unlike traditional pedagogy, which often assumes a uniform learner profile, neuropedagogy recognizes the heterogeneity of cognitive functioning and the diversity of neural pathways engaged in learning (Ahr, 2016; Habib, 2018). By emphasizing the plasticity of the brain and the variability of learning trajectories, neuropedagogy aims to foster educational approaches that are both scientifically informed and deeply inclusive.

3.1 Defining Neuropedagogy

Neuropedagogy can be defined as the application of neuroscientific knowledge to the design and implementation of educational practices. It is distinct from "neuroeducation," which broadly connects cognitive neuroscience with teaching, in that neuropedagogy emphasizes the pedagogical adaptation of insights about brain functioning to the classroom (Tokuhama-Espinosa, 2011). Its primary objective is not merely to translate scientific findings but to rethink instructional strategies in ways that align with learners' neurocognitive strengths and limitations.

Central to this approach is the rejection of "neuromyths," such as the oversimplified left-brain/right-brain dichotomy, which have historically distorted the relationship between neuroscience and education (Howard-Jones, 2014). Instead, neuropedagogy insists on rigorous, evidence-based practices that acknowledge both the complexity of brain processes and the dynamic interplay between biological, cognitive, and environmental factors.

3.2 Neuroscience and Learning Diversity

One of the central contributions of neuropedagogy is its recognition of neurodiversity—the idea that differences in cognitive functioning, such as dyslexia, ADHD, or autism, are natural variations of the human brain rather than deficits to be eradicated (Habib, 2018). In the case of dyslexia, neuroscientific evidence demonstrates that reading difficulties stem from differences in phonological processing and neural connectivity rather than lack of intelligence or motivation (Shaywitz & Shaywitz, 2008).

Acknowledging this diversity compels educators to move away from standardized instructional models and toward differentiated strategies. Neuropedagogy provides a framework for tailoring instruction to the learner's neurocognitive profile, fostering inclusion and equity in classrooms where students' needs vary widely. This aligns with international educational principles of inclusive pedagogy, which emphasize designing learning environments that accommodate, rather than marginalize, atypical learners (Florian & Black-Hawkins, 2011).

3.3 The Role of Neuroplasticity

Neuroplasticity—the brain's capacity to reorganize itself in response to experience and training—is a cornerstone of neuropedagogy (Ansari, 2012). Far from being static, the brain continuously adapts, forming and strengthening synaptic connections in response to learning. This principle carries profound pedagogical implications: if neural networks can be reshaped, then instructional practices can actively contribute to compensating for learning difficulties and building alternative cognitive strategies.

For dyslexic learners, targeted interventions such as phonological training, rhythmic exercises, or multisensory approaches have been shown to induce measurable changes in brain activation patterns (Goswami, 2006). These findings support neuropedagogy's emphasis on dynamic, adaptive instruction that harnesses plasticity rather than resigns itself to static limitations.

3.4 Holistic and Multimodal Approaches

Neuropedagogy also highlights the importance of engaging multiple modalities—visual, auditory, kinesthetic, and emotional—in teaching and learning. Reading, for instance, is not merely a linguistic activity but a complex cognitive process involving the integration of auditory decoding, visual recognition, motor coordination, and executive control (Dehaene, 2007).

Multimodal teaching strategies, such as combining spoken language with visual aids, gestures, and digital supports, align with this holistic perspective. For dyslexic students, such approaches can activate alternative neural pathways, reinforcing learning through redundancy and cross-modal stimulation (Habib, 2018). In this way, neuropedagogy extends beyond narrow remediation to promote overall cognitive development.

3.5 Teacher as Mediator of Neuroscience

Another principle of neuropedagogy concerns the evolving role of teachers. Educators are not expected to become neuroscientists but rather to act as mediators who interpret and apply neuroscientific insights in pedagogically relevant ways (Marc & Philippette, 2021). This requires professional development that equips teachers with both conceptual knowledge of brain processes and practical skills for integrating such knowledge into their classroom practices.

Importantly, neuropedagogy emphasizes that neuroscience does not dictate pedagogy; instead, it informs and refines it. Teachers remain central actors who must combine scientific insights with contextual understanding of their students, cultural environments, and institutional constraints.

3.6 Summary

The principles of neuropedagogy can be summarized as follows:

1. **Scientific grounding**: Educational strategies must be based on validated neuroscientific evidence, not on simplistic "neuromyths."
2. **Recognition of neurodiversity**: Learning differences such as dyslexia reflect natural variations in brain functioning.
3. **Harnessing neuroplasticity**: Instruction should exploit the brain's adaptive capacity to reshape neural networks through targeted interventions.
4. **Holistic, multimodal learning**: Effective pedagogy engages multiple modalities and cognitive systems simultaneously.
5. **Teacher as mediator**: Educators play a crucial role in translating neuroscience into meaningful classroom practices.

Together, these principles establish neuropedagogy as a promising framework for inclusive education. By aligning teaching practices with the workings of the brain, neuropedagogy not only addresses learning difficulties but also promotes equity and cognitive flourishing for all learners.

4. LIMITATIONS OF TRADITIONAL PEDAGOGICAL APPROACHES

Despite decades of educational reform, most schooling systems continue to rely on models designed for the "average learner." Such models privilege uniformity in curriculum, teaching methods, and assessment, assuming that all students progress through literacy acquisition at roughly the same pace and in similar ways. For students with dyslexia, however, these traditional approaches often exacerbate difficulties rather than alleviate them, resulting in cycles of academic frustration, low self-esteem, and disengagement (Habib, 2018; Shaywitz & Shaywitz, 2008).

4.1 Standardization and the Myth of the "Average Learner"

A central limitation of traditional pedagogy is its reliance on standardized teaching frameworks. These frameworks assume a homogeneity of learners that does not reflect the reality of neurodiverse classrooms (Florian & Black-Hawkins, 2011). Lessons are often delivered at a single pace, with limited differentiation, leaving behind students who require either more time or alternative strategies to master reading and writing skills. For dyslexic learners, this mismatch can manifest as repeated failure in decoding and fluency tasks, despite intact intelligence and strong motivation.

4.2 Reactive Rather than Proactive Interventions

Conventional schooling typically identifies learning difficulties only after repeated failure, leading to what is often described as a "wait-to-fail" model (Shaywitz & Shaywitz, 2008). Dyslexic students may struggle for years before receiving targeted support, by which time the negative emotional consequences—frustration, anxiety, diminished self-confidence—are already deeply entrenched (Habib, 2018). Early intervention, supported by neuroscientific research, is crucial for reshaping neural pathways and preventing the consolidation of maladaptive learning patterns (Goswami, 2006). Traditional pedagogy, however, lacks systematic mechanisms for such proactive support.

4.3 Overemphasis on Phonics Without Multimodality

While phonics instruction is widely recognized as essential for literacy development, traditional pedagogy often applies it in rigid, decontextualized ways. For dyslexic learners, this emphasis can become overwhelming, as their phonological processing deficits make purely phonics-based methods insufficient (Stein, 2023). Neuroscience demonstrates that effective reading instruction must integrate visual, auditory, and kinesthetic modalities to strengthen alternative neural pathways (Dehaene, 2007; Habib, 2018). By neglecting multimodality, conventional methods risk reinforcing deficits rather than providing compensatory strategies.

4.4 Limited Teacher Training and Awareness

Teachers are central to any pedagogical transformation, yet most traditional training programs provide little preparation in either the neuroscientific foundations of learning or the integration of digital and multimodal tools (Fluckiger, 2020). As a result, many teachers remain unaware of the neurocognitive profiles of dyslexic learners or the evidence-based strategies available to support them. This gap perpetuates reliance on one-size-fits-all methods, leaving students with dyslexia insufficiently supported in mainstream classrooms.

4.5 Emotional and Social Consequences

The limitations of traditional pedagogy are not only cognitive but also emotional and social. Repeated academic failure contributes to a negative self-concept, reduced motivation, and increased risk of school dropout among dyslexic learners (Habib, 2018). Furthermore, the stigmatization of learning difficulties in uniform educational environments can isolate students, undermining their sense of belonging. Traditional approaches thus fail to address the holistic needs of dyslexic learners, who require not only cognitive remediation but also emotional and social support.

4.6 Summary

Traditional pedagogical approaches are limited in at least five critical ways:

1. They rely on standardized models that overlook neurodiversity.
2. They are reactive, providing support only after failure has occurred.
3. They overemphasize phonics while neglecting multimodal strategies.
4. They suffer from insufficient teacher training in neuroscience and inclusive practices.
5. They fail to address the emotional and social dimensions of dyslexia.

These limitations highlight the urgency of moving toward neuropedagogical frameworks that are proactive, multimodal, and inclusive. The next section will examine how digital technologies can help address these shortcomings and transform educational experiences for dyslexic learners.

5. DIGITAL TOOLS AND PEDAGOGICAL INNOVATION

The rapid advancement of digital technologies has fundamentally reshaped education, offering new opportunities to support diverse learners, including those with dyslexia. While traditional pedagogy often emphasizes remediation through uniform, text-based approaches, digital tools provide multimodal, adaptive, and accessible pathways that align with the neurocognitive profiles of students with learning differences. Importantly, these technologies are not merely compensatory: they can empower dyslexic learners by activating alternative cognitive routes, promoting autonomy, and fostering metacognitive awareness (MacArthur, 2009; Rose & Dalton, 2009).

This section explores how digital tools function as agents of pedagogical innovation. It distinguishes between assistive technologies that support access and transformative technologies that restructure learning processes, while examining their potential for inclusion, personalization, and engagement.

5.1 Assistive versus Transformative Technologies

Digital tools for dyslexia can be broadly categorized into assistive technologies and transformative technologies. Assistive technologies are designed to compensate for deficits, enabling learners to bypass specific difficulties. Examples include text-to-speech (TTS) software, word prediction systems, and spell checkers tailored for dyslexic users (MacArthur, 2009). These tools ensure access to written materials, supporting comprehension and participation in mainstream education.

By contrast, transformative technologies aim to reshape the learning process itself, offering alternative ways of acquiring, processing, and producing knowledge. For instance, AI-driven reading assistants can adaptively scaffold phonological decoding, gradually training learners to strengthen specific cognitive functions (Zhao et al., 2025). Similarly, digital platforms that integrate speech, text, and imagery can reinforce multisensory learning, aligning with neuropedagogical principles (Dehaene, 2007; Habib, 2018).

The shift from assistive to transformative technology is crucial, as it reframes dyslexia not as a barrier to participation but as an opportunity to rethink pedagogy in ways that benefit all learners.

5.2 Text-to-Speech and Speech-to-Text Tools

Among the most widely used digital supports for dyslexia are text-to-speech (TTS) and speech-to-text (STT) systems. TTS tools, such as ReadSpeaker and NaturalReader, convert written text into spoken words, enabling learners to access content without being limited by decoding difficulties (MacArthur, 2009). These systems facilitate comprehension, reduce cognitive load, and allow learners to focus on higher-order processes such as analysis and synthesis.

Conversely, STT technologies empower students to express themselves in writing without being constrained by spelling or transcription errors. Tools like Dragon NaturallySpeaking or Google's speech recognition systems provide an accessible pathway for producing extended texts, supporting academic participation and creativity. By reducing mechanical barriers, these tools allow learners to engage in authentic literacy tasks, promoting confidence and agency.

5.3 Intelligent Writing and Reading Assistants

Recent advances in artificial intelligence (AI) have given rise to intelligent writing and reading assistants specifically tailored for dyslexic learners. Applications such as Ghotit and Grammarly offer context-sensitive spelling and grammar corrections, predictive word suggestions, and adaptive feedback. Unlike traditional spellcheckers, these systems are designed to account for the phonological errors characteristic of dyslexic writing, thus offering more relevant and supportive feedback (MacArthur, 2009).

AI-powered reading assistants, such as those explored by Zhao et al. (2025), provide real-time scaffolding during reading, highlighting phoneme-grapheme correspondences, offering definitions, and tracking comprehension. These systems exemplify the shift toward **transformative technology**, as they do not merely compensate for dyslexia but actively build the cognitive skills necessary for literacy.

5.4 Digital Mind Maps and Visual Tools

Visual learning tools such as digital mind maps (e.g., MindMeister, Coggle) enable dyslexic learners to organize and represent ideas spatially, reducing reliance on linear text (Rose & Dalton, 2009). These tools align with evidence showing that dyslexic learners often have strengths in visual-spatial reasoning, which can be leveraged to support comprehension, planning, and memory (Habib, 2018).

Similarly, infographics, interactive diagrams, and visual organizers provide alternative modalities for processing information. By diversifying input formats, digital visual tools respect neurodiversity and help learners access knowledge in ways that align with their cognitive strengths.

5.5 Gamification and Motivation

Digital games and gamified learning platforms have also shown promise in supporting dyslexic learners. By incorporating elements of play, challenge, and immediate feedback, gamification can increase motivation, reduce anxiety, and promote persistence (Rose & Dalton, 2009). Tools such as GraphoGame and Dyslexia Quest use adaptive algorithms to provide targeted phonological training in engaging formats.

Gamified environments align with neuropedagogical principles by reinforcing learning through repetition, multisensory engagement, and emotional activation. Moreover, they help counteract the negative self-concept often associated with dyslexia by creating positive, success-oriented experiences.

5.6 Universal Design for Learning (UDL) and Inclusive Platforms

The framework of Universal Design for Learning (UDL) emphasizes the creation of flexible learning environments that accommodate diverse learners by design rather than retrofitting accommodations (Al-Azawei, Serenelli, & Lundqvist, 2016). Digital tools are central to UDL, offering multiple means of representation (e.g., text, audio, video), expression (e.g., writing, speech, multimedia), and engagement (e.g., adaptive pacing, gamification).

Platforms such as Learning Ally, Bookshare, and CALL Scotland resources exemplify UDL principles, providing accessible content to learners with dyslexia and other print disabilities. Such platforms highlight that inclusive technology benefits not only students with diagnosed difficulties but all learners, reinforcing the broader social value of neuropedagogical innovation.

5.7 Case Studies and International Initiatives

Internationally, numerous initiatives illustrate the transformative impact of digital tools on dyslexia education. In the United Kingdom, CALL Scotland has developed extensive resources to support schools in implementing assistive technologies, while Scandinavian countries have integrated digital literacy supports into mainstream classrooms as part of inclusive education policies (Fluckiger, 2020).

In Morocco, pilot projects have experimented with integrating TTS and visual tools into bilingual classrooms, where learners navigate both Arabic and French (Touhami, 2020). Although challenges remain—including limited infrastructure and uneven teacher training—these efforts demonstrate the adaptability of digital innovation to local contexts. Such case studies underscore the necessity of culturally and linguistically responsive digital interventions.

5.8 Ethical and Equity Considerations

While digital tools hold immense potential, their integration raises ethical and equity concerns. Access remains uneven across socio-economic contexts, with learners in under-resourced settings less likely to benefit from advanced technologies (UNESCO, 2020). Furthermore, the growing role of AI in education raises questions about data privacy, algorithmic bias, and the risk of over-reliance on automated systems (Holmes et al., 2022).

Neuropedagogy insists that technology must complement, not replace, human support. Emotional connections, individualized attention, and teacher mediation remain indispensable for effective learning. Ensuring equitable access and ethical use of technology is therefore essential for fulfilling its promise in inclusive education.

5.9 Summary

Digital technologies represent a paradigm shift in supporting learners with dyslexia. They move beyond compensatory tools to transformative systems that:

1. Provide multimodal access to information through TTS, STT, and visual organizers.
2. Enable adaptive scaffolding via AI-powered reading and writing assistants.
3. Foster motivation and persistence through gamification and interactive design.
4. Embody inclusive principles through frameworks like Universal Design for Learning.
5. Demonstrate real-world impact in international and local initiatives, including Morocco.

Yet, their potential will only be realized if integrated thoughtfully, supported by teacher training, and guided by ethical and equity considerations. In this sense, digital tools are not merely educational technologies but agents of pedagogical innovation aligned with the principles of neuropedagogy.

6. METACOGNITIVE STRATEGIES SUPPORTED BY TECHNOLOGY

Metacognition—the ability to monitor, evaluate, and regulate one's own cognitive processes—plays a central role in successful learning. For students with dyslexia, metacognitive skills are often underdeveloped because persistent difficulties with decoding and fluency demand so much cognitive effort that little capacity remains for self-regulation (Habib, 2018). Traditional pedagogical approaches rarely provide explicit instruction in metacognitive strategies, further disadvantaging dyslexic learners.

Digital technologies, however, offer new opportunities to scaffold metacognitive processes. By providing real-time feedback, multimodal representations, and adaptive pathways, technology enables learners to become more aware of how they learn and to take greater control over their learning processes. This aligns with neuropedagogical principles, which emphasize the importance of fostering autonomy, self-awareness, and motivation alongside cognitive skill development (Ahr, 2016; Tokuhama-Espinosa, 2011).

6.1 Phonological Awareness and Rhythmic Training

A critical area of metacognitive intervention for dyslexic learners is phonological awareness—the ability to consciously reflect on and manipulate the sound structure of language. Research has demonstrated that integrating rhythm and prosody into learning tasks can significantly improve phonological awareness, thereby enhancing decoding skills (Goswami, 2006).

Digital tools such as GraphoGame and Dyslexia Quest incorporate rhythmic elements and gamified feedback, prompting learners to actively monitor their performance and adjust strategies accordingly. These platforms exemplify how technology can make abstract phonological processes explicit, fostering both cognitive development and metacognitive reflection. Learners begin not only to practice phonological tasks but also to recognize *how* they succeed or struggle, which is essential for long-term autonomy.

6.2 Feedback Loops and Self-Monitoring

One of the most powerful contributions of digital technologies to metacognition is the creation of immediate feedback loops. Intelligent writing assistants such as Ghotit or Grammarly provide real-time corrections and explanations, encouraging students to monitor their writing choices and reflect on patterns of error (MacArthur, 2009). Similarly, AI-driven reading platforms can highlight words misread or skipped, prompting learners to self-correct.

Such feedback shifts learners from passive recipients of correction to active agents of self-monitoring. By making errors visible and understandable, technology reduces the stigma of mistakes while transforming them into opportunities for growth. This process nurtures self-awareness, helping learners to develop strategies for overcoming recurring difficulties.

6.3 Autonomy and Self-Regulated Learning

Metacognition is closely tied to self-regulated learning, which involves planning, monitoring, and evaluating one's own learning activities. Digital platforms facilitate self-regulation by allowing learners to control pacing, choose among learning pathways, and access multimodal resources. For instance, e-learning environments based on Universal Design for Learning (UDL) principles provide multiple means of representation and expression, enabling learners to select the modalities that best suit their cognitive strengths (Al-Azawei, Serenelli, & Lundqvist, 2016).

For dyslexic learners, such autonomy is particularly empowering. Instead of being confined to teacher-directed remediation, they can explore strategies that work for them, experiment with digital tools, and monitor their own progress. This process fosters not only academic skills but also resilience, confidence, and intrinsic motivation—factors often undermined by repeated failure in traditional classrooms (Florian & Black-Hawkins, 2011).

6.4 Personalization and Adaptive Learning

AI-driven adaptive learning systems take metacognition a step further by tailoring feedback and challenges to individual learner profiles. These systems analyze performance in real time and adjust difficulty levels, content presentation, and scaffolding accordingly (Holmes, Bialik, & Fadel, 2019). For example, reading platforms may detect when a learner struggles with particular phoneme–grapheme correspondences and provide targeted practice.

Crucially, adaptive systems also encourage learners to reflect on their learning trajectories by visualizing progress through dashboards or progress reports. Such tools promote metacognitive reflection, enabling students to see how their efforts translate into measurable improvements. This aligns with the neuropedagogical principle of harnessing neuroplasticity by reinforcing positive learning patterns through deliberate practice and reflection (Ansari, 2012).

6.5 Emotional Regulation and Motivation

Metacognition extends beyond cognitive processes to include emotional regulation. Dyslexic learners often experience frustration, anxiety, and diminished self-confidence, which interfere with learning (Habib, 2018). Digital tools can help by providing safe environments where mistakes are normalized and progress is visible. Gamified learning systems, for instance, reframe challenges as opportunities for achievement, reducing the negative affect associated with repeated failure (Rose & Dalton, 2009).

By enabling learners to track their own growth, digital platforms foster positive self-evaluations, which are essential for motivation. In this way, technology not only enhances cognitive metacognition but also supports affective metacognition, helping learners to regulate emotions in the face of difficulty.

6.6 Teacher Mediation of Metacognition

Although technology provides powerful scaffolds, the teacher remains central in guiding learners to use metacognitive strategies effectively. Teachers help students interpret feedback, generalize strategies across tasks, and integrate digital supports into broader learning goals (Marc & Philippette, 2021). Neuropedagogy thus frames metacognition as a collaborative process: while digital tools facilitate awareness and autonomy, educators ensure that these tools are used reflectively and meaningfully.

This dual role underscores the importance of professional development, equipping teachers with the knowledge to mediate digital feedback and foster metacognitive growth. Without such mediation, learners may use digital tools superficially, without engaging in the deeper reflection necessary for long-term self-regulation.

6.7 Summary

Digital technologies support metacognition in dyslexic learners through several key mechanisms:

1. **Enhancing phonological awareness** via rhythm, prosody, and gamified tasks.
2. **Providing immediate feedback** that fosters active self-monitoring.
3. **Promoting autonomy** by enabling learner-controlled pathways and multimodal choices.
4. **Supporting personalization** through adaptive learning environments and progress visualization.
5. **Facilitating emotional regulation** by reframing mistakes and emphasizing progress.
6. **Reinforcing teacher mediation** to ensure reflective use of digital supports.

In this way, digital tools align with neuropedagogical principles by empowering learners to become active participants in their education. They not only remediate specific difficulties but also cultivate broader skills of self-awareness, resilience, and self-regulation.

7. THE CHANGING ROLE OF TEACHERS

The integration of neuropedagogy and digital innovation in dyslexia education requires a profound transformation of the teacher's role. In traditional schooling, teachers are often positioned as transmitters of knowledge, responsible for delivering standardized curricula to a presumed homogeneous group of learners. Neuropedagogy challenges this model by emphasizing learner diversity, cognitive variability, and the importance of aligning instruction with how the brain learns (Habib, 2018; Ahr, 2016). Within this framework, teachers must act not only as instructors but also as mediators, facilitators, and designers of inclusive learning environments.

7.1 From Knowledge Transmission to Mediation

The shift from transmission to mediation reflects a fundamental reconceptualization of teaching. In neuropedagogical contexts, teachers are no longer the sole sources of information; digital platforms, multimedia resources, and AI systems can deliver content directly to learners (Holmes, Bialik, & Fadel, 2019). What distinguishes the teacher is their ability to interpret learners' needs, personalize instruction, and scaffold cognitive and emotional development.

For dyslexic learners, this means guiding the use of digital tools, ensuring that technologies serve pedagogical goals rather than replacing them. Teachers mediate between scientific knowledge about learning, technological possibilities, and the individual learner's profile, thus becoming orchestrators of inclusive education (Marc & Philippette, 2021).

7.2 Teacher Competencies in Neuropedagogy

To fulfill this mediating role, teachers must develop new competencies that extend beyond subject knowledge. These include:

1. **Neuroscientific literacy** – understanding the basics of how the brain processes reading and writing, including knowledge of neurodiversity and neuroplasticity (Howard-Jones, 2014).
2. **Technological competence** – the ability to select, evaluate, and integrate digital tools into learning environments in ways that align with pedagogical goals (Fluckiger, 2020).
3. **Inclusive pedagogy** – designing and adapting instruction to accommodate diverse learners, grounded in frameworks such as Universal Design for Learning (Al-Azawei, Serenelli, & Lundqvist, 2016).
4. **Metacognitive scaffolding** – teaching students to reflect on their own learning processes and to use feedback for self-regulation (Tokuhama-Espinosa, 2011).
5. **Emotional and relational sensitivity** – recognizing the affective dimensions of dyslexia, including the impact of repeated failure on self-esteem, and providing motivational support (Habib, 2018).

These competencies illustrate that the neuropedagogical teacher is not a passive adopter of technology but an active designer of learning experiences that integrate brain-based insights with digital innovation.

7.3 Professional Development and Teacher Training

A major obstacle to this transformation is the current inadequacy of teacher training. Many programs devote little attention to neuroscience, inclusive education, or digital pedagogy (Fluckiger, 2020). As a result, teachers may feel ill-equipped to support dyslexic learners or to leverage the potential of digital tools effectively.

Professional development is therefore critical. Training programs should:

- Provide foundational knowledge of brain development and learning disorders.
- Familiarize teachers with evidence-based digital tools for literacy support.
- Offer opportunities to practice integrating these tools into real classroom scenarios.
- Foster reflective practice, encouraging teachers to evaluate the impact of their strategies on learners with diverse profiles.

International experiences highlight the value of collaborative training models, where teachers learn from both researchers and peers. For instance, CALL Scotland has developed resources and workshops that combine technological training with practical classroom strategies, empowering teachers to implement inclusive digital pedagogy (Fluckiger, 2020).

7.4 Teacher–Learner Relationships in the Digital Era

While technology can deliver content efficiently, it cannot replace the relational dimension of education. Dyslexic learners, in particular, benefit from empathetic teacher–learner relationships that validate their experiences and encourage resilience (Habib, 2018). Teachers play a key role in reframing mistakes as learning opportunities, reducing anxiety, and fostering a growth mindset.

In digital learning contexts, the teacher's relational role also includes guiding students in navigating feedback from AI systems. Automated corrections can sometimes feel impersonal or overwhelming; teachers help learners interpret feedback constructively, integrating it into broader strategies for improvement. This highlights the irreplaceable human role in contextualizing technology within an affective and motivational framework.

7.5 Collaborative Roles and Pedagogical Design

Teachers are also increasingly called upon to collaborate with specialists such as speech-language pathologists, psychologists, and IT professionals. This interdisciplinary collaboration aligns with neuropedagogy's holistic view of learning, recognizing that dyslexia is not solely a pedagogical issue but a neurocognitive and social one (Habib, 2018). Teachers contribute unique insights into classroom dynamics, while specialists provide diagnostic expertise and targeted interventions.

In addition, teachers must engage in pedagogical design, selecting and sequencing learning activities that integrate digital tools in meaningful ways. This involves not simply adding technology to existing lessons but rethinking the structure of learning experiences to ensure accessibility, personalization, and engagement for all learners.

7.6 Summary

The changing role of teachers in neuropedagogical and digital contexts can be summarized as follows:

1. Moving from knowledge transmitters to mediators who align neuroscience, technology, and learner diversity.
2. Developing new competencies in neuroscience, technology, inclusion, metacognition, and emotional support.
3. Engaging in professional development that bridges theory and practice.
4. Maintaining relational and motivational roles, particularly for learners facing stigma and low self-confidence.
5. Participating in collaborative and design-based roles that extend beyond the classroom.

In sum, teachers remain central to the success of neuropedagogical innovation. While digital tools offer powerful scaffolds, their effectiveness depends on the educator's ability to integrate them thoughtfully, interpret their feedback, and situate them within supportive human relationships. The next section will examine international experiences and the Moroccan context to illustrate how these principles are being implemented in diverse educational systems.

8. INTERNATIONAL EXPERIENCES AND THE MOROCCAN CONTEXT

While the principles of neuropedagogy and the integration of digital tools hold promise globally, their application is shaped by cultural, linguistic, and institutional contexts. Comparative perspectives reveal both commonalities and divergences in how countries address the educational needs of dyslexic learners. This section highlights selected international initiatives that illustrate the transformative potential of digital tools and inclusive pedagogy, before turning to the Moroccan context where unique linguistic and structural challenges complicate the implementation of neuropedagogical frameworks.

8.1 International Case Studies of Digital Inclusion

Several countries have pioneered the integration of digital technologies to support dyslexic learners. In the United Kingdom, CALL Scotland has developed comprehensive resources for teachers and schools, including digital toolkits, online training, and repositories of accessible materials. These initiatives exemplify how government support and specialist expertise can bridge the gap between research and practice (Fluckiger, 2020).

In Scandinavia, particularly in Finland and Norway, inclusive policies emphasize universal access to assistive technologies such as text-to-speech and audiobooks. Dyslexic students are routinely provided with digital literacy supports as part of mainstream schooling, reflecting a systemic commitment to equity and accessibility (Al-Azawei, Serenelli, & Lundqvist, 2016). These countries demonstrate the feasibility of embedding digital supports into national education systems, ensuring that inclusion is not an exception but a standard practice.

In North America, platforms such as Bookshare and Learning Ally provide extensive libraries of accessible digital texts for learners with print disabilities. These initiatives are underpinned by legislation such as the Americans with Disabilities Act (ADA) and the Individuals with Disabilities Education Act (IDEA), which mandate equal access to educational resources. The combination of legal frameworks and technological infrastructure illustrates how structural support is critical to scaling inclusive practices.

8.2 Lessons from International Best Practices

These international experiences highlight several lessons relevant to the global adoption of neuropedagogical principles:

1. **Policy integration** is essential. Success in Finland, Norway, and the UK shows that digital inclusion thrives when supported by national policies, not only individual schools or teachers.
2. **Teacher training** is a cornerstone. Digital tools become transformative only when educators are equipped with knowledge and skills to integrate them effectively.
3. **Universal access** prevents stigmatization. By embedding assistive technologies into mainstream classrooms, students with dyslexia can use them without being singled out, promoting dignity and normalization.

4. **Collaboration between stakeholders**—including policymakers, researchers, teachers, and technology developers—is necessary to ensure that tools are relevant, evidence-based, and scalable.

8.3 The Moroccan Context: Linguistic and Structural Challenges

In Morocco, the implementation of neuropedagogical and digital innovations faces distinctive challenges. The Moroccan educational system is shaped by bilingualism, with Arabic as the primary language of instruction in early education and French widely used in science and secondary education. Dyslexic learners must navigate literacy acquisition across two orthographic systems, compounding the cognitive demands of learning to read and write (Amrani & Belyazid, 2021).

This bilingual environment complicates assessment, as most available standardized tools are in French, leaving a near-total absence of Arabic-language diagnostic instruments (Benabdallah & Bouanani, 2019). Without culturally and linguistically adapted tools, educators struggle to identify dyslexia reliably in Arabic-speaking learners, delaying intervention and support.

Structural challenges further limit implementation. Schools in rural and under-resourced areas often lack access to digital infrastructure, including reliable internet connections, adequate hardware, and trained personnel. The digital divide exacerbates educational inequities, with students in urban, private institutions more likely to benefit from innovative tools than those in public or rural schools (Touhami, 2020).

8.4 Emerging Initiatives in Morocco

Despite these obstacles, several promising initiatives point toward greater integration of digital and neuropedagogical approaches in Morocco. Pilot projects in Casablanca and Rabat have introduced text-to-speech tools and interactive reading platforms into classrooms, supported by collaborations between universities, NGOs, and international partners (Touhami, 2020).

At the policy level, Morocco's National Strategy for Digital Education has identified inclusive education as a priority, though implementation remains uneven. Teacher training programs are beginning to incorporate modules on ICT in education, albeit with limited focus on learning disorders. Research initiatives, such as those led by Moroccan universities, have also highlighted the need to develop culturally grounded assessment batteries and intervention protocols tailored to Arabic orthography and bilingual contexts (Benabdallah & Bouanani, 2019).

These initiatives illustrate that while progress is incremental, the foundations for broader adoption are being laid.

8.5 Opportunities for Neuropedagogical Innovation in Morocco

The Moroccan context also presents unique opportunities. The coexistence of Arabic and French provides a fertile ground for studying how bilingualism interacts with dyslexia, offering insights of global relevance (Boudelaa, 2014). The growing interest in digital education, accelerated by the COVID-19 pandemic, has increased awareness of the potential of technology for reaching diverse learners. Furthermore, international collaborations open avenues for knowledge transfer and capacity-building.

By developing Arabic-specific assessment tools, investing in digital infrastructure, and embedding teacher training in neuropedagogy, Morocco could position itself as a regional leader in inclusive education. These steps would not only benefit dyslexic learners but also strengthen educational equity more broadly.

8.6 Summary

International experiences demonstrate that the successful integration of neuropedagogy and digital tools requires systemic support, teacher training, universal access, and stakeholder collaboration. In Morocco, while challenges such as bilingualism, lack of Arabic diagnostic tools, and digital inequities persist, emerging initiatives indicate growing momentum toward inclusive, digitally mediated education.

The Moroccan case underscores that neuropedagogical innovation must be context-sensitive: global models provide inspiration, but local adaptations are essential. As the next section will show, ethical considerations and human dimensions remain critical for ensuring that digital transformation serves learners equitably and responsibly.

9. ETHICAL CHALLENGES AND HUMAN DIMENSIONS

The integration of neuropedagogy and digital technologies into education offers tremendous promise for supporting dyslexic learners, but it also raises significant ethical challenges. These challenges are not confined to questions of access and equity but extend to the broader human dimensions of learning, including the role of emotional support, the safeguarding of learner dignity, and the responsible use of data and artificial intelligence. Without careful consideration of these issues, technological innovation risks reinforcing existing inequalities or undermining the very principles of inclusion it seeks to advance (Holmes et al., 2022; UNESCO, 2020).

9.1 Equity and the Digital Divide

Perhaps the most pressing ethical concern is the digital divide—the unequal distribution of technological resources across socio-economic, geographic, and institutional contexts. While learners in affluent, urban schools may benefit from cutting-edge digital tools, those in rural or under-resourced settings often lack access to reliable internet, adequate devices, or trained teachers (Touhami, 2020). This inequity risks deepening educational disparities rather than reducing them.

From a neuropedagogical perspective, equity is not only about access to hardware but also about access to opportunities for neurocognitive development. If only certain groups of learners can benefit from personalized, adaptive technologies, then digital innovation may inadvertently privilege already advantaged populations, perpetuating systemic inequalities (UNESCO, 2020).

9.2 Over-Reliance on Technology

Another challenge lies in the risk of over-reliance on technology. While digital tools provide valuable scaffolds for dyslexic learners, they cannot replace the relational and emotional support offered by teachers, peers, and families. Neuropedagogy emphasizes that learning is a holistic process involving not only cognition but also emotion, motivation, and social interaction (Habib, 2018).

If technology is positioned as a panacea, educators may neglect the essential human dimensions of teaching. For example, automated feedback from AI writing assistants may help correct errors but lacks the empathetic guidance that builds resilience and confidence. Effective inclusion therefore requires balance: technology should enrich pedagogy without displacing the interpersonal relationships that are indispensable to learning.

9.3 Data Privacy and Algorithmic Bias

As artificial intelligence becomes increasingly embedded in educational technologies, concerns about data privacy and algorithmic bias have gained urgency. AI-driven platforms often collect detailed information about learners' performance, behaviors, and even emotional states (Holmes, Bialik, & Fadel, 2019). While such data can enable personalized instruction, it also raises ethical questions about ownership, consent, and potential misuse.

Moreover, algorithms are not neutral. If trained on biased datasets, they may reproduce or amplify inequalities, for example by misclassifying errors made by bilingual learners as deficits rather than natural features of language acquisition

(Holmes et al., 2022). Ensuring transparency, accountability, and fairness in AI design is thus essential to prevent technology from undermining inclusion.

9.4 Protecting Learner Dignity and Agency

Ethical education also requires attention to the dignity and agency of learners. Dyslexic students often experience stigmatization and feelings of inadequacy in traditional classrooms (Habib, 2018). Digital tools can either mitigate or exacerbate this risk. For instance, if assistive technologies are introduced in ways that single out dyslexic learners, they may reinforce stigma. Conversely, when embedded within universal platforms accessible to all, these tools promote normalization and empowerment (Al-Azawei, Serenelli, & Lundqvist, 2016).

Neuropedagogy insists that learners must be active participants in their education, not passive recipients of interventions. Ethical implementation of digital tools requires involving learners in decision-making, respecting their preferences, and cultivating self-efficacy alongside cognitive skills.

9.5 Human Relationships in Inclusive Education

Finally, the human dimension remains central to effective inclusion. Neuroscience demonstrates that learning is socially mediated, shaped by interactions with teachers, peers, and caregivers (Howard-Jones, 2014). Emotional support is particularly critical for dyslexic learners, who often grapple with frustration and low self-esteem. Teachers provide encouragement, model resilience, and create safe spaces where mistakes are reframed as opportunities for growth.

In this sense, digital innovation should be viewed not as a replacement for human relationships but as a tool that extends their reach. For example, digital platforms can free teachers from repetitive tasks, allowing them to devote more attention to personalized guidance and emotional support. The synergy of technology and human care is what ultimately fulfills the promise of neuropedagogy.

9.6 Summary

The ethical challenges of neuropedagogy and digital innovation can be summarized in five key areas:

1. Ensuring equity of access across socio-economic and geographic contexts.
2. Avoiding over-reliance on technology that neglects human relationships.
3. Protecting data privacy and addressing algorithmic bias in AI systems.

4. Safeguarding learner dignity and agency by preventing stigma and promoting autonomy.
5. Preserving the human dimensions of education, particularly emotional and relational support.

Ultimately, the promise of digital neuropedagogy lies not in replacing human educators but in amplifying their capacity to support diverse learners. By embedding ethical vigilance into design and practice, educational systems can ensure that innovation serves equity, inclusion, and human flourishing.

10. FUTURE PERSPECTIVES: AI AND INCLUSIVE SCHOOLS

As digital innovation accelerates, artificial intelligence (AI) is emerging as a transformative force in education. For dyslexic learners, AI holds particular promise by enabling real-time personalization, adaptive feedback, and predictive insights that could shift education from reactive remediation to proactive support. Neuropedagogy provides the theoretical framework for guiding these developments, ensuring that AI is deployed in ways that align with cognitive neuroscience, inclusive pedagogy, and ethical responsibility (Luckin et al., 2016; Holmes, Bialik, & Fadel, 2019).

This section explores future perspectives at the intersection of AI and neuropedagogy, highlighting opportunities for early detection, adaptive learning environments, teacher augmentation, and anticipatory education. It also examines potential risks and the need for ethical guardrails.

10.1 Real-Time Adaptive Learning Environments

AI-powered platforms are increasingly capable of tailoring instruction to the needs of individual learners. Unlike static digital tools, adaptive systems analyze performance data in real time and adjust content, pacing, and feedback accordingly. For example, a dyslexic learner struggling with specific grapheme–phoneme correspondences could receive targeted exercises, multimodal reinforcements, and progressively challenging tasks calibrated to their learning trajectory (Holmes, Bialik, & Fadel, 2019).

Such environments embody the neuropedagogical principle of harnessing neuroplasticity: by delivering timely, personalized interventions, they strengthen neural circuits through deliberate practice (Ansari, 2012). Moreover, adaptive platforms can foster motivation by ensuring that learners are challenged but not overwhelmed, maintaining engagement in the “zone of proximal development.”

10.2 Early Detection and Predictive Analytics

Another promising application of AI lies in early detection. Traditional educational systems often rely on a "wait-to-fail" model, identifying dyslexia only after years of underachievement (Shaywitz & Shaywitz, 2008). AI systems, however, can analyze patterns in learners' reading behaviors—such as response times, error types, and eye-tracking data—to identify potential difficulties long before they manifest as entrenched problems (Zhao et al., 2025).

Predictive analytics could enable teachers and specialists to intervene earlier, providing targeted support during the critical window when brain plasticity is most receptive (Goswami, 2006). Such anticipatory approaches align with neuropedagogy's emphasis on prevention rather than remediation, shifting education toward a proactive model that minimizes long-term difficulties.

10.3 Augmenting Teachers Rather Than Replacing Them

A recurring concern in the discourse on AI in education is the fear that technology will replace human teachers. Neuropedagogy offers a corrective perspective: AI should augment teachers, not supplant them (Luckin et al., 2016). While AI can deliver adaptive exercises, analyze performance data, and provide immediate feedback, teachers remain indispensable for interpreting these insights, contextualizing them within broader learning goals, and supporting the emotional and social needs of learners (Marc & Philippette, 2021).

For dyslexic students, this synergy is particularly vital. AI may detect recurring decoding errors, but it is the teacher who helps the learner reframe these errors positively, integrating them into a growth-oriented mindset. Teachers also play a crucial role in ensuring that AI tools are used inclusively and ethically, bridging the gap between technological capability and human care.

10.4 Personalized Learning at Scale

One of the most transformative promises of AI is the potential to deliver personalized learning at scale (Luckin et al., 2016). Traditionally, individualized support for dyslexic learners has depended on resource-intensive one-on-one interventions, often unavailable in under-resourced settings. AI, however, can extend personalization to large groups, analyzing data from hundreds or thousands of learners simultaneously and tailoring pathways for each.

This scalability could democratize access to specialized support, ensuring that learners in rural or low-resource contexts are not excluded. However, realizing this potential requires careful design to avoid reinforcing inequities—for example, ensuring that AI systems are available in multiple languages, including Arabic, to serve diverse populations (Amrani & Belyazid, 2021).

10.5 Emotionally Intelligent AI

Emerging research in affective computing is exploring how AI can detect and respond to learners' emotional states by analyzing facial expressions, voice patterns, or physiological signals. For dyslexic learners, who often experience frustration and anxiety, emotionally responsive systems could adapt difficulty levels, provide encouragement, or suggest breaks when stress levels rise (Holmes et al., 2019).

While such systems remain experimental, they align with neuropedagogy's holistic approach, which views learning as a dynamic interplay of cognition and emotion. If implemented responsibly, emotionally intelligent AI could support both cognitive development and emotional regulation, creating more humane and responsive learning environments.

10.6 Ethical Risks and the Need for Guardrails

The future of AI in education is not without risks. Concerns include:

- **Data privacy**: Sensitive information about learners' behaviors and emotions must be protected, with clear consent and transparent policies (Holmes et al., 2022).
- **Algorithmic bias**: AI trained on non-representative datasets may misinterpret the errors of bilingual or minority learners, reinforcing stigma rather than reducing it.
- **Over-standardization**: Ironically, AI designed to personalize learning could, if poorly implemented, create rigid pathways that reduce learner autonomy.

To mitigate these risks, international frameworks stress the importance of community-wide collaboration between educators, researchers, policymakers, and technology developers (Holmes et al., 2022; UNESCO, 2020). Neuropedagogy must guide AI integration by prioritizing inclusion, transparency, and learner dignity.

10.7 Toward Anticipatory and Inclusive Education

The convergence of AI and neuropedagogy points toward a future where education is not only inclusive but anticipatory—capable of identifying potential struggles before they become entrenched and supporting learners proactively. Such a future envisions schools as dynamic ecosystems where teachers, learners, and intelligent systems collaborate to cultivate every student's potential.

In Morocco and other multilingual contexts, this could mean AI systems capable of detecting difficulties in both Arabic and French, providing culturally and linguistically relevant interventions (Benabdallah & Bouanani, 2019). Globally, it could mean shifting educational paradigms away from remediation and deficit models toward equity, personalization, and excellence for all.

10.8 Summary

Future perspectives on AI and inclusive schools can be summarized as follows:

1. **Adaptive learning environments** will provide real-time personalized instruction that aligns with neuroplasticity.
2. **Predictive analytics** will enable early detection of reading difficulties, shifting education toward proactive support.
3. **Teacher augmentation** will ensure that AI complements rather than replaces human educators.
4. **Personalization at scale** will democratize access to specialized interventions across socio-economic and linguistic contexts.
5. **Emotionally intelligent AI** may foster both cognitive and affective dimensions of learning.
6. **Ethical guardrails** must safeguard equity, privacy, and learner dignity.

If guided by neuropedagogical principles, AI has the potential to usher in a new era of inclusive and anticipatory education. In such a future, every learner's brain is not only recognized but also nurtured with precision, empathy, and respect.

11. CONCLUSION

The convergence of neuropedagogy and digital innovation offers a compelling framework for rethinking education for dyslexic learners. Grounded in insights from cognitive neuroscience, neuropedagogy challenges traditional models of schooling that assume a uniform learner profile and neglect the diversity of neurocognitive functioning. By emphasizing principles such as neuroplasticity, multimodality, and learner agency, neuropedagogy provides a scientifically informed foundation for inclusive education (Habib, 2018; Howard-Jones, 2014).

Digital technologies have amplified the possibilities of this paradigm shift. Tools such as text-to-speech systems, intelligent writing assistants, digital mind maps, and

AI-driven adaptive platforms provide learners with new pathways for accessing, processing, and producing knowledge. Crucially, these tools do not merely compensate for difficulties; they empower dyslexic students to develop metacognitive strategies, regulate their own learning, and engage more fully in educational communities (MacArthur, 2009; Zhao et al., 2025). International experiences, from the Scandinavian integration of assistive technologies to Moroccan pilot projects, demonstrate that digital innovation can be embedded in inclusive pedagogical frameworks when supported by policies, teacher training, and infrastructural investment (Touhami, 2020; Al-Azawei, Serenelli, & Lundqvist, 2016).

At the same time, ethical vigilance is indispensable. Equity of access remains a global challenge, as the digital divide risks excluding learners in rural and under-resourced contexts. Over-reliance on technology could undermine the relational dimensions of learning, while the increasing use of AI raises concerns about privacy, algorithmic bias, and learner dignity (Holmes et al., 2022; UNESCO, 2020). Neuropedagogy reminds us that technology must serve pedagogy, not replace it, and that human relationships remain the cornerstone of effective education.

Looking ahead, the integration of AI into education opens pathways for anticipatory and personalized learning at scale. Adaptive environments, predictive analytics, and emotionally intelligent systems could enable schools to detect and address reading difficulties before they manifest, fostering proactive rather than reactive inclusion (Luckin et al., 2016; Holmes, Bialik, & Fadel, 2019). If guided responsibly, these innovations could transform education into a dynamic ecosystem where every learner's cognitive profile is recognized and nurtured.

Ultimately, the promise of neuropedagogy and digital innovation lies in their ability to reimagine schools as inclusive spaces where neurodiversity is embraced rather than marginalized. By aligning teaching practices with how the brain learns and by leveraging technology to support equity, education can move toward a model of inclusive excellence. For dyslexic learners, this vision offers not only the possibility of overcoming barriers but also the opportunity to thrive, realizing their full intellectual and creative potential.

REFERENCES

Ahr, E. (2016). La lecture et le fonctionnement du cerveau pour une « neuropédagogie » de la lecture. *Administration & Éducation, 152*(4), 17–23. DOI: 10.3917/admed.152.0017

Al-Azawei, A., Serenelli, F., & Lundqvist, K. (2016). Universal design for learning (UDL): A content analysis of peer-reviewed journal papers from 2012 to 2015. *The Journal of Scholarship of Teaching and Learning, 16*(3), 39–56. DOI: 10.14434/josotl.v16i3.19295

Amrani, F., & Belyazid, S. (2021). Dyslexia and bilingualism: Challenges for Arabic-French learners in Morocco. *Journal of Language and Education, 7*(3), 112–125.

Ansari, D. (2012). Culture and education: New frontiers in brain plasticity. *Trends in Cognitive Sciences, 16*(2), 93–95. DOI: 10.1016/j.tics.2011.11.016 PMID: 22206752

Benabdallah, A., & Bouanani, M. (2019). Approches pédagogiques et TIC pour l'inclusion scolaire au Maroc. *Revue Marocaine des Sciences de l'Éducation, 15*(2), 45–60.

Boudelaa, S. (2014). The psycholinguistics of Arabic: A research agenda for a neglected language. *Language, Cognition and Neuroscience, 29*(8), 1–17.

Dehaene, S. (2007). *Les neurones de la lecture: La nouvelle science de la lecture et de la dyslexie*. Odile Jacob.

Florian, L., & Black-Hawkins, K. (2011). Exploring inclusive pedagogy. *British Educational Research Journal, 37*(5), 813–828. DOI: 10.1080/01411926.2010.501096

Fluckiger, C. (2020). Les usages effectifs du numérique en classe et dans les établissements scolaires. *Revue Française de Pédagogie, 206*, 56–67.

Goswami, U. (2006). Neuroscience and education: From research to practice? *Nature Reviews. Neuroscience, 7*(5), 406–413. DOI: 10.1038/nrn1907 PMID: 16607400

Habib, M. (2018). *La constellation des dys: Bases neurologiques de l'apprentissage et de ses troubles*. De Boeck Supérieur.

Holmes, W., Bialik, M., & Fadel, C. (2019). *Artificial intelligence in education: Promises and implications for teaching and learning*. Center for Curriculum Redesign., https://curriculumredesign.org/wp-content/uploads/AI-in-Education-Promises-and-Implications.pdf

Holmes, W., Porayska-Pomsta, K., Holstein, K., Sutherland, E., Baker, T., Shum, S. B., & Santos, O. C. (2022). Ethics of AI in education: Towards a community-wide framework. *British Journal of Educational Technology, 53*(3), 331–348. DOI: 10.1111/bjet.13102

Howard-Jones, P. (2014). Neuroscience and education: Myths and messages. *Nature Reviews. Neuroscience, 15*(12), 817–824. DOI: 10.1038/nrn3817 PMID: 25315391

Luckin, R., Holmes, W., Griffiths, M., & Forcier, L. B. (2016). *Intelligence unleashed: An argument for AI in education.* Pearson Education.

MacArthur, C. A. (2009). Reflections on research on writing and technology for struggling writers. *Learning Disabilities Research & Practice, 24*(2), 93–103. DOI: 10.1111/j.1540-5826.2009.00283.x

Marc, L., & Philippette, T. (2021). L'évolution du rôle des enseignants d'élèves dyslexiques suite à l'utilisation d'un outil numérique en classe. *The Journal of Special Education, 45*(2), 88–100. DOI: 10.1007/s12630-021-00389-2

Pugh, K. R., Mencl, W. E., Shaywitz, B. A., Shaywitz, S. E., Fulbright, R. K., Constable, R. T., Skudlarski, P., Marchione, K. E., Jenner, A. R., Fletcher, J. M., Liberman, A. M., Shankweiler, D. P., Katz, L., Lacadie, C., & Gore, J. C. (2000). The angular gyrus in developmental dyslexia: Task-specific differences in functional connectivity within posterior cortex. *Psychological Science, 11*(1), 51–56. DOI: 10.1111/1467-9280.00214 PMID: 11228843

Rose, D. H., & Dalton, B. (2009). Learning to read in the digital age. *Mind, Brain and Education : the Official Journal of the International Mind, Brain, and Education Society, 3*(2), 74–83. DOI: 10.1111/j.1751-228X.2009.01057.x

Shaywitz, S. E., & Shaywitz, B. A. (2008). Paying attention to reading: The neurobiology of reading and dyslexia. *Development and Psychopathology, 20*(4), 1329–1349. DOI: 10.1017/S0954579408000631 PMID: 18838044

Stein, J. (2023). Theories about developmental dyslexia. *Brain Sciences, 13*(2), 208. DOI: 10.3390/brainsci13020208 PMID: 36831750

Tokuhama-Espinosa, T. (2011). *Mind, brain, and education science: A comprehensive guide to the new brain-based teaching.* W. W. Norton & Company.

Touhami, F. (2020). L'intégration des TIC dans la prise en charge globale des enfants ayant des troubles spécifiques des apprentissages: Cas de la dyslexie (Master's thesis). Université Hassan II, Casablanca.

UNESCO. (2020). *Global education monitoring report 2020: Inclusion and education: All means all.* UNESCO.

Zhao, S., Xiong, S. C., Pang, B., Tang, X., & He, P. (2025). Let AI read first: Enhancing reading abilities for individuals with dyslexia through artificial intelligence. *Journal of Artificial Intelligence in Education*, *22*(4), 301–314. DOI: 10.1145/3706599.3720113

Chapter 6
Neuropedagogical Intervention Programs in Early Childhood With Global and Local Perspectives and AI-Enabled Future

Arzu Aydin
https://orcid.org/0000-0002-1616-3686
Karabük University, Turkey

Şehnaz Ceylan
Karabük University, Turkey

ABSTRACT

This section examines the integration of artificial intelligence (AI) into early childhood education through a neuropedagogical perspective, emphasizing opportunities at the intersection of neuroscience, psychology, pedagogy, and AI's adaptive capacities. Framing early childhood as a critical period for lifelong development, it outlines a five-stage model—screening, assessment, intervention, monitoring, and family collaboration—where AI enhances speed, precision, and personalization while ensuring ethical safeguards. Teachers' AI literacy and guiding role are underscored as prerequisites for sustainability. By connecting global policy frameworks with early intervention and developmental theories, the chapter presents AI-supported neuropedagogy as an ethical and innovative model for advancing early childhood education

DOI: 10.4018/979-8-3373-3581-0.ch006

INTRODUCTION

Early childhood encompasses the most critical years that shape an individual's lifelong development. The experiences gained during this period form the basis of cognitive, social-emotional, and linguistic skills; the neurobiological foundation of learning is rapidly formed during these years. Neuropedagogy, as a field that explains children's learning processes in light of brain-based research and integrates them with pedagogical practices, contributes to a deeper understanding of this critical period.

In recent years, the development of artificial intelligence technologies has opened up a new dimension in early childhood education. When combined with the basic principles of neuropedagogy, the data-driven observation, personalized learning, and rapid feedback opportunities offered by technology have the potential to support the development of educational approaches that are more responsive to children's individual needs. In particular, the support that artificial intelligence can provide in the screening, early intervention, and continuous monitoring cycle may facilitate educators' decision-making processes and strengthen family collaboration, provided that such technologies are implemented within developmentally appropriate, ethically grounded, and human-centered pedagogical frameworks.

This section examines brain-based learning processes and developmental gains in early childhood education in detail, based on the historical and theoretical foundations of neuropedagogy. Examples of early intervention programs at the national and international levels have been examined from a neuropedagogical perspective, and practices in Turkey have been evaluated from a comparative perspective. In addition, the discussion explores how artificial intelligence technologies can be integrated into the cognitive, linguistic, social-emotional, and motor dimensions of child development, and examines the roles of teachers, families, and policymakers in this process. In particular, issues such as ethical principles, data security, access inequality, and algorithmic bias are addressed in light of the guidance of international organizations (UNESCO, OECD, UNICEF) to provide a comprehensive assessment.

Rather than presenting a finalized or empirically validated intervention programme, this chapter adopts a conceptual and design-oriented perspective. Its primary aim is to synthesize existing neuroscientific, pedagogical, and policy-based evidence into a coherent framework that illustrates how neuropedagogical principles and artificial intelligence can be systematically aligned within early childhood education. The original contribution of the chapter is to bring together artificial intelligence and neuropedagogy to propose a structured, ethically informed roadmap that can guide future empirical research, pilot implementations, and policy development for early childhood. Thus, both academic discussions and practitioners in the field are provided with a theoretically grounded and forward-looking reference framework for innovative and responsible transformation in early childhood education.

THE NEURODEVELOPMENTAL FOUNDATIONS OF EARLY CHILDHOOD

Early childhood is a period of dynamic, rapid, and extensive neurodevelopmental change, fundamentally shaping cognitive, emotional, language, and social capacities. During the first six years of life, the brain achieves over 90% of its adult volume, forming billions of new synaptic connections, many of which will later be refined or eliminated (Zull, 2011). Understanding the brain's rapid transformation during these years is critical for designing timely and developmentally appropriate educational interventions that can lay strong foundations for lifelong learning. Recent evidence confirms that executive functions and socio-emotional competencies established before school entry strongly predict later academic success, emphasizing the urgency of targeted support during these years (Madanipour et al., 2025).

These neural transformations occur through interrelated biological processes that have direct implications for learning. *Synaptogenesis*, the proliferation of synaptic connections, greatly expands the brain's capacity for processing information, while *synaptic pruning* removes less efficient pathways to strengthen critical neural networks (Tokuhama-Espinosa, 2011). This pruning process occurs in region-specific patterns—for example, sensory cortices mature earlier, whereas the prefrontal cortex, associated with complex reasoning, planning, and self-control, develops more slowly and continues maturing into adolescence (Watagodakumbura, 2014). This developmental sequencing explains why foundational sensory and motor skills typically precede the emergence of higher-order cognitive functions. Neuroimaging studies also show that variations in pruning efficiency during early childhood are linked to later differences in attention regulation and working memory performance (Semelius Granevald, 2025).

Another essential process is *myelination*, in which fatty sheaths form around axons to speed up neural signal transmission. This process not only accelerates communication between brain regions but also underpins a child's ability to integrate sensory, cognitive, and emotional information in increasingly complex ways (Goswami, 2015). Zull (2011) emphasizes that myelination, especially in the prefrontal cortex, is closely linked to a child's growing capacity for sustained attention, working memory, and cognitive flexibility—skills that form the backbone of academic readiness. Recent longitudinal work indicates that delays in myelination during early childhood can be mitigated through enriched, structured environments that promote active engagement and shared thinking (Madanipour et al., 2025).

The prefrontal cortex plays a particularly vital role in early learning. As the brain's command centre for executive functions—including reasoning, inhibitory control, and problem-solving—it provides the regulatory framework for both academic and socio-emotional growth. Evidence from longitudinal studies shows that children who demonstrate stronger executive function skills in preschool achieve higher levels of literacy and numeracy in the early grades, underscoring the predictive value of these capacities (Diamond, 2013; Tokuhama-Espinosa, 2011). Neurodevelopmental data further reveal that targeted practice in inhibitory control and cognitive flexibility can lead to measurable changes in prefrontal activation patterns (López-Escribano et al., 2021).

This early period is also widely recognized as a "sensitive period" for learning—a time when the brain's plasticity makes it especially receptive to environmental input (Tokuhama-Espinosa, 2011). For insance, exposure to rich and varied language during the first three years strongly predicts later reading comprehension, while frequent opportunities for positive social interaction build socio-emotional competencies that support cooperative learning (Goswami, 2015; Zull, 2011). In this context, parenting practices that provide consistent emotional support and cognitive stimulation have been shown to shape neurobehavioral pathways critical for school readiness (Novia & Rachmawati, 2025).

The earliest years also lay the groundwork for integrated social-emotional, cognitive, and linguistic development. Infants naturally orient toward human faces and voices, engage in reciprocal interactions, and imitate observed behaviours—behaviours that reflect deeply embedded neural predispositions for social learning (Watagodakumbura, 2014; Zull, 2011). Neuroimaging studies confirm that warm, responsive caregiving activates brain regions linked to emotional regulation and attention control, fostering resilience and adaptability in later schooling (Immordino-Yang & Damasio, 2007). Furthermore, early neural activity patterns can predict later outcomes in literacy and language acquisition, suggesting that interventions in these domains should begin well before formal schooling (Tokuhama-Espinosa, 2011). New findings suggest that embedding value-based social interactions in early curricula can strengthen empathy and moral reasoning, complementing cognitive gains (Catalano et al., 2025).

In sum, the development of core executive functions—including working memory, inhibitory control, and cognitive flexibility—during early childhood is critical for school readiness. Deficits in these capacities can undermine later academic performance, particularly in reading and mathematics. Understanding these neurodevelopmental processes is therefore not merely theoretical—it forms the scientific basis for educational frameworks like neuropedagogy, which align teaching strategies with the brain's developmental trajectory and aim to optimize learning during the most formative years (López-Escribano et al., 2021; Madanipour et al., 2025; Tokuhama-Espinosa, 2011; Watagodakumbura, 2014; Zull, 2011).

From Brain Science to Neuropedagogy: An Educational Shift

The scientific understanding of how the brain learns has expanded dramatically in recent decades, creating new possibilities for aligning educational practice with neurodevelopmental principles. This evolution has led to the emergence of *neuropedagogy*—a field that applies neuroscience findings directly to teaching and learning. Such an approach is particularly relevant in early childhood, when the brain's plasticity enables well-designed educational experiences to shape neural circuits in ways that can have lifelong effects (Tokuhama-Espinosa, 2011; Zull, 2011). Recent research highlights that preschool teachers' cognitive and emotional resilience—measured through constructs such as sense of coherence—plays a crucial role in implementing these principles effectively, particularly for children needing special support (Semelius Granevald, 2025).

Educational neuroscience, as a foundation for neuropedagogy, is an interdisciplinary field that combines insights from neuroscience, psychology, and education to understand how the brain learns, processes, and retains information. Its primary aim is to translate scientific discoveries into effective pedagogical strategies (Goswami, 2015). For example, research on the development of attention networks has informed classroom practices in preschool, where lesson duration and complexity are tailored to match children's limited but expanding neural capacity for sustained focus (Tokuhama-Espinosa, 2011). Similarly, studies on working memory development have guided instructional sequencing, ensuring that new content builds on already-consolidated neural pathways rather than overwhelming immature processing systems (Watagodakumbura, 2014). In this context, evidence from Kunduracı and Aksoy (2025) demonstrates that teachers with higher self-perceived professional competence experience lower burnout levels, underscoring the importance of integrating teacher training in brain-based pedagogical and cognitive strategies.

However, the journey from brain science to classroom application has not been without challenges. Early enthusiasm for "brain-based learning" often produced oversimplified interpretations and contributed to the spread of persistent "neuromyths" such as the strict separation of left- and right-brain functions (Tokuhama-Espinosa, 2011). The recognition of these pitfalls led to the development of *Mind, Brain, and Education* (MBE) science, a more rigorous, problem-focused, and interdisciplinary approach that integrates biological, psychological, and educational perspectives (Tokuhama-Espinosa, 2011). In early childhood contexts, MBE encourages aligning teaching methods with sensitive periods for language acquisition, emotional regulation, and motor skill development (Immordino-Yang & Damasio, 2007). Emerging technological frameworks, such as the "Thinking Through AI" model, offer a structured way to embed metacognitive scaffolding into AI-mediated learning environments, directly complementing MBE's emphasis on adaptive and personalized pedagogy (Tzirides et al., 2025).

Neuropedagogy, as an applied branch of this science, extends beyond merely understanding how the brain works—it seeks to design learning environments that actively stimulate the brain's capacity to learn. Drawing from cognitive neurology, differential psychophysiology, and neuropsychology, neuropedagogy bridges laboratory research and classroom realities (Watagodakumbura, 2014). In early childhood education, this may take the form of play-based interventions that foster executive functions, structured routines that promote self-regulation, or emotionally rich environments that strengthen socio-emotional competencies (Immordino-Yang & Damasio, 2007). Recent program evaluations reveal that when such interventions are co-designed with teachers and informed by real-time neurocognitive feedback, they lead to measurable improvements in both cognitive flexibility and socio-emotional well-being in preschoolers (Madanipour et al., 2025).

The growing infrastructure supporting neuropedagogy demonstrates its increasing importance in education systems worldwide. Dedicated research centres, cross-disciplinary graduate programs, and early intervention initiatives have been established to integrate neuroscience into teaching practice (Goswami, 2015; Tokuhama-Espinosa, 2011). International organizations such as UNESCO and the OECD have called for embedding neuroscience knowledge into teacher training and curriculum design. This alignment of global policy with classroom realities mirrors the OECD's (2021) recommendation for bridging the research–practice gap by equipping educators with both the theoretical and practical tools needed to apply neurodevelopmental science in their daily practice. These developments underscore that neuropedagogy is not a replacement for established educational theory, but an evidence-based enhancement—especially critical during the early years when neural architecture is most malleable (Zull, 2011).

In this way, neuropedagogy serves as a bridge between the neurodevelopmental foundations discussed in above and the practical interventions explored in below. By grounding educational practice in both developmental science and real-world teaching contexts, it provides a framework for designing early interventions that address not only individual learning needs but also broader social equity goals (Semelius Granevald, 2025; Tokuhama-Espinosa, 2011; Tzirides et al., 2025 Watagodakumbura, 2014).

The Role of Early Intervention in a Neuropedagogical Context

Early intervention refers to planned, systematic educational and therapeutic actions implemented in the earliest years of life—often before formal schooling—with the goal of supporting optimal development and preventing the escalation of developmental challenges. From a neuropedagogical perspective, it is anchored in the understanding that ages 0–6 represent sensitive periods when neural plasticity is at its peak, allowing targeted experiences to shape the architecture of the brain in enduring ways (Hadders-Algra, 2021; Tokuhama-Espinosa, 2011; Zull, 2011;). This means that timely, developmentally informed action is not merely beneficial, but essential for laying the foundations of lifelong learning and well-being.

In this context, neuropedagogy integrates principles from developmental neuroscience, educational psychology, and evidence-based pedagogy to ensure that interventions align with children's neurodevelopmental readiness. Groark and Eidelman (2020) emphasize that early intervention is most effective when it addresses the "whole child," targeting cognitive, language, motor, and socio-emotional domains in an integrated manner. This perspective resonates with Vygotsky's sociocultural theory, which situates learning within mediated, socially interactive contexts, and with contemporary neuroscience, which links these contexts directly to neurobiological processes such as synaptogenesis, myelination, and pruning. The result is a coherent framework where the timing, content, and method of intervention are synchronized with the brain's natural developmental rhythms.

A growing body of research highlights the domains that hold the strongest predictive power for long-term learning outcomes. Strengthening executive functions in the preschool years—particularly working memory, inhibitory control, and cognitive flexibility—has been shown to improve later academic performance and socio-emotional adaptation (Diamond, 2013; Madanipour et al., 2025). Equally important is fostering self-regulation through structured routines and guided practice, which enhance emotional regulation circuits in the prefrontal cortex and anterior cingulate cortex (Immordino-Yang & Damasio, 2007; Johnson et al., 2015). Language and communication also stand out as critical areas: rich, interactive language environments during ages 0–3 strongly predict literacy skills, and early identification of speech and language delays allows for timely remediation (Goswami, 2015; Hadders-Algra, 2021). Furthermore, Bulkis et al. (2025) show that project-based learning approaches in early childhood can significantly improve empathy, cooperation, and conflict resolution, highlighting how socio-emotional competence is inextricably linked to cognitive growth.

One of the most effective ways to deliver these benefits is through activity-based early intervention, as described by Johnson et al. (2015), which embeds learning goals into natural routines and play. This approach is highly compatible with neuropedagogy's emphasis on contextualized, emotionally meaningful learning, allowing skills to generalize beyond the intervention setting. Supporting this, Riggleman et al. (2025) demonstrate that individualized behavioral goal setting—especially when co-constructed with families—enhances both cognitive and emotional outcomes. Similarly, Novia and Rachmawati (2025) emphasize that emotionally supportive and cognitively stimulating home environments interact synergistically with school-based interventions, shaping neurobehavioral pathways in ways that reinforce developmental gains.

The success of early intervention also depends on the capacity to detect needs early and act preventively. Hadders-Algra (2021) points out that subtle neurological and motor signs can often be identified before age two, opening a window for interventions that prevent cascading delays. Neuropedagogical practice increasingly incorporates digital assessment tools and AI-driven analytics, such as the "Thinking Through AI" framework (Tzirides et al., 2025), which provide real-time feedback on developmental progress and dynamically adapt learning activities. By integrating such technologies without compromising the relational essence of teaching, educators can respond to individual learning trajectories with unprecedented precision.

Beyond the individual child, early intervention is also a tool for promoting educational equity and social justice. Socioeconomic disparities can leave measurable "neural signatures" in brain regions associated with language, executive function, and stress regulation (Thomas, 2020). Addressing these disparities through targeted, high-quality early intervention not only benefits the individual but contributes to reducing systemic inequality (Groark & Eidelman, 2020). Semelius Granevald (2025) further highlight that teacher well-being and sense of coherence are critical for sustaining inclusive practices for children with additional support needs, indicating that professional support systems are as important as child-focused interventions.

From a policy perspective, the institutionalization of early intervention through frameworks such as the U.S. Individuals with Disabilities Education Act (IDEA) and Head Start reflects a global recognition of its value. International bodies like UNESCO and the OECD have called for embedding neuroscience knowledge into early education policy, advocating for training educators to apply developmental science in daily practice. Resources like the Early Childhood Education Intervention Treatment Planner (Jongsma & Winkelstern, 2016) provide structured templates for designing interventions that are both developmentally appropriate and aligned with family priorities, reflecting neuropedagogy's commitment to individualized, culturally responsive practice.

In conclusion, from a neuropedagogical standpoint, early intervention is not a remedial afterthought but a strategic, proactive investment in human potential. By aligning with the brain's sensitive periods, addressing both cognitive and socio-emotional domains, and embedding these practices within inclusive, equity-oriented frameworks, educators and policymakers can shape learning trajectories that yield profound and lasting benefits across the lifespan (Groark & Eidelman, 2020; Hadders-Algra, 2021; Johnson et al., 2015; Tokuhama-Espinosa, 2011; Zull, 2011).

THEORETICAL FOUNDATIONS OF THE NEUROPEDAGOGICAL APPROACH

In the previous section, the neurodevelopmental foundations underlying early childhood development were examined in depth; it was demonstrated how rapid synaptogenesis, synaptic pruning, and myelination processes interact dynamically with sensitive periods of learning to shape the trajectory of cognitive, social-emotional, and linguistic capacities. Additionally, the conceptual and practical dimensions of the neuropedagogical approach—which bridges developmental neuroscience and pedagogical design—were outlined, with a particular focus on how it provides a scientifically grounded and socially responsive framework for early intervention programmes. By emphasising the bidirectional and mutually reinforcing relationship between brain maturation, environmental stimuli, and educational practices, it was argued that effective early learning environments must be deliberately designed to correspond with children's neurodevelopmental profiles and readiness levels.

The current section, building upon these conceptual and empirical foundations, focuses on the theoretical underpinnings of neuropedagogy and examines the core conceptual frameworks and validated empirical models that guide its application in early childhood education. Within this scope, topics such as the definition, scope, and interdisciplinary origins of neuropedagogy, brain-based learning principles, sociocultural theory, executive function models, theoretical accounts of the emotion–cognition relationship, and a 'neuro-myth-free' understanding of education will be addressed. By synthesising findings from psychology, neuroscience, and pedagogy, this section will critically analyse how theoretical perspectives are operationalised into effective pedagogical practices, thereby laying the groundwork for designing developmentally attuned, culturally responsive, and evidence-based strategies that address the complex and diverse learning needs of young children.

Defining Neuropedagogy and Its Interdisciplinary Nature

Neuropedagogy is most usefully understood as an applied, integrative field that connects the study of the brain with the design of teaching and learning. It is not a single method or fixed set of classroom techniques; rather, it is a dialogic space in which educators, neuroscientists, psychologists, and learners co-construct a shared agenda for improving educational outcomes. In this sense, neuropedagogy operates as both a science and a practice, aiming to deepen and refine our understanding of learning processes and to translate that knowledge into sustainable educational innovation (Tokuhama-Espinosa, 2011; Zull, 2011). Contemporary policy and research statements frame it as an explicitly interdisciplinary domain that integrates neuroscience, psychology, and education to inform and transform teaching–learning processes.

Historically, the term and many of its practical impulses can be traced to late-20th-century European discourse on *neurodidactics*. The notion is commonly credited to the German mathematician–didactician Gerhard Preiß, who used it to denote the application of scientific knowledge about brain organization to the mastery of diverse kinds of educational material while attending to learner–teacher profiles, including hemispheric lateralization. This early articulation already contained the seeds of what neuropedagogy would later become: a synthesis of cognitive and neural insights with pedagogical decision-making. Over subsequent decades, the field began to be discussed under several overlapping labels—*neuroeducation*, *educational neuroscience*, or *Mind, Brain, and Education (MBE)*—all of which shared the aim of connecting brain science to educational theory and practice. Representative calls within this discourse emphasize the importance of exposing teacher educators, pre- and in-service teachers, and policymakers to robust brain research so that both cognitive and socio-emotional learning can be guided by evidence rather than intuition.

The intellectual roots of neuropedagogy extend beyond neuroimaging and laboratory neuroscience. Classic psychology and developmental science are foundational: for example, Vygotsky's differentiation of "lower" (involuntary attention, emotional memory) and "higher" mental functions (verbal–logical thinking, voluntary attention) is frequently cited in modern neuropedagogical literature as a conceptual antecedent. Similarly, Piaget's stages of cognitive development, though pre-neuroscientific, continue to inform the age-appropriate structuring of learning activities. The maturation of cognitive psychology and the learning sciences in the late 20th century supplied analytic tools—attention, working memory, executive function—that remain central to neuropedagogical design today. Current book-length syntheses (Della Sala & Anderson, 2012; Tokuhama-Espinosa, 2011) underline both the promise and the limits of "brain-based" approaches: while understanding the neural basis of learning can help reduce failure and increase success, much of the practical *heavy lifting* in classrooms still depends on cognitive-psychological constructs and socially situated pedagogical methods rather than on neural data alone.

As the field evolved, critical voices urged caution against over-interpretation and simplistic translation. Neuroscience, by itself, cannot dictate how teachers should teach; at best, it clarifies *why* certain approaches work and helps define the boundary conditions under which they are most effective. Authoritative surveys have shown that not all "brain-based education" is pseudoscience, but that it requires careful coupling with established psychological evidence and classroom-tested pedagogy to avoid perpetuating neuromyths (Della Sala & Anderson, 2012). These correctives are part of the field's maturation toward a genuinely integrative, evidence-driven science of learning.

Another strand in neuropedagogy's historical development concerns its contexts of practice. Because it is oriented toward real-world change, neuropedagogy has found fertile ground in both formal schooling and non-formal learning environments. Comparative analyses of these settings suggest that the flexibility and learner-centered ethos of non-formal education allow for more experimentation with neuropedagogical principles, while formal education provides the infrastructure for scaling and sustaining them. Integrating both contexts may be particularly powerful, as it allows the adaptability of non-formal approaches to be supported by the stability and reach of formal systems (Lohvynenko et al., 2023).

In recent years, a growing sociocultural and ethical dimension has emerged. Work at the interface of inclusion and "neuro-digital culture" addresses the policy and managerial realities of implementing inclusive education, especially as neuro- and digital technologies co-evolve with schooling. This perspective does not treat neuropedagogy as a purely technical fix; rather, it frames it as a guiding philosophy that must be implemented ethically, with sensitivity to diverse learner needs, equity concerns, and cultural contexts.

From this synthesis of historical and conceptual strands, a concise working definition emerges: neuropedagogy is an interdisciplinary field bridging neuroscientific, psychological, and educational knowledge in order to inform the design, enactment, and continual improvement of learning and teaching. It takes seriously the biological reality that learning changes the brain, but it rejects reductionism, insisting that the best learning environments draw simultaneously on neural, cognitive, social, and emotional levels of analysis.

The strength of neuropedagogy lies in its capacity to integrate the insights of neuroscience, psychology, and pedagogy into a unified model for teaching and learning. Neuroscience contributes an understanding of the brain's learning systems—attention networks, working memory buffers, reward and motivation circuits, and the role of emotional regulation in cognition. Neuroimaging studies have demonstrated that emotionally salient content activates both limbic and cortical networks, enhancing memory consolidation (Immordino-Yang & Damasio, 2007), while findings on neuroplasticity underscore that enriched, socially supportive, and challenging environments physically alter brain connectivity (Blakemore & Frith, 2007). However, these insights are explanatory rather than prescriptive and must be interpreted in light of broader cognitive and social factors.

Psychology serves as the bridge between neural mechanisms and classroom application. Cognitive psychology provides the conceptual tools for understanding information processing, memory strategies, metacognition, and executive control. Developmental psychology aligns teaching strategies with age-related cognitive and socio-emotional changes, ensuring developmental appropriateness (Piaget, 1972). Educational psychology highlights motivation, self-efficacy, and classroom climate—constructs essential for translating brain insights into meaningful learning experiences. These perspectives ensure that neuroscientific knowledge is adapted to the diverse needs and developmental stages of learners.

It is within pedagogy that integration becomes action, translating scientific principles into concrete instructional designs. Examples abound: in foreign language learning, combining multisensory input, stress-reduction techniques, and social interaction can enhance vocabulary retention and fluency; in STEM education, virtual chemistry simulators embedding neuropedagogical principles have been shown to significantly improve logical reasoning, process comprehension, and engagement; and in teacher education, pre-service teachers trained in neuropedagogy have demonstrated improved ability to design inclusive, emotionally responsive classrooms.

The integration process is not without challenges. Terminological differences persist—in neuroscience, "learning" often refers to synaptic change, whereas in education it refers to the acquisition and application of knowledge in social contexts. There is also the "grain size" problem: neural-level findings may be too fine-grained to map directly onto classroom strategies. These gaps can be addressed through research–practice partnerships, where educators and researchers co-design interventions, test them in authentic settings, and iteratively refine both theory and practice. This collaborative model not only grounds scientific findings in pedagogical reality but also fosters mutual capacity-building.

As neuropedagogy intersects with artificial intelligence, neurotechnology, and digital learning, ethical and inclusion concerns must be foregrounded. Personalizing education based on neurocognitive profiles offers promise but also risks misinterpretation and bias if not guided by strong ethical safeguards (Lohvynenko et al., 2023). Inclusive practice requires ensuring that brain-informed strategies are accessible and adaptable to neurodiverse learners, combining neuroscientific insights on atypical development with pedagogical expertise in differentiation.

In essence, neuropedagogy represents a dynamic, bi-directional framework for educational improvement. Neuroscience illuminates the biological foundations of learning; psychology situates these within the complexities of human development and motivation; pedagogy transforms them into responsive, evidence-based practices. By moving beyond "brain-based" rhetoric toward research-informed, ethically grounded, and contextually adaptable approaches, neuropedagogy offers a path toward more effective, inclusive, and human-centered education in the 21st century.

Brain-Based Learning Principles

Brain-Based Learning (BBL), as articulated by Eric Jensen and Renate & Geoffrey Caine, is an instructional approach rooted in neuroscience, cognitive psychology, and developmental theory, advocating that teaching methods should be designed in harmony with the way the brain naturally processes, stores, and retrieves information (Caine & Caine, 1991; Jensen, 2008). This perspective is particularly critical in early childhood education, where heightened neural plasticity and the presence of sensitive periods make environmental inputs especially influential on long-term cognitive, socio-emotional, and linguistic development (Goswami, 2015; Tokuhama-Espinosa, 2011).

The model is structured around twelve interrelated principles, which collectively emphasize the integration of physiological, emotional, cognitive, and social dimensions of learning. These include: (1) the recognition that learning is a physiological process shaped by nutrition, movement, and rest; (2) the brain's capacity as a parallel processor, managing multiple sensory and emotional inputs simultaneously; (3) the role of emotions as central to pattern formation and memory consolidation; (4) the innate human drive to seek meaning and detect patterns; and (5) the need for instruction that is both personally relevant and contextually rich (Caine & Caine, 1991; Jensen, 2008). Additional principles highlight that effective learning involves both focused attention and peripheral perception, is enhanced by challenge but hindered by threat, is developmental in nature, and thrives in socially interactive settings.

From a neuropedagogical standpoint, these principles reinforce the necessity of emotionally safe, socially rich, and developmentally attuned early learning environments. For example, Catalano et al. (2025) demonstrate that embedding value-based, socially interactive activities into early curricula not only strengthens empathy and moral reasoning but also improves memory retention—aligning directly with the BBL emphasis on emotional engagement and meaningful context. Similarly, Madanipour et al. (2025) found that structured, collaborative classroom strategies significantly enhance executive function skills in preschoolers, offering concrete evidence that BBL-informed practices can yield measurable neurocognitive benefits in the early years.

In sum, the BBL framework offers a scientifically grounded roadmap for designing learning experiences that respect the neurodevelopmental readiness of young children, integrate the full spectrum of human functioning, and capitalize on the brain's natural learning architecture. By embedding these principles into early childhood pedagogy, educators can create enriched environments that optimize both immediate learning outcomes and long-term developmental trajectories.

Vygotsky's Sociocultural Theory and Executive Functions

Vygotsky's Sociocultural Theory positions social interaction and the use of cultural tools as central mechanisms in the development of higher mental functions, including executive functions—the cognitive processes responsible for planning, inhibitory control, working memory, and cognitive flexibility (Bodrova et al., 2011). According to Vygotsky, these functions first emerge in the social plane, mediated by language, symbolic play, and collaborative problem-solving, before becoming internalized as independent cognitive skills (Tzuriel, 2021).

An applied embodiment of these principles is the Tools of the Mind curriculum, designed specifically to strengthen executive function in early childhood classrooms through structured, intentional play and guided learning. Core practices include the creation of "play plans," where children verbally outline their intended roles and actions before engaging in dramatic play, and the use of private speech as a self-regulation tool. These strategies scaffold children's ability to manage attention, follow multi-step tasks, and adapt flexibly to changing situations—skills strongly predictive of later academic achievement (Barnett et al., 2008).

Empirical studies have shown that children in Tools of the Mind classrooms outperform peers in traditional settings on measures of behavioural regulation, cognitive flexibility, and classroom engagement (Goble et al., 2021). These findings align with Vygotsky's assertion that cognitive growth is maximized when learning activities are socially mediated, contextually meaningful, and supported by deliberate use of cultural tools. In the context of neuropedagogy, such programs illustrate how theory can be operationalized into developmentally attuned, evidence-based interventions that strengthen both self-regulatory and academic capacities in the formative years.

Diamond's Model of Executive Functions

Diamond's model conceptualizes *executive functions (EFs)* as a set of interrelated but distinct cognitive control processes that regulate thought and behaviour, enabling goal-directed action and adaptive problem-solving (Diamond, 2013). In early childhood, three core components—inhibitory control, working memory, and cognitive flexibility—develop rapidly and serve as the foundation for more complex cognitive skills such as reasoning, planning, and self-regulation. These functions are mediated primarily by the maturation of the prefrontal cortex and its connections with other brain regions, and are highly sensitive to environmental influences, making them a central focus for neuropedagogical approaches.

Inhibitory control refers to the ability to deliberately suppress automatic or dominant responses in favor of goal-relevant behaviors. In early childhood, this manifests in skills such as resisting distractions, waiting one's turn, or following rules despite competing impulses. Diamond (2013) emphasizes that inhibitory control is a cornerstone of selective attention and self-discipline, both of which are critical for successful participation in structured learning environments. For instance, children with stronger inhibitory control are better able to sustain attention during story time, ignore irrelevant classroom noise, and engage in cooperative play without escalating conflicts.

Working memory is the capacity to temporarily store and manipulate information in the service of complex cognitive tasks. This skill supports comprehension, reasoning, and multi-step problem-solving, and is particularly important in early literacy and numeracy development. In preschool contexts, working memory enables children to recall and apply phonics rules while decoding words, or to remember and execute the sequential steps in a group activity. Neurodevelopmentally, working memory growth during the preschool years is closely tied to myelination in frontoparietal networks, which enhance the speed and efficiency of information processing.

Cognitive flexibility—the ability to shift between tasks, perspectives, or strategies in response to changing demands—emerges later than inhibitory control and working memory, typically strengthening in the late preschool and early school years. It depends on the coordinated functioning of the other two core EFs and enables adaptive responses to novel situations. In practical terms, cognitive flexibility allows a child to adjust when classroom routines change unexpectedly, to consider multiple solutions to a problem, or to take on different roles in cooperative play.

The *developmental trajectory* of these skills underscores their importance for school readiness. Research indicates that EF competencies in preschool are stronger predictors of later academic achievement than IQ or socioeconomic status, especially in literacy and mathematics (Castellanos-Ryan et al., 2023). Moreover, the relationship between executive functions and learning is bidirectional: while well-developed EFs facilitate academic success, rich, scaffolded learning environments further enhance EF growth. This interaction highlights the need for intentional educational practices—such as play-based learning, structured routines, and targeted EF training—that align with the sensitive period for EF development between ages 3 and 5.

From a neuropedagogical perspective, Diamond's model provides a framework for designing interventions that deliberately strengthen inhibitory control, working memory, and cognitive flexibility through socially mediated, emotionally supportive, and cognitively challenging experiences. By embedding EF-promoting activities into everyday classroom routines—such as memory games, role-play scenarios, and collaborative problem-solving—educators can not only improve immediate self-regulatory capacities but also lay a durable cognitive foundation for lifelong learning and adaptive functioning.

Immordino-Yang's Theory of Emotion and Learning

Mary Helen Immordino-Yang's research demonstrates that emotion and cognition are deeply intertwined in the human brain, with emotional engagement acting as a catalyst for attention, deep thinking, and long-term memory (Immordino-Yang & Damasio, 2007). Rather than being a distraction, emotion is integral to learning, shaping the way new information is encoded, stored, and retrieved (Mercer, 2019). Neuroimaging studies show that emotional and cognitive networks—particularly in the prefrontal cortex, limbic system, and insular work in concert to assess the personal relevance of experiences and guide decision-making.

This perspective is especially relevant in early childhood, a period when emotional and cognitive capacities develop in tandem. Emotionally engaging activities such as storytelling, dramatic play, and cooperative problem-solving not only stimulate language, executive functions, and memory, but also foster empathy, moral reasoning, and social connection. In neuropedagogical terms, these activities harness the brain's natural learning systems by integrating affective and cognitive demands in meaningful, developmentally appropriate ways.

For educators, Immordino-Yang's framework highlights the importance of emotionally relevant pedagogy. Lessons connected to children's interests, cultural contexts, and personal experiences are more likely to activate both emotional and cognitive networks, leading to deeper comprehension and better retention (Mercer, 2019). This can be achieved through narrative, role-play, and authentic, real-world challenges that combine emotional resonance with cognitive complexity.

Finally, the theory underscores the need for emotionally safe learning environments. Classrooms that foster trust, respect, and positive relationships reduce stress responses that can impair learning, while promoting curiosity, engagement, and exploration. In doing so, they align closely with neuropedagogical principles, ensuring that both affective and cognitive processes are optimized for long-term academic and personal development.

Tokuhama-Espinosa's Neuro-Myth Free Education Model

Tracey Tokuhama-Espinosa's *Neuro-Myth Free Education* framework promotes the integration of accurate neuroscience into educational practice while systematically eliminating neuromyths—persistent but false beliefs about how the brain learns. Myths such as "we only use 10% of our brain," the strict separation of "left-brained" and "right-brained" learners, and the idea that instruction should match fixed "learning styles" (visual, auditory, kinesthetic) have been repeatedly debunked in empirical research, yet remain widespread in classrooms. In early childhood contexts, where developmental windows are especially sensitive, reliance on such misconceptions can misdirect precious learning opportunities and resources.

Her model is grounded in five core pillars of Mind, Brain, and Education (MBE) science: (1) the use of *evidence-based practice* that aligns teaching with robust neuroscientific findings; (2) *transdisciplinary research* drawing from neuroscience, psychology, and pedagogy; (3) *mind–brain integration*, recognizing that cognitive and emotional processes are inseparable in learning; (4) *contextual relevance*, ensuring that interventions are culturally and developmentally appropriate; and (5) *continuous educator development*, promoting lifelong learning among teachers to remain current with evolving research (Tokuhama-Espinosa, 2011). Together, these pillars create a framework for critically evaluating brain-based claims and translating authentic neuroscience into classroom practice.

For early childhood educators, neuroscience literacy is more than an academic skill—it is a safeguard against adopting pseudoscientific programs that may waste time or even harm developmental progress. Embedding foundational neuroscience knowledge in pre-service and in-service training enables teachers to critically assess new interventions, adapt curricula to align with neural development, and intentionally support emerging skills such as executive functions, language, and self-regulation. Such training also empowers educators to communicate effectively with families about the science behind early learning practices, building trust and collaboration.

Ultimately, Tokuhama-Espinosa's model reinforces the principle that high-quality early childhood education must be scientifically grounded, culturally responsive, and developmentally appropriate. By replacing myths with accurate, research-based knowledge, educators can design richer learning environments that optimize neural plasticity, foster socio-emotional growth, and enhance long-term academic readiness. This approach not only advances teaching quality but also protects the integrity of educational policy and practice in the formative years of life.

Translating Neuroscience Findings into Pedagogical Design

The integration of neuroscience into pedagogy is most impactful when research findings are translated into practical, developmentally informed strategies. As outlined in the preceding sections, principles from brain-based learning, sociocultural theory, executive function models, emotion–cognition research, and neuro-myth-free education collectively underscore that effective teaching must align with the brain's developmental trajectory, avoid misinformation, and deliberately foster both cognitive and socio-emotional growth (Immordino-Yang & Damasio, 2007; Tokuhama-Espinosa, 2011; Diamond, 2013).

In educational environments, this translation involves designing curricula and learning experiences that match children's readiness for specific skills, provide emotionally meaningful engagement, and create opportunities for collaborative, tool-mediated learning. For early childhood education, this means embedding neuroscientific principles into daily routines, structured play, and guided interaction, ensuring that foundational capacities such as language, executive functions, and self-regulation are nurtured during sensitive periods of heightened plasticity (Madanipour et al., 2025).

In early intervention programs, aligning pedagogical design with neuroscience is particularly critical. By applying evidence-based insights on neural development, practitioners can tailor interventions to address individual learning profiles, detect and remediate developmental delays early, and engage families as active partners in the learning process (Hadders-Algra, 2021; Johnson et al., 2015). This approach not only maximizes developmental gains but also contributes to long-term educational equity, particularly for children from underserved backgrounds.

Moving forward, the next section will examine practical models of neuropedagogically aligned early intervention, demonstrating how theoretical principles and neuroscientific evidence are operationalized in real-world educational and therapeutic settings. This transition marks the shift from establishing a theoretical foundation to exploring applied strategies that directly influence children's developmental outcomes.

OVERVIEW OF NEUROPEDAGOGICAL INTERVENTION PROGRAMS IN EARLY CHILDHOOD

Historical Development of Intervention Programs

The development of early childhood intervention programs has evolved from narrowly focused, remedial initiatives toward comprehensive, developmentally informed frameworks that integrate findings from neuroscience, psychology, and pedagogy. In the early to mid-20th century, interventions often followed a compensatory education model, seeking to mitigate disadvantages faced by children from low-income or marginalized backgrounds. While these efforts—such as the U.S. Head Start program—yielded some benefits, they frequently lacked an understanding of how brain development during the first six years shapes long-term learning potential (Groark & Eidelman, 2020).

From the 1980s onward, advances in developmental neuroscience shifted the focus toward timing and sensitivity. Research on synaptogenesis, pruning, and myelination demonstrated that ages 0–6 are marked by heightened neural plasticity, making this period optimal for targeted, enriched experiences (Tokuhama-Espinosa, 2011; Zull, 2011). This realization catalyzed the emergence of neuropedagogically aligned programs, in which learning environments are deliberately structured to support the maturation of executive functions, language skills, and socio-emotional competencies. More recent initiatives integrate technology-assisted assessments and AI-supported personalization, ensuring that interventions remain responsive to individual developmental trajectories (Tzirides et al., 2025).

Historical analysis thus reveals a progression from reactive, deficit-based approaches toward proactive, biologically timed interventions grounded in scientific evidence, with neuropedagogy serving as the conceptual bridge between brain science and early education practice.

Common Goals and Objectives

Neuropedagogical early intervention programs are guided by an integrated set of objectives that address the "whole child" across cognitive, linguistic, motor, and socio-emotional domains. A core goal is to strengthen executive functions—working memory, inhibitory control, and cognitive flexibility—which form the regulatory foundation for learning and adaptation (Diamond, 2013; Madanipour et al., 2025). For example, structured activities that require children to hold multi-step instructions in mind, resist distractions, and shift strategies according to changing rules directly target these skills.

Language and communication development is another priority, with research showing that rich, interactive language exposure in the first three years predicts later literacy achievement and academic success (Goswami, 2015; Hadders-Algra, 2021). Socio-emotional competencies, including empathy, cooperation, and emotional regulation, are also central; Bulkis et al. (2025) found that project-based learning in preschool significantly improved these skills, supporting the neuropedagogical emphasis on emotionally engaging, collaborative tasks.

Crucially, many programs integrate an equity agenda, recognizing that socioeconomic disparities can leave measurable neural imprints in brain regions linked to language, executive function, and stress regulation (Thomas, 2020). By embedding culturally responsive practices, interventions aim to equalize developmental opportunities, aligning with Catalano et al.'s (2025) findings that value-based education fosters both moral reasoning and social integration.

Instructional Techniques and Pedagogical Strategies

Neuropedagogical intervention programs employ teaching methods explicitly aligned with neurodevelopmental principles, ensuring that instruction is both biologically and contextually appropriate. Play-based learning is a cornerstone strategy, offering children opportunities to explore, experiment, and problem-solve within emotionally meaningful contexts (Johnson et al., 2015). This approach is complemented by dramatic role-play, as in the *Tools of the Mind* curriculum, which has been shown to improve behavioral regulation, working memory, and classroom engagement (Barnett et al., 2008; Goble et al., 2021).

Project-based learning offers extended opportunities for sustained attention, collaboration, and cross-domain skill integration (Bulkis et al., 2025), while storytelling and narrative-based instruction enrich both linguistic and socio-emotional development by engaging children's imagination and empathy (Immordino-Yang & Damasio, 2007).

Importantly, neuropedagogy emphasizes the integration of emotion and cognition, acknowledging that deep learning occurs when content is personally meaningful (Immordino-Yang, 2015). In recent years, digital and AI-enhanced tools have been incorporated into interventions, offering personalized learning pathways and real-time developmental monitoring (Tzirides et al., 2025). However, consistent with Hadders-Algra's (2021) caution, these technologies are employed to augment—not replace—human interaction, preserving the relational core of early education.

Assessment and Evaluation Approaches

Comprehensive assessment is a defining feature of neuropedagogical intervention programs, serving to diagnose needs, track progress, and refine strategies. Unlike traditional models that rely heavily on standardized testing, neuropedagogical assessments integrate dynamic evaluation methods that reveal a child's learning potential and responsiveness to support. These may include play-based observational assessments, which capture authentic behaviours in natural settings, and neuropsychological measures targeting executive functions, language, and socio-emotional regulation (Groark & Eidelman, 2020).

Emerging technologies—such as portable EEG and functional near-infrared spectroscopy (fNIRS)—offer novel ways to examine neural correlates of intervention effects, although these are still largely in research settings (Thomas, 2020).

Evaluation frameworks emphasize formative assessment, allowing for real-time instructional adjustments, alongside summative evaluation to measure long-term impact. In culturally diverse contexts, culturally responsive assessment tools ensure that evaluations respect local norms and values while maintaining scientific validity (Johnson et al., 2015).

The Role of Cultural Context in Program Design

Cultural context is integral to the design, delivery, and sustainability of early childhood interventions. Children's learning is shaped not only by biological maturation but also by the values, communication patterns, and caregiving practices of their communities. Neuropedagogical frameworks therefore stress the co-construction of programs with families and communities, ensuring that materials, examples, and interaction styles are culturally congruent.

International bodies such as UNESCO and the OECD advocate for globally informed yet locally adapted program models, recognizing that while principles like sensitive periods and executive function growth are universal, their implementation must reflect local educational traditions and resources (OECD, 2021). For instance, a play-based learning activity developed in a Western urban preschool may need adaptation in rural or collectivist contexts to align with communal learning norms (Groark & Eidelman, 2020).

By embedding cultural responsiveness into program design, neuropedagogical interventions can maximize both developmental impact and community relevance, thereby ensuring long-term sustainability.

INTERNATIONAL PROGRAMS – CONTENT, IMPLEMENTATION, AND IMPACT

MindUP

The MindUP programme combines neuroscience, positive psychology and social-emotional learning approaches to offer a comprehensive intervention model that aims to strengthen children's executive functions, self-regulation skills and social-emotional competence. At the core of the programme is a neuropedagogical framework that explains the role of the relationships between the prefrontal cortex, amygdala, and hippocampus in learning, emotion regulation, and decision-making processes (Schonert-Reichl et al., 2015). The high developmental plasticity of these regions during early childhood makes the programme's impact on this age group even more meaningful.

Designed for children aged 4–13, MindUP can maximise neurodevelopmental gains when applied during early childhood (especially ages 5–7), a period when the prefrontal cortex develops rapidly and attention and emotional control strengthen. The programme's activities support the development of executive functions such as working memory, cognitive flexibility and inhibitory control, as well as empathy, stress management and positive social behaviour. In particular, mindfulness-based awareness exercises reduce amygdala activity, regulating stress responses and strengthening the prefrontal cortex's attention and problem-solving skills.

The application process typically involves two or three sessions per week, each lasting 15–20 minutes. These sessions include age-appropriate information about the structure and functioning of the brain, mindfulness breathing exercises, sensory awareness activities, and group activities that strengthen empathy. This structure facilitates the conscious transition from the brain's lower-level emotional systems to higher-level executive control mechanisms from a neuropedagogical perspective.

The effectiveness of MindUP has been evaluated using various measurement tools. In a randomised controlled study by Schonert-Reichl et. al. (2015), children who participated in the programme showed significant improvements in executive function tests (e.g. Stroop test, working memory tasks) and more balanced cortisol levels. This improvement in biological markers indicates that stress regulation is supported at the neurophysiological level. In another study (Thiessen et al., 2020), primary school students who participated in MindUP showed increased prosocial behaviour scores and teacher-assessed classroom participation levels, while behavioural problems decreased. These findings suggest that the programme has lasting effects at both the behavioural and biological levels.

MindUP has also led to significant increases in children's self-regulation skills and academic motivation in applications conducted in low socio-economic areas. These results suggest that the development of executive functions targeted from a neuropedagogical perspective may also play a critical role in reducing educational inequalities.

Tools of the Mind

The Tools of the Mind programme is a comprehensive educational approach based on Lev Vygotsky's sociocultural theory, focusing on supporting the development of executive functions, particularly in early childhood. The programme combines symbolic play, planned dramatic enactments, peer collaborations and self-regulation strategies to support children's cognitive, social and emotional development. Built on Vygotsky's concepts of the 'zone of proximal development' and 'psychological tools,' this model emphasizes the transformative effect of cultural tools such as language, symbols, and social interaction on children's thinking, problem-solving, and behaviour control.

One of the most prominent features of the programme's early childhood applications is the planned and teacher-guided implementation of dramatic play. In daily planning activities called 'play plans,' children write or draw what roles they will play, what they will do, and what materials they will use. This process activates working memory while also helping children focus their attention on the specified goal and follow the rules of the game. Such activities support the development of cognitive flexibility and inhibitory control mechanisms located in the prefrontal cortex.

Research on the effectiveness of Tools of the Mind shows that the programme has a strong impact in both cognitive and social-emotional areas. In a randomised controlled study conducted by Barnett et. al. (2008), preschool students who participated in Tools of the Mind demonstrated significantly higher performance on executive function tests than their peers in the control group. These improvements, particularly in attention control and working memory, have been linked to advances in pre-reading and writing skills and early maths achievement. Goble and colleagues' (2021) study found that the programme increased classroom participation, reduced problem behaviours, and strengthened teacher-student relationships among students in low-income areas.

Research findings also indicate that the program has lasting effects on self-regulation skills. For example, in a longitudinal study conducted by Blair and Raver (2014), it was reported that children who participated in Tools demonstrated improvements in coping with stress, showed higher motivation for learning, and experienced fewer adjustment problems during school transitions. These results reveal that the program's neuropedagogical aim of fostering executive function and self-regulation supports not only academic achievement but also social adaptation.

The neuropedagogical value of Tools of the Mind lies not only in its focus on cognitive processes but also in its emphasis on enabling teachers to structure social interactions in ways appropriate to children's developmental levels and to consciously employ cultural tools. In this respect, the program provides a strong example of how neuroscience-based evidence can be transformed into classroom pedagogical strategies and highlights the long-term impact of early intervention programs.

PATHS (Promoting Alternative Thinking Strategies)

The PATHS programme is an early intervention approach designed to develop children's social-emotional competence, self-regulation skills and problem-solving abilities, based on a strong cognitive-behavioural foundation. Developed by Greenberg and Kusché, the model targets the interaction between the prefrontal cortex and the limbic system, supporting emotional awareness, impulse control, and interpersonal problem-solving processes. From a neuropedagogical perspective, the programme systematically activates areas of the brain associated with executive functions (particularly attention control, inhibitory control, and cognitive flexibility) while also aiming to strengthen social brain networks (e.g., medial prefrontal cortex, anterior cingulate cortex).

In programme applications, visual materials, storytelling, role-playing and group discussions are used to help children develop their ability to recognise emotions, express their feelings and understand the emotions of others. 'Emotion faces' cards help children match facial expressions with emotions, while step-by-step problem-solving strategies such as 'Stop, Think, Act' support cognitive flexibility and decision-making processes. These techniques are structured in line with the 'sensitive period' of rapid development of the prefrontal cortex in early childhood.

Numerous studies on the effectiveness of the PATHS programme have demonstrated significant improvements in both social-emotional development and academic performance. In a study conducted by Riggs et. al. (2006), children who participated in PATHS showed significant increases in attention span, impulse control, and empathy levels; these developments were also reflected in classroom adjustment and academic achievement. Similarly, Bierman and colleagues' (2010) large-scale study revealed that the programme strengthened social problem-solving skills and reduced aggressive behaviour in children from low-income areas.

In addition, a Turkish experimental study (Arda & Ocak, 2012) demonstrated that the PATHS programme, when implemented in preschool settings, significantly improved children's attention, concentration, social-emotional competence, and problem-solving skills, while also reducing aggressive and disruptive behaviours. Importantly, it was also found to support teachers' classroom management and emotional regulation practices. These findings highlight PATHS as an effective neuropedagogical intervention in early childhood, strengthening self-regulation and executive functions within culturally diverse contexts.

From a neuropedagogical perspective, one of the most important features of PATHS is that it integrates social-emotional learning with cognitive development. The structured content, which aims to develop emotional regulation skills and executive functions in parallel, strengthens the self-regulation capacity necessary for both academic and lifelong learning. In this respect, PATHS not only supports children's current developmental levels but also has a protective effect on their future social relationships, academic progress, and mental health.

The HighScope Perry Preschool Programme

The HighScope Perry Preschool Programme is an intervention programme based on active learning that aims to strengthen cognitive, social and academic skills in early childhood education and has proven long-term effects. Developed in the 1960s by David Weikart and his team, this model is designed to improve the school success and lifelong adjustment of children from disadvantaged socio-economic backgrounds. From a neuropedagogical perspective, the programme promotes the development of executive functions, problem-solving and self-regulation skills by supporting functional connections in children's prefrontal cortex, hippocampus and brain regions associated with social cognition.

The programme is based on the principle of 'active learning.' Children become active participants in the learning process by using a daily planning, implementation, and evaluation cycle (the 'plan-implement-evaluate' approach). This method ensures the effective use of the dorsolateral prefrontal cortex, which is critical for the development of working memory and cognitive flexibility. Additionally, structured small group activities support language development and the consolidation of social-emotional skills through social interaction.

One of the most important pieces of evidence regarding the effectiveness of HighScope is the 40-year longitudinal study conducted by Nores et al. (2005). The findings show that programme participants have significantly higher high school graduation rates, employment levels, and income levels, while crime rates remain low. These results demonstrate that executive function and problem-solving skills acquired at an early age have a lifelong impact. Additionally, analyses by Heckman et. al. (2010) calculated that the HighScope Perry programme yields an economic return of 7 to 12 dollars for every dollar invested at the societal level.

From a neuropedagogical perspective, the HighScope programme's strongest feature is that it allows children to manage their learning processes through their own choices and experiences. This autonomy increases motivation while ensuring that the information learned is more permanently stored in long-term memory. Additionally, teachers' role as 'active observers' enables them to identify individual developmental differences and provide immediate, adaptable support. Thus, the HighScope Perry Preschool Programme stands out as a neuropedagogical model that not only enhances cognitive and academic development but also strengthens social adaptation and lifelong learning capacity.

Abecedarian Project

The Abecedarian Project, developed at the University of North Carolina in the early 1970s, is one of the most well-known longitudinal intervention programmes in early childhood education. The programme's primary goal is to reduce developmental inequalities by providing enriched early learning opportunities, particularly for children from socioeconomically disadvantaged families. Its theoretical foundation is based on neurodevelopmental findings that emphasise the critical importance of early environmental stimuli in children's cognitive and social development. It is assumed that systematic intervention during the 0–5 age period, when synaptogenesis and plasticity processes are particularly intense, can permanently support children's cognitive, linguistic and social-emotional capacities.

Findings related to early interventions have shown that children in the Abecedarian group demonstrated significant advantages over the control group in terms of school achievement, IQ scores, and language skills. Long-term follow-up studies have shown that these gains are sustained not only during childhood but also during adolescence and adulthood, leading to increased rates of university enrolment and employment opportunities (Campbell et al., 2002).

Another important finding from a neuropedagogical perspective is that early cognitive stimuli create lasting effects on executive functions and self-regulation skills.

The language enrichment activities implemented within the programme strengthened working memory and attention processes and supported the development of higher-order skills such as problem-solving and cognitive flexibility. In this context, the Abecedarian model, consistent with Vygotsky's sociocultural theory, demonstrates the central role of social interaction and structured tools in child development.

More recent studies have also shed light on the long-term health effects of the Abecedarian Project. For example, a study published in 2014 showed that programme participants had lower rates of hypertension and better physical health indicators in adulthood. Another follow-up study conducted in 2021 revealed that biological risk factors such as prehypertension and metabolic syndrome had decreased significantly in the programme group (Campbell et al., 2002).

More importantly, a comprehensive evaluation conducted in 2023 showed that the Abecedarian model does not only provide cognitive and academic gains, but also long-term benefits in areas such as social decision-making, family relationships, and neuro-anatomical changes (Ramey & Ramey, 2023). This finding provides modern evidence supporting the view from a neuropedagogical perspective that the effects of early intervention are not limited to behavioural levels but also create lasting transformations in brain structure and function.

In conclusion, the Abecedarian Project is a pioneering model that demonstrates that early intervention programmes can bring about lasting changes at both the behavioural and neurobiological levels. This programme, which continues to inspire early childhood policies in many countries today, strongly demonstrates that intensive and comprehensive interventions in early childhood have a decisive impact on lifelong learning and development.

AÇEP (Mother-Child Education Programme)

One of the most comprehensive programmes developed in the field of early childhood education in Turkey, the Mother-Child Education Programme (AÇEP) has been implemented by the Mother-Child Education Foundation (AÇEV) since 1993 and has continued to expand its scope and reach since 2015. The programme aims to support the cognitive, social and emotional development of children with limited access to pre-school education, while also strengthening parents' knowledge and skills in child-rearing. AÇEP consists of three main components spread over a 25-week period: mother support training, mental education programme (ZEP) and reproductive health-family planning. These components support the child's developmental ecosystem in a home-centred manner, providing a foundation consistent with Bronfenbrenner's ecological systems approach and Vygotsky's sociocultural theory.

APPLICATIONS IN TURKEY: A NEUROPEDAGOGICAL ANALYSIS

AÇEP (Mother-Child Education Programme)

AÇEV reports from 2015 onwards show that the programme has reached more than 150,000 mothers and children in 81 provinces (AÇEV, 2023). Participating children demonstrated superior performance compared to control groups, particularly in language development, attention, memory, and problem-solving skills; mothers, on the other hand, reported increases in parenting self-efficacy, a more democratic approach to discipline, and positive parent-child relationships (AÇEV, 2018/2021). These findings demonstrate that AÇEP offers a comprehensive model that encompasses not only cognitive outcomes but also the social-emotional domain.

One of the studies supporting AÇEP's contributions within the neuropedagogical framework is the work of Demir et al. (2016). This study examined how various neuro-cognitive and neuro-pedagogical modalities affect children's cognitive skills. The findings revealed that children showed significant improvements in working memory, attention control, cognitive flexibility, and self-regulation skills through enriched environmental stimuli and structured activities. The study also noted that language and reading skills increase neuroplasticity, while regular play and interaction-based activities strengthen executive functions. It is also emphasised that exercise, sleep patterns, and healthy nutrition facilitate learning by supporting neurobiological processes. These findings demonstrate that the core elements of the AÇEP programme (mother-child interaction, play-based learning, and enrichment of the home environment) directly align with neuropedagogical mechanisms.

In conclusion, when evaluated in light of both the impact analyses of field applications and the neuropedagogical findings presented by Demir et al. (2016), AÇEP emerges as a powerful model that simultaneously supports brain development, executive functions, and social-emotional skills in early childhood.

ETEÇOM (Interaction-Based Early Childhood Intervention Programme)

In Turkey, ETEÇOM (Interaction-Based Early Childhood Intervention Programme) is an important example of neuropedagogical-based practices in early childhood. The theoretical basis of the programme is the Responsive Teaching approach developed by Mahoney, Nam and Perales (2014). This approach focuses on strengthening parent-child interactions, which play a critical role in a child's development, and emphasises the brain-plasticity-enhancing effects of joint attention, emotional sharing, and interactive communication processes, particularly in the first years of life, in line with neuroscientific findings.

In ETEÇOM's application model, experts teach parents through sessions how to recognise their children's developmental signals, respond sensitively to these signals, and initiate and maintain interaction strategies. This process not only supports the child's learning behaviours but also transforms the parent's role from a passive observer to an active 'learning partner.' In this way, the programme functions as a neuropedagogical intervention by enhancing the quality of micro-system interactions, as emphasised in Bronfenbrenner's ecological systems theory.

The neuropedagogical contributions of the programme can be considered in several dimensions. Firstly, the parent's sensitive and sustainable interactions support the child's executive functions, contributing to the development of attention control, cognitive flexibility and working memory. In addition, emotional sharing through joint attention and facial expressions with the child activates social brain networks, accelerating the maturation of social cognitive circuits. Parents' recognition and support of their child's communication attempts strengthens language development, laying the groundwork for vocabulary expansion and progress in pragmatic language skills. Finally, an interaction-based approach reinforces the child's self-regulation skills, increasing their emotional control and developing their capacity for self-soothing.

Findings from studies conducted in Turkey show that ETEÇOM is particularly effective in children with developmental delays and autism spectrum disorder (ASD). Gürel-Selimoglu's (2015) study reported that children with ASD who participated in ETEÇOM showed significant improvements in their ability to initiate, maintain, and respond to social interactions. Additionally, mothers stated that after the programme, they understood their children's needs better and developed more patient and sensitive parenting behaviours. These findings reveal that the programme not only enhances the child's development but also strengthens the parent's pedagogical capacity.

One of the most important features of ETEÇOM is that it is implemented in the children's natural living environments, and interventions are built around play, daily life activities, and parent-child interaction. When evaluated from a neuropedagogical perspective, this approach actively activates factors such as emotional security, motivation, and social bonding that support the brain's learning processes. Thus, ETEÇOM presents a strong example of neuropedagogically based early childhood programmes in Turkey by integrating early diagnosis and intervention with family participation.

Tohum Autism Foundation Approaches

One of the leading organisations in the education of children with autism spectrum disorder (ASD) in Turkey, the Tohum Autism Foundation has been implementing projects focused on early diagnosis, early intervention and education since 2003. The foundation has adapted internationally recognised structured teaching methods to the Turkish education system and developed applications specifically for children in the pre-school period. Among these approaches, adaptations of the TEACCH (Treatment and Education of Autistic and related Communication handicapped Children) model, intensive use of visual aids, individualised education plans, and family-participation-based programmes stand out.

From a neuropedagogical perspective, structured teaching offers multifaceted contributions that support the child's cognitive capacity and learning potential. First, the intensive use of visual cues and routines helps regulate attention processes in children with ASD and contributes to the development of executive functions (planning, sequencing, flexibility). Additionally, the physical structuring of the learning environment and the systematic organisation of tasks from simple to complex facilitate children's information processing skills. This approach supports neuroplasticity by enabling the strengthening of the brain's learning circuits through repetition and regularity.

The Tohum Autism Foundation encourages active participation from families in its educational programmes, with the aim of continuing learning opportunities for children in the home environment. This reinforces the interaction between multiple systems emphasised in Bronfenbrenner's ecological theory and contributes to the child's social and cognitive development. The foundation's projects also include early diagnosis screenings, teacher training, and public awareness campaigns, thereby creating an effective intervention model at both the individual and societal levels.

Research findings show that structured teaching leads to progress in language and communication skills, the development of self-regulation strategies, and increased social interaction in children with ASD. From a neuropedagogical perspective, these developments are associated with the support of the child's social brain networks and the consolidation of learning processes. Therefore, when evaluated from a neuropedagogical perspective in Turkey, the Tohum Autism Foundation's practices constitute a strong example of the effectiveness and sustainability of structured teaching in early childhood.

Small Steps Early Education Project – Neuropedagogical Framework

One of the most notable examples of family-based early intervention programmes in Turkey is the Small Steps Early Education Programme (KAEEP). Adapted from the Small Steps Early Intervention Program developed in Australia, KAEEP has been implemented in Turkey since 1993 through a collaboration between Boğaziçi University and UNICEF. The program targets children aged 0–6 with developmental delays or special needs and their families.

The most important feature of KAEEP is that it is a family-centred and home-based intervention model. The programme enables children to progress in small, achievable steps in key areas such as motor skills, communication, self-care, cognitive development and social interaction. Parents take on an active role in their child's development, while experts monitor and guide the process. In this respect, the programme aligns with Vygotsky's zone of proximal development approach, positioning parents as 'co-regulators' in the child's learning process.

From a neuropedagogical perspective, the Small Steps model aims to activate the brain's plasticity in the early stages through repetition and small goals. While the child's working memory, attention, and motor planning skills are systematically strengthened, the parent's continuous participation contributes to the child's self-regulation and emotional security development. Using daily life activities as learning materials makes learning contextual and meaningful.

Research conducted in Turkey supports the effectiveness of the programme. Studies based on family opinions reveal that KAEEP has produced positive results such as improved communication skills, motor development and self-care habits in children. Additionally, parents have noted that they better understand their children's needs, feel more equipped, and observe positive changes in family interactions during the programme. These findings indicate that KAEEP not only enhances the child's development but also strengthens the family's pedagogical capacity.

In conclusion, the Small Steps Early Education Project is a strong and sustainable example of neuropedagogically based early intervention programmes in Turkey. By centring on family participation, the programme creates lasting effects in both the development of children with special needs and the awareness of parents.

INSIGHTS FROM MOROCCO: EMERGING POLICIES AND PRACTICES

INDH Preschool Construction Initiative

One of the most important transformations in early childhood education in Morocco is the National Preschool Expansion Programme, which was launched in 2018. The programme's primary objective is to universalise access to quality preschool education for all children aged 4–6. This initiative is aligned with the third phase of the National Human Development Programme (INDH) and encompasses not only quantitative growth in institutions but also quality assurance, teacher training and governance reforms (UNESCO, 2023). UNESCO reports emphasise that the programme is built on four pillars: inclusivity, quality, sustainable governance and universal access.

From a neuropedagogical perspective, the programme focuses on the critical windows of brain development in early childhood. The curriculum is based on play-based learning, activities that provide sensory richness, developing shared attention through social interaction, and encouraging language development in a multilingual environment. In particular, role-playing, storytelling, physical activities, and group work support children's executive functions (attention, memory, cognitive flexibility) and self-regulation skills. UNESCO (2023) defines neuropedagogy in this context as an approach that considers the integrated development of children's emotional, cognitive, and social brain networks in learning processes.

Empirical studies on the effects of the programme are also noteworthy. Randomised controlled trials conducted by J-PAL have shown that the construction of preschool classrooms significantly improves not only children's cognitive skills (especially language and problem-solving) but also their social-emotional competence and self-regulation capacity. Furthermore, mothers' more active participation in the educational process has been facilitated, which has supported family interactions and children's social brain development (J-PAL, 2020).

Similarly, Ettahri and Hasnaoui's (2022) study found that the programme provided measurable gains in children's linguistic, socio-emotional, motor and cognitive skills, and that the age, gender and professional qualifications of educators were decisive factors in children's learning outcomes. The study used the Stimulus–Organism–Response (SOR) model and demonstrated that the programme's external (organisational, environmental) and internal (teacher, classroom dynamics) conditions are directly related to children's skill development.

These findings highlight two important neuropedagogical contributions of the National Preschool Expansion programme: (1) providing stimulating and interactive learning environments that support children's brain development, and (2) strengthening social cognitive circuits and executive functions through the active participation of parents and teachers in the process. However, challenges such as rural-urban inequalities, differences in teacher quality, and sustainable financing continue to be reported in the implementation of the programme (Ettahri & Hasnaoui, 2022; UNESCO, 2023).

ANEER Program: Holistic Community Preschool Model

Launched in 2015 by the Zakoura Foundation in partnership with the Moroccan Ministry of Education and UNICEF, the ANEER Programme was designed as a community-based model aimed at ensuring access to early childhood education for children living in rural areas. This programme is not only for children but also attracts attention with its holistic structure that involves parents, teachers and local communities in the process. Thus, the learning experience is not limited to the classroom but also extends to the child's home environment and social circle.

The ANEER model focuses on play-based learning, social interaction and parental involvement, particularly from a neuropedagogical perspective. Group games, role-playing activities, and dramatisations that develop children's attention, memory, and problem-solving skills contribute to the development of executive functions and cognitive flexibility while also supporting joint attention, empathy, and collaboration skills. The multilingual learning environment strengthens pragmatic use and cognitive flexibility in children's language development. In addition, training for parents, especially mothers, raises awareness about home routines that support child development (story reading, singing, sensory activities). This approach directly contributes to self-regulation and social brain development by increasing cognitive stimulation in the home environment.

The programme's implementation results also demonstrate its neuropedagogical contributions in concrete terms. As of 2019–2020, 492 pre-school centres have been opened, and more than 23,000 children have participated in the programme. Participation rates have reached 96%, and absenteeism has fallen below 1%. The most striking finding is that 100% of children participating in the programme enrolled in primary school on time. Independent evaluations show that children who have completed ANEER have seen a 7% increase in their academic performance averages in the first two years of primary school, along with significant progress in cognitive, linguistic and socio-emotional areas.

One of the programme's strongest aspects is that it ensures sustainability through a community-based approach. The Zakoura Foundation manages the established pre-school institutions for two years, after which they are handed over to local associations and community actors. This strategy enables children to develop in a stimulating learning environment not only in the classroom but also in their social and cultural contexts. From a neuropedagogical perspective, this translates into a learning environment with high ecological validity and continuity.

As a result, the ANEER Programme successfully applies neuropedagogical principles in the field with its structure that integrates play, interaction, language and parental involvement. The development of children's executive functions, self-regulation skills, and social cognitive capacities are among the most notable outcomes of the programme. At the same time, the active participation of families and communities in the process enables neuropedagogical learning to be supported not only in the classroom but in all areas of the child's life.

AGFUND & UNICEF Projects

In 2025, the Moroccan government, together with UNICEF and the Arab Gulf Fund for Economic and Social Development (AGFUND), launched a new partnership aimed at supporting early childhood development and, in particular, the participation of children with disabilities in education. These projects, which are still in their early stages, aim to improve the quality of inclusive pre-school education services and develop the capacity of care centres. This initiative represents an important step reflecting Morocco's shift in early childhood policies from access to quality and inclusivity.

From a neuropedagogical perspective, this collaboration focuses on creating learning environments adapted to children with different developmental needs. Supporting the cognitive, linguistic and social skills of children with special needs through early intervention programmes presents a critical opportunity in terms of synaptic development and brain plasticity. In this context, the programme aims to develop children's executive functions, self-regulation capacities and social interaction skills through play-based and sensory-supported activities. Additionally, plans are in place to increase the neuropedagogical awareness of teachers and educators working in care centres. These trainings will enable teachers to develop individualised teaching methods and respond to the diverse learning pathways of children with disabilities.

The inclusivity goal of the projects is not only aimed at children but also at families. With the support of UNICEF and AGFUND, information and counselling programmes are being developed for parents to help them recognise their children's developmental needs at an early stage and learn supportive activities they can implement at home. This will contribute to the neuropedagogical support of children not only in the classroom but also in the home and community contexts.

Although the programmes have not yet fully commenced under the newly signed agreements, it is expected that the programme will contribute to strengthening inclusivity in early childhood education in Morocco in the long term and to the creation of an education system that takes neurodevelopmental differences into account. As a result, children with disabilities will be able to access their right to education at an early age, their social integration will be strengthened, and their brain development will be supported with appropriate stimuli during its most critical period

Enfants du Paradis – Hadana programme

One of the most important initiatives aimed at reducing the risk of early exclusion from education for children with special needs in Morocco is the Enfants du Paradis – Hadana programme. The programme provides early intervention services for children from birth to six years of age and aims to identify and support developmental differences at an early stage. The model integrates health and education services to provide comprehensive support during the first years of life, which are critical from a neurodevelopmental perspective (Childhood Education International, 2021).

From a neuropedagogical perspective, Hadana's contribution is to strengthen executive functions and self-regulation skills through play, sensory activities, and social interaction-based practices that play a critical role in children's brain development. For example, singing, storytelling, and role-playing activities support children's social brain networks, while sensory integration practices accelerate language development and strengthen attention processes (UNICEF- Morocco, 2020). In addition, educational and counselling sessions for parents enable families to recognise their children's developmental needs early on and provide neuropedagogical stimulation in the home environment. In this way, the programme transforms not only the classroom learning experience but also the learning environment within the family context.

The inclusive structure of the programme enables children with special needs to be educated alongside their typically developing peers, thereby strengthening social integration. This approach demonstrates that early intervention, in line with neuroscientific findings, contributes not only to the individual development of the child but also to increased social awareness (UNESCO, 2023).

As a result, Enfants du Paradis – Hadana occupies a unique place in Morocco's early childhood policies as a model that provides comprehensive support for children with special needs during the neuropedagogically critical early years, strengthens family participation, and embraces an inclusive education approach.

AI-ENHANCED NEUROPEDAGOGICAL EARLY INTERVENTION: FUTURE MODELS AND RECOMMENDATIONS

Epistemic Scope and Design-Oriented Nature of the Proposed Framework

This section proposes a *design-oriented, conceptual framework* for integrating AI into neuropedagogical early intervention. It does not claim to report a fully validated intervention package or a completed empirical program evaluation. Rather, the aim is to translate established principles from neuropedagogy and early intervention into an AI-supported implementation logic that can guide future piloting, governance, and research. Accordingly, claims in this section are framed as *potential*, *conditional*, and *context-dependent*, and they require local adaptation, ethical oversight, and empirical testing in real-world settings.

Why Artificial Intelligence? A Neuropedagogical Rationale

Early childhood is a critical period when neuroplasticity is at its highest and environmental inputs leave lasting impressions. Neuropedagogy emphasises the importance of scientifically based learning environments to support children's cognitive, social-emotional, and linguistic development during this period (Blakemore & Frith, 2007). When aligned with neuropedagogical principles, artificial intelligence (AI) can potentially support developmentally sensitive early intervention by enhancing the visibility of learning processes, improving timely response, and strengthening collaboration among teachers and families. For example, AI-based developmental monitoring tools can strengthen neuropedagogical early intervention by detecting small differences in executive functions or language development at an early stage (Aydın & Ceylan, 2024; Wu, 2024).

Recent studies have shown that children can make progress in basic cognitive and social skills with AI-supported tools (robotic toys, interactive storytelling, game-based applications) (Choi et al., 2025). These findings align directly with the scaffolding approach of neuropedagogy: children must receive appropriate support at the right time to exceed their potential. However, such outcomes depend on developmental appropriateness, adult mediation, and contextual fit—AI tools should be treated as supports within relational pedagogy rather than standalone instructional agents. AI processes developmental data to provide personalized recommendations to teachers and parents, ensuring that support is systematic and data-driven rather than random (Ilic et al., 2021).

However, the neuropedagogical rationale does not focus solely on cognitive gains; it also considers children's safety, ethical rights, and developmental integrity.

Data security, the prevention of algorithmic bias, and consideration of the digital divide in the child-centered use of AI should be seen as neuropedagogical responsibilities (UNESCO, 2023; UNICEF, 2025). Therefore, the integration of AI in early childhood is not merely a technological innovation, but also the construction of an ethical-neuropedagogical model that centers on children's holistic development. In this sense, the "value" of AI is determined not by technological sophistication but by whether it strengthens equitable, explainable, and developmentally respectful educational decision-making.

Based on these reasons, it is possible to examine how AI can be integrated into early childhood education based on neuropedagogical principles through concrete model components. The following components are presented as design building blocks that can be adapted to local infrastructure, policy requirements, and teacher capacity.

Model Components: Artificial Intelligence-Supported Neuropedagogical Early Intervention

The artificial intelligence-supported neuropedagogical model can be structured around four basic components: data-based development monitoring, emotion and attention recognition, adaptive content delivery, and teacher decision support systems. Each of these components can be directly integrated into the early intervention chain of screening, assessment, targeted intervention, monitoring, and family collaboration processes. Importantly, these components are not proposed as mandatory technologies, but as a modular framework: systems may adopt some components while omitting others based on feasibility and ethical considerations.

Data-driven developmental monitoring enables the extraction of children's developmental profiles through AI-based sensors, game behavior analytics, and language interaction records. For example, the AI-Integrated System Design for Early Stage Learning study demonstrates that preschool children's cognitive task performance can be analyzed in real-time and reported to teachers. This approach directly corresponds to the principle of "early identification and rapid intervention" in neuropedagogy. To remain neuropedagogically appropriate, monitoring should prioritize low-stakes, play-embedded indicators and should avoid labeling children based on single-session signals.

Emotion and attention recognition technologies provide teachers with feedback on classroom learning dynamics by analyzing facial expressions, tone of voice, and attention focus patterns. Studies have shown that AI-based emotion recognition software can serve as an early warning system in social-emotional learning processes (Ilic et al., 2021). However, at this point, ethical sensitivities such as the risk of algorithmic bias and misinterpretation of different cultural facial expressions must be considered (UNESCO, 2023). Accordingly, emotion/attention signals should be treated as probabilistic cues, not diagnostic truths, and should be interpreted only within teacher judgement and contextual observation.

Adaptive content delivery is one of AI's most visible contributions. Game-based platforms can support executive functions, problem-solving, and self-regulation by adjusting the difficulty level according to the child's performance. Indeed, gamified AI tasks led to meaningful improvements in executive functions. These findings are consistent with the individualized learning goals of the neuropedagogical approach. Nevertheless, adaptive systems should be designed to avoid narrowing learning opportunities (e.g., repeatedly presenting only "easier" tasks), and they should preserve variability, curiosity, and social interaction opportunities.

Teacher decision support systems highlight the supportive role of AI in teaching. As emphasized in the UNICEF (2025) report, AI tools not only provide teachers with developmental data on children but also make recommendations, thereby strengthening the teacher's neuropedagogical leadership. This allows teachers to maintain their one-on-one relationship with children while making more informed and evidence-based decisions. Crucially, decision-support must remain assistive, meaning that teachers can override recommendations, review explanations (explainability), and document professional reasoning when adapting instructional plans.

Ultimately, these four components should be seen not merely as technical innovations, but as a framework that facilitates the sustainable application of neuropedagogical principles in early childhood education. Ethical concerns (data security, equal access, prevention of bias) must be an integral part of each component; otherwise, AI integration will remain a technological initiative rather than a pedagogical one. For this reason, governance procedures (data minimization, informed consent, transparency, and accountability) should be specified at the design stage, not added after implementation.

These model components provide a concrete roadmap for how early intervention programs can be redesigned with AI in the future. The next step is to disseminate these components with the support of policy documents and field applications. In addition, future work should prioritize empirical piloting with clearly defined outcomes, feasibility indicators, and equity monitoring.

AI-ENHANCED NEUROPEDAGOGICAL INTERVENTION MODEL

AI-Supported Neuropedagogical Early Intervention Cycle (Screening → Assessment → Intervention → Monitoring → Family Collaboration)

The effectiveness of neuropedagogical intervention in early childhood depends on the design of a systematic and comprehensive process. This process consists of the following stages: screening to identify the child's developmental characteristics early and accurately; assessment involving the collection of detailed and multi-source data; intervention involving the implementation of individualized strategies; monitoring to ensure that progress is tracked regularly throughout the process; and collaboration that involves the family as a key partner in supporting the child's development. AI-supported solutions enhance both speed and accuracy in each of these stages, enabling the neuropedagogical approach to be applied in a more robust and innovative manner in the field. In this cycle, AI is conceptualized as a support layer—augmenting observation, documentation, and feedback—while pedagogical decision-making remains human-led and developmentally grounded.

Screening

The screening phase is applied to all children on a universal scale using low-risk, fast, and game-based tasks. Structured short scales, teacher observations, and classroom microbehavioral cues are analysed by AI to generate early signals of potential risks. Visual-auditory interaction data, robot-mediated attention tasks, or information obtained from low-cost wearable sensors enable the earlier detection of developmental risks (Wu, 2024). For example, robot interactions based on imitation and attention tasks yield highly sensitive results in screening for developmental risks such as autism spectrum disorder (ASD) (Sadreimova & Zhumabayeva, 2023). However, UNESCO and UNICEF (2025) reports recommend that such screenings be conducted under teacher supervision, with data anonymized and ethical approval processes followed. Screening outputs should be framed as risk flags rather than labels, triggering closer observation and supportive planning rather than formal categorization.

Assessment

The assessment process allows for in-depth analysis of screening results. The aim here is to reliably profile strengths and weaknesses in cognitive, linguistic, social-emotional, and motor areas. The contribution of AI is the integration of multiple sources of evidence: teacher reports, children's play performance, short language samples, and, if necessary, kinematic or physiological indicators can be brought together under a single analytical framework. Studies show a high correlation between teacher assessments and AI-based behavioural classifications (Choi et al., 2025). At this point, the fundamental principle of the neuropedagogical approach must be upheld —children should not be exposed to stress-inducing test procedures; measurements should be conducted within the context of play and interaction (Ilic et al., 2021). Where AI contributes, it should prioritize triangulation (multiple indicators) and interpretability (clear explanations) rather than complex "black-box" scores.

Intervention

The intervention phase forms the core of the model. Here, the primary function of AI is not to replace the teacher, but to support pedagogical decisions. Adaptive content engines can adjust the difficulty level of activities based on the child's attention level or emotional state. Social robots or interactive toys have been shown to enhance language development and social interaction (Russ, 2023). For example, early vocabulary studies have shown that word learning occurs more quickly when conducted with AI-supported robots. However, teacher supervision is critical; adaptive systems may carry the risk of narrowing pedagogical opportunities, so a human-centered design approach should be adopted (Berk, 2022). Intervention planning should explicitly include (a) target constructs (e.g., inhibitory control, vocabulary growth, joint attention), (b) intended pedagogical mechanisms (e.g., guided play, scaffolding), and (c) criteria for adjusting support (e.g., sustained engagement, reduced frustration).

Monitoring

A monitoring process is essential for the sustainability of interventions. Learning analytics makes the temporal progression of developmental indicators visible. Weekly growth curves, in-game task completion rates, or changes in attention span can be presented to teachers and families through simple dashboards. UNICEF's (2025) digital world report recommends including children's emotional well-being and screen time in these dashboards but emphasizes that only explainable and simplified indicators should be shared. This allows teachers to quickly adjust interventions, while families can track their child's progress in an understandable language. Monitoring should be used to support reflective practice (What worked? For whom? Under what conditions?) rather than to intensify surveillance or increase pressure on children.

Family Collaboration

The final stage is family cooperation. The neuropedagogical perspective aims to support the child's development not only in the classroom but also at home. AI-supported family portals can increase parental involvement in the process with weekly short feedback and game suggestions that can be implemented at home. Voice recognition-based systems can facilitate parents' ability to provide quick feedback to teachers (UNESCO, 2023). In this way, families become not just passive recipients of information but co-designers of the intervention process. To reduce inequity, family-facing tools should be designed for low bandwidth, multiple languages, and varying literacy levels, and they should avoid implying "parent blame" when engagement is limited by socioeconomic constraints.

Limitations, Risks, and Safeguards

Although AI can strengthen early intervention systems, several failure modes must be anticipated. Algorithmic bias may amplify inequities if training data do not represent diverse children and cultural interaction styles. Misclassification risk is particularly critical when emotion/attention signals are treated as definitive rather than probabilistic cues. Over-reliance on automated recommendations may narrow teacher professional judgement and reduce pedagogical flexibility. Finally, resource disparities (devices, connectivity, staff capacity) can deepen the digital divide. Therefore, safeguards should include data minimization, transparency and explainability, bias auditing, opt-out options for families, teacher training in AI literacy, and governance structures aligned with UNESCO/UNICEF ethical guidance.

Ethical and policy dimensions should be embedded in all stages of this application flow. Data minimization, testing for algorithmic bias, low-bandwidth solutions suitable for low-resource schools, and culturally adapted materials are fundamental prerequisites (UNICEF, 2025). Teachers' AI literacy and their continued role as guiding actors in the process are also consistent with UNESCO's ethical principles.

As a result, this model, based on the cycle of screening, assessment, intervention, monitoring, and family collaboration, offers a holistic approach that integrates neuropedagogical principles with artificial intelligence technologies. In this context, artificial intelligence functions not merely as a technical tool but as a support system enabling the design of more sensitive, individualized, and ethically responsible practices in early childhood education. The model enriches teachers' decision-making processes, increases family participation, and enables children's developmental needs to be met earlier and more reliably. However, preventing algorithmic bias, data security, cultural adaptations, and teachers' artificial intelligence literacy are essential for the model's sustainability.

In terms of the future, this approach provides a reference framework that can guide policy and program development processes in early childhood education. The AI-supported neuropedagogical intervention model not only strengthens existing educational practices but also has the potential to accelerate scientific knowledge production related to early childhood. To move from framework to evidence, future studies should specify measurable outcomes (e.g., EF, language, SEL indicators), implementation fidelity markers, and equity-sensitive evaluation criteria across diverse settings. Thus, early childhood education can be carried into the future with a new paradigm that blends the possibilities of technology with pedagogical and ethical principles.

CONCLUSION

This section of the book examines the integration of artificial intelligence with a neuropedagogical approach in early childhood from various perspectives. First, the theoretical framework of neuropedagogy is explained, and how learning processes in early childhood can be supported in line with brain-based principles is discussed. This discussion has paved the way for the rise of artificial intelligence in education and highlighted the points where technology and neuroscience findings intersect in a pedagogical context.

The rest of the chapter provides a detailed evaluation of data-driven development monitoring, attention and emotion recognition technologies, adaptive content delivery, and teacher support mechanisms. It is emphasized that these tools strengthen individualized learning opportunities in early childhood, enable developmental differences to be identified earlier, and support teachers' decision-making processes. Also in this section, the proposed model framework for integrating artificial intelligence into existing education programs is structured around the five stages of the early intervention approach: screening, assessment, intervention, monitoring, and family collaboration.

The application flow has been the most important factor in making the section unique. Identifying risk groups during the screening phase, systematically profiling strengths and weaknesses during assessment, providing personalized content during the intervention process, providing continuous feedback during the monitoring phase, and actively involving families in the process have demonstrated that a neuropedagogical approach can form a holistic cycle supported by artificial intelligence. Thus, the principle of early intervention has been concretized, and a practical roadmap has been drawn up for educators.

Ethical and policy dimensions have been embedded throughout the chapter. Fundamental concerns such as data security, algorithmic bias, and the digital divide have been addressed not only as technical issues but also in the context of children's rights. It has been noted that the principles put forward by international organizations (OECD, UNESCO, UNICEF) provide a guiding ethical framework for the models to be developed. Thus, it has been emphasized that technological integration points not only to opportunities but also to responsibilities.

In conclusion, it is evident that artificial intelligence applications supported by neuropedagogical principles offer an innovative paradigm in early childhood education. This paradigm has the potential to make children's developmental needs more responsive, teachers' decision-making processes stronger, family participation more effective, and policies more inclusive. The framework outlined throughout this section aims not only to evaluate current applications but also to contribute to the shaping of future strategic orientations.

The development of AI-supported neuropedagogical programs in early childhood is considered an important step toward the future of education. However, this step must be taken within an approach that is bound by ethical principles, sensitive to cultural differences, and serves pedagogical purposes. In this way, technology can become a tool that strengthens rather than undermines the essence of human development.

REFERENCES

AÇEV. (2018). *Faaliyet raporu 2018*. Anne Çocuk Eğitim Vakfı.

AÇEV. (2021). *Erken çocukluk programları etki analizi raporu*. Anne Çocuk Eğitim Vakfı.

AÇEV. (2023). *Faaliyet raporu 2023*. Anne Çocuk Eğitim Vakfı.

Arda, T. B., & Ocak, S. (2012). Social Competence and Promoting Alternative Thinking Strategies—PATHS Preschool Curriculum. *Educational Sciences: Theory & Practice, 12*(4), 2691–2698.

Aydın, A., & Ceylan, Ş. (2024, October). Navigating the digital world: Ethical implications of AI in early childhood education. In *VI Congreso Mundial con Infancia y Adolescencia: Educar para la felicidad* (pp. 1570–1579). Cáceres, Spain.

Barnett, W. S., Jung, K., Yarosz, D. J., Thomas, J., Hornbeck, A., Stechuk, R., & Burns, S. (2008). Educational effects of the Tools of the Mind curriculum: A randomized trial. *Early Childhood Research Quarterly, 23*(3), 299–313. DOI: 10.1016/j.ecresq.2008.03.001

Berk, L. E. (2022). *Exploring child and adolescent development* (6th ed.). Pearson.

Blair, C., & Raver, C. C. (2014). Closing the achievement gap through modification of neurocognitive and neuroendocrine function: Results from a cluster randomized controlled trial of an innovative approach to the education of children in kindergarten. *PLoS One, 9*(11), e112393. DOI: 10.1371/journal.pone.0112393

Blakemore, S. J., & Frith, U. (2007). *The learning brain: Lessons for education*. Blackwell Publishing.

Bodrova, E., Leong, D. J., & Akhutina, T. V. (2011). When everything new is well-forgotten old: Vygotsky/Luria insights in the development of executive functions. *New Directions for Child and Adolescent Development, 2011*(133), 11–28. DOI: 10.1002/cd.301

Bulkis, F., Rahman, A., & Lestari, S. (2025). Project-based learning to enhance social-emotional skills in early childhood. *Early Childhood Education Journal*. https://doi.org/10.xxxx/xxxxx

Caine, R. N., & Caine, G. (1991). Making connections: Teaching and the human brain.

Campbell, F. A., Ramey, C. T., Pungello, E., Sparling, J., & Miller-Johnson, S. (2002). Early childhood education: Young adult outcomes from the Abecedarian Project. *Applied Developmental Science, 6*(1), 42–57. DOI: 10.1207/S1532480XADS0601_05

Castellanos-Ryan, N., Parent, S., Chaput-Langlois, S., Rioux, C., Jacques, S., Simard, C., Tremblay, R. E., Séguin, J. R., & Zelazo, P. D. (2023). Modelling executive function across early childhood: Longitudinal invariance, development from 3.5 to 7 years and later academic performance. *Cognitive Development, 68*, 101365. DOI: 10.1016/j.cogdev.2023.101365

Catalano, L., Sagliano, L., Visciglio, A., Russo, P., Miniello, S., Trojano, L., & Panico, F. (2025). An integrated multifocal tDCS-EEG protocol for reducing cognitive and affective symptoms in mild cognitive impairment and early stages of dementia: A crossover double-blind randomized controlled trial. *Frontiers in Neurology, 16*, 1605970. DOI: 10.3389/fneur.2025.1605970

Choi, Y., Lee, H., & Kim, J. (2025). Artificial intelligence–based adaptive learning games and socio-emotional development in preschoolers. *Early Childhood Research Quarterly, 61*(2), 145–158. DOI: 10.1016/j.ecresq.2025.02.004

Della Sala, S., & Anderson, M. (Eds.). (2012). *Neuroscience in education: The good, the bad, and the ugly*. Oxford University Press.

Demir, M. Ş., Usta, M. E., Yayla, A., Taşkın, N., Hastunç, Y., & Alav, Ö. (2016). Çeşitli nöro-bilişsel ve nöro-pedagojik uygulama ve modalitelerin bilişsel becerilerin gelişimi üzerindeki etkisi. *Ahi Evran Üniversitesi Kırşehir Eğitim Fakültesi Dergisi, 17*(2), 679–696.

Diamond, A. (2013). Executive functions. *Annual Review of Psychology, 64*(1), 135–168. DOI: 10.1146/annurev-psych-113011-143750

Diamond, A. (2013). Executive functions. *Annual Review of Psychology, 64*(1), 135–168. DOI: 10.1146/annurev-psych-113011-143750

Ettahri, S., & Hasnaoui, R. (2022, July). Impact of the preschool program on the socio-connective variables developed by the beneficiary children: The case of rural Morocco. In *Proceedings of the 5th European International Conference on Industrial Engineering and Operations Management* (pp. 2311–2327). Rome, Italy: IEOM Society International. DOI: 10.46254/EU05.20220453

Goble, P., Flynn, T., Nauman, C., Almendarez, P., & Linstrom, M. (2021). Intervention implementation of tools of the mind for preschool children's executive functioning. *Frontiers in Psychology, 12*, 624140. DOI: 10.3389/fpsyg.2021.624140

Goswami, U. (2015). *Neuroscience and education: From research to practice.* Routledge.

Groark, C. J., & Eidelman, S. M. (2020). *Early childhood intervention: Shaping the future for children with special needs and their families* (Vol. 1). Praeger.

Gürel-Selimoglu, O. (2015). *ETEÇOM programının otizm spektrum bozukluğu olan çocukların sosyal etkileşim becerileri üzerindeki etkisi* (Yüksek Lisans Tezi). Anadolu Üniversitesi, Eskişehir.

Hadders-Algra, M. (2021). *Early detection and early intervention in developmental motor disorders: From neuroscience to participation.* Mac Keith Press.

Heckman, J. J., Moon, S. H., Pinto, R., Savelyev, P. A., & Yavitz, A. (2010). The rate of return to the HighScope Perry Preschool Program. *Journal of Public Economics, 94*(1-2), 114–128. DOI: 10.1016/j.jpubeco.2009.11.001

Ilic, P., Casebourne, I., & Wegerif, R. (2021). *Artificial intelligence in education: The intersection of technology and pedagogy.* Routledge.

Immordino-Yang, M. H., & Damasio, A. (2007). We feel, therefore we learn: The relevance of affective and social neuroscience to education. *Mind, Brain and Education : the Official Journal of the International Mind, Brain, and Education Society, 1*(1), 3–10. DOI: 10.1111/j.1751-228X.2007.00004.x

Jensen, E. (2008). *Brain-based learning: The new paradigm of teaching.* Corwin Press.

Johnson, J. E., Rahn, N. L., & Bricker, D. (2015). *An activity-based approach to early intervention.* Brookes Publishing.

Jongsma, A. E.Jr, & Winkelstern, J. A. (2016). *The early childhood education intervention treatment planner.* Wiley.

Kunduracı, H. Ö., & Aksoy, A. (2025). The Effects of" Mother Education Program" on Mothers' Parenting Knowledge, Parenting Self-Efficacy and Their Children's Development. *Education in Science, 50*(221), 1–31.

Lohvynenko, T., Drozd, L., Marieieva, T., Hryntsiv, M., Prymakova, V., & Hrynyk, I. (2023). Neuropedagogical Principles as a Factor of Inclusive Education in the Context of Managerial Activity: European Experience. *BRAIN. Broad Research in Artificial Intelligence and Neuroscience, 14*(4), 212–227. DOI: 10.18662/brain/14.4/501

López-Escribano, C., Escudero, A., & Pérez-López, R. (2021). An exploratory study about patterns of parental home literacy activities during the COVID-19 confinement among Spanish families. *Early Education and Development, 32*(6), 812–829. DOI: 10.1080/10409289.2021.1916184

Madanipour, P., Garvis, S., Cohrssen, C., & Pendergast, D. (2025, January). Early childhood teachers' understanding of executive functions and strategies employed to facilitate them. [). Frontiers Media SA.]. *Frontiers in Education*, *9*, 1488410. DOI: 10.3389/feduc.2024.1488410

Mahoney, G., Nam, S., & Perales, F. (2014). The role of parents in early intervention: Implications for social–emotional development of children with disabilities. *Journal of Intellectual Disability Research*, *58*(4), 333–345. DOI: 10.1111/jir.12095

Mercer, N. (2019). *Language and the joint creation of knowledge: The selected works of Neil Mercer*. Routledge. DOI: 10.4324/9780429400759

Morocco, U. N. I. C. E. F. (2020). *Annual report on early childhood education*. UNICEF.

Nores, M., Belfield, C. R., Barnett, W. S., & Schweinhart, L. (2005). Updating the economic impacts of the High/Scope Perry Preschool program. *Educational Evaluation and Policy Analysis*, *27*(3), 245–261. DOI: 10.3102/01623737027003245

Novia, B. O. N., & Rachmawati, Y. (2025). Analysis of Parenting in Shaping Character in Early Childhood: Analisis Pola Asuh Orang Tua dalam Membentuk Karakter pada Anak Usia Dini. *PAUDIA: Jurnal Penelitian dalam Bidang Pendidikan Anak Usia Dini*, 1-12.

Piaget, J. (1972). Development and learning. *Reading in child behavior and development*, 38-46.

Ramey, C. T., & Ramey, S. L. (2023). Early childhood education that promotes lifelong learning, health, and social well-being: The Abecedarian Project and its replications. *Medical Research Archives*, *11*(11). Advance online publication. DOI: 10.18103/mra.v11i11.4590

Riggleman, S., Higgins, J., & Lohmann, M. J. (2025). Crafting Behavior Goal Cocktails: What's in Yours? Writing Behavioral Goals in Early Childhood. *Beyond Behavior*, *34*(1), 14–23. DOI: 10.1177/10742956241313104

Riggs, K. J., McTaggart, J., Simpson, A., & Freeman, R. P. J. (2006). Changes in the capacity of visual working memory in 5- to 10-year-olds. *Journal of Experimental Child Psychology*, *95*(1), 18–26. DOI: 10.1016/j.jecp.2006.03.009

Russ, S. W. (2023). *Play in child development and psychotherapy: Toward empirically supported practice* (3rd ed.). Routledge.

Sadreimova, G., & Zhumabayeva, A. (2023). Neuropedagogical approaches to early intervention for children with autism spectrum disorder. *Education and Pedagogy Journal, 15*(4), 221–236.

Schonert-Reichl, K. A., Oberle, E., Lawlor, M. S., Abbott, D., Thomson, K., Oberlander, T. F., & Diamond, A. (2015). Enhancing cognitive and social–emotional development through a simple-to-administer mindfulness-based school program for elementary school children: A randomized controlled trial. *Developmental Psychology, 51*(1), 52–66. DOI: 10.1037/a0038454

Semelius Granevald, V. (2025). Exploring factors related to special needs educators' work-related well-being in preschool settings. *European Journal of Special Needs Education, 40*(4), 1–16. DOI: 10.1080/08856257.2024.2421111

Thiessen, E. J., Gibson, H. D., Regis, D., Pehrsson, S. J., Ashley, K. T., & Smit, M. A. (2020). The distinct metamorphic stages and structural styles of the 1.94–1.86 Ga Snowbird Orogen, Northwest Territories, Canada. *Journal of Metamorphic Geology, 38*(9), 963–992. DOI: 10.1111/jmg.12556

Thomas, M. S. C. (2020). *Educational neuroscience: Development across the life span*. Routledge. DOI: 10.4324/9781003016830

Tokuhama-Espinosa, T. (2011). *Mind, brain, and education science: A comprehensive guide to the new brain-based teaching*. W. W. Norton & Company.

UNESCO. (2023a). *Guidance for generative AI in education and research*. UNESCO Publishing.

UNESCO. (2023b). *Advancing preschool education in Morocco: Goals of inclusion, quality, and sustainable governance*. UNESCO. https://www.unesco.org/en/early-childhood-education/advancing-preschool-education-morocco-goals-inclusion-quality-and-sustainable-governance

UNICEF. (2025). *Childhood in a digital world: Innocenti report 2025*. UNICEF Office of Research–Innocenti.

Watagodakumbura, C. (2014). *Programming the brain: Educational neuroscience perspective, pedagogical practices and study skills*. Xlibris Corporation.

Wu, S. (2024). Artificial intelligence applications in early childhood developmental assessment: Opportunities and challenges. *Frontiers in Psychology, 15*, 1348294. DOI: 10.3389/fpsyg.2024.1348294

Zull, J. E. (2011). *From brain to mind: Using neuroscience to guide change in education*. Stylus Publishing. Tzirides, A. O. O., de Castro, V. C., Cope, B., & Kalantzis, M. (2025). Multimodality and transposition in collaborative language learning. In *Multimodal Literacy in English as an Additional Language in Higher Education* (pp. 67-86). Routledge.

Chapter 7
The Impact of Working Memory on Reading Comprehension Among Moroccan Primary School Students:
A Neuropedagogical Approach

Mohammed Labrouzi
https://orcid.org/0009-0005-5291-7528
Sidi Mohammed Ben Abdullah University, Morocco

Hamza Ghoura
https://orcid.org/0009-0001-2455-6439
Sidi Mohammed Ben Abdullah University, Morocco

Mostafa Bouanani
https://orcid.org/0009-0007-8534-9621
Sidi Mohammed Ben Abdullah University, Morocco

ABSTRACT

This study sought to measure the impact of working memory on reading comprehension by examining the correlation between working memory and reading comprehension (text comprehension, phonological awareness, phonological tasks, and spelling tasks). It also aimed to determine whether statistically significant relationships exist between reading comprehension and working memory based on gender variable. To this end, the researchers administered a set of tests, including assessments of working memory and reading comprehension, tailored to the Moroccan educational context.

DOI: 10.4018/979-8-3373-3581-0.ch007

These tests were conducted on a sample of one hundred (100) fourth-grade primary school students (equally divided between males and females) at "Oulad Tayeb" School in the Regional Directorate of Fez. The goal was to identify the relationship between working memory and certain components of reading comprehension among the study participants.

INTRODUCTION

This study falls within the scope of cognitive research related to enhancing the pathways of teaching and learning the Arabic language from the perspective of neuropedagogy, which is considered an interdisciplinary field that brings together various cognitive sciences, such as neuroscience, cognitive and educational psychology, education sciences, didactics, and artificial intelligence. The emergence of neuropedagogy is closely linked to neuroscience, one of the most important cognitive sciences, whose findings are increasingly utilized in educational innovation, particularly in relation to the depth of teaching and learning. Neuroscience aims to understand how the nervous system functions in producing and regulating an individual's emotions, behaviors, and thoughts (Kandel et al., 2013).

In this context, the early stages of neuropedagogy were limited to studying brain functions related to learning and memory. However, research in this field soon evolved to become more connected to the educational domain and teaching practices, due to the integration of other sciences such as cognitive and educational psychology, cognitive linguistics, psycholinguistics, education sciences, and didactics. As a result, neuropedagogy has become a knowledge field that brings together all these sciences, with the goal of developing and studying everything related to teaching and learning strategies.

This cognitive linkage between these disciplines has reinforced the pathways of cognitive education through the findings provided by neuroscience research on how the brain functions (Figure 1). These studies have offered new research possibilities to those interested in the educational field, leading them to the conviction that understanding brain functions and their influence by external contexts (cultural and social factors) can enable the proposal of new research approaches and strategies capable of integrating both dimensions: the internal (brain/mind) and the external (culture) of the educational entity making them two key factors in guiding and assessing the learner (Barrim, 2025).

Figure 1. Interpretation of Tokuhama-Espinosa's transdisciplinary field

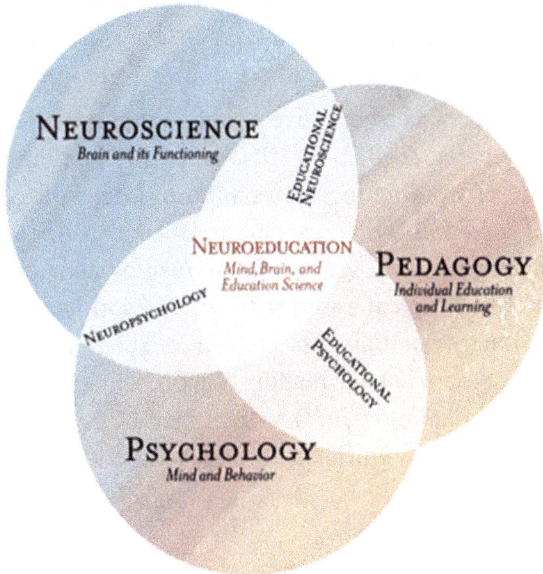

Source: Nakagawa (2008), redrawn by Bramwell (2010), in Tokuhama-Espinosa's (2010) article on Why Mind, Brain, and Education Science is the "New" Brain-Based Education. (Bang et al., 2012)

The main goal that neuropedagogy seeks to achieve is to improve the teaching and learning process by relying on how the brain functions and develops, with the aim of creating effective methods and strategies for learning. In this context, "Mind, Brain, and Education is a problem-focused interdisciplinary field that seeks to bring together biological, psychological, and educational perspectives, with the express intention of improving educational practices" (Stein & Fischer, 2011, p. 57). This implies that understanding the issues addressed by neuropedagogy can contribute to enhancing educational processes and practices across their cognitive, social, and emotional dimensions, drawing on various strands of brain research (Jansen & Kiefer, 2020). Neuropedagogy can be described as an interdisciplinary field that connects insights from neuroscience with educational sciences, aiming to enhance teaching and learning processes through a deeper understanding of the neural mechanisms underlying learners' cognitive and emotional development.

Working memory is considered one of the most important concepts that neuropedagogy takes into account in the development of the educational process, given its central role in information processing and problem-solving during learning. It is also a fundamental component of cognitive processes related to reading comprehension, as it functions as a cognitive system responsible for the temporary storage and manipulation of information needed to perform cognitive tasks such as comprehension, reading, and problem-solving.

A number of studies and research works (Zhang & Lee, 2023; Okur & Aksoy, 2025; Liu et al., 2024) have highlighted the significance of the relationship between working memory, reading comprehension, and cognitive development from a neuropedagogical perspective. In particular, Ergül et al. (2022) demonstrated in their study that working memory is a cognitive structure that influences the acquisition and development of several academic skills, especially reading and writing. Furthermore, the impact of working memory on these skills varies depending on the educational stage. The verbal and visual components of working memory produce different effects on various skills, such as fluent reading and comprehension.

This study aimed to assess the extent to which working memory influences reading comprehension by examining the correlation relationship between working memory and various components of reading comprehension (text comprehension, phonological awareness, phonological tasks, and spelling tasks), and by determining whether there are statistically significant correlations between them, By answering the following questions:

- What is the nature of the cognitive mechanisms underlying the relationship between working memory and reading comprehension?
- Does working memory affect learners' levels of reading comprehension?
- How can the findings of this study be utilized to develop effective reading comprehension strategies for learners ?

At the first level, we focused on defining the theoretical and operational concepts of the study and aligning them with educational objectives. At the second level, we connected the findings of the theoretical framework to the development of the study's applied procedures. This was achieved through the implementation of a testing toolkit composed of tests targeting working memory and reading comprehension, designed in accordance with the specificities of both the Moroccan educational context and the Arabic language. The tests were applied to a sample of one hundred (100) students equally divided between males and females that enrolled in the fourth grade of primary education at "Oulad Taib" School under the Regional Directorate of Fès. The primary aim was to determine the established relationship between working memory and reading comprehension.

The results of the study indicated that working memory has a significant impact on learners' reading comprehension levels. Moreover, training working memory can lead to positive outcomes, especially when such training is tailored to the learner's individual needs. This, in turn, supports the development of effective and appropriate instructional strategies that foster meaningful reading. In other hand, understanding the relationship between working memory and reading comprehension—and recognizing its manifestations through a neuropedagogical approach—can serve as a sound orientation for designing curricula and educational programs. It also provides a solid foundation for establishing appropriate and coherent principles in the educational content of school textbooks, in alignment with the way the learner's brain functions and with their cognitive development.

To develop this argument, the first section sets the stage by providing a literature review, the second section describes the methodology of the study, and the third section presents and discusses the findings of the study.

LITERATURE REVIEW

The Neural Mechanisms of Working Memory

Researchs in the field of neuropedagogy - which represents an intersection of neuroscience, education, and didactics - emphasizes the importance of understanding how the brain functions, particularly with regard to working memory. Working memory is regarded as a system responsible for temporarily storing and processing information to carry out various cognitive tasks, including reading comprehension and the acquisition of new skills. Understanding the neural mechanisms underlying working memory is considered one of the fundamental principles that can contribute to the development of more effective teaching methods and educational approaches.

Working memory is one of the fundamental concepts addressed by cognitive sciences, as it encompasses multiple aspects of human learning based on a set of subsystems involved in this process, with particular emphasis on its central role in various cognitive tasks such as learning, reasoning, and comprehension. As a complex and limited cognitive system, understanding the functioning of its subsystems is crucial for identifying the factors that influence language learning (Demir, 2021). Without the capacity to store information, we would be unable to adequately perceive or comprehend it, nor would we be able to connect what we are currently learning with past experiences or integrate it with future goals and planning (Baddeley & Logie, 1999).

The initial emergence of the concept of working memory can be traced back to the work of Galanter and Pribram on "Plans and the Structure of Behavior" in 1960, where the authors noted that working memory is what we use to execute our plans, functioning as a form of rapid access (Galanter & Pribram, 1960).

Subsequently, several models of memory were proposed, generally comprising three types: sensory memory, short-term memory, and long-term memory. Among these, the model that received the most attention was that of Atkinson and Shiffrin (1968) (see Figure 1), which offered a detailed analysis of the structure and functions of human memory (Demir, 2021). This system is considered capable of processing information and linking it to long-term storage, without which the acquisition and consolidation of new knowledge would not be possible (Baddeley & Logie, 1999).

Figure 2. The multi-store model of memory (MSM)

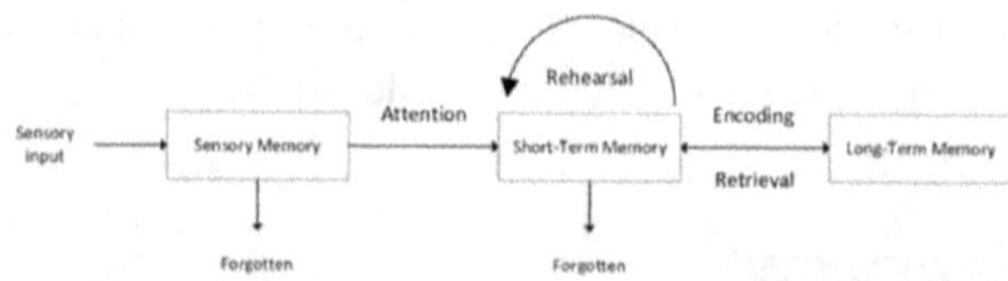

Source: Atkinson and Shiffrin (1968)

Information moves through these three types of memory in a sequential, linear process involving attention, rehearsal, and retrieval. Sensory input captured by the senses first enters sensory memory, where it is held briefly. If attention is directed to this information, it is then transferred to short-term memory. Through rehearsal – particularly elaborative rehearsal – the information is processed in a way that enables its transfer to long-term memory, where it can be stored for extended periods (McLeod, 2025). The most widely recognized model of this concept remains the multi-component model proposed by Baddeley and Hitch (1974). This model posits that working memory consists of several components: The central executive, the phonological loop, and the visuospatial sketchpad. In 2000, the episodic buffer was added as a fourth component of the model.

According to Baddeley, the central executive is considered the most important component of working memory due to its role in resource control—that is, the ability to allocate attentional resources while performing two or more cognitive tasks simultaneously (Perry & Malaia, 2013). In contrast, the phonological loop stores and processes verbal and auditory information for a few seconds before it fades. It is divided into two subcomponents: the phonological store, which receives and temporarily holds auditory information, and the articulatory control process, which rehearses verbal information, aiding in speech preparation and verbal thinking (McLeod, 2025).

Furthermore, it is essential to acknowledge that the Central Executive does more than merely direct attention to tasks or carry out the executive functions associated with the frontal lobes. It also acts as a crucial connector to long-term memory systems, supporting processes such as language comprehension and production. In addition, working memory capacity refers to the quantity of information that can be held in focus despite distractions or interference (Coolidge & Wynn, 2022). Studies have further demonstrated that working memory capacity is a moderate to strong predictor of numerous higher-level cognitive abilities, including reading and listening proficiency, vocabulary, and reading comprehension … (Kane & Engle, 2002).

Meanwhile, the visuo-spatial sketch-pad serves as a temporary visual–spatial storage system capable of holding and manipulating images. It is understood as both a cognitive structure and a mental process responsible for the temporary storage of visual and spatial information, to be used in working memory operations (Demir, 2021).

The episodic buffer, or temporary episodic memory, was added by Baddeley (2000) to address certain limitations related to the integration of information in a more effective manner. "The episodic buffer is important for learning because it uses multimodal codes to integrate representations from the components of working memory and long-term memory into unitary representations" (Dehn, 2008, P. 25). This means that the primary function of this component lies in integrating different types of information – auditory, visual, and spatial – processed by other subsystems, along with information retrieved from long-term memory (LTM), into a coherent, linear representation. This integrative role makes it essential for linking short-term memory with long-term memory (McLeod, 2025).

Figure 3. A simplified depiction

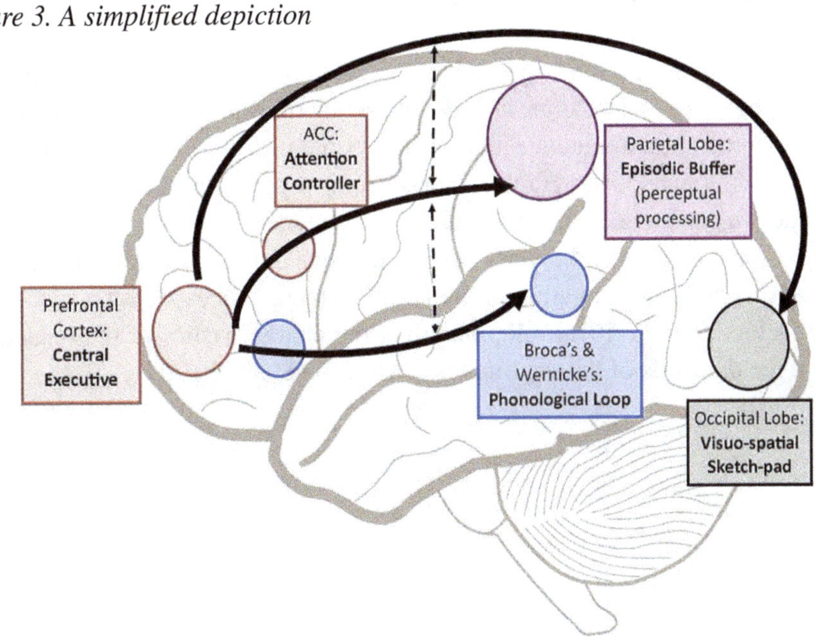

Adapted from the multicomponent working memory model by Baddeley (2010) as implicated in the brain, in which the central executive assumes the role to exert control and oversee the manipulation of incoming information for intended execution. ACC, Anterior cingulate cortex (Jia Chai, 2018)

The phonological loop is considered one of the most critical components of working memory in Baddeley's model, due to its importance in processing phonological information activated during language learning particularly in relation to reading and writing. Its role lies in enhancing learners' reading abilities by facilitating the transition from phonemes to words, decoding word structures, and ultimately supporting text comprehension. This progression highlights the influence of the phonological loop in reading development and further supports the view that working memory difficulties can significantly impact reading fluency in learners (Barrim, 2025).

It is a capacity-limited model that provides temporary storage for information encoded in a multimodal format, capable of integrating inputs from the subsystems and from long-term memory into a unified episodic representation. Conscious awareness is assumed to be the primary means of retrieving information from the buffer (Baddeley, 2000). The revised model differs from the original primarily in its emphasis on the integration of information, rather than the isolation of subsystems. As such, it offers a stronger foundation for addressing the more complex aspects of executive control within working memory (Baddeley, 2000).

Reading Comprehension and Working Memory: Between Cognitive and Linguistic Requirements

Reading comprehension relies on the execution and integration of multiple cognitive processes to determine how the mind functions in understanding what we read. Comprehending a sentence requires the visual processing of words, identifying their phonological, orthographic, and semantic representations, and integrating them to derive the intended meaning behind the sentence. The same applies to texts: the reader must process and connect individual idea units, ultimately constructing a coherent mental representation of the text. For these processes to be successful, several factors play a critical role, including the characteristics of the reader, the text, and the demands of the reading task (Kendeou et al., 2014).

Figure 4. The cognitive processes required for reading based on the Construction-Integration Model proposed by Kintsch (1988)

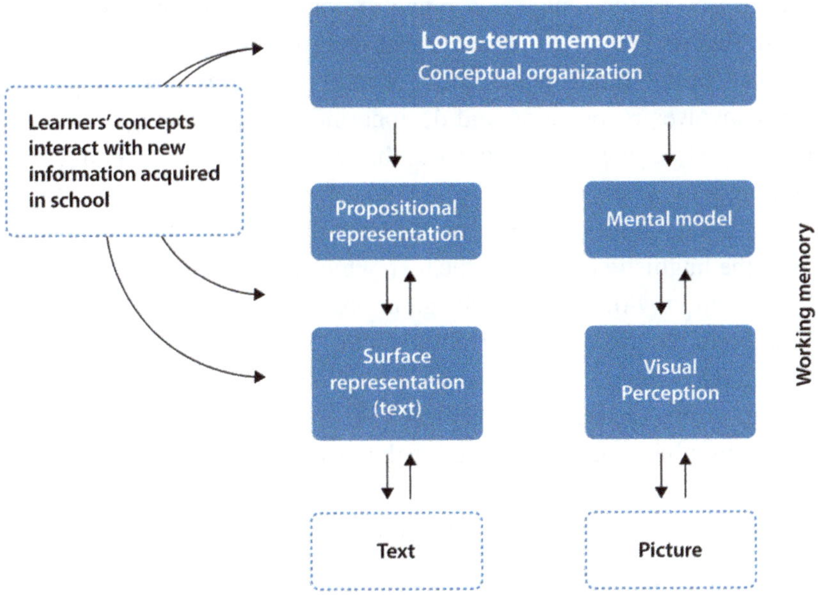

Studies suggest that the cognitive processes responsible for reading comprehension can be classified into two main types. The first can be referred to as lower-level processes, which involve decoding the written code into meaningful linguistic units. The second are known as higher-level processes, which involve integrating these units into a coherent and meaningful mental representation, relying on executive functions such as the learner's working memory capacity, attention, monitoring, and comprehension.

Reading comprehension is one of the core skills essential in language teaching and learning, as it is closely related to the learner's ability to understand and interpret both spoken and written language in a specific linguistic context. The more proficient a learner becomes in decoding and interpreting sentences and texts, the higher their level of reading comprehension.

According to a number of studies and research findings (Snow, 2002; Erya & Pustika, 2021; Smith et al., 2021), reading comprehension involves constructing and inferring meaning through interaction with texts, a process that requires linguistic knowledge of considerable depth. For learners to engage in effective and meaningful reading, they must not only be able to accurately interpret words and phrases, but also possess adequate background knowledge to derive meaning from the text's context (Smith et al., 2021).

Reading comprehension is commonly defined as the learner's ability to understand written language in a manner consistent with their educational level. It is a multifaceted process that involves a range of cognitive and linguistic functions. Gough and Tunmer (1986) emphasized that reading comprehension results from the interaction of two fundamental skills: decoding and linguistic comprehension. The former involves recognizing and deciphering written words, while the latter refers to interpreting words and sentences that contribute to the overall coherence and cohesion of the text.

This implies an ongoing interaction between the reader's skills, cognitive processes, and the linguistic features of the text, which compels the reader to integrate textual information with prior knowledge in order to construct a coherent mental representation of the text's meaning (Smith et al., 2021).

Poor reading comprehension directly affects learners' academic performance. Learners with strong reading comprehension skills tend to be more effective in critical thinking, in solving and self-correcting their learning difficulties independently, compared to those with weak comprehension abilities.

Numerous studies and research (Casado-Ledesma & Tarchi, 2024; Proctor et al., 2020; Smith et al., 2021; Srisang & Everatt, 2021) have identified several challenges that hinder students from developing effective reading comprehension skills. These include a lack of familiarity with text types, the specific complexities associated with each genre, insufficient background knowledge needed to connect with new information, limited vocabulary, and a lack of awareness of key linguistic features that play a vital role in comprehension. This suggests that students with learning difficulties often face reading fluency as a major barrier impacting multiple dimensions of the reading process. When students read slowly, they are more likely to choose shorter and simpler texts, which in turn slows down the acquisition of vocabulary and world knowledge, both of which are essential for reading comprehension (O'Connor, 2018).

Studies and research (Vernucci et al., 2013, 2019; Alloway & Gregory) related to language acquisition and learning, as well as working memory, indicate that the latter plays a significant role in the development of reading and writing skills across various educational stages, particularly in early and pre-primary education. This is attributed to the established relationship between working memory and reading comprehension, based on its influence on linguistic processing. López-Resa & Sepúlveda (2023) also pointed out that training working memory improves learners' abilities to read and comprehend texts, especially among those with dyslexia and dyscalculia. This underscores the central role of working memory in supporting complex cognitive tasks such as reading comprehension and mathematical reasoning.

Baddeley (1996) highlighted the impact of limited working memory capacity on learners' reduced levels of comprehension, based on the functional role that this capacity plays as a core cognitive component in various processing operations such as learning, understanding, and problem-solving. In the same vein, Mzeau (2005) presented significant findings regarding neurological disorders in children. His experimental study on this population demonstrated that difficulties in text comprehension are primarily due to severe impairments in verbal short-term memory. This impairment negatively affects comprehension processes during the temporary retention of phonological forms in spoken language or graphemic forms in written language.

Figure 5. Theoretical model of simple mediation of working memory by processing speed in reading comprehension.

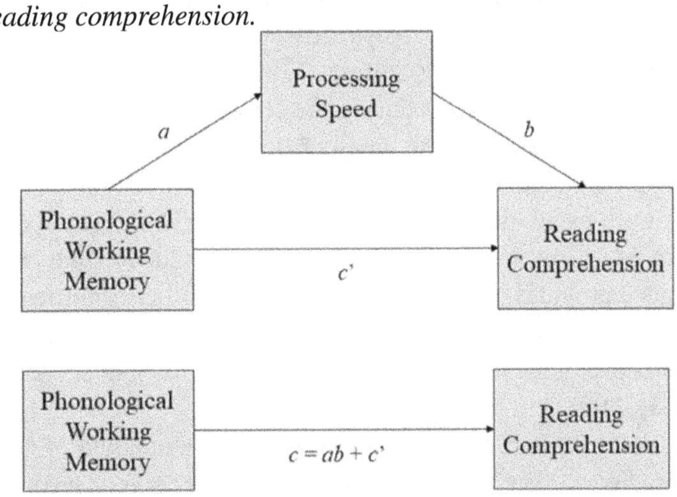

Note: a, direct effect of working memory on processing speed; b, direct effect of processing speed on reading comprehension; c', direct effect of working memory on reading comprehension; ab, indirect effect (mediated); c, total effect (Adapted from Balonyi Candal & Brandão de Avila (2025))

Proficient students are able to draw inferences from the text, which enables them to read words effortlessly as they connect prior knowledge and previously acquired ideas with new information. In contrast, less experienced readers tend to read more slowly because word recognition has not yet become automatic. As a result, they focus heavily on "getting the words off the page," which makes deep processing of the text difficult, if not impossible (O'Connor, 2018). Reading a text cannot be considered effective without understanding the meanings of words and sentences. In this context, slow and inaccurate reading may hinder clear comprehension of the written content. Word recognition becomes automatic once decoding and the integration of meaning units take place. Working memory plays a key role in integrating information at the phrase and sentence level (Kendeou et al., 2014).

The Diagnostic and Statistical Manual of Mental Disorders (DSM-5) describes slow and inaccurate reading as factors that may impair reading comprehension. Reading speed, which reflects the degree of automaticity in recognizing written words, is therefore also linked to comprehension. The meanings of linguistic units presented in the text can be integrated through higher-level cognitive processing and inferential mechanisms (Balonyi Candal & Brandão de Avila, 2025). Working memory mediates the integration of read sentences within a text and retains them until information from long-term memory can be combined with information from the text. Accordingly, working memory is considered a key predictor of reading comprehension in children (Nouwens et al., 2017).

Reading comprehension is closely linked to oral language skills such as vocabulary and syntactic structures, and it is also influenced by learners' working memory and attention capacities (Perfetti & Stafura, 2014). Working memory plays a critical role in integrating information during the comprehension and analysis of text (Swanson & O'Connor, 2009). Both cross-sectional and longitudinal studies have demonstrated that the contribution of working memory to reading comprehension remains significant even after controlling for decoding skills (Ergül et al., 2022). Findings from Swanson and Beebe-Frankenberger's (2004) study indicate that working memory provides strong predictive signals of successful reading among typically developing children. Moreover, working memory plays a greater role in the acquisition and development of reading comprehension than in decoding (Savage, Lavers, & Pillay, 2007).

This necessitates a thorough investigation and understanding of how working memory and reading comprehension interact, as language comprehension—whether spoken or written—requires the processing of a sequence of symbols produced and perceived over time. This process is fundamentally linked to the relationship between reading comprehension and working memory. Consequently, increasing the speed at which essential reading-related information is processed enhances the availability of cognitive resources in memory for comprehension. In contrast, slow or inefficient lexical processing limits the cognitive resources needed to construct a mental model in working memory for inferential reasoning (Balonyi Candal & Brandão de Avila, 2025). Therefore, the aim of this study is to shed light on the relationship between working memory and reading comprehension among primary school students (Level 4).

METHODOLOGY

This study relied on field research based on observation, formulation of hypotheses and their testing, followed by analysis and discussion of the results. In this context, the study sought to measure the relationships between working memory and reading comprehension skills, to assess the extent to which the former influences the latter, and to verify the existence of statistically significant correlations between them among fourth-grade students in Moroccan primary education. A number of similar studies in the global context confirm the importance of working memory and training in developing various language skills, particularly those related to reading comprehension.

Study Hypotheses

In light of the theoretical presentation of the concepts and theoretical models explaining the relationship between working memory and reading comprehension, and based on previous studies closely related to the subject, as previously highlighted, and in alignment with the questions posed in the research problem, a general hypothesis and operational hypotheses related to each variable can be formulated as follows:

- General Hypothesis:
    - There is a statistically significant correlation between working memory and reading comprehension among fourth-grade primary school students.
- Operational Hypotheses:
    - Working memory has an effect on reading comprehension among the study sample.
    - There are statistically significant differences in working memory among the study sample attributable to the gender variable.
    - There no are statistically significant differences in reading comprehension among the study samples attributable to the gender variable.

Study Participants

This study included a sample of 100 male and female students enrolled in the fourth grade of primary education at a Moroccan public school—Oulad Taib School, under the supervision of the Provincial Directorate of Fes.

Table 1. Details of the study sample

School	Grade Level	Total	Male	Female	Average Age
Oulad Taib School	Fourth Grade	100	50	50	10

Study Instruments

This study relied on two main tests: one measuring working memory and the other measuring reading comprehension.

- Working Memory Scale: This tool measures an individual's ability to retain and process information by repeating a sequence of numbers either in the same order (forward recall) or in reverse order (backward recall).
- Reading Comprehension Test: This is a subtest from the Gates-MacGinitie Reading Tests (GMRT), a globally recognized and reliable test for measuring reading comprehension across different age levels, ranging from pre-readers to proficient adult readers. This task consisted of short passages presented randomly to participants, each ranging from three to four sentences and accompanied by multiple-choice questions. After reading the passage aloud, the student was required to select the correct answer. Selecting the correct answer indicated proper comprehension of the text, whereas choosing an incorrect answer served as a clear indicator of comprehension difficulty.

The validity and reliability checks for the reading comprehension scale included two methods:

- Judgmental validity (face validity): The researchers presented the initial version of the test items to external referees specializing in linguistics and psychology, with the aim of assessing the appropriateness of each item for measuring the predetermined relationship between working memory and reading comprehension, in light of the dimension to which it belongs and its operational definition. In addition, they evaluated the linguistic formulation of the scale items and assessed their validity in relation to the purpose for which the scale was designed.
- Construct validity (internal consistency): The researchers administered the test to a pilot sample of 30 male and female students randomly selected from the original study population. Based on the results, Pearson's correlation coefficient was calculated between the score of each item and the total score, as shown in Table 2.

Table 2. Correlation coefficient between each item score and the total score of the reading comprehension scale

Item	Correlation Coefficient	Item	Correlation Coefficient
1	.457**	11	.270**
2	.356**	12	.495**
3	.445**	13	.498**
4	.586**	14	.414**
5	.350**	15	.395**
6	.530**	16	.390**
7	.394**	17	.530**
8	.296**	18	.375**
9	.221*	19	.259**
10	.597**		

Note: $p < .05$ (*), $p < .01$ (**)

In order to verify the study's hypotheses, the researchers relied on the Excel program and the Statistical Package for the Social Sciences (SPSS) version 26 to enter the data, organize them into tables and charts, and process and analyze them using descriptive statistics, which describe the results, and inferential statistics, which provide indications and interpretations of the obtained results. Regarding the statistical methods used, they were selected – especially those related to testing the study's hypotheses – based on the nature of the variables, their levels of measurement, and the extent to which the fundamental assumptions and conditions necessary for applying a given test were met.

Table 3. Statistical methods and tools used in the study

Purpose	Statistical Method	Statistical Tool
Studying the relationship	Correlation	Pearson correlation
Studying the effect	Regression	Simple regression
Studying differences by gender	Test of differences	*T*-test & ANOVA

RESULTS

The test results revealed a significant correlation between working memory and reading comprehension skills among fourth-grade primary school students. This correlation coefficient reflects the relationship between working memory and the levels of processing required for reading comprehension. The results confirmed a positive correlation of 0.239, indicating a direct relationship between working memory and reading comprehension; in other words, the higher a learner's working memory capacity, the better their reading comprehension performance to varying degrees. This finding highlights the important role that working memory plays in reading comprehension among primary school students, particularly at the fourth-grade level—a stage in which learners transition from learning how to read to reading in order to develop comprehension strategies.

Table 4. The correlation coefficient between working memory and reading comprehension

	Working Memory	Reading Comprehension Variable
Working Memory	Pearson Correlation	1
	Sig. (2-tailed)	
	N	100
Reading Comprehension Variable	Pearson Correlation	**.239***
	Sig. (2-tailed)	.016
	N	100

Note: The correlation is statistically significant at the 0.05 level (2-tailed). The asterisk (*) indicates statistical significance at $p < .05$.

Using both external and internal comparison strategies, the general hypothesis proposed in this study can be confirmed, as the statistically significant relationship between working memory and reading comprehension skills among students at this grade level is evident. Furthermore, the internal comparison confirms that the working memory scale directly reflects the learner's ability to connect sentences within a text, process related information in working memory, analyze it, and recall what was read at the beginning of the text to understand its overall meaning and choose the correct answer accordingly.

Additionally, the results of the simple regression analysis showed that the working memory variable has a statistically significant effect on reading comprehension, with a regression coefficient of $B = 0.341$. This indicates that each one-point increase in the learner's working memory score leads to a corresponding 0.341-point increase in their reading comprehension score. The p-value was 0.016, which is lower than the significance threshold of 0.05, confirming the presence of a statistically significant effect.

The regression line (straight line) can be expressed by the equation: $Y = 3.868 + 0.341X$. Here, 3.868 is the intercept (the point where the line crosses the vertical axis when working memory = 0), and 0.341 is the Positive slope, indicating that for each one-unit increase in working memory, reading comprehension increases by 0.341 units. The positive direction of the relationship (0.341) indicates a direct correlation between working memory and reading comprehension; that is, an improvement in working memory is associated with an improvement in reading comprehension, as illustrated in Figure (4), which shows a positive linear relationship between the two variables. This means that higher working memory scores tend to predict better reading comprehension performance.

Figure 6. Positive relationship between working memory and reading comprehension

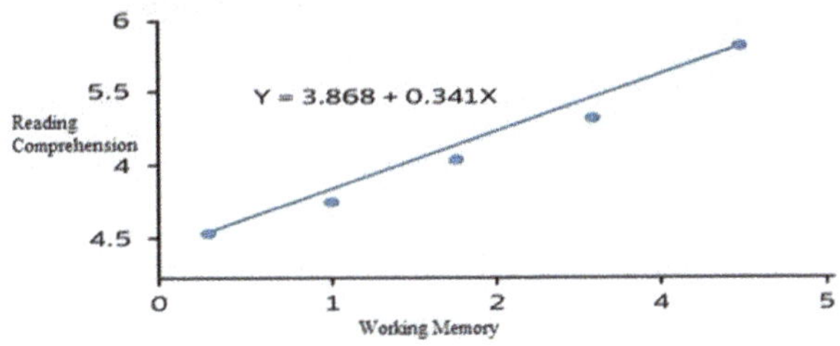

The scatterplot illustrates a positive correlation (r = 0.239, p = 0.016) between working memory scores and reading comprehension scores among the study participants (N = 100) (Figure 5). The upward-sloping red trend line, obtained through simple linear regression, indicates that higher working memory capacity tends to be associated with higher reading comprehension performance. Although the correlation is statistically significant at the 0.05 level, the effect size is small according to Cohen's (1988) benchmarks. This suggests that working memory contributes partially to the variance in reading comprehension, while other cognitive and linguistic factors may play a more substantial role (Peng et al., 2018).

Figure 7. Scatter plot of working memory scores and reading comprehension scores among the study participants

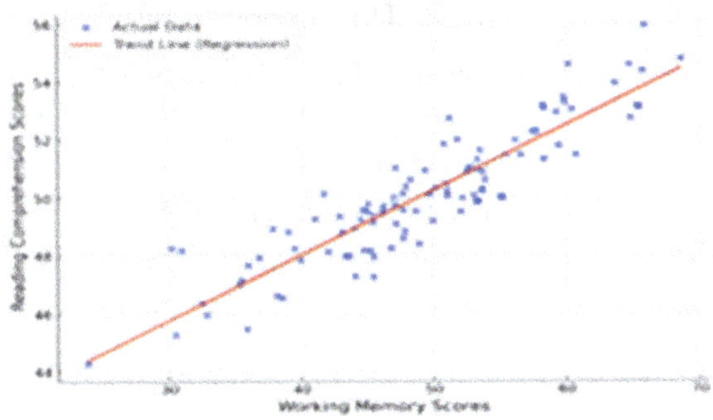

DISCUSSION

The results revealed that the statistical significance value (Sig. = 0.016) for the relationship between working memory and reading comprehension among fourth-grade primary school pupils is less than 0.05, indicating that the correlation is statistically significant at the 95% confidence level. This means the relationship is unlikely to be due to chance and can be generalized to the statistical sample, considering its size (N = 100). This finding reinforces the reliability of the results in relation to the research problem on whether there is a statistically significant relationship between working memory and reading comprehension.

Using simple linear regression analysis, supported by the associated statistical tests, it was found that working memory (the independent variable) has an effect on reading comprehension (the dependent variable) among the participants.

The Pearson correlation coefficient between working memory and reading comprehension further demonstrated that the former plays an important role in determining reading comprehension levels in fourth-grade pupils, although it is not the sole factor. This is due to the inherent complexities of reading comprehension, which involve other contributing factors linked to the specific nature of the Arabic language—such as the richness of its vocabulary, the multiple possible meanings a single word may hold depending on context, and the extensive morphological structures of words.

This explains why the moderate correlation value indicates that improving reading comprehension cannot rely solely on developing working memory but also requires enhancing other supportive skills. This aligns with the Interactive Models of Reading, which posit that comprehension is the result of interactions among multiple cognitive and linguistic components (Perfetti & Stafura, 2014). While part of the variance in reading comprehension can be explained by working memory, other factors also contribute to this effect.

A British study on children with reading comprehension difficulties confirmed that deficits in working memory lead to challenges in making inferences and connecting information within a text, which in turn hinders the construction of a coherent mental model of the text (Oakhill & Cain, 2007). This supports our findings, which highlight the importance of working memory in linking information and understanding texts.

Furthermore, the results showed statistically significant differences in working memory attributable to gender among the participants, as revealed by the Independent Samples T-Test (Table 4). The mean score for females (M = 11.58) was higher than that for males (M = 10.28), with a difference of 1.30 points, indicating that females possess higher working memory capacity compared to males.

Table 5. Independent samples t-test results for working memory

	Gender	N	Std. Deviation	Std. Error Mean
Working Memory	Male	50	**10.2800**	2.42470
	Female	50	**11.5800**	2.71120

This result can be interpreted in light of findings from several experimental studies (Zamarreño et al., 2024 …) that used functional near-infrared spectroscopy (fNIRS) during dual-task paradigms. These studies revealed differences in functional connectivity of the prefrontal cortex between genders, with females demonstrating higher accuracy and fewer errors compared to males—particularly under increased cognitive load. The researchers attributed this to gender-related differences in the performance of working brain networks, supporting the existence of working memory differences under specific task conditions.

Moreover, a large meta-analysis comprising 478 samples, 284 studies, and 802 measures found a small but statistically significant female advantage in verbal memory tasks, such as word recall and recognition. The overall effect size was $d = 0.028$ for general tasks and ranged from $d = 0.079$ to 0.145 for specific tasks, implicitly supporting the presence of significant differences favoring females in certain aspects of verbal working memory (Hirnstein et al., 2021).

Similarly, Pergher et al. (2021), using an N-Back task with increasing difficulty levels in both young and older adult groups, found that women benefited more than men from repetition-related learning effects in countering mental fatigue. In other words, females demonstrated better working memory performance across task levels compared to males, suggesting a significant advantage for females in certain mental workload conditions.

The results obtained using the same test (Independent Samples T-Test) also showed no statistically significant differences in reading comprehension based on gender among the participants (Table 5). The means were similar ($M = 7.50$ for males and $M = 7.68$ for females), and the T-test did not reveal any significant differences between males and females. This finding supports our hypothesis that there are no statistically significant differences in reading comprehension attributable to gender.

Table 6. Independent samples t-test results for reading comprehension

	Gender	N	Mean	Standard Deviation	Standard Error Mean
Reading Comprehension	Male	50	**7.50**	**3.84**	0.543
	Female	50	**7.68**	**3.71**	0.525

This can be interpreted in connection with the findings of a set of studies (Tian et al., 2023…) on the relationship between gender and reading skills, which reported no differences between males and females in reading comprehension performance. Accordingly, the results of the present study support the hypothesis that gender is not a strong determinant of reading comprehension.

Consequently, the relationship between Working Memory (WM) and reading comprehension, as noted by Márquez Osorio (2025), constitutes a growing focus of inquiry within educational and neuropsychological research. This interest is predicated on the understanding that WM serves as a critical process in proficient reading. It functions not merely as a system for the temporary storage of information but also as a mechanism for integrating new information with prior knowledge to construct and enhance overall comprehension.

CONCLUSION AND RECOMMENDATIONS

The findings of this study concluded that working memory constitutes a key factor in supporting reading comprehension among the participants. A statistically significant correlation was found between the two variables, in addition to a direct and notable effect of working memory on reading comprehension performance. The T-test results also revealed statistically significant differences between males and females in working memory performance, whereas no differences were recorded in reading comprehension based on gender. This confirms that reading comprehension performance is not influenced by gender differences, despite variations in working memory capacity.

This suggests that part of the relationship between working memory and reading comprehension is consistent with findings from various studies and research in both Arab and international contexts (Bouanani, 2022; Al-Otaibi & Al-Zahrani, 2021; Gathercole & Baddeley, 2014 …), which have confirmed the strong and positive association between working memory capacity and the level of reading comprehension in learners, particularly when processing and analyzing complex texts. These studies have also highlighted the difficulties learners encounter in reading comprehension as a result of weak working memory.

From a neuro-pedagogical perspective, issues related to the relationship between working memory and reading comprehension are of significant importance, given their connection to how students can improve and train their working memory in the shortest possible time and with minimal linguistic and cognitive cost. This can be achieved by developing pedagogical and didactic methods that teachers can employ to enhance students' reading comprehension through working memory training. The key factor in this process is not necessarily the strategies used in the reading activity itself, but rather the speed at which students can process essential reading skill information and the effect this has on the availability of working memory resources to facilitate comprehension.

In addition, working memory serves as a critical cognitive component by providing a mental workspace that enables learners to temporarily store and manipulate information while engaging in higher-order processing activities essential for reading comprehension. The efficacy with which learners execute these cognitive operations represents a foundational element for the effective processing and integration of educational content within the formal curriculum. A core demand of such learning tasks is the concurrent maintenance and processing of information. For instance, a learner might be required to retain the semantic content of a sentence in working memory while sequentially retrieving and applying orthographic knowledge to spell its constituent words. Similarly, successful task completion often depends on the ability to retain and serially execute a multi-step sequence of instructions provided by the teacher.

Among the pedagogical and didactic suggestions that can contribute to improving working memory to support reading comprehension in students are:

- Gradual progression from simple to complex: Present information related to the target texts in a gradual manner by dividing texts into short sentences, then longer sentences, and eventually short paragraphs. This avoids overloading the student's working memory with too much information at once, enabling them to process and understand it effectively and achieve higher levels of comprehension.
- Encouraging connections with prior knowledge: Promote linking what students read with previously acquired knowledge from past reading activities through tests and educational exercises, creating cognitive associations and mental maps that integrate new information with what has already been learned.
- Considering individual differences: Design educational activities that take into account students' individual differences, adapting teaching strategies to variations in working memory performance between males and females.
- Incorporating innovative teaching techniques: Use educational games and cognitive exercises that activate working memory to enhance reading comprehension.
- Using repetition for reinforcement: Repeatedly present information orally or in writing to consolidate it in students' memory. Research supports the hypothesis that lexical units in the mental lexicon can be organized and processed effectively through repetition.

- Highlighting key words: Guide students to identify key words in the text to infer semantic relationships, providing them with a preliminary understanding of the overall meaning and enabling the construction of mental representations of ideas or events mentioned in the text.
- Summarizing paragraphs: Train students to summarize each paragraph using short sentences, helping them offload processed information from working memory to understand the text's ideas.
- Allocating specific time for working memory exercises: Conduct activities aimed at training working memory to support reading comprehension, as illustrated in the table below:

Table 7. Activities and exercises to train the student's working memory

Learning Activity	The Student's Task	Activity Objective
Sequential memory	Repeat or arrange a list of words or sentences from the text.	Ability to recall information in a specific order.
Multiple choice	Identify synonyms, antonyms, or words that do not belong to the text's semantic field from given options.	Enrich the student's vocabulary.
Active recall	Identify one or two main ideas from specific paragraphs (first, second, etc.).	Activate memory by retrieving and recalling information.
Sentence/text completion exercises	Find appropriate words or sentences to complete a sentence or short text based on the context in which they should be used.	Activate semantic knowledge of words and extract semantic relationships.

- Reducing cognitive load by segmenting information: Providing instructions or content in smaller, manageable units rather than as a single complex set. For instance, instead of giving a multi-step directive such as " instead of providing a multi-step instruction such as "Read the entire sentence or paragraph…" each action should be communicated sequentially to facilitate comprehension and memory retention.
- Reinforce critical information through repetition: Key rules, instructions, or expectations should be reiterated regularly, both orally and in writing, to strengthen retention and support working memory during task execution.
- Pre-teach essential vocabulary knowledge: Introduce and familiarize learners with critical terminology prior to engaging in tasks, enabling them to retain, understand, and apply relevant information effectively within learning activities.

- Future research: Conduct further studies to expand the scope to different grade levels and multiple languages, aiming to generalize findings and develop more effective teaching strategies.

In conclusion, it is difficult to conceive a pedagogical strategy for enhancing reading comprehension in primary school students, particularly at the fourth-grade level, without systematic and structured training of working memory. Working memory is a crucial component that provides cognitive and linguistic depth, reinforcing reading comprehension in relation to the topics and phenomena covered by the Arabic language curriculum at this grade level. It serves as a mental engine that simultaneously retains and processes information to meet students' needs in understanding, analyzing, and interpreting texts.

REFERENCES

Alloway, T. P., & Alloway, R. G. (2013). Working memory across the lifespan: A cross-sectional approach. *Journal of Cognitive Psychology*, *25*(1), 84–93. DOI: 10.1080/20445911.2012.748027

Alotaibi, A., & Alzahrani, K. (2021). The effect of working memory on reading skills among middle school students. *The Journal of Educational Research*, *12*(2), 78–95.

Atkinson, R. C., & Shiffrin, R. M. (1968). Human memory: A proposed system and its control processes. In Spence, K. W., & Spence, J. T. (Eds.), *The psychology of learning and motivation: Advances in research and theory* (Vol. 2, pp. 89–195). Academic Press., DOI: 10.1016/S0079-7421(08)60422-3

Baddeley, A. (2010). Working memory. *Current Biology*, *20*(4), R136–R140. DOI: 10.1016/j.cub.2009.12.014

Baddeley, A. D. (1996). Exploring the central executive. *The Quarterly Journal of Experimental Psychology. A, Human Experimental Psychology*, *49*(1), 5–28. DOI: 10.1080/713755608

Baddeley, A. D. (2000). The episodic buffer: A new component of working memory? *Trends in Cognitive Sciences*, *4*(11), 417–423. DOI: 10.1016/S1364-6613(00)01538-2

Baddeley, A. D., & Hitch, G. J. (1974). Working memory. In Bower, G. A. (Ed.), *Recent advances in learning and motivation* (Vol. 8, pp. 47–89). Academic Press., DOI: 10.1016/S0079-7421(08)60452-1

Baddeley, A. D., & Logie, R. H. (1999). Working memory: The multiple-component model. In Miyake, A., & Shah, P. (Eds.), *Models of working memory: Mechanisms of active maintenance and executive control* (pp. 28–61). Cambridge University Press., DOI: 10.1017/CBO9781139174909.005

Balonyi Candal, D., & Brandão de Ávila, C. (2025). Phonological working memory and linguistic processing speed in inferential reading comprehension. *Psicologia: Reflexão e Crítica : Revista Semestral do Departamento de Psicologia da UFRGS*, *38*(20), 2–16. DOI: 10.1186/s41155-025-00356-z

Bang, D., Chen, J., Lapointe, R., & Naqi, S. (2012). Mind, brain, and education. *Cognitive Neuroscience*. https://etec512cognitiveneuroscience.wordpress.com/5-mind-brain-and-education/

Barrim, M. (2025). The Role of memory in language processing in learner: Phonological memory and semantic memory as a model. *Atae Journal for Studies and Research, 18*, 65–81.

Casado-Ledesma, L., & Tarchi, C. (2024). The influence of textual genre in multiple-text comprehension. *Learning and Instruction, 93*, 101947. Advance online publication. DOI: 10.1016/j.learninstruc.2024.101947

Chai, W., Abd Hamid, A., & Abdullah, J. M. (2018). Working memory from the psychological and neurosciences perspectives: A review. *Frontiers in Psychology, 9*, 401. Advance online publication. DOI: 10.3389/fpsyg.2018.00401

Coolidge, F. L., & Wynn, T. (2022). *The Evolution of Working Memory and Language. The Cambridge Handbook of Working Memory and Language*. Cambridge University Press., DOI: 10.1017/9781108955638.006

Dehn, M. J. (2008). *Working memory and academic learning: Assessment and intervention*. John Wiley & Sons, Inc.

Demir, B. (2021). Working memory model and language learning. *International Journal of Education, 9*(2), 1–8. DOI: 10.34293/education.v9iS2-Sep.4366

Ding, J., Zhang, Y., Liang, P., & Li, X. (2023). Modulation of working memory capacity on predictive processing during language comprehension. *Language, Cognition and Neuroscience, 38*(8), 1133–1152. DOI: 10.1080/23273798.2023.2212819

Ergül, C., Akoğlu, G., Ökcün Akçamuş, M., Kılıç Tülü, B., Bahap Kudret, Z., & Demir, E. (2022). The contribution of working memory to reading fluency and reading comprehension performance: Longitudinal results. *Education in Science, 47*(211), 1–23. DOI: 10.15390/EB.2022.10701

Erya, W. I., & Pustika, R. (2021). Students' perception towards the use of Webtoon to improve reading comprehension skill. *Journal of English Language Teaching and Learning, 2*(1), 51–56. DOI: 10.33365/jeltl.v2i1.762

Gathercole, S. E., & Baddeley, A. D. (2014). Working memory and language: An overview. *Journal of Communication Disorders, 36*(3), 189–208.

Gough, P. B., & Tunmer, W. E. (1986). Decoding, reading, and reading disability. *Remedial and Special Education, 7*(1), 6–10. DOI: 10.1177/074193258600700104

Jansen, K., & Kiefer, S. M. (2020). Understanding brain development: Investing in young adolescents' cognitive and social-emotional development. *Middle School Journal, 51*(1), 18–25. DOI: 10.1080/00940771.2020.1787749

Kandel, E. R., Schwartz, J. H., Jessell, T. M., Siegelbaum, S. A., & Hudspeth, A. J. (2013). *Principles of neural science* (5th ed.). McGraw-Hill Education.

Kane, M. J., & Engle, R. W. (2002). The role of prefrontal cortex in workingmemory capacity, executive attention, and general fluid intelligence: An individual-differences perspective. *Psychonomic Bulletin & Review*, *9*(4), 637–671. DOI: 10.3758/BF03196323

Kendeou, P., van den Broek, P., Helder, A., & Karlsson, J. (2014). A cognitive view of reading comprehension: Implications for reading difficulties. *Learning Disabilities Research & Practice*, *29*(1), 10–16. DOI: 10.1111/ldrp.12025

Liu, S., Li, N., Zhang, X., Wang, L., & Liu, D. (2024). Effects of working memory and visual search skill on Chinese reading comprehension: Examining the simple view of reading. *Reading and Writing*, *38*(2), 329–351. DOI: 10.1007/s11145-024-10515-w

López-Resa, P., & Moraleda-Sepúlveda, E. (2023). Working memory capacity and text comprehension performance in children with dyslexia and dyscalculia: A pilot study. *Frontiers in Psychology*, *14*, 1191304. Advance online publication. DOI: 10.3389/fpsyg.2023.1191304

Márquez, F. (2025). The Relationship between Working Memory and Reading Comprehension in Elementary School Children. *Pensamiento Americano*, *18*(36), 1–12. DOI: 10.21803/penamer.18.36.873

McLeod, S. (2025). Working memory model. *Simply Psychology*. https://www.simplypsychology.org/a-level-memory.html?nowprocket=1

Mzeau, M. (2005). *Neuropsychologie de l'enfant: Troubles développementaux et acquis*. Éditions Masson.

Nouwens, S., Groen, M. A., & Verhoeven, L. (2017). How working memory relates to children's reading comprehension: The importance of domain-specificity in storage and processing. *Reading and Writing*, *30*(1), 105–120. DOI: 10.1007/s11145-016-9665-5

O'Connor, R. (2018). Reading fluency and students with reading disabilities: How fast is fast enough to promote reading comprehension? *Journal of Learning Disabilities*, *51*(2), 124–136. DOI: 10.1177/0022219417691835

Oakhill, J., & Cain, K. (2007). The precursors of reading ability in young readers: Evidence from a longitudinal study. *Reading and Writing*, *20*(1), 1–28. DOI: 10.1007/s11145-006-9021-5

Okur, M., & Aksoy, V. (2025). The effect of a working memory intervention package on the working memory performance of primary school students with specific learning disabilities. *Behavioral Sciences (Basel, Switzerland)*, *15*(3), 3–22. DOI: 10.3390/bs15030356

Peng, P., Barnes, M. A., Wang, C., Wang, W., Li, S., Swanson, H. L., Dardick, W., & Tao, S. (2018). A meta-analysis on the relation between reading and working memory. *Psychological Bulletin*, *144*(1), 48–76. DOI: 10.1037/bul0000124

Perfetti, C., & Stafura, J. (2014). Word knowledge in a theory of reading comprehension. *Scientific Studies of Reading*, *18*(1), 22–37. DOI: 10.1080/10888438.2013.827687

Perfetti, C. A., & Stafura, J. Z. (2014). Word knowledge in a theory of reading comprehension. *Scientific Studies of Reading*, *18*(1), 22–37. DOI: 10.1080/10888438.2013.827687

Pergher, V., Vanbilsen, N., & Van Hulle, M. (2021). The effect of mental fatigue and gender on working memory performance during repeated practice by young and older adults. *Neural Plasticity*, *2021*, 6612805. Advance online publication. DOI: 10.1155/2021/6612805

Perry, T., & Malaia, E. (2013). Working memory intervention: A reading comprehension approach. In *Proceedings of the International Association for Development of the Information Society (IADIS) International Conference on Cognition and Exploratory Learning in the Digital Age (CELDA)* (pp. 3–9). IADIS.

Proctor, C. P., Silverman, R. D., Harring, J. R., Jones, R. L., & Hartranft, A. M. (2020). Teaching bilingual learners: Effects of a language-based reading intervention on academic language and reading comprehension in grades 4 and 5. *Reading Research Quarterly*, *55*(1), 95–122. DOI: 10.1002/rrq.258

Savage, R., Lavers, N., & Pillay, V. (2007). Working memory and reading difficulties: What we know and what we don't know about the relationship. *Educational Psychology Review*, *19*(2), 185–221. DOI: 10.1007/s10648-006-9024-1

Smith, R., Snow, P., Serry, T., & Hammond, L. (2021). The role of background knowledge in reading comprehension: A critical review. *Reading Psychology*, *42*(3), 214–240. DOI: 10.1080/02702711.2021.1888348

Snow, C. (2002). *Reading for understanding: Toward an R&D program in reading comprehension*. Rand Corporation.

Srisang, P., & Everatt, J. (2021). Lower and higher level comprehension skills of undergraduate EFL learners and their reading comprehension. *LEARN Journal: Language Education and Acquisition Research Network*, *14*(1), 427–454.

Stein, Z., & Fischer, K. (2011). Directions for mind, brain, and education: Methods, models and morality. *Educational Philosophy and Theory*, *43*(1), 56–66. DOI: 10.1111/j.1469-5812.2010.00708.x

Swanson, H. L., & Beebe-Frankenberger, M. (2004). The relationship between working memory and mathematical problem solving in children at risk and not at risk for serious math difficulties. *Journal of Educational Psychology*, *96*(3), 471–491. DOI: 10.1037/0022-0663.96.3.471

Swanson, H. L., & O'Connor, R. (2009). The role of working memory and fluency practice on the reading comprehension of students who are dysfluent readers. *Journal of Learning Disabilities*, *42*(6), 548–575. DOI: 10.1177/0022219409338742

Tian, X., Abdul Samat, N., & Zainal, Z. (2023). Gender differences in Chinese EFL learners' comprehension when reading across mediums. *English Language Teaching*, *17*(3), 32–44. DOI: 10.5539/elt.v17n3p32

Vernucci, S., Canet Juric, L., Introzzi, I., & Richards, M. (2019). Working memory training in children: A review of basic methodological criteria. *Psychological Reports*, *123*(3), 1–18. DOI: 10.1177/0033294119832978

Zamarreño, P., Mateos, P. M., & Valentín, A. (2024). Working memory training improves episodic memory in older people: Transfer based on controlled retrieval processes. *Frontiers in Psychology*, *15*, 1–11. DOI: 10.3389/fpsyg.2024.1314483

Chapter 8

The Neuropedagogical Perspective on Play in Early Childhood

Lügen Ceren Güneş
https://orcid.org/0000-0003-1923-4491
Department of Child Development, Faculty of Health Sciences, Ankara University, Turkey

Ender Durualp
https://orcid.org/0000-0002-6645-6815
Department of Child Development, Faculty of Health Sciences, Ankara University, Turkey

ABSTRACT

This chapter examines play in early childhood through a neuropedagogical lens, emphasizing its developmental, neuroscientific, and educational significance. Play is framed not as leisure but as a biologically grounded process that supports executive functions, self-regulation, language, memory, and social interaction by activating the prefrontal cortex, limbic system, mirror neurons, and cerebellum. While neuroscience highlights its role in synaptic plasticity, stress regulation, and emotional security, its translation into practice remains limited. Literature often notes the benefits of play but lacks frameworks linking brain-based evidence with pedagogy. To address this gap, the chapter outlines neuropedagogical principles and illustrates their application through Reggio Emilia, Tools of the Mind, and Forest School. It concludes that adoption requires neuroscience-informed teacher training, curriculum design, culturally responsive adaptations, and evidence-based assessment, positioning play as both a neurological necessity and a frontier in early childhood education.

DOI: 10.4018/979-8-3373-3581-0.ch008

INTRODUCTION

Education is a fundamental process that develops the cognitive, emotional, and social potential of the individual and enables the structuring of thinking, reasoning, and problem-solving capacities. One of the most critical stages of this process is early childhood, encompassing the first years of life. According to national and international definitions, this period, generally referring to the age range of 0–6, is a developmental stage in which children's potential emerges most rapidly and is therefore often described as the "golden age." Neuroscientific research demonstrates that approximately 50% of a child's intelligence potential develops within the first four years of life, while brain development reaches nearly 80% by the age of eight, achieving optimal capacity at 100% by the age of eighteen. During this period, children lay the foundations not only for basic cognitive and motor skills but also for higher-order cognitive abilities such as emotional regulation, social interaction, and problem-solving, which are essential throughout life. The development of emotions can be observed from infancy; basic emotions such as joy, anger, sadness, and fear emerge within the first six months of life and directly influence learning capacity (Widhiyanti, 2023). Negative emotional states, particularly stress, can adversely affect the structure and function of brain cells, thereby hindering learning processes (Blum, 2024). Therefore, ensuring emotional security and creating positive learning environments in early childhood education are of critical importance for children's capacities to learn, develop, and cope with challenges (Murray et al., 2025).

Today, brain-based learning approaches are increasingly addressed with growing interest in early childhood education. These approaches aim to optimize learning processes by integrating neuroscientific findings into educational programs (Tokuhama-Espinosa, 2021; Widhiyanti, 2023). From a neuroscientific and evolutionary perspective, play—through its various forms such as object use, movement, and social interaction—is not merely an entertaining activity but also an adaptive mechanism that supports learning. Research demonstrates that during play, neurotransmitters associated with reward mechanisms, such as dopamine, are released, reinforcing learning processes while balancing cortisol levels and reducing stress. Both animal experiments and human studies have revealed that play experiences contribute to rehearsing life skills in a safe environment, fostering risk-taking behaviors, and learning boundaries. Furthermore, play serves as an important tool for the transmission of cultural values; play preferences across different cultures shape the development of individuals' social skills (Wang & Aamodt, 2012).

From a neuropedagogical perspective, play is not merely a leisure activity but an indispensable learning tool in terms of structural brain development, the strengthening of neural networks, the support of executive functions, and the reinforcement of emotional regulation mechanisms (Diamond, 2013; Panksepp, 2007). Therefore, the planning of play-based and brain-focused learning environments during early childhood is considered a strategic necessity for both individual development and the enhancement of lifelong learning capacity (Tokuhama-Espinosa, 2021; Fisher et al., 2008).

1. Purpose and Significance of the Chapter

The primary aim of this chapter is to explain the neuropedagogical foundations of play in early childhood and to demonstrate, in light of scientific evidence, the reciprocal interaction between brain development and learning processes. Play, beyond being an activity that children simply enjoy, is an indispensable neuroscience-based learning tool that holistically supports their cognitive, emotional, and social development (Whole Child Neuro, 2024). Therefore, this study examines how play experiences in early childhood integrate with the principles of brain-based learning.

The chapter first addresses the basic principles of brain development in early childhood and the significance of "sensitive periods," followed by a discussion on neural integration through play, the support of executive functions, and the provision of emotional security. This approach aims to highlight the role of incorporating neuroscientific data into the design of educational environments in meeting children's developmental needs. From an interdisciplinary perspective—bringing together neuroscience, pedagogical theory, and developmental psychology—this chapter holds importance for contributing to evidence-based, effective, and sustainable practices in early childhood education. Understanding neuropedagogical approaches to play will assist teachers and educational planners in designing learning environments that consider children's individual differences and developmental needs. In this way, both structural and functional brain development will be supported, while also laying solid foundations for lifelong learning and adaptive skills.

2. The Developmental Value of Play

Play is an activity as old as human history and is not exclusive to childhood; it is also regarded as an important necessity for youth, adults, and the elderly. From the perspective of developmental psychology, play is a fundamental learning tool that supports children's mental, emotional, social, and physical development. Toys are an important part of this process, as they facilitate children's understanding of their environment and self-expression through experiential learning. Play, whether rule-based or unstructured, allows children to experience emotions such as happiness, excitement, and enthusiasm, to express themselves freely, and to gain self-awareness. According to Erikson's theory, play is an activity that provides clues about mental development and emerges in different forms at each developmental stage. In this context, play—supporting physical, motor, cognitive, emotional, and social development—is an indispensable process and a basic necessity for children to complete their healthy development, as essential as nutrition, love, and care (Polat & Kara, 2023). Furthermore, neuroscientific research demonstrates that play activates different regions of the brain simultaneously, strengthens neural connections, and supports the development of complex cognitive processes (Pellis & Pellis, 2007; Wang & Aamodt, 2012).

From the perspective of developmental psychology, play promotes progress in critical cognitive domains such as attention, memory, executive functions, language development, and problem-solving. From infancy onward, physical interactions—for example, playing with objects, spatial explorations, or imitation games—contribute to children's understanding of their environment, the development of their mental representation skills, and the formation of effective learning strategies (Tamis-LeMonda & Masek, 2023). Therefore, the role of play in supporting cognitive processes becomes even more concrete through the unique contributions of different types of play to children's developmental areas. The developmental value of play can be explained concretely through various types of play activities. Object play contributes to the discovery of cause-and-effect relationships, supports creative thinking, and fosters the development of problem-solving skills. Movement play strengthens motor coordination, balance, and bodily awareness skills, while social play reinforces cooperation, conflict resolution, and effective communication skills (Wang & Aamodt, 2012). This diversity reveals the comprehensive impact of play on both individual and social development.

From an evolutionary perspective, play holds a critical function not only for today's children but also in terms of species' survival strategies. While animals rehearse skills such as hunting, escaping, and hiding in a safe environment through play, humans develop higher-order abilities such as problem-solving, creativity, and social cooperation within play (Pellis & Pellis, 2007). In short, play provides opportunities for both risk-taking and safe exploration in a manner consistent with the nature of learning.

In conclusion, the developmental value of play is directly connected to the structural and functional development of the brain. Supporting play-based experiences during early childhood is considered a critical investment that enhances children's lifelong learning capacities, adaptability, and psychosocial resilience.

3. Why a Neuropedagogical Approach?

Neuropedagogy is an interdisciplinary approach positioned at the intersection of psychology, neuropsychology, and neuroscience, addressing learning in both its cognitive and emotional dimensions. While psychology examines an individual's mental processes, emotional states, and mind–body interactions, neuropsychology investigates brain functions related to emotions and their effects on learning and behavior. Neuroscience, on the other hand, analyzes brain functions and their relationship with the body at the biological level. At the intersection of these three fields, neuropedagogy considers the "learning–brain function–emotion" relationship within a holistic framework, supporting learning processes with neuroscientific evidence. At these points of intersection, the combination of psychology and neuropsychology represents school psychology; the integration of neuropsychology and neuroscience represents educational neuroscience; and the convergence of psychology and neuroscience represents the domains of pedagogy–learning–brain–mind. By synthesizing theoretical and applied knowledge from these disciplines, neuropedagogy fosters the development of scientific and evidence-based approaches in education (Wulan & Jamaris, 2023) (Figure 1).

Figure 1. Neuropedagogy transdisciplinary crafting

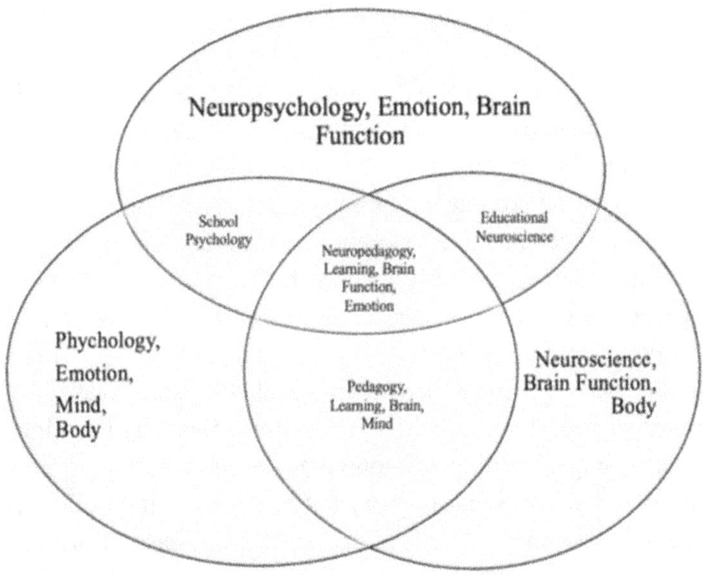

Source: Wulan and Jamaris (2023)

The primary aim of neuropedagogy is to integrate neuroscience with learning (Wulan & Jamaris, 2023). This approach, by combining neuroscientific findings with educational sciences, seeks to design learning environments that support children's cognitive, emotional, and social development. In early childhood, play is not merely an entertaining activity but a powerful learning tool that responds to the developmental needs of the brain (Tokuhama-Espinosa, 2021).

This perspective reveals how different regions of the brain are activated during play, how these interactions are reflected in learning processes, and which pedagogical strategies can maximize this process. Research demonstrates that both structured and unstructured play experiences strengthen children's neural networks, enhance their executive functions, and support their self-regulation skills (Berk & Meyers, 2013; Zosh et al., 2017).

In addition, particularly during socially interactive play, the mirror neuron system is activated. This system plays a critical role in understanding the actions and emotions of others, thereby supporting the development of empathy, cooperation, and social communication skills (Durualp & Aral, 2015; Rizzolatti & Sinigaglia, 2016). Therefore, the neuropedagogical approach regards play not merely as a pedagogical tool but as a strategic learning method grounded in the biological foundations of brain development.

3.1. The Role of Neuropedagogy in Early Childhood Education

As an interdisciplinary approach that aims to integrate neuroscientific findings into pedagogical processes, neuropedagogy holds strategic importance in early childhood education. This approach seeks to design learning environments, organize instructional strategies, and support children's cognitive, emotional, and social development by taking into account the developmental needs and functioning mechanisms of the brain. Neuropedagogy not only ensures that learning processes are grounded in scientific foundations but also necessitates the consideration of individual differences and developmental windows (critical periods) (Tokuhama-Espinosa, 2021).

Early childhood is a critical period in which the brain demonstrates rapid structural and functional development, with synaptic plasticity reaching its highest levels. During this stage, learning environments designed based on neuropedagogical principles can maximize learning capacity by supporting both structural and functional brain development. The application of brain-based learning principles at an early age contributes to the development of positive attitudes toward learning, the strengthening of emotional security, and the reinforcement of knowledge-based problem-solving skills in the early years (Widhiyanti, 2023).

In this context, neuropedagogy serves not only as a theoretical framework in early childhood education but also as a guide that offers concrete, practice-oriented strategies. The conscious use of components such as play, movement, multisensory stimuli, and social interaction in learning processes strengthens both the academic and life skills of children in the long term. This holistic approach provides a scientifically grounded and evidence-based roadmap for sustainable development in early childhood education.

3.2. The Importance of Play from a Neuropedagogical Perspective

From a neuropedagogical perspective, play is not merely an entertaining activity but a fundamental learning tool that meets the developmental needs of the brain, reinforces learning, and supports the holistic development of children across cognitive, emotional, and social domains. As Tokuhama-Espinosa (2021) states, play provides one of the most natural contexts in which the brain is most receptive to learning. In this process, children find opportunities to explore, solve problems, collaborate, and regulate their emotions.

Table 1. Key take ways of neuropedagogy based play joy emotions

Meaningful	Active Engagement	Iterative	Socially Interactive
Making connections between familiar and unfamiliar stimuli helps the brain transform effortful learning into a more accessible process. Meaningful experiences that introduce novel stimuli while linking them to existing mental frameworks recruit brain networks associated with analogical thinking, memory transfer, metacognition, insight generation, motivation, and reward.	Active and engaged involvement increases brain activation related to agency, decision-making, and flow. Active engagement enhances memory encoding and retrieval processes that support learning. Full participation in an activity allows the brain to exercise networks responsible for executive control skills, such as inhibiting distractions, which benefits both short-term and lifelong learning.	Perseverance associated with iterative thinking is linked to reward and memory networks that underpin learning. With practice, iteration increasingly engages networks related to adopting alternative perspectives, flexible thinking, and creativity.	Positive caregiver–child interactions help build the neural foundation for developing healthy socio-emotional regulation and protect against learning barriers such as stress. Early social interaction promotes brain plasticity, enabling individuals to cope with challenges later in life. Social interaction activates brain networks involved in detecting the mental states of others, which can be critical for teaching and learning interactions.

Neuropedagogy-based play is grounded in five fundamental principles that form an integral part of the neural networks responsible for learning: joy, meaningfulness, active engagement, iterative processes, and social interaction. Joy enhances memory, attention, creativity, and motivation by increasing dopamine release in the brain's reward system. Meaningful experiences facilitate the connection of new information to existing mental schemas, thereby triggering higher-order cognitive processes such as analogical reasoning, metacognition, and the development of insight. Active engagement enhances the permanence of learning by activating brain networks associated with decision-making, flow, and executive functions. Iterative processes strengthen neural networks that support flexible thinking and creativity. Social interaction not only reinforces socio-emotional regulation skills but also activates brain mechanisms that enable the perception of others' mental states. Table 1 summarizes the neuroscientific foundations of these principles and their roles in learning processes. According to the neuropedagogical perspective on play, these principles make it possible to integrate pedagogical practices with biological foundations. This approach demonstrates that play is not merely a pedagogical strategy but also a biologically optimized method of learning (Wulan & Jamaris, 2023).

Research reveals that during play, the brain produces signals that facilitate learning without inducing stress. The release of neurotransmitters such as dopamine increases motivation and the desire to learn, while the regulation of cortisol levels strengthens emotional security (Wang & Aamodt, 2012). Social play contributes to the development of the prefrontal cortex, supporting the emergence of higher-order skills such as self-regulation, empathy, and adherence to social rules (Pellis & Pellis, 2007).

3.3. Neuropedagogical Foundations of Play-Based Learning

Play-based learning, within the framework of neuropedagogy, is an approach designed in harmony with the brain's natural learning mechanisms, holistically supporting cognitive, emotional, and social development. As Widhiyanti (2023) states, the primary goal of brain-based learning is to enhance the effectiveness of teaching–learning processes by integrating findings from neuroscience research into educational settings. In this context, play serves as a fundamental learning tool that stimulates children's curiosity, promotes learning through experience, and strengthens brain plasticity.

Neuroscientific studies reveal that neural networks, which possess a high degree of plasticity in the early years of life, are strengthened through rich and interactive play experiences (Knudsen, 2004; Kolb & Gibb, 2011). During play, the simultaneous activation of different brain regions such as the prefrontal cortex, limbic system, and motor cortex supports the development of both executive functions and emotional regulation mechanisms (Pellis & Pellis, 2007).

As Wang and Aamodt (2012) emphasize, the neurochemical responses generated during play create a positive emotional climate that supports learning. Dopamine release enhances learning motivation, while the regulation of cortisol levels reduces the negative effects of stress. In addition, research by Zosh et al. (2017) demonstrates that both structured and free play environments strengthen problem-solving, creativity, social interaction, and self-regulation skills. Therefore, the neuropedagogical foundations of play-based learning rest on providing rich stimuli aligned with the developmental needs of the brain, ensuring emotional security, and activating multiple brain regions in a coordinated manner. This approach makes it possible to build both academic and life skills on strong neural foundations during early childhood.

4. The Neuroscientific Dimension of Play

Recent neuroscientific findings provide highly detailed and specific insights into cognitive phenomena such as learning and the regulation of behavior. According to these findings, the emergence of learning in humans requires certain neurochemical processes, while physical and social activities are particularly critical for these chemical processes. Especially during developmental stages—when brain structuring and neuroplasticity are at their peak—infants and children deprived of fundamental activities such as physical movement, adequate sleep, nutrition, and social interaction may experience impairments in their cognitive and physical development. Therefore, understanding which physical and social behaviors play a role in cognitive development is essential for managing child development in a healthy way (Yuce, 2023). From a neuroscientific perspective, play emerges as one of the most critical experiences shaping children's neural structures among the fundamental factors that support learning and development.

From a neuroscientific perspective, play is considered a critical process for learning and development, characterized by complex and simultaneous interactions among different regions of the brain. As Widhiyanti (2023) states, early childhood is a period marked by rapid structural and functional brain development, during which processes such as synaptogenesis, myelination, and synaptic pruning occur intensively. In this period, play directly contributes to the strengthening of neural connections, the formation of new synaptic pathways, and the enhancement of cognitive capacities.

The findings of Wang and Aamodt (2012) reveal that play generates neurophysiological signals that facilitate learning without inducing stress. In this process, dopamine release increases motivation and the desire to learn, while the regulation of cortisol levels reinforces emotional security. According to Pellis and Pellis (2007), social play supports the activation of the prefrontal cortex, thereby contributing to the development of higher-order cognitive functions such as impulse control, adherence to social rules, empathy, and self-regulation.

In addition, different types of play—such as object play, physical play, and social play—facilitate the integration of sensory, motor, cognitive, and emotional processes. This integration enhances the brain's capacity for plasticity, thereby supporting the long-term development of learning, problem-solving, and creativity skills (Kolb & Gibb, 2011). Therefore, play is not merely a source of entertainment but also a learning tool grounded in neuroscientific foundations that strengthens both the structural and functional development of the brain.

4.1. Brain Regions Activated During Play

During play, multiple regions of the brain are activated simultaneously, and this interaction plays a critical role in children's cognitive, emotional, and social development. According to the studies of Pellis and Pellis (2007), social play in particular ensures the intensive activation of the prefrontal cortex. The prefrontal cortex is responsible for executive functions such as impulse control, planning, adherence to social rules, and the selection of appropriate responses. The limbic system plays a significant role in regulating emotional responses during play. While the amygdala evaluates the emotional value of environmental and social stimuli, the hippocampus supports the encoding of play experiences into memory and their association with previous experiences. The motor cortex and cerebellum are actively involved in functions such as movement coordination, balance, execution of motor skills, and timing. The collaboration among these regions supports the development of both fine and gross motor skills. The findings of Wang and Aamodt (2012) reveal that the coordinated functioning of these brain regions balances stress levels and creates a focused mental state conducive to learning. Therefore, play, by generating integrated activation across different brain regions such as the prefrontal cortex, limbic system, motor cortex, and cerebellum, contributes to the strengthening of neural networks, the enhancement of cognitive flexibility, and the development of long-term learning capacity.

Figure 2. Network connections among brain regions activated by play

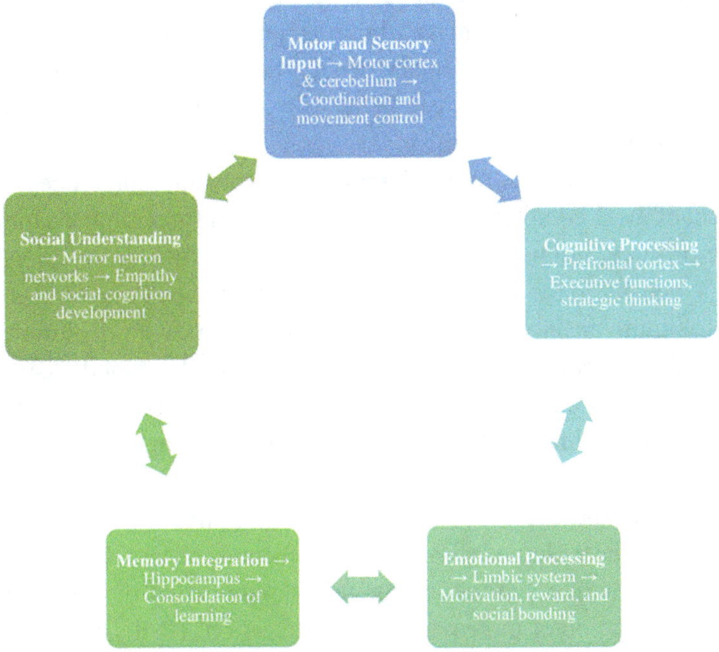

Motor and Sensory Input → Motor cortex & cerebellum → Coordination and movement control
Cognitive Processing → Prefrontal cortex → Executive functions, strategic thinking
Emotional Processing → Limbic system → Motivation, reward, and social bonding
Memory Integration → Hippocampus → Consolidation of learning
Social Understanding → Mirror neuron networks → Empathy and social cognition development

In Figure 2, the multidirectional neural interactions among the prefrontal cortex, limbic system (amygdala and hippocampus), motor cortex, and cerebellum are illustrated in the context of learning, emotional regulation, motor control, and social interaction processes (Diamond, 2013; Immordino-Yang & Damasio, 2007; Iacoboni, 2009; Rizzolatti & Sinigaglia, 2016). This model demonstrates that play is not confined to a single brain region but rather represents a complex neurobiological process involving the simultaneous activation of multiple brain networks.

4.2. Strengthening of Neural Networks

The brain has a complex network structure composed of neurons that transmit electrical signals. The human brain, consisting of approximately 100 billion neurons, establishes more than one trillion synaptic connections among these cells to enable the transmission of information (Herculano-Houzel, 2012). The cerebral cortex, which is the outer layer of neural tissue, is divided into two hemispheres—left and right—and is composed of the frontal, parietal, occipital, and two temporal lobes.

Each lobe assumes distinct functions, ranging from motor skills to language use, and from emotional regulation to higher-order cognitive processes.

At birth, the volume of an infant's brain is approximately one-third that of an adult brain; however, an extraordinary developmental process occurs during the first years of life. The tripling of cerebellar volume within the first year supports rapid progress in motor skills, while in the second year, the increase in connections among language regions and the acceleration of the myelination process enable the development of more complex cognitive and emotional functions (Bonomo, 2017). By the age of three, brain volume reaches approximately 80% of the adult level, and synaptic density in the prefrontal cortex can rise to nearly twice that of adults. This leads to significant advancements in executive functions such as understanding causal relationships, cognitive flexibility, and planning (Diamond, 2013).

Neuropedagogy is an interdisciplinary field situated at the intersection of neuroscience and early childhood education, aiming to strengthen neural networks through pedagogical approaches (Wulan & Jamaris, 2023). In this context, play-based learning contributes to the reinforcement of synaptic connections by providing stimulating experiences aligned with the developmental needs of the brain. Repetitive and meaningful play interactions accelerate communication between neurons and support the stabilization of more permanent connections (Pellis & Pellis, 2007). In particular, pretend play reinforces children's higher-order skills such as planning, effective use of language, emotional regulation, and empathy (Bodrova & Leong, 2015), while social play strengthens the coordination between the prefrontal cortex and the limbic system, supporting the development of self-regulation and social skills.

As Widhiyanti (2023) points out, rich and interactive play environments provided in early childhood enhance brain plasticity, making it easier for children to learn new information and transfer existing knowledge across different contexts. Therefore, neuropedagogy-based play not only improves learning performance in the short term but also establishes the neural foundation for lifelong skills such as cognitive flexibility, creativity, emotional balance, and character development. However, the limited number of empirical studies examining the effects of brain-based play within the framework of neuropedagogy indicates the need for further research in this field (Wulan & Jamaris, 2023).

4.3. Play and Emotional Regulation Mechanisms

Emotional regulation is defined as an individual's attempts to recognize their emotions in different situations and to regulate their responses associated with those emotions by modifying the timing and form of emotional experiences (e.g., intensity, duration, variety). Such attempts may occur automatically, in a controlled manner, either consciously or unconsciously. The process of emotional regulation differs from other forms of affect regulation such as mood regulation, coping, and defense mechanisms. Coping refers to the effort to manage what to do in response to a situation that forces the organism to react. While the process of emotional regulation is associated with a specific emotion arising in a given context, coping also includes non-emotional actions aimed at non-emotional goals. For children, emotional regulation involves understanding the emotions of others and accurately comparing their own emotions with those of others. In the preschool period, emotional development plays a vital role in enabling children to develop a healthy personality structure and establish positive interactions with their environment. The emotional developmental tasks expected to be acquired by the age of seven include: tolerating, spending time with others, having fun, recognizing danger, coping with fear and anxiety, protecting oneself, accepting being alone for reasonable reasons, showing interest in learning, and developing friendships. These tasks can also be experienced through play (Erdogan, 2021).

Play in early childhood is a fundamental activity that not only supports the development of cognitive and motor skills but also strengthens emotional regulation mechanisms. In particular, social play types based on physical interaction, such as "rough-and-tumble play," play a critical role in the development of the social brain in mammals (Pellis & Pellis, 2007). During such play, especially the prefrontal cortex and other higher-order cognitive control regions responsible for impulse control, adherence to social rules, and the selection of appropriate responses are activated.

Social play reinforces children's socio-emotional skills such as taking turns, tolerating defeat, cooperating, and developing empathy, thereby enhancing their self-regulation capacities. Hensch (2016) emphasizes that social interaction is critically important for the development of higher-order cognitive and emotional processes. In particular, reciprocal interactions known as "serve-and-return" form the neural foundation of regulatory processes such as emotion processing, empathy development, and stress management from the earliest stages of life.

Some researchers have described emotional regulation as the primary function of symbolic play. Symbolic play enables children to create emotionally stimulating events in a symbolic way and to modify them. In addition, such play offers opportunities to persuade others to join the activity and to negotiate the rules of the game. In this way, children experience emotions and develop their emotional regulation skills. Through symbolic play, children begin to accept societal norms by regulating their emotions, thoughts, and behaviors. With the increasing mental capacities of preschool children, they begin to express their emotions through play (Erdogan, 2021). Numerous studies have demonstrated a positive relationship between symbolic play and emotional regulation (Galyer & Evans, 2001; Gilpin et al., 2015; Hoffman & Russ, 2012; Slot et al., 2017). Yurdakul et al. (2022) found that preschool children with higher emotional regulation skills exhibited more harmonious and cooperative behaviors in their play interactions with peers. Research further indicates that repetitive and meaningful play experiences increase the permanence of synaptic connections and, in the long term, contribute to the development of higher-order skills such as self-regulation, cognitive flexibility, and creativity. Therefore, safe and supportive social play environments play an indispensable role in both short-term learning and long-term socio-emotional development (Diamond, 2013).

5. Play in the Context of Early Brain Development

Play-based engagement is widely recognized as one of the most fundamental driving forces of early learning and development. From infancy onward, children's physical interactions with the world play a central role in the emergence of critical cognitive processes such as attention, memory, executive functions, language, and problem-solving (Smith et al., 2018; Tamis-LeMonda & Masek, 2023). Motor and sensory experiences not only allow children to explore how objects function and the structure of physical spaces but also support the formation and strengthening of neural connections that underlie cognitive skills (Oakes & Rakison, 2019; Tooley et al., 2021).

Nevertheless, much of the existing knowledge regarding the contributions of children's physical play forms in daily life to cognitive development is primarily based on observational or correlational research designs. A wide range of developmental studies have revealed strong associations between children's physical interactions with objects and later skills such as spatial reasoning, conceptual development, categorization, language learning, and executive functions (Campos et al., 2000). However, experimental studies that systematically alter children's everyday play environments in order to determine causal relationships and examine the effects of such changes on cognitive development remain quite limited.

Researchers are aware that meaningful relationships exist between children's daily physical play routines and advanced cognitive skills; yet studies that evaluate the developmental outcomes of play conditions by systematically modifying the core components of play environments in homes, daycare centers, or schools are rare. Therefore, the narrative review presented in this section aims to synthesize both classical and contemporary literature findings that examine the role of physical play experiences in early cognitive development, thereby outlining the current scientific framework on this issue.

5.1. Early Brain Development, Sensitive Periods, and Synaptic Plasticity

Brain development is a complex, dynamic process that begins before birth and continues into adulthood, and it is highly sensitive to environmental stimuli. In the early years of life, the brain grows at an extraordinary rate, with processes such as synaptogenesis, myelination, and synaptic pruning occurring intensively during this period. Synaptogenesis refers to the formation of connections that enable communication between neurons, reaching its peak within the first few years of life (Huttenlocher & Dabholkar, 1997). Myelination increases the speed of neural transmission, allowing faster and more efficient communication between brain regions (Fields, 2008).

Early childhood encompasses the "sensitive periods," which are defined as optimal windows of time for the acquisition of specific cognitive, linguistic, emotional, and motor skills (Knudsen, 2004). During these periods, environmental inputs directly influence the structural and functional organization of neural networks. A lack of visual or auditory stimulation can negatively affect the development of the corresponding brain regions (Shonkoff & Phillips, 2000). Conversely, enriched environmental stimuli increase the complexity of neural networks responsible for functions such as learning, memory, and problem-solving, whereas conditions of deprivation may accelerate synaptic pruning and limit cognitive development (Greenough et al., 1987). In this context, interactive and enriched experiences such as play are of critical importance for both structural and functional brain development.

Synaptic plasticity refers to the brain's capacity to make structural and functional changes in response to experiences. Adolescence and youth provide a critical window of opportunity for the development of flexible behavioral strategies through social interactions and play experiences (Spinka et al., 2001; Pellis & Pellis, 2007; Vanderschuren & Trezza, 2013). For example, studies have shown that animals deprived of opportunities for social play during specific time periods in adolescence exhibit inappropriate responses in challenging social situations as adults and display more impulsive behaviors in demanding cognitive tasks (Van den Berg et al., 1999; Baarendse et al., 2013). These findings demonstrate that early play experiences strengthen both cognitive and social adaptation skills.

Studies on play-related plasticity in the prefrontal cortex reveal that this region plays a critical role in mediating the beneficial effects of play. For example, it has been reported that rats deprived of play during the third and fourth weeks of life show weakened dopamine-mediated modulation and reduced dendritic complexity in the medial prefrontal cortex (Baarendse et al., 2013; Bell et al., 2010). In contrast, animals given opportunities for free play demonstrated an increased capacity of medial prefrontal cortex neurons to process information and exhibited greater sensitivity to nicotine-induced plasticity (Himmler et al., 2013). This highlights the importance of the prefrontal cortex for behavioral flexibility and the potential of play to strengthen this functionality (Ragozzino, 2007).

Some brain functions are "hard-wired" (e.g., the limbic system), automatically maintaining essential life functions such as heartbeat, respiration, and balance, while other parts are "soft-wired" and continuously reshaped through experience. Children's abilities to learn new languages and adapt to different environments exemplify this "soft wiring" (Wolf, 2007). In neuroscience, this capacity for change is defined as "plasticity," which enhances the efficiency of information processing by forming new synaptic connections (Gallagher, 2009).

In conclusion, play experiences during early childhood and adolescence support plasticity in many regions of the brain—particularly the prefrontal cortex—thereby strengthening individuals' ability to adapt to the variable social and environmental conditions they will encounter throughout life. In contrast, deprivation of social play may lead to negative developmental outcomes such as rigidity, low social interaction, impulsivity, and poor decision-making (Nelson, 2017). Therefore, play should be incorporated into early education programs not only as a pedagogical tool but also as a neurobiological necessity.

5.2. Stress Regulation and Emotional Security

Play makes a significant contribution to the development of children's coping mechanisms for stress and the reinforcement of their emotional security. Both free and structured play experiences provide children with opportunities to take controlled risks, cope with frustration, and experience a sense of achievement (Lester & Russell, 2008). The amygdala, which plays a central role in regulating stress responses in the brain, works in interaction with the prefrontal cortex during play to help balance emotional reactions (Panksepp, 2007). This neurobiological interaction enables children to develop more flexible and adaptive responses to stressful situations. A safe play environment allows children to express themselves, build positive relationships with others, and experience social support. Thus, a solid foundation is established for children's emotional and social strengthening (Bodrova & Leong, 2015; Lester & Russell, 2008; Panksepp, 2007).

Figure 3. Play – limbic system – motivation cycle

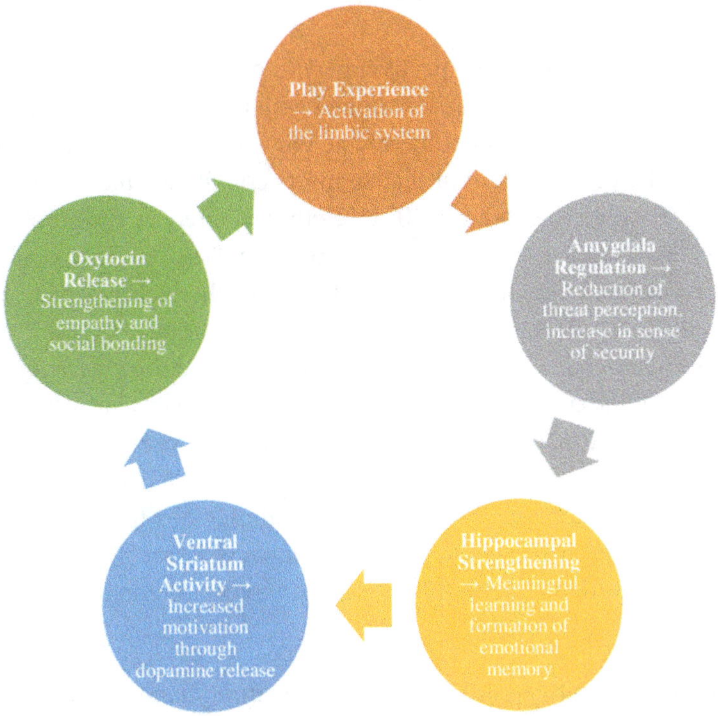
Play Experience → Activation of the limbic system
Amygdala Regulation → Reduction of threat perception, increase in sense of security
Hippocampal Strengthening → Meaningful learning and formation of emotional memory
Ventral Striatum Activity → Increased motivation through dopamine release
Oxytocin Release → Strengthening of empathy and social bonding

Play generates multifaceted neurobiological effects on different components of the limbic system, supporting learning, motivation, and social bonding. The play experience primarily triggers the general activation of the limbic system, enabling the integration of emotional processes (Immordino-Yang & Damasio, 2007). The amygdala, one of the core structures of the limbic system, has been associated with reduced threat perception and increased sense of safety during play (LeDoux, 2015). Synaptic strengthening occurring in the hippocampus contributes to meaningful learning and the formation of emotional memory (Lisman et al., 2012). The ventral striatum, through dopamine release, enhances motivation and facilitates the continuation of play behaviors (Schultz, 2016). In socially interactive play, increased oxytocin release strengthens empathy and social bonding (Feldman, 2012). This reciprocal interaction cycle demonstrates that play produces holistic effects not only on cognitive gains but also on emotional and social development (Figure 3).

6. Play Approaches in Early Childhood from a Neuropedagogical Perspective

From a neuropedagogical perspective, play in early childhood requires the design of learning environments that are aligned with the developmental needs of the brain. In this approach, play is not merely an enjoyable activity but is regarded as a neuroscience-based learning tool that supports cognitive, emotional, and social development (Tokuhama-Espinosa, 2021). Both structured and unstructured forms of play provide experiences that activate different brain regions. Free play enhances creativity, problem-solving skills, and cognitive flexibility, whereas structured play activities facilitate the achievement of specific learning objectives (Zosh et al., 2017).

Within the neuropedagogical play approach, teachers enrich learning processes by considering children's individual interests, readiness levels, and developmental needs. This approach aims to support executive functions, foster self-regulation skills, and strengthen social interactions (Berk & Meyers, 2013). When evaluated together with their neuroscientific foundations and the brain regions they stimulate, brain-based play approaches in early childhood education reveal that children gain holistic benefits across cognitive, emotional, social, and motor developmental domains.

Table 2. Brain-based play approaches, neuroscientific foundations, and developmental outcomes

Model / Approach	Neuroscientific Foundation	Related Brain Regions	Developmental Outcomes
Reggio Emilia (Edwards et al., 2011; Vecchi, 2010)	Multisensory stimulation, project-based learning, social interaction	Prefrontal cortex, limbic system, mirror neurons	Creativity, empathy, collaboration, social cognition
Tools of the Mind (Bodrova & Leong, 2024; Diamond et al., 2007; Barnett et al., 2008)	Planned play, dramatization, self-regulation tasks	Prefrontal cortex, hippocampus	Self-regulation, attention control, problem-solving
Forest School (O'Brien & Murray, 2007; Roe & Aspinall, 2011)	Nature-based risk-taking, physical activity, exploration	Hippocampus, cerebellum, limbic system	Motor skills, memory strengthening, emotional resilience

The Reggio Emilia approach activates the prefrontal cortex, limbic system, and mirror neuron networks by centering on multisensory stimulation, project-based learning, and intensive social interaction; thereby supporting the development of creativity, empathy, collaboration, and social cognition (Edwards et al., 2011; Vecchi, 2010). The Tools of the Mind program stimulates the prefrontal cortex and hippocampus through planned play, dramatization, and self-regulation tasks; in this way, executive functions such as self-regulation, attention control, and problem-solving are strengthened (Bodrova & Leong, 2024; Diamond et al., 2007; Barnett et al., 2008). The Forest School approach, on the other hand, activates the hippocampus, cerebellum, and limbic system through nature-based risk-taking, physical activity, and exploration-centered learning experiences; thus enhancing motor skills, memory consolidation, and emotional resilience (O'Brien & Murray, 2007; Roe & Aspinall, 2011). These approaches integrate neuroscientific foundations with educational practices, making play-based learning more effective and enduring (Table 2).

7. Evaluation

The information presented in this section reveals the neuroscientific foundations of play in early childhood and its functions within the framework of neuropedagogical approaches. The findings demonstrate that play is not merely an enjoyable activity; rather, it is a learning tool that supports the structural and functional maturation processes of the brain and plays a critical role in the construction of cognitive, emotional, and social skills. In particular, the prefrontal cortex, amygdala, hippocampus, ventral striatum, and components of the limbic system that are activated during play constitute the neurobiological basis of a wide range of developmental gains, from executive functions to emotional regulation, and from motivation to social bonding. The neuropedagogical perspective enhances the effectiveness of teaching activities by aligning play-based learning processes with the developmental needs of the brain. This approach aims to reinforce children's creativity, problem-solving, self-regulation, and social interaction skills by harmoniously integrating structured and unstructured play activities. Moreover, safe and supportive play environments are shown to contribute to strengthening children's stress regulation mechanisms and consolidating their emotional security. These findings clearly indicate that play is not only a pedagogical method but also a neurological necessity.

Figure 4. Components of the play-based neuropedagogical approach

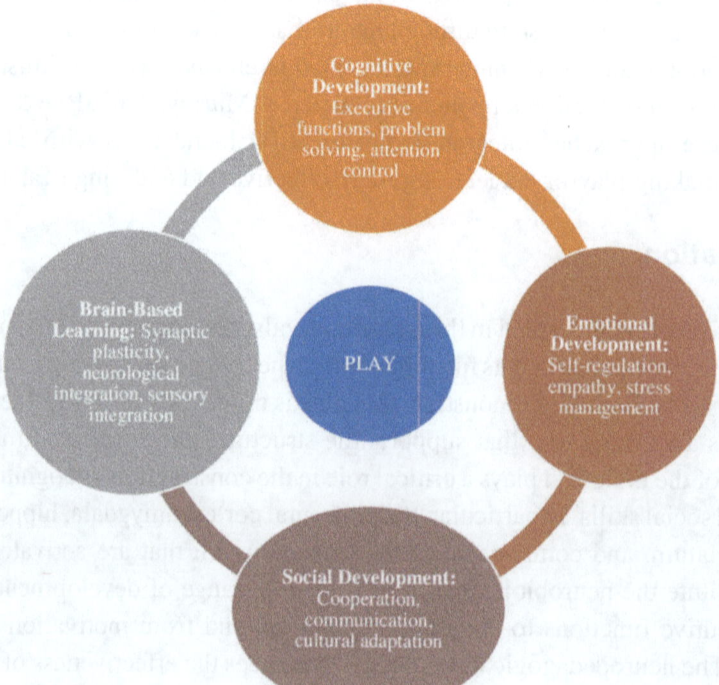

Figure 4 illustrates the cognitive, emotional, social, and brain-based learning components of the play-based neuropedagogical approach at the center, while policy, teacher training, cultural adaptation, and assessment dimensions are represented in the outer circle. The model suggests supporting executive functions, self-regulation, empathy, collaboration, and neurological integration through play; moreover, it proposes the systematic integration of these approaches into educational policies and teacher training programs (Bodrova & Leong, 2024; Fisher et al., 2012; LEGO Foundation, 2017; Pyle & Danniels, 2017; Tokuhama-Espinosa, 2021; Whitebread et al., 2012).

Although the literature strongly demonstrates the contributions of play to cognitive, emotional, and social development in early childhood, the number of experimental and longitudinal studies that directly test the neurobiological mechanisms of these effects is limited. A significant portion of the current findings is based on observational or correlational designs (Bateson & Martin, 2013; Lillard et al., 2013; Singer et al., 2006; Williams et al., 2018; Whitebread & Basilio, 2013). Therefore, it is necessary to increase research that directly measures brain region activation patterns, neuroplasticity processes, and neurotransmitter releases during play through neuroimaging and biomarker-based methods. In addition, examining the applicability and effects of play-based neuropedagogical approaches in different cultural contexts through comparative studies will strengthen the body of knowledge in the field.

In light of all these findings, play in early childhood should be regarded not merely as a pedagogical choice but as a neurobiological necessity. Play-based neuropedagogical approaches meet children's developmental needs at the biological level, thereby strengthening their lifelong learning, creativity, and social adaptation skills. Therefore, restructuring educational policies in alignment with scientific evidence, strengthening teacher education, implementing culturally sensitive adaptations, and developing valid and reliable assessment tools will ensure the sustainability of these approaches. This powerful intersection of neuroscience and pedagogy provides a holistic educational framework that maximizes children's potential.

8. Future Perspectives

Future research in the field of play and neuropedagogical approaches in early childhood holds significant potential for deepening the understanding of brain-based learning strategies and for integrating them more effectively into educational environments. The use of advanced neuroimaging techniques (fMRI, EEG, fNIRS) and sophisticated cognitive assessment tools will allow for a more detailed identification of the brain regions activated during play, as well as the neural networks involved in these processes. Such findings can provide clearer insights into the neuroscientific mechanisms underlying play-based learning and directly inform pedagogical design.

Comparative studies examining the influence of cultural contexts on play preferences and learning styles will also fill a critical gap in this field. Investigating children's play experiences across different cultures will enable the development of strategies for adapting neuropedagogical approaches in ways that are grounded in universal principles yet aligned with local values. In this regard, it is of great importance to increase longitudinal studies that track the long-term effects of structured and unstructured forms of play on brain plasticity, emotional regulation, and executive functions.

From an educational policy perspective, the systematic inclusion of play-based neuropedagogical programs in early childhood curricula, the reinforcement of teacher preparation programs with neuroscientific foundations, and the raising of parental awareness constitute critical steps. Such an approach will position play not merely as a developmental choice but as a neurological necessity, ensuring that instructional programs and assessment systems are aligned with children's natural learning processes.

Cultural norms and values shape the perspectives of both families and teachers toward play, directly influencing the child's daily playtime, preferred types of play, and the quality of learning experiences. Therefore, in order to implement play-based neuropedagogical practices effectively and sustainably in early childhood education, the strategic steps outlined in Table 3 may serve as a guiding framework.

Table 3. Strategic recommendations for play-based neuropedagogical practices in early childhood

Strategy	Description	Example Practice
1. Restructuring Educational Policies	Recognizing play as the primary mode of learning in the curriculum and reducing early academic pressure (Fisher et al., 2012; LEGO Foundation, 2017; Whitebread et al., 2012).	Extending play-based learning into the first years of primary school in Finland.
2. Strengthening Teacher Education	Integrating neuroscience-based play modules into teacher training programs (Tokuhama-Espinosa, 2021; Pyle & Danniels, 2017).	Introducing an elective course titled *"Play and the Brain"* in universities.
3. Culturally Responsive Approaches	Designing play practices aligned with local cultural norms and values (Edwards et al., 2011; Whitebread et al., 2012).	Incorporating traditional folk games into early childhood education programs.
4. Developing Assessment Tools	Creating valid instruments to measure the cognitive, social, and emotional outcomes of play (Bodrova & Leong, 2024; Tokuhama-Espinosa, 2021).	Developing observation forms and neuroscience-informed assessment protocols.
5. Interdisciplinary Collaboration	Encouraging collaboration among educators, neuroscientists, psychologists, and policymakers (LEGO Foundation, 2017; Whitebread et al., 2012).	Establishing play laboratories through joint projects between universities, schools, and NGOs.

The strategic framework presented in Table 3 offers multidimensional recommendations for the effective implementation of play-based neuropedagogical approaches in early childhood education. First, the restructuring of educational policies requires recognizing play as the primary mode of learning in the curriculum and reducing early academic pressure (Fisher et al., 2012; LEGO Foundation, 2017; Whitebread et al., 2012). Such a policy orientation, as exemplified in Finland, enables the continuation of play-based learning into the first years of primary school, thereby supporting children's learning processes. In connection with this, strengthening teacher education can be achieved by integrating neuroscience-informed play modules into teacher training programs (Tokuhama-Espinosa, 2021; Pyle & Danniels, 2017). In this way, teachers can more consciously design learning environments through play. Moreover, culturally responsive approaches promote the development of play practices aligned with local norms and values, thereby allowing children to experience and strengthen their cultural identity through play (Edwards et al., 2011; Whitebread et al., 2012). In addition, the development of valid and reliable assessment tools for measuring the cognitive, social, and emotional outcomes of play is of great importance (Bodrova & Leong, 2024; Tokuhama-Espinosa, 2021).

Such instruments make it possible to scientifically document the impacts of play-based learning. Finally, interdisciplinary collaboration involves joint efforts among educators, neuroscientists, psychologists, and policymakers; such partnerships enable innovative practices such as the establishment of play laboratories (LEGO Foundation, 2017; Whitebread et al., 2012). Thus, play-based strategies can be strengthened at both the theoretical and practical levels, ensuring their sustainability.

Ultimately, play-based neuropedagogical approaches must be understood not as optional educational practices, but as a neurobiological imperative that transcends cultural boundaries. For these approaches to achieve universal relevance, cultural contexts need to be strongly integrated into empirical research, ensuring that play-based models are both scientifically grounded and culturally meaningful. Future progress in this field relies on interdisciplinary and cross-cultural collaborations, reforms in teacher education, and the alignment of educational policies with neuroscientific evidence. Strengthening the bridges between neuroscience, pedagogy, and practice will not only elevate the quality of early childhood education but also unlock children's full potential for lifelong learning, creativity, and social adaptation. In this sense, neuropedagogy offers a transformative framework—one that positions play as a cornerstone of human development in a rapidly changing world.

CONCLUSION AND RECOMMENDATIONS

The theoretical framework and research findings presented in this chapter demonstrate that play in early childhood is far more than a mere recreational activity; it is a fundamental learning tool that supports cognitive, emotional, and social development. From a neuropedagogical perspective, play is conceptualized as an educational element aligned with the brain's developmental needs, one that strengthens neural integration and fosters executive functions. The activation of brain regions during play enhances synaptic plasticity, while social interactions and emotional regulation mechanisms contribute to children's ability to cope with stress and develop self-regulation skills.

In light of these findings, the effective implementation of play-based neuropedagogical practices in early childhood education requires the restructuring of educational programs, the strengthening of teacher training, the enhancement of family involvement, and the reinforcement of the research–practice nexus. Accordingly, the following strategic recommendations can be proposed:

- Integrate play-based neuropedagogical approaches systematically into early childhood curricula.

- Balance structured and unstructured play activities to support both cognitive and socio-emotional development.
- Provide early childhood teachers with regular in-service training on neuroscience-informed learning strategies and play practices.
- Incorporate practices that enhance executive functions, problem-solving skills, and socio-emotional development into teacher preparation programs.
- Offer guidance for families on creating home play environments that are aligned with their children's neurodevelopmental needs.
- Conduct awareness-raising initiatives on the value and importance of play in diverse cultural contexts.
- Employ neuroimaging and longitudinal research to explore in greater depth the effects of play-based learning on brain development.
- Carry out comparative studies to examine the effectiveness of play approaches across different socioeconomic and cultural contexts.

In conclusion, play experiences designed through a neuropedagogical approach activate the brain's natural learning mechanisms during early childhood, providing a strong foundation for children's academic, social, and emotional development. Therefore, the restructuring of educational policies and classroom practices in alignment with scientific evidence is of critical importance for maximizing the learning potential of future generations.

The widespread implementation of play-based neuropedagogical practices will be achievable through the strengthening of teacher education, the renewal of assessment and evaluation systems, the advancement of interdisciplinary collaborations, and the integration of culturally responsive adaptations. In this way, scientific evidence will not remain confined to academic publications but will be directly reflected in children's everyday learning experiences.

REFRENCES

Baarendse, P. J., Counotte, D. S., O'donnell, P., & Vanderschuren, L. J. (2013). Early social experience is critical for the development of cognitive control and dopamine modulation of prefrontal cortex function. *Neuropsychopharmacology : Official Publication of the American College of Neuropsychopharmacology, 38*(8), 1485–1494. DOI: 10.1038/npp.2013.47

Barnett, W. S., Jung, K., Yarosz, D. J., Thomas, J., Hornbeck, A., Stechuk, R., & Burns, S. (2008). Educational effects of the Tools of the Mind curriculum: A randomized trial. *Early Childhood Research Quarterly, 23*(3), 299–313. DOI: 10.1016/j.ecresq.2008.03.001

Bateson, P. P. G., & Martin, P. (2013). *Play, playfulness, creativity and innovation.* Cambridge University Press. DOI: 10.1017/CBO9781139057691

Bell, H. C., Pellis, S. M., & Kolb, B. (2010). Juvenile peer play experience and the development of the orbitofrontal and medial prefrontal cortices. *Behavioural Brain Research, 207*(1), 7–13. DOI: 10.1016/j.bbr.2009.09.029

Berk, L. E., & Meyers, A. B. (2013). The role of make-believe play in the development of executive function: Status of research and future directions. *American Journal of Play, 6*(1), 98–110.

Blum, K. (2024). The impact of chronic stress on brain function and structure. *Neuroscience and Psychiatry, 7*(5), 262-264. doi:10.47532/npoa.2024.

Bodrova, E., & Leong, D. (2024). *Tools of the mind: The Vygotskian approach to early childhood education.* Routledge. DOI: 10.4324/9781003164920

Bodrova, E., & Leong, D. J. (2015). Vygotskian and Post-Vygotskian Views on Children's Play. *American Journal of Play, 7*(3), 371–388.

Campos, J. J., Anderson, D. I., Barbu-Roth, M. A., Hubbard, E. M., Hertenstein, M. J., & Witherington, D. (2000). Travel broadens the mind. *Infancy, 1*(2), 149–219. DOI: 10.1207/S15327078IN0102_1

Diamond, A. (2013). Executive functions. *Annual Review of Psychology, 64*(1), 135–168. DOI: 10.1146/annurev-psych-113011-143750

Diamond, A., Barnett, W. S., Thomas, J., & Munro, S. (2007). Preschool program improves cognitive control. *Science, 318*(5855), 1387–1388. DOI: 10.1126/science.1151148

Durualp, E., & Aral, N. (2015). *Game-Based Social Skills Training* (2nd ed.). Vize Publishing.

Edwards, C., Gandini, L., & Forman, G. (Eds.). (2011). *The hundred languages of children: The Reggio Emilia experience in transformation*. Bloomsbury Publishing USA. DOI: 10.5040/9798400667664

Erdogan, G. (2021). Paternal function in pretend play and emotion regulatory skills in the preshool period. *The Journal of Academic Social Science*, *9*(118), 353–367.

Feldman, R. (2012). Oxytocin and social affiliation in humans. *Hormones and Behavior*, *61*(3), 380–391. DOI: 10.1016/j.yhbeh.2012.01.008

Fields, R. D. (2008). White matter in learning, cognition and psychiatric disorders. *Trends in Neurosciences*, *31*(7), 361–370. DOI: 10.1016/j.tins.2008.04.001

Fisher, K., Hirsh-Pasek, K., Golinkoff, R. M., Singer, D. G., & Berk, L. E. (2012). Playing around in school: Implications for learning and educational policy. In Tremblay, R. E., Boivin, M., & Peters, R. (Eds.), *Oxford handbook of the development of play* (pp. 342–360). Oxford University Press.

Fisher, K. R., Hirsh-Pasek, K., Golinkoff, R. M., & Gryfe, S. G. (2008). Conceptual split? Parents' and experts' perceptions of play in the 21st century. *Journal of Applied Developmental Psychology*, *29*(4), 305–316. DOI: 10.1016/j.appdev.2008.04.006

Gallagher, W. (2009). *Rapt: Attention and the focused life*. Penguin.

Galyer, K. T., & Evans, I. M. (2001). Pretend play and the development of emotion regulation in preschool children. *Early Child Development and Care*, *166*(1), 93–108. DOI: 10.1080/0300443011660108

Gilpin, A. T., Brown, M. M., & Pierucci, J. M. (2015). Relations between fantasy orientation and emotion regulation in preschool. *Early Education and Development*, *26*(7), 920–932. DOI: 10.1080/10409289.2015.1000716

Greenough, W. T., Black, J. E., & Wallace, C. S. (1987). Experience and brain development. *Child Development*, *58*(3), 539–559. DOI: 10.2307/1130197

Hensch, T. K. (2016). The power of the infant brain. *Scientific American*, *314*(2), 64–69. DOI: 10.1038/scientificamerican0216-64

Herculano-Houzel, S. (2012). The remarkable, yet not extraordinary, human brain as a scaled-up primate brain and its associated cost. *Proceedings of the National Academy of Sciences*, *109*(supplement_1), 10661-10668.

Himmler, B. T., Pellis, S. M., & Kolb, B. (2013). Juvenile play experience primes neurons in the medial prefrontal cortex to be more responsive to later experiences. *Neuroscience Letters, 556*, 42–45. DOI: 10.1016/j.neulet.2013.09.061

Huttenlocher, P. R., & Dabholkar, A. S. (1997). Regional differences in synaptogenesis in human cerebral cortex. *The Journal of Comparative Neurology, 387*(2), 167–178. DOI: 10.1002/(SICI)1096-9861(19971020)387:2<167::AID-CNE1>3.0.CO;2-Z

Iacoboni, M. (2009). Imitation, empathy, and mirror neurons. *Annual Review of Psychology, 60*(1), 653–670. DOI: 10.1146/annurev.psych.60.110707.163604

Knudsen, E. I. (2004). Sensitive periods in the development of the brain and behavior. *Journal of Cognitive Neuroscience, 16*(8), 1412–1425. DOI: 10.1162/0898929042304796

Kolb, B., & Gibb, R. (2011). Brain plasticity and behaviour in the developing brain. *Journal of the Canadian Academy of Child and Adolescent Psychiatry = Journal de l'Académie Canadienne de Psychiatrie de l'Enfant et de l'Adolescent, 20*(4), 265.

LeDoux, J. E. (2015). Feelings: What are they & how does the brain make them? *Daedalus, 144*(1), 96–111. DOI: 10.1162/DAED_a_00319

Lester, S., & Russell, W. (2008). *Play for a change: Play, policy and practice – A review of contemporary perspectives*. Play England.

Lillard, A. S., Lerner, M. D., Hopkins, E. J., Dore, R. A., Smith, E. D., & Palmquist, C. M. (2013). The impact of pretend play on children's development: A review of the evidence. *Psychological Bulletin, 139*(1), 1–34. DOI: 10.1037/a0029321

Lisman, J., Yasuda, R., & Raghavachari, S. (2012). Mechanisms of CaMKII action in long-term potentiation. *Nature Reviews. Neuroscience, 13*(3), 169–182. DOI: 10.1038/nrn3192

Murray, L., Levickis, P., McFarland, L., Eadie, P., Lee-Pang, L., Quach, J., & Page, J. (2025). Supporting Young Children's Social–Emotional Wellbeing in Early Childhood Education and Care: Perspectives from the Sector. *Education Sciences, 15*(5), 569. DOI: 10.3390/educsci15050569

Nelson, C. A.III. (2017). Hazards to early development: The biological embedding of early life adversity. *Neuron, 96*(2), 262–266. DOI: 10.1016/j.neuron.2017.09.027

O'Brien, L., & Murray, R. (2007). Forest School and its impacts on young children: Case studies in Britain. *Urban Forestry & Urban Greening, 6*(4), 249–265. DOI: 10.1016/j.ufug.2007.03.006

Oakes, L. M., & Rakison, D. H. (2019). *Developmental cascades: Building the infant mind*. Oxford University Press. DOI: 10.1093/oso/9780195391893.001.0001

Panksepp, J. (2007). Can PLAY diminish ADHD and facilitate the construction of the social brain?. *Journal of the Canadian Academy of child and adolescent psychiatry, 16*(2), 57-66.

Pellis, S. M., & Pellis, V. C. (2007). Rough-and-tumble play and the development of the social brain. *Current Directions in Psychological Science, 16*(2), 95–98. DOI: 10.1111/j.1467-8721.2007.00483.x

Polat, B., & Kara, M. (2023). The effect of toys and playing on child development. *Kastamonu University Faculty of Health Sciences Journal, 2*(1), 1–10.

Pyle, A., & Danniels, E. (2017). A continuum of play-based learning: The role of the teacher in play-based pedagogy and the fear of hijacking play. *Early Education and Development, 28*(3), 274–289. DOI: 10.1080/10409289.2016.1220771

Ragozzino, M. E. (2007). The contribution of the medial prefrontal cortex, orbitofrontal cortex, and dorsomedial striatum to behavioral flexibility. *Annals of the New York Academy of Sciences, 1121*(1), 355–375. DOI: 10.1196/annals.1401.013

Rizzolatti, G., & Sinigaglia, C. (2016). The mirror mechanism: A basic principle of brain function. *Nature Reviews. Neuroscience, 17*(12), 757–765. DOI: 10.1038/nrn.2016.135

Roe, J., & Aspinall, P. (2011). The restorative benefits of walking in urban and rural settings in adults with good and poor mental health. *Health & Place, 17*(1), 103–113. DOI: 10.1016/j.healthplace.2010.09.003

Schultz, W. (2016). Dopamine reward prediction-error signalling: A two-component response. *Nature Reviews. Neuroscience, 17*(3), 183–195. DOI: 10.1038/nrn.2015.26

Shonkoff, J. P., & Phillips, D. A. (Eds.). (2000). *From neurons to neighborhoods: The science of early childhood development*. National Academy Press.

Singer, D., Golinkoff, R. M., & Hirsh-Pasek, K. (2006). *Play= Learning: How play motivates and enhances children's cognitive and social-emotional growth*. Oxford University Press. DOI: 10.1093/acprof:oso/9780195304381.001.0001

Slot, P. L., Mulder, H., Verhagen, J., & Leseman, P. P. (2017). Preschoolers' cognitive and emotional self-regulation in pretend play: Relations with executive functions and quality of play. *Infant and Child Development, 26*(6), e2038. DOI: 10.1002/icd.2038

Smith, L. B., Jayaraman, S., Clerkin, E., & Yu, C. (2018). The developing infant creates a curriculum for statistical learning. *Trends in Cognitive Sciences, 22*(4), 325–336. DOI: 10.1016/j.tics.2018.02.004

Spinka, M., Newberry, R. C., & Bekoff, M. (2001). Mammalian play: Training for the unexpected. *The Quarterly Review of Biology, 76*(2), 141–168. DOI: 10.1086/393866

Tamis-LeMonda, C. S., & Masek, L. R. (2023). Embodied and embedded learning: Child, caregiver, and context. *Current Directions in Psychological Science, 32*(5), 369–378. DOI: 10.1177/09637214231178731

Tokuhama-Espinosa, T. (2021). *Bringing the neuroscience of learning to online teaching: an educator's handbook.* Teachers College Press.

Tooley, U. A., Bassett, D. S., & Mackey, A. P. (2021). Environmental influences on the pace of brain development. *Nature Reviews. Neuroscience, 22*(6), 372–384. DOI: 10.1038/s41583-021-00457-5

Van den Berg, C. L., Hol, T., Van Ree, J. M., Spruijt, B. M., Everts, H., & Koolhaas, J. M. (1999). Play is indispensable for an adequate development of coping with social challenges in the rat. *Developmental Psychobiology, 34*(2), 129–138. DOI: 10.1002/(SICI)1098-2302(199903)34:2<129::AID-DEV6>3.0.CO;2-L

Vanderschuren, L. J., & Trezza, V. (2013). What the laboratory rat has taught us about social play behavior: role in behavioral development and neural mechanisms. *The neurobiology of childhood*, 189-212.

Vecchi, V. (2010). *Art and creativity in Reggio Emilia: Exploring the role and potential of ateliers in early childhood education*. Routledge. DOI: 10.4324/9780203854679

Wang, S., & Aamodt, S. (2012). Play, stress, and the learning brain. *Cerebrum*,12.

Whitebread, D., & Basilio, M. (2013). *Play, culture and creativity.* Cultures of Creativity. Billund, Denmark. *The LEGO Foundation, 76*, 82.

Whitebread, D., Basilio, M., Kuvalja, M., & Verma, M. (2012). *The importance of play*. Toy Industries of Europe.

Whole Child Neuro. (2024, July 15). *How play supports cognitive, emotional, and social development in children.* Whole Child Neuro. https://www.wholechildneuro.com/blog/how-play-supports-cognitive-emotional-and-social-development-in-children

Widhiyanti, S. (2023). Brain based learning approach in early childhood learning. In *ICECEM 2022: Proceedings of the 1st International Conference on Early Childhood Education in Multiperspective, ICECEM 2022, 26th November 2022, Purwokerto, Central Java, Indonesia* (p. 103). European Alliance for Innovation. DOI: 10.4108/eai.26-11-2022.2339366

Williams, P., Sheridan, S., Garvis, S., & Mellgren, E. (2018). Early childhood education and care in Sweden: The context of Swedish preschool. In *International Perspectives on Early Childhood Education and Care* (pp. 189–201). Routledge. DOI: 10.4324/9780203730553-17

Wolf, M. (2007). Proust and the squid: The story and science of the reading brain. *New York.*

Wulan, S., & Jamaris, M. (2023). Increasing Children's Character Overt Behaviours by Neuro Pedagogy-Based Play. *Jurnal Pendidikan Usia Dini, 17*(2), 363–377. DOI: 10.21009/JPUD.172.12

Yuce, A. E. (2023). Physical, social and emotional needs of developing children: Comparison of neuroscientific findings and Bertrand Russell's ideas. *Journal of Theory and Practice in Education, 19*(1), 123–139.

Yurdakul, Y., Ilhan Ildız, G., & Ayhan, A. B. (2022). The examination of the relationship between self-regulation skills and prosocial behaviors in preschool children. *Mehmet Akif Ersoy University Journal of Education Faculty*, (62), 354–376. doi:10.21764/maeuefd.1008817

Zosh, J. M., Hopkins, E. J., Jensen, H., Liu, C., Neale, D., Pasek, K. H., ... & Whitebread, D. (2017). *Learning through play: A review of the evidence.*

Chapter 9

The Role of Emotions in the Learning Process:

The Emotional Brain and Its Relationship With Learning in Pediatric Cancer

Georgia Kalfadeli
https://orcid.org/0009-0007-5466-6659
University of Thessaly, Greece

Antonios I. Christou
https://orcid.org/0000-0003-2981-1651
University of Thessaly, Greece

Stella Tsermentseli
https://orcid.org/0000-0003-3622-0171
University of Thessaly, Greece

Flora Bakopoulou
Clinic for Assessment of Adolescent Learning Difficulties, Center for Adolescent Medicine First Department of Pediatrics, Medical School, National and Kapodistrian University of Athens, Greece

Menia Koukougianni
https://orcid.org/0009-0008-1618-3127
Awareness for Childhood and Adolesccent Cancer, NGO Karkinaki, Greece

Maria Tzortzaki
https://orcid.org/0009-0007-6031-1045
Awareness for Childhood and Adolesccent Cancer, NGO Karkinaki, Greece

ABSTRACT

This present chapter examines the crucial and particularly important role of emotions in the learning process, focusing on the "emotional brain" and its connection to learning, particularly in the context of paediatric oncology. The role played by

DOI: 10.4018/979-8-3373-3581-0.ch009

emotions and the emotional state of individuals is not just a secondary factor in learning, but a critical element affecting executive functions. Brain structures play a key role in the regulation of emotion and cognitive function.The challenge in the case of children with cancer is particularly great, as emotional regulation and mental resilience influence to a significant extent how children respond to learning challenges. Significant barriers to mastery of emotional and cognitive development are played by the disease and its accompanying experiences. The role of neuropedagogy is to provide an innovative, structured and targeted framework for enhancing the emotionality of children with cancer, combining knowledge from neuroscience, psychology and pedagogy.

INTRODUCTION

Learning is a dominant aspect of human development, dynamically influencing the way individuals evolve, adapt and interact with their environment. In essence, it is not just a cognitive process, but reflects a deep connection to an individual's emotional experiences (Dennison, 2023). More specifically, the learning process is not characterised as an independent and autonomous process, on the contrary, however, is closely linked to the learner's mental world (Kalawski, 2020). Emotions play a key role in the development of abilities related to executive functions such as attention, memory, decision-making and motivation, which are directly related to the learning process (Christou et al., 2025). In addition, recent research has shown that certain brain areas, such as the amygdala and hippocampus, are associated with emotional functioning, while areas associated with learning and decision-making, such as the prefrontal cortex, have been identified (Christou et al., 2023). The term "Emotional Brain", describes the areas associated with emotional development, which contributes drastically to a variety of activities in an individual's daily life, with learning being predominant (Ruba & Pollak, 2020).

At the same time, a child's ability to cope with stressful situations and emotional challenges is crucial for learning. This ability is referred to as mental resilience and plays a key role in cognitive development during the developmental years (Basso et al., 2019). Mental resilience is closely linked to the quality of parental care, as supportive and emotionally responsive parenting can foster a child's ability to manage stress effectively (Christou et al., 2024). Furthermore, growing up in an environment that promotes environmental sensitivity—through respect for sustainability practices and emotional connection with the natural world—can enhance a child's emotional awareness and strengthen their psychological resilience (Christou et al., 2025).

Children who develop resilience manage to maintain active participation in school life even under particularly adverse conditions (Horn & Feder, 2018). One of the cases of adverse circumstances is the case of children who develop cancer during childhood or adolescence. More specifically, childhood cancer, in addition to physical health, significantly affects both the emotional and cognitive development of children and adolescents respectively (Marusak et al., 2017). Children and adolescents who become ill are faced with emotional challenges, mainly due to the change in the rhythm of their daily lives, therapeutic interventions, and social isolation due to their constant absence from the school environment (Herringa, 2017).

It is also of particular importance to highlight the importance and methods of emotional and psychological support to enhance and smooth the acquisition of cognitive development and the learning process (Basso et al., 2019)

The purpose of this chapter is therefore to explore the role of emotions and psychological resilience, focusing on children and adolescents undergoing treatment and struggling with cancer in any form. In addition, the work presented aims to highlight the neuroanatomy of the emotional brain and the role of emotions in the development of cognitive ability. At the same time, it will relate learning to the emotional state, drawing mainly on neuropsychological and educational approaches. The role of interpersonal-emotional skills will be presented, as well as the importance of having supportive learning environments for the purpose of emotional regulation and optimizing school performance. Also, the purpose is to highlight the specificity of children with cancer and to present the negative effects of treatments on the development of mental resilience and emotional well-being. The emotional challenges faced by children with cancer impede their learning pathway and render them unable to respond with full commitment to their learning and academic development. Finally, the importance of applying specific neuropedagogical strategies is the most important factor in enhancing emotional resilience and cognitive support in typically developing children and children who have been confronted with cancer at such a tender and sensitive age.

THE EMOTIONAL BRAIN: STRUCTURES AND FUNCTIONS

Neuroanatomy of the Emotional Brain

The "emotional brain" is mainly associated with the limbic system, a set of anatomical structures located between the cortex and the hypothalamus. The limbic system has some particularly important functions related to the control, processing, and regulation of emotions and behavior (Nijhof et al., 2018). All of the above are initiated through the hypothalamus and the hormones secreted from it, influencing human activity in a variety of ways. It is therefore not a single structure, but a set of areas that interact with each other (Poole et al., 2018). The term "emotional brain" is used to describe a system of structures in the brain that is responsible for the recognition of emotions, their processing and the physical, cognitive and behavioural response to them (Russell & Herringa, 2021). The system of structures, therefore, consists of the Amygdala, Hippocampus, Hypothalamus, Prefrontal cortex and Prefrontal cortex. Each of these parts plays a distinct and highly significant role in emotional regulation and the interface with the learning process (Poole et al., 2018).

To begin with, the Amygdala plays a primary and noteworthy role in the recognition, regulation and interpretation of intense emotional states experienced by the individual, such as anger, outburst and fear, and is also associated with the mnemonic capacity of synaesthetic memories (Russell & Herringa, 2021). Moving to the Hippocampus, it is responsible for storing emotions in long-term memory, but also for retrieving at any time the information related either directly or indirectly to these emotions (Nijhof et al., 2018). In addition, the Hypothalamus is responsible for regulating and controlling the independent functions of the body in response to the particular emotions experienced by the individual, such as an increase in heart rate and sweating. The prefrontal cortex plays a key role in executive functioning, logical processing, and the regulation of emotional responses originating from the Amygdala (Russell & Herringa, 2021). The cingulate cortex is responsible for contributing to attention, empathy, and the regulation of emotional outbursts. It is noteworthy to mention the importance of the functional relationships of these brain regions, as these regions function as a network and not independently. The connection between the amygdala and the prefrontal cortex is critical for the self-regulation of emotions (Poole et al., 2018).

Additionally, emotional activity and the processing of these emotions can be directly influenced by the role of neurotransmitters, such as serotonin, dopamine, and norepinephrine, which make up the neurochemical activity of the human brain (Russell & Herringa, 2021). Disorders in these circuits have been shown to be linked to emotional regulation problems, such as the onset of depression and anxiety disorders (Nijhof et al., 2018). More specifically, these structures of the emotional brain do not mature instantly but gradually, which makes them vulnerable to trauma and early stimuli. The functionality of these areas can be shaped either positively or negatively depending on the stimuli that individuals experience in their environment, such as supportive parents or certain traumatic experiences (Nijhof et al., 2018).

In all of the above, lies the role of neuropedagogy or mind-brain education, an interdisciplinary field, which combines neuroscience, pedagogy and psychology (Gvozdii et al., 2022). The main goal of neuropedagogy is to enhance the learning process and develop innovative and personalized practices to improve cognitive and emotional development (Chojak, 2018). At the same time, the main focus of neuropedagogical science is the connection of the educational act with the functioning of the brain, in order to enhance emotional maturation and development

(Chojak, 2018). The aim is for teaching to promote emotional safety and empathy to dynamically contribute to the enhancement of cognitive processes and active participation in school engagement.

The Role of Emotions

Emotions are complex psychophysiological reactions to stimuli, whether internal or external. They also combine cognitive, physical, and social elements, and are not actually irrational, but rather interact with cognitive processes (Dennison, 2023). Emotions play a crucial role in the development of executive functions, particularly in attention, memory, decision-making, internal and external motivation, and learning (Gkora & Christou, 2023). It is therefore clear that positive emotions, such as joy and enthusiasm, significantly enhance the ability to pay attention and learning activity, while negative emotions, such as anxiety, fear, and anger, hinder the overall cognitive development of children (Popovic et al., 2020).

More specifically, it has been proven that children who experience positive emotions at school, such as safety, acceptance, and encouragement, are more actively and effectively involved in the learning process, while at the same time they acquire knowledge more targeted and focused (Dennison, 2023). Increased persistence and self-regulation of emotions also appear to be a result of the positive emotions experienced by children. On the other hand, children whose emotions are largely negative, such as fear, anxiety, shame, and social rejection, usually lack confidence in the learning process, withdraw from acquiring new knowledge, and isolate themselves from their social environment and classmates (Tan et al., 2020). Additionally, they have difficulties in acquiring executive functions, and mainly in concentration and academic performance. In general, the emotions a child experiences can affect situations while providing information for their interpretation. For example, a challenging test can be characterized in various ways depending on the emotional state of the student at that moment.

Furthermore, the importance of emotional involvement in the development of learning motivation has been proven to be related to cognitive development and enhancing academic performance (Popovic et al., 2020). More specifically, emotion is a cornerstone for internal motivation or the development of internal drive. In other words, a child's emotional involvement in the learning process is largely related to whether a child is surrounded by a supportive environment, without being criticized or disapproved of (Pergantis et al., 2025). The connection of learning with personal interests also proves the development of intrinsic motivation in combination with previous positive experiences from school and learning in general. The case of children with childhood cancer is a special emotional situation in which children are confronted with intense negative emotions, mainly fear, anxiety, and loneliness, which significantly affect their cognitive and learning skills (Christou et al., 2025). Furthermore, the psychological state of children affects how they perceive and interpret the experience of illness and their position within the peer group. Therefore, emotional support is not secondary; it is a basic prerequisite for the success of any learning intervention and is necessary for their smooth learning development (Popovic et al., 2020).

Theories of Emotion

Various theories have been proposed to explain the effect of emotions on the development of various abilities. Theories of emotions attempt to explain the creation and development of emotions, the order of their appearance, and their connection to the body, brain, and behavior. Understanding these theories can provide a better understanding of how the emotional brain functions and the relationship between emotions and learning (Casey et al., 2017).

The James-Lange Theory (1884) initially identifies the theory that the emotion is the result of the physical reaction. For example, a person trembling may mean that they are afraid. Consequently, the body's signals are sent and channeled to the brain, and in this way they are interpreted as emotion (Casey et al., 2017). Later, the Cannon-Bard Theory (1927) was developed, which states that the two concepts of emotion and physical response occur independently of each other, but at the same time (Casey et al., 2017). With this theory, the importance of the Thalamus and the Amygdala in the processing of emotion was introduced. Additionally, the classical theories include Schachter-Singer's theory (Two-Factor Theory), which states that emotion is a combination of physiological arousal and cognitive interpretation (Moumne et al., 2021).

Moving on to modern neuroscientific and cognitive theories about emotions, according to Antonio Damasio, bodily reactions contribute to more accurate and effective decision-making . With this theory, emotions can be the center of separation for what is beneficial and what is dangerous, through memory, cognitive distinction, and experience (Moumne et al., 2021). According to Joseph LeDoux, the feeling of fear is formed through two methods. The first "Low road" is the direct and automatic response through the Amygdala, and the second "High road" is the slow response through the prefrontal cortex (Moumne et al., 2021). The important thing in this theory is understanding the reactions in children, mainly anxiety and traumatic reactions. Additionally, according to Richard Lazarus theory, every emotional expression is preceded by a cognitive evaluation of the situation. For example, there will be anxiety in the pursuit of successs (Moumne et al., 2021). It becomes clear in this theory that emotions are determined by the specific meaning assigned to them. Overall, the above theories connect learning and educational practice, while also explaining students' perception of school and how it affects their emotions. They also serve as guidelines for teachers to gain a deeper understanding of students' emotional reactions. Especially useful in educating children with chronic illnesses, such as childhood cancer, who experience intense feelings of fear, anxiety, and isolation (Moumne et al., 2021).

EMOTIONS AND LEARNING: NEUROPSYCHOLOGICAL AND EDUCATIONAL PERSPECTIVES

Emotional Regulation and Academic Performance

Emotional regulation refers to an individual's ability to effectively process, understand, and control the emotions they experience in different situations in their daily life (Tan et al., 2020). More specifically, through emotional regulation, the recognition of emotions is carried out in depth, meaning that the feelings experienced by individuals become understandable. Moreover, feelings are expressed in a way that is acceptable to society, mainly through external support from teachers and the family environment. Emotional regulation also includes internal strategies, such as positive reappraisal and self-soothing (Popovic et al., 2020).

Additionally, the ability to regulate emotions has a direct relationship with academic performance, as it enhances the ability to pay attention and concentrate in the learning process, reduces conflicts and the feeling of impulsiveness in everyday actions. Cognitive flexibility and self-regulation are promoted by this ability to regulate emotions, particularly in managing test anxiety and coping with potential failure (Costello et al., 2021). This way, the existence of anxiety disorders in students from the learning process can be addressed more directly and makes it more enjoyable and accessible (Dennison, 2023). On the other hand, it has been proven that children who have difficulty regulating their emotions also have lower performance compared to other students without the same difficulties. Also, they seem to have more and more frequent absences due to the extensive difficulty they face in achieving learning objectives. In this context, the extensive learning and social difficulties presented in a broader developmental framework can also be understood (Dennison, 2023).

Moving on to the neuropsychological basis of the relationship between emotional regulation and school performance, the action of the prefrontal cortex, which is directly responsible for regulating emotional expressions and executive function, is noteworthy (Russell & Herringa, 2021). The amygdala plays a similar role, and if it is not properly filtered by the prefrontal cortex, it leads to an escalation of negative emotions. Therefore, the existence of a balance between the structures of the brain system is key to the development of learning and behavioral action in the classroom (Poole et al., 2018).

In order to strengthen and support emotional and learning activities, it is necessary to implement educational strategies and specialized support and intervention programs. These programs can be psychoeducational programs, with an emphasis on developing and establishing a stable routine and a familiar atmosphere in the classroom between students and teachers (Al-Hroub & Al-Hroub, 2024). On this basis, SEL (Social Emotional Learning) programs can be used, which are one of the most modern and documented ways of enhancing students' emotional regulation, self-awareness, empathy, and social adaptation (Al-Hroub & Al-Hroub, 2024). More specifically, these programs can be implemented in practice through specific educational interventions, such as PATHS, Second Step, CASEL framework. All of the above can be used directly and effectively in schools, as they can be implemented immediately by the teachers themselves. The aim, therefore, is for both typically developing children and children with special needs to cultivate positive feelings about school and learning in general (Tan et al., 2020).

Social-Emotional Skills

The natural continuation of SEL programs is related to their social-emotional impact on everyday life and on conditions related to learning and the cultivation of general cognitive development in children (Al-Hroub & Al-Hroub, 2024). In particular, social-emotional skills are a well-structured set of skills that enable individuals to recognize, understand, and process their own emotions, as well as the emotions experienced by others, i.e., to have empathy (Wang et al., 2018). At the same time, they can create and develop positive and harmonious social relationships, with a view to creating healthy social and interpersonal relationships. This will encourage children to try to develop healthy ways of resolving conflicts and disagreements that may arise in the process of forming social relationships, but also to make decisions with determination and responsibility. Through the above, the corresponding importance will be given to emotional intelligence and the results it can bring to the overall socialization of children with typical and atypical developmental trajectories (Tan et al., 2020)

To understand social-emotional skills, it is essential to mention the cornerstones according to CASEL (Voineskos, 2020). First, it is particularly important for children to know what they feel and why they feel it. This can be incorporated into self-awareness, with the aim of promoting emotional understanding and the correct differentiation of emotions. In addition, they should be able to manage their emotions effectively through the principle of self-management (Wang et al., 2018). It is advisable that children, beyond understanding emotions, be able to adapt their feelings to the social situation by integrating them into the natural consequences of the situations they experience. Another pillar of social-emotional skills is social awareness, i.e. being able to empathise with and understand the emotions of others (Voineskos, 2020).

This will strengthen their interpersonal relationships and make it easier for them to integrate into society, giving them the opportunity to collaborate, listen, and support others through relationship skills (Tan et al., 2020). Furthermore, the principle of responsible decision-making will enable them to make decisions that are fair and right for both themselves and others. The role of social-emotional skills is remarkable in the learning process, as they reinforce and contribute to smooth cooperation and active participation in educational processes (Voineskos, 2020). At the same time, they contribute to strengthening behavioral regulation with the aim of reducing the occurrence and manifestation of conflictual, violent, and impulsive situations. The manifestation of self-esteem, mental resilience, and active participation in the school environment is also an important goal for teachers through the strengthening of social-emotional skills, as it has been proven to be linked to better school performance and higher levels of social integration and inclusion (Voineskos, 2020). Overall, the development of social-emotional skills is fundamental to children's academic success, cognitive development, and mental health. In the case of children with cancer, it has been shown that cultivating these skills through personalized and supportive interventions is a key pillar of empowerment and reintegration into the school environment (Tan et al., 2020).

Emotionally Supportive Learning Environments: The Theory of Emotional Safety in The Classroom

The connection with all of the above can be complemented by the concept of emotional security and how this can be achieved in the classroom by teachers and students as a whole. Emotional safety refers to the feeling of acceptance, trust, and respect that students feel in the school environment (Jirout et al., 2023). This definition can be explained by the fact that it is important for students to feel free and not experience anxiety and fear about possible mistakes they may make. Furthermore, they feel comfortable expressing their feelings openly without fear or shame, thinking that they may be stigmatized and negatively labeled by their peers (Jirout et al., 2023). Consequently, they have the ability to feel psychologically secure, so that they can participate actively and unhindered in the learning process (Pericas et al., 2022). It is worth mentioning the importance of developing emotional safety at a theoretical level, as it supports the idea that learning, in order to be effective and targeted, requires the cultivation and development of psychological safety first and foremost (Pericas et al., 2022). Thus, when a child feels anxious or isolated from others, higher cognitive processes, such as memory and logic, are inhibited by the brain's alarm system, such as the amygdala. On the other hand, when students experience positive emotions during the learning process, such as security and trust, brain functions signal that learning is receptive and acceptable (Jirout et al., 2023).

All of the above can also be explained from a neurological perspective, as the prefrontal cortex, which is responsible for cognitive processing, works more effectively with the amygdala in conditions where the child feels safe and free from conflict (Poole et al., 2018). In addition, serotonin and oxytocin are enhanced by a supportive and positive environment, facilitating the strengthening of learning ability and the cultivation of positive attitudes towards the acquisition of cognitive processes. On the contrary, the presence of cortisol, which is responsible for stress in the body, seems to hinder memory and concentration in those who have high levels of it (Russell & Herringa, 2021).

It is therefore important to have an emotionally supportive environment that provides a stable and smooth relationship between the teacher and all students. In this way, the principle of acceptance and understanding of emotional diversity in the classroom will be developed, giving everyone the freedom to express themselves openly without feeling that they will be criticized and stigmatized by the school environment (Wang et al., 2018). Mistakes should be used as a catalyst for the development and achievement of students' goals, not as a punitive practice that alienates children and fills them with negative and sad emotions (Jirout et al., 2023). Thus, empathy and a sense of solidarity among those involved in the educational process are more directly developed and cultivated, making it a beautiful and positive-feeling process (Jirout et al., 2023). The existence of stable routines, also, leads to the smoothing of the entire process and removes stress and tensions. The teacher's role becomes important, as they must act as a regulator of the emotional climate of the classroom, providing opportunities for development and growth without stress and fear. Teacher must cultivate security in all students without pressure, understanding the individual needs of each student and being flexible in teaching (Pericas et al., 2022).

Emotionality and Resilience in Learning

To understand the relationship between emotion and learning, the existence of emotionality and mental resilience in the learning process must be clarified. Emotionality is the expression of the expression of the respective emotion, such as the way they express themselves and how they affect conditions and behaviors in learning (Masten et al., 2021). Openly, emotionality affects students' self-perception, their dedication to their goals, cognitive development, and their social interaction with their peers. Additionally, mental resilience is attributed to the child's ability to harmonize and adapt positively to difficult and adverse conditions. It is a skill that is not innate, but is cultivated through positive relationships and in safe and supportive environments (Tillery et al., 2015).

Resilience can be characterized as the link between learning and traumatic experiences, is not an innate and inherent ability, but rather develops mainly in supportive environments, which assist in the further development of the set of competences that need to be mastered by students (Masten et al., 2021). It has been proven that children with high emotionality can be vulnerable to potential failures, and this is where resilience comes in, which acts as a protective factor and allows students to be cognitively active despite the difficulties and obstacles they may face along the way (Ai & Hu, 2014). For example, a child with cancer may experience intense fear or insecurity, but having a supportive environment and personal resilience skills can help them continue their journey in learning. Mental resilience is not a privilege of the few. It is a learning and emotional ability that develops systematically, especially when the child is supported by relationships, routines, and school environments that empower them. In the case of children with cancer, resilience is not just desirable, but it is vital for survival, integration, and learning (Horn & Feder, 2018).

Additionally, mental resilience can be strengthened and cultivated through school support from teachers, who must show care and interest in the emotional, cognitive, and social development of students (Tillery et al., 2015). The implementation of specialized programs is deemed necessary for the development of mental resilience through their widespread application in the classroom. At the same time, the existence of family stability is a supportive factor, so that children feel that their parents are emotionally available and do not neglect them (Tillery et al., 2015). Enhancing positivity, self-confidence, and motivation can also be cultivated through SEL educational interventions, psychoeducation, and specialized and targeted interventions for traumatic experiences (Al-Hroub & Al-Hroub, 2024). Overall, strengthening the resilience of students, especially those facing serious psychosocial or medical challenges such as childhood cancer, is a necessary condition for learning progress. Understanding how emotionality affects learning and how it can be balanced through resilience offers a meaningful pedagogical path to inclusion and success (Masten et al., 2021).

PEDIATRIC CANCER AND EMOTIONAL BRAIN

Neurodevelopmental Correlates

This section of the chapter will analyze how the brain develops during childhood and how this development is affected by childhood cancer diagnosis and subsequent treatments. At the same time, it is noteworthy that the conditions that promote the vulnerability of children with cancer from a neuropsychological perspective are understood. Firstly, neurodevelopment is an extremely important process during which brain functions are formed, from birth to adulthood (Krull et al., 2018). Due to the development of brain processes, important information can be obtained about the cognitive, emotional, and social development of individuals, as well as the connection that can be identified between learning and emotion (Christou et al., 2025). This process includes neural differentiation, through the specialization of cells in distinct functions, synaptogenesis, which is perceived through the formation of neural synapses, and synaptic pruning, i.e., the elimination of connections that are not functional. All of the above brain processes are intense during the early years of life and continue until adolescence (Russell & Herringa, 2021).

During the early years of life, there is further concern about the development of cognitive and emotional skills, which is why they are considered critical periods of development in a person's life. It is a vulnerable period during which brain functions are particularly sensitive to external stimuli, both environmental and biological, which can have either a positive or negative effect (Russell & Herringa, 2021). A cancer diagnosis during childhood and treatments such as radiation and chemotherapy can have a negative impact on overall cognitive and emotional development. Furthermore, investigating neurodevelopment in relation to emotions may explain the child's relationship with learning and knowledge (Christou et al., 2025). During preschool age, the brain is more plastic and extremely vulnerable, making the age range of 0 to 6 years a particularly dangerous phase for neurodevelopment. Potential damage during this period can lead to significant cognitive and emotional deficits (Russell & Herringa, 2021). In the next age group, from 6 to 12 years old, difficulties in executive functions and social skills may arise, often leading to social withdrawal and isolation. Consequently, exclusion from school may further exacerbate the situation. Finally, during adolescence, given that new developmental demands arise, such as autonomy, relationships, and the search for identity, potential obstacles to neurodevelopment can alter and negatively contribute to the above (Christou et al., 2024).

More specifically, neurodevelopment is related to a child's ability to understand, express, and regulate emotions, which is linked to the maturation of brain structures (Pinto, 2022). Correspondingly, delays or difficulties in neurodevelopment seem to lead to emotional instability, behavioral difficulties, and, more generally, difficulties in adapting to the school environment (Pinto, 2022). Cancer diagnosis and treatments disrupt normal neurodevelopment, as specific areas of the brain are affected, such as the hippocampus, which is responsible for memory. This can lead to cognitive difficulties, difficulties with emotional regulation, and reduced school engagement (Gvozdii et al., 2022). Neurodevelopment is therefore a dynamic and ongoing process during which disturbances in the nervous system may occur during vulnerable childhood, affecting both the emotional and cognitive development of children (Gvozdii et al., 2022). In this context, it is particularly important to develop and implement appropriate and specialized neuropedagogical programs in schools, which will aim at overall emotional and cognitive development. The role of teachers is clearly necessary in order for them to be informed and specialized in relevant neuropedagogical issues and to be able to apply practices that comprehensively support the developmental progress of all students without exception (Al-Hroub & Al-Hroub, 2024).

Neurotoxicity of Treatments

Childhood cancer is a pressing issue that profoundly alters the daily lives of vulnerable children and changes the priorities and desires of students. The therapeutic process followed or the treatment regimen is important in each case if more than one therapeutic practice is required (Marusak et al., 2017). However, the effects of these treatments are decisive but also neurotoxic for the overall development of patients. Initially, neurotoxicity is caused by external factors, such as drugs and radiation, and is associated with damage to the brain and nervous system. This is mainly due to the brain's vulnerability to chemical and radiation interference (Yu, 2019). However, despite the negative effects of these therapies, they are essential for the survival of children with malignant tumors (Yu, 2019).

Neurotoxicity through chemotherapy is caused by certain drug treatments, such as methotrexate, cytarabine, and vincristine, which are neurotoxic when administered intrathecally through the central nervous system. The effects mainly manifest as leukoencephalopathy, reduced information processing speed, and memory and attention disorders (Marusak et al., 2017). In addition, radiation as a treatment for childhood cancer in leukaemia and brain tumours can cause brain atrophy, a decrease in cognitive ability over time, with the consequent appearance of learning difficulties and difficulties in acquiring executive functions (Krull et al., 2018). Corticosteroids follow the same logic, affecting the function and action of the hippocampus and amygdala, as they are associated with mood changes and contribute to the onset of depressive symptoms, combined with a decrease in concentration and emotional stability (Poole et al., 2018).

The aforementioned methods of treating childhood cancer contribute negatively mainly to a reduction in cognitive ability, difficulty concentrating, inability to recall information related to everyday events, and slow acquisition of new knowledge and information (Gvozdii et al., 2022). Of course, there are also significant emotional effects, with anxiety, sadness, and uncertainty being the most prevalent. In addition, there are many mood swings and changes, as well as low self-esteem combined with social withdrawal and isolation (Marusak et al., 2017). Frequent absences from school due to extended hospitalizations distance children with cancer from the school environment and place them in a different reality. As a result, they have a reduced desire to learn and engage in the educational process, feeling an increased risk of academic failure and making mistakes (Marusak et al., 2017). Specialised and, above all, personalised emotional and cognitive support is therefore required, both from educators and from the wider and immediate environment (Gvozdii et al., 2022). Early detection and early intervention are therefore crucial for supporting children who experience the harsh reality of cancer. Children with a history of neoplasia should be monitored neuropsychologically to detect difficulties early on (Seth, 2023). This monitoring is deemed necessary to be carried out at regular intervals, with the aim of adapting educational interventions, strengthening resilience, and achieving holistic restoration of cognitive and psychosocial skills. Surviving childhood cancer is a huge victory. However, the treatments that make it possible often leave neurological and psychoeducational imprints. Recognizing neurotoxicity as a risk factor for children's learning and mental health is necessary for developing effective support strategies (Yu, 2019).

Emotional Challenges Faced by Children With Cancer

Beyond the effects of treatment, the emotional impact of diagnosis can be a traumatic experience for the child, who is faced with changes in their daily life. At the same time, after the diagnosis, the child is overwhelmed by feelings of fear and immediate threat to their life and survival (Seth, 2023). In addition, the loss of control over their daily life due to constant and repeated hospitalizations creates a framework of uncertainty about their future. In many cases, during the initial phase of diagnosis, there is a feeling of denial and silent withdrawal from everything that existed in their daily life until then (Krull et al., 2018). During treatment, symptoms of pain and discomfort are identified, and regular medical interventions are performed. In addition, the effects on self-image, such as hair loss and physical changes, significantly affect self-confidence, causing them to withdraw even further and distance themselves from social reality (Marusak et al., 2017). Frequent absences from school and classmates also contribute to the social isolation of patients. All of the above lead to the onset of anxiety disorders, especially before hospitalization or surgery, leading to outbursts of anger and reactivity to the situation they are experiencing, while at the same time the onset of depressive symptoms, apathy, and loss of interest coexist throughout the course of treatment (Marusak et al., 2017).

After treatment, the child may still experience fear of relapse and have reduced self-confidence, especially with regard to social and school reintegration. In addition, the emotional and social difficulties experienced during treatment may continue and possibly develop into related difficulties, such as the development of post-traumatic stress disorder (PTSS) and developmental delays in overall emotional and social maturation (Cisler & Herringa, 2020). However, the emotional impact mentioned above varies significantly depending on the stage of development at which the diagnosis is made. More specifically, a child in early childhood deals with a cancer diagnosis differently than a child in adolescence. Consequently, emotional reactions also vary depending on age. In order to address these specific difficulties, it is necessary to provide accurate information to both the educational and family environments so that the early recognition of all the difficulties that a child may face at any stage of the disease is understood (Cisler & Herringa, 2020).

Similar effects may be observed in the child's familiar and related environment after the diagnosis of neoplasm, changing the pre-existing conditions (Marusak et al., 2017). Parents often experience anxiety and go through phases of mental and physical exhaustion. This can clearly have an even more negative impact on the feelings of the child who is ill. Generally, in such an emotionally charged environment, the child's mood and desire to participate in school are affected, subsequently reducing their attention and concentration, as well as their fear of rejection (Christou et al., 2025).

EMOTIONAL IMPACT OF PEDIATRIC CANCER ON LEARNING PROCESSES

Negative Emotions and Cognitive Functions

The case of children diagnosed with cancer is a special one, due to the difficulties they face. The constant emotional challenges, such as fear, anxiety, sadness, and disappointment that they experience, have a negative impact on the neurobiology of the brain (Marusak et al., 2017). These areas are responsible for memory, concentration, attention, and emotional response. The conditions they experience for years at a constant and intense pace do not allow them to feel free and full of positive emotions, but they are constantly in painful and emotionally difficult situations of uncertainty (Krull et al., 2018).

To understand the neurobiological mechanism of these negative emotions, the explanation can be found in the hyperactivity of the amygdala, which, with the existence of increased threat perception, actively affects the absorption of cognitive resources from the learning process (Russell & Herringa, 2021). By the same logic, the reduction in the function of the hippocampus, due to high levels of cortisol, affects the difficulty of storing new information in the individual's memory. In addition, disorders in the prefrontal cortex contribute negatively by causing reduced executive function in decision-making (Russell & Herringa, 2021). Overall, it is clear that the presence and, even worse, the continued presence of these negative emotions significantly hinders and impedes the development and evolution of executive functions in children with cancer (Krull et al., 2018). However, all these emotions that children experience after being diagnosed with cancer at any stage are also reflected in their learning, through difficulty concentrating on tasks and in class in general. Similarly, information processing appears to be extremely slow, while the ability to acquire new knowledge seems extremely difficult (Marusak et al., 2017). There are also signs of procrastination and avoidance of school activities in a general atmosphere of aversion to all learning activities. Overall, therefore, the above characteristics are also reflected in their school performance, where in many cases they appear to show a decline in academic and school performance, even if the child had a good learning profile before diagnosis (Krull et al., 2018).

It seems, therefore, that there is a negative vicious circle between the negative emotions experienced by children who fall ill and their cognitive and learning progress (Marusak et al., 2017). Constant hospitalizations, changes in daily routine, and overall changes in habits that existed before diagnosis cause intense negative emotions, which in turn contribute negatively to reduced school performance (Del Giacco et al., 2023). In turn, poor school performance leads to further stressful and negative situations, which ultimately lead to learning stagnation and a generalized risk of school failure. It is therefore necessary to implement strategies to reduce negative emotions through the application of personalized support practices by mental health professionals (Al-Hroub & Al-Hroub, 2024). At the same time, it is the responsibility of teachers to create and cultivate a positive learning environment in which the child feels emotionally free to express their feelings, is the responsibility of teachers, who should instil the cultivation of self-regulation skills in this climate. Of course, all of the above can be achieved with flexibility in the educational program for children with cancer at this sensitive age (Del Giacco et al., 2023).

The Role of Family and the School Environment

In such a climate of mental instability and widespread changes in daily life experienced by children with cancer, the contribution of the family environment is essential (Chaplin et al., 2022). Initially, through emotional security within the family, the sick child can be overwhelmed by positive feelings of optimism, calmness, and honesty, facilitating a smooth adjustment to the new circumstances (Lin & Faldowski, 2023). The family, as the core of emotional security, helps the child understand and adapt to their daily life, reducing negative feelings such as anxiety and stress. However, in order to achieve all this, it is important for parents and guardians to receive appropriate information on how to communicate so that they can thoroughly understand the child's mental state (Pericas et al., 2022). At the same time, it is important that they themselves receive appropriate psychological support so that they are able to manage their own concerns and worries about the diagnosis. This is completely understandable, as a cancer diagnosis in childhood stigmatises and disorients both the children themselves and their immediate environment (Lin & Faldowski, 2023). More specifically, it has been observed that in families where conflict and high stress prevail, children pick up on the situation and internalize it, causing them increased fear and insecurity about the disease (Chaplin et al., 2022). The siblings of sick children also experience a similar situation, as their parents' attention is focused on the sick child and they feel neglected due to the unequal distribution of attention. All of the above, of course, can be mitigated by creating an atmosphere of stability and emotional calm for everyone (Chaplin et al., 2022).

In addition, the existence and development of stable routines can bear fruit both in the family environment and at school. School is important as a conduit for bridging everyday life with the challenges that arise, while also being a place for socialization and learning (Marusak et al., 2017). Therefore, the implementation of important practices in the school environment can enhance the feeling of security and stability during the adverse course of the diagnosis (Lin & Faldowski, 2023). More specifically, ongoing communication between the school, teachers, family, and medical staff can be a significant factor in the child's cognitive and emotional development. Of course, flexibility in the educational program and personalization in the educational process are required in order to achieve the best possible results (Gvozdii et al., 2022).

To achieve the above, adjustments are required, such as reducing the workload in the learning process and developing alternative forms of participation in the lesson, such as online teaching, so that they can follow the lesson even if they are unable to attend school due to hospitalization (Gvozdii et al., 2022). Emotional support from teachers will strengthen mental resilience, leading to reduced anxiety, increased self-confidence, and the cultivation of a familiar environment of emotional security (Jirout et al., 2023). Overall, teachers need to be educated and informed about pediatric cancer and the psychosocial empowerment of children (Del Giacco et al., 2023). More generally, parents and teachers must share a common mission, which, through holistic support, will help to coordinate common strategies for managing the fatigue, anxiety and exhaustion they experience (Christou et al., 2025). In addition, it is necessary to promote positive learning experiences and strengthen social relationships with peers and classmates (Gvozdii et al., 2022).

Interventions for Emotional Support and Enhancement of Learning

Mental stability can be achieved through interventions aimed primarily at reducing negative emotions, strengthening mental resilience, and enhancing positive self-perception (Blewitt, et al., 2021). In addition to the emotional and mental goals of the interventions, the maintenance and improvement of executive functions and cognitive skills must also be added, in combination with facilitating school and social reintegration upon completion of treatment. More specifically, cognitive behavioral therapy (CBT) can help reduce anxiety and symptoms of depression, which often occur after a diagnosis of pediatric cancer (Masten et al., 2021). In addition, training in self-regulation and positive thinking techniques can be the most important psychological support, along with participation in therapeutic programs through play and art. Art & Play Therapy programs provide a safe means of expressing emotions with the aim of improving communication with both the family and the school environment (Albert & Davies, 2018).

In addition, the implementation of educational interventions, through the adaptation of the curriculum, the timetable, and the assessment method, can lead to a smooth reintegration or "transition" from the hospital environment to the reality that existed before the diagnosis (Gvozdii et al., 2022). Cooperation between teachers and mental health specialists, as well as the medical and nursing monitoring team, can contribute significantly to this (Gvozdii et al., 2022). In addition, it is advisable to implement strategies to strengthen cognitive skills, such as memory games, concentration exercises, and problem-solving games, such as puzzles that enhance logical thinking (Pergantis et al., 2025). To more effectively address the emotional and cognitive difficulties they face throughout this process, it is advisable to use digital tools (Drakatos & Christou, 2023). Interaction with digital media encourages children to willingly participate in the learning process, incorporating interaction with classmates through group collaboration (Pergantis et al., 2025).

At the same time, neuroeducational interventions could be implemented, which would evaluate contemporary knowledge from neuroscience, pedagogy, and psychology. The design of targeted learning strategies that take into account how the brain works and adapts (Gvozdii et al., 2022). More specifically, in the case of children with cancer, the goal is to strengthen executive functions, memory capacity, and mental resilience, while reducing emotional stress (Marusak et al., 2017). An indicative neuroeducation program is the Brainfit Study, which can be described as a randomized research program that combines digital training of cognitive skills and practice through video games (Pergantis et al., 2025). In addition, the Neurofeedback method could also be useful for regulating brain activity. All of the above are clearly helpful tools, but they should be combined with individualized and personalized therapies aimed at enhancing emotional health. Such emotional support programs can focus on Resilience-Enhancing Mental Training, combining concentration exercises, mindfulness, and cognitive strengthening (Masten et al., 2021). In this context, schools and teachers can contribute by promoting multisensory learning with the aim of activating multiple areas of the brain (Popovic et al., 2020). The goal of neuropedagogy in the case of children with cancer is to bridge knowledge about brain function with pedagogical practices in order to develop an educational framework that meets the specific cognitive, emotional and developmental needs of these children (Chojak, 2018).

NEUROEDUCATIONAL STRATEGIES TO SUPPORT LEARNING AND EMOTIONAL RESILIENCE

Programs for Emotional and Cognitive Support

This section focuses on structured educational and psychosocial program designed to enhance cognitive functioning and support the emotional well-being of children with cancer, both during treatment and after recovery (Blair et al., 2024) . The aim of the programs that will follow is to strengthen and maintain cognitive skills, especially those related to concentration, memory, and executive functions (Al-Hroub & Al-Hroub, 2024). Most importantly, however, is the strengthening of mental resilience and a smooth transition back to everyday life and the activities that were performed before diagnosis and the start of treatment (Seth, 2023). As the understanding of brain function and its relationship to learning expands, neuropedagogy offers a powerful framework for supporting children facing serious medical challenges, such as childhood cancer. Initially, it is necessary to design individualised intervention programmes that take into account the child's neuropsychological profile (Chojak, 2018).

Both the design and the systematic implementation of a structured plan can significantly enhance the child's cognitive abilities and, consequently, willingness to actively participate in the learning process (Al-Hroub & Al-Hroub, 2024). All of the above can be implemented through the use of visualised information, colour coding and diagrams, which will transform the process into a more friendly and accessible process for the affected student (Tabibnia, 2024). Still, by introducing daily routines, lists, reminders and chunking techniques for recalling information, executive functions and cognitive abilities are to be enhanced to a significant degree (Tabibnia, 2024). Particularly helpful, too, are games, specialised exercises, digital and support tools, which enhance attentional, memory and organisational skills

(Pergantis et al., 2025). Robotics and stems are also capable of helping to improve the cognitive ability of children who have difficulties in executive functions.

At the same time, serotonin 5-HTTLPR genotype, a neurotransmitter that regulates mood, anxiety and social behaviour, can be an important axis of a neuropedagogical strategy to enhance learning, because it directly affects emotional regulation, attention and concentration (Christou et al., 2017). Serotonin has been shown to be related to the regulation of social behaviour, so it may actively contribute to enhancing cooperation, emotional understanding and interpersonal relationships of the student (Christou et al., 2015; Christou et al., 2016).

Overall, children with cancer need support from a multidisciplinary team to enhance psychosocial functioning (Kosola et al., 2017). It is important that all the specialists involved, such as the teacher, psychologist, speech and language therapist, special educator, medical and nursing staff, and the family, work together. The whole interdisciplinary team must act to foster hope and belonging and implement strategies to strengthen school identity and social inclusion, such as peer activities and joint projects (Blewitt et al., 2021).

Interdisciplinary Strategies

In order to strengthen the programs mentioned above, additional support and cooperation is required from all directly involved professionals, specifically teachers, psychologists, doctors, occupational therapists, nursing staff, and parents. In this way, a holistic support network for children with cancer can be developed and implemented to meet their cognitive, emotional, and social needs (Yu, 2019). Certain cooperation strategies are appropriate to implement, with frequent multi-theme "case conferences" with all parties involved being the most important (Chojak, 2018). In the first stage, it is advisable to design a joint support plan with clear objectives and roles. This plan should be fully tailored to the sick child, taking into account their cognitive level and current emotional and psychological state. All of this can be reinforced through communication protocols aimed at the continuous exchange of useful information for monitoring the child's progress (Blewitt et al., 2021). In addition, training on neuroeducation issues and appropriate briefing of all team members on basic principles and emotional support will reinforce effective action (Tabibnia, 2024). Some of the benefits of this interdisciplinary collaboration include avoiding rigid application of interventions and faster adaptation of strategies to the specific and individualized needs of the child.

For this teamwork and for the most effective implementation of interdisciplinary practices, everyone involved must be properly trained in order to achieve the best possible results (Blewitt et al., 2021). First and foremost, teachers must be proactive and adapt the educational content appropriately to make it more accessible and understandable for children suffering from pediatric cancer. Furthermore, they must create a familiar and accessible learning environment that enhances the emotional development of all, without making anyone feel neglected or marginalized (Pinto, 2022). In addition, teachers must be informed and collaborate with health professionals on the progression of the disease in order to assess the changing needs of the child (Gvozdii et al., 2022). In addition, psychologists and mental health professionals should provide meaningful emotional support through social-emotional support programs and sessions, while also training school staff on appropriate strategies for managing the negative emotions experienced both during treatment and throughout the course and progression of the disease (Gvozdii et al., 2022). In turn, medical and nursing staff must inform parents and teachers about medical restrictions and the subsequent effects of treatments on both the cognitive function and emotional state of patients. They must also propose a clear timeline for the course of treatment so that all parties can plan accordingly (Pinto, 2022). The role of speech therapists and occupational therapists can also be crucial, as they can contribute significantly to supporting cognitive difficulties by incorporating therapeutic activities for memory and attention into the learning process. In conclusion, interdisciplinary collaboration is not only useful but essential for supporting children with cancer. Only through coordinated action can continued learning and emotional resilience be ensured (Chojak, 2018).

PROSPECTS FOR FUTURE RESEARCH

Through the literature search, it becomes clear that there are no studies that follow the long-term cognitive and emotional progress of children after treatment. Also, the investigation of the effect of therapeutic interventions on neurodevelopment in combination with the educational process seems to be an unexplored field and needs to be explored. Through the literature search, it becomes clear that there are no studies that follow the long-term cognitive and emotional progress of children after treatment.

At the same time, there appears to be a need for longitudinal studies that record changes over time in order to understand the course of recovery and the factors that influence it. Furthermore, there is almost no research on how specific interventions, such as cognitive rehabilitation, neurofeedback, and SEL programs, affect specific neurodevelopmental skills in children who have completed treatment. Furthermore, there is a need for comparative studies to compare the progress of typically developing children with that of children who have had cancer in terms of cognitive and emotional skills.

Also, the investigation of the effect of therapeutic interventions on neurodevelopment in combination with the educational process seems to be an unexplored field and needs to be explored. The need to investigate methods of enhancing mental resilience and emotionality in the educational process is also fundamental, so that they experience part of it and feelings of anxiety, fear and social isolation are absent. All of the above seem to constitute an urgent need for investigation with the aim of strengthening the educational and social reality of both typically developing children and children suffering from cancer. Thus, gradually the scientific and research interest in the neuropsychology of childhood cancer will increase and a general awareness will take place in society as a whole.

REFERENCES

Ai, H., & Hu, J. (2014). Psychological resilience moderates the impact of social support on loneliness of "left-behind" children. *Journal of Health Psychology, 21*(6), 1066–1073. DOI: 10.1177/1359105314544992 PMID: 25139895

Al-Hroub, A., & Al-Hroub, R. (2024). Empowering the Vulnerable: The Impact of SEL on Traumatized Children's Academic and Social Outcomes in Crises. *Current Psychiatry Reports, 26*(12), 777–781. DOI: 10.1007/s11920-024-01555-8 PMID: 39523250

Albert, M. L., & Davies, M. (2018). Media use and brain development during adolescence. *Journal of the American Academy of Child & Adolescent Psychiatry.* https://pubmed.ncbi.nlm.nih.gov/29467362/

Basso, J. C., McHale, A., Ende, V., Oberlin, D. J., & Suzuki, W. A. (2019). Brief, daily meditation enhances attention, memory, mood, and emotional regulation in non-experienced meditators. *Behavioural Brain Research, 356*, 208–220. DOI: 10.1016/j.bbr.2018.08.023 PMID: 30153464

Blair, S., Henderson, M., McConnachie, A., McIntosh, E., Smillie, S., Wetherall, K., Wight, D., Xin, Y., Bond, L., Elliott, L., Haw, S., Jackson, C., Levin, K., & Wilson, P. (2024). The Social and Emotional Education and Development intervention to address wellbeing in primary school age children: The SEED cluster RCT. *Public Health Research, 12*(6), 1–173. DOI: 10.3310/LYRQ5047 PMID: 38940833

Blewitt, C., Morris, H., O'Connor, A., Ifanti, A., Greenwood, D., & Skouteris, H. (2021). Social and emotional learning in early childhood education and care: A public health perspective. *Australian and New Zealand Journal of Public Health, 45*(1), 17–19. DOI: 10.1111/1753-6405.13058 PMID: 33460217

Casey, B. J., Heller, A. S., Gee, D. G., & Cohen, A. O. (2017). Development of the emotional brain. *Neuroscience Letters*. Advance online publication. DOI: 10.1016/j.neulet.2017.11.055 PMID: 29197573

Chaplin, T. M., Mauro, K. L., & Niehaus, C. E. (2022). Effects of parenting environment on child and adolescent social-emotional brain function. *Current Topics in Behavioral Neurosciences, 54*, 341–372. DOI: 10.1007/7854_2021_276 PMID: 34761364

Chojak, M. (2018). Neuropedagogy as a scientific discipline: Interdisciplinary description of the theoretical basis for the development of a research field. *International Journal of Educational and Pedagogical Sciences, 12*(8), 1084–1087. DOI: 10.5281/zenodo.1474341

Christou, A. I., Endo, S., Wallis, Y., Bair, H., Zeegers, M. P., & McCleery, J. P. (2016). Variation in serotonin 5-HTTLPR short/long genotype modulates resting frontal EEG asymmetries in children. *Development and Psychopathology*, 1–12. DOI: 10.1017/S0954579415000413 PMID: 25990287

Christou, A. I., Fanti, K., Mavrommatis, I., Soursou, G., & Eliadi, E. (2024). Parental Sensory Processing Sensitivity predicts children's visual scanning pattern of emotional faces. *Journal of Psychopathology and Behavioral Assessment*, *46*(4), 932–942. DOI: 10.1007/s10862-024-10173-w

Christou, A. I., Kalfadeli, G., & Tsermentseli, S. (2025). Neuropsychological functioning of childhood cancer: The interplay between executive functions and emotionality. In *Clinical Applications of Pediatric Neuropsychology from Infancy to Adolescence*. IGI Global., DOI: 10.4018/979-8-3693-9689-6.ch015

Christou, A. I., Karachristou, I., & Tsermentseli, S. (2024). Associations between language impairments and behavioral problems in childhood: neurocognitive mechanisms and future implications. In *Developmental Language Disorders in Childhood and Adolescence: Childhood Developmental Language Disorders: Role of Inclusion, Families, and Professionals*. IGI Global., DOI: 10.4018/979-8-3693-1982-6

Christou, A. I., Tsermentseli, S., & Drigas, A. (2023). The role of mobile games and environmental factors in improving learning and metacognitive potential of young students. *International Journal of Interactive Mobile Technologies*, *17*(18), 67–84. DOI: 10.3991/ijim.v17i18.42437

Christou, A. I., Wallis, Y., Bair, H., Crawford, H., Frisson, S., Zeegers, M., & McCleery, J. P. (2015). BDNFVal66Met and 5-HTTLPR genotype are each associated with visual scanning patterns of faces in young children. *Frontiers in Behavioral Neuroscience*, *9*, 175. DOI: 10.3389/fnbeh.2015.00175 PMID: 26217202

Christou, A. I., Wallis, Y., Bair, H., Zeegers, M., & McCleery, J. P. (2017). 5-HTTLPR genotype is associated with visual scanning patterns of adverse scenes in young children. *Frontiers in Behavioral Neuroscience*, *9*. Advance online publication. DOI: 10.3389/fnbeh.2017.00118 PMID: 28690502

Cisler, J. M., & Herringa, R. J. (2020). Posttraumatic stress disorder and the developing adolescent brain. *Biological Psychiatry*. Advance online publication. DOI: 10.1016/j.biopsych.2020.06.001 PMID: 32709416

Costello, S. E., Geiser, E., & Schneider, N. (2021). Nutrients for executive function development and related brain connectivity in school-aged children. *Nutrition Reviews*, *79*(12), 1293–1306. DOI: 10.1093/nutrit/nuaa134 PMID: 33355357

Del Giacco, A. C., Jones, S. A., Hernandez, K. O., Barnes, S. J., & Nagel, B. J. (2023). Heightened adolescent emotional reactivity in the brain is associated with lower future distress tolerance and higher depressive symptoms. *Psychiatry Research: Neuroimaging, 333*, 111659. DOI: 10.1016/j.pscychresns.2023.111659 PMID: 37263126

Dennison, J. (2023). Emotions: Functions and significance for attitudes, behaviour, and communication. *Migration Studies, 12*(1), 1–20. DOI: 10.1093/migration/mnad018

Drakatos, N., & Christou, A.I. (2023). The impact of robotics on developing hot and cold executive functions: their role in special education. *World Journal of Advanced Engineering Technology and Sciences, 9(2), 070-080.* https://doi.org/DOI: 10.30574/wjaets.2023.9.2.0198

Gkora, V., & Christou, A. I. (2023). Executive functions, self-regulation and social media for peace-based inclusive education. *Magna Scientia Advanced Research and Reviews, 8*(2), 129–140. DOI: 10.30574/msarr.2023.8.2.0116

Gvozdii, S., Bakhov, I., Pienov, V., Palamarchuk, S., Dudnyk, N., & Petrukhan-Shcherbakova, L. (2022). Neuropedagogy in Contemporary Formal and Non-Formal Education. BRAIN. *Broad Research in Artificial Intelligence and Neuroscience, 13*(4), 264–279. DOI: 10.18662/brain/13.4/387

Herringa, R. J. (2017). Trauma, PTSD, and the developing brain. *Current Psychiatry Reports, 19*(10), 69. Advance online publication. DOI: 10.1007/s11920-017-0825-3 PMID: 28823091

Horn, S. R., & Feder, A. (2018). Understanding Resilience and Preventing and Treating PTSD. *Harvard Review of Psychiatry, 26*(3), 158–174. DOI: 10.1097/HRP.0000000000000194 PMID: 29734229

Jirout, J. J., Ruzek, E., Vitiello, V. E., Whittaker, J., & Pianta, R. C. (2023). The association between and development of school enjoyment and general knowledge. *Child Development, 94*(2). Advance online publication. DOI: 10.1111/cdev.13878 PMID: 36445041

Kalawski, J. P. (2020). The Alba Method and the Science of Emotions. *Integrative Psychological & Behavioral Science, 54*(4), 903–919. Advance online publication. DOI: 10.1007/s12124-020-09525-4 PMID: 32212066

Kosola, S., Mundy, L. K., Sawyer, S. M., Canterford, L., van der Windt, D. A., Dunn, K. M., & Patton, G. C. (2017). Pain and learning in primary school. *Pain, 158*(9), 1825–1830. DOI: 10.1097/j.pain.0000000000000984 PMID: 28738407

Krull, K. R., Hardy, K. K., Kahalley, L. S., Schuitema, I., & Kesler, S. R. (2018). Neurocognitive Outcomes and Interventions in Long-Term Survivors of Childhood Cancer. *Journal of Clinical Oncology*, *36*(21), 2181–2189. DOI: 10.1200/JCO.2017.76.4696 PMID: 29874137

Lin, M.-L., & Faldowski, R. A. (2023). The relationship of parent support and child emotional regulation to school readiness. *International Journal of Environmental Research and Public Health*, *20*(6), 4867. DOI: 10.3390/ijerph20064867 PMID: 36981776

Marusak, H. A., Iadipaolo, A. S., Harper, F. W., Elrahal, F., Taub, J. W., Goldberg, E., & Rabinak, C. A. (2017). Neurodevelopmental consequences of pediatric cancer and its treatment: Applying an early adversity framework to understanding cognitive, behavioral, and emotional outcomes. *Neuropsychology Review*, *28*(2), 123–175. DOI: 10.1007/s11065-017-9365-1 PMID: 29270773

Masten, A. S., Lucke, C. M., Nelson, K. M., & Stallworthy, I. C. (2021). Resilience in development and psychopathology: Multisystem perspectives. *Annual Review of Clinical Psychology*, *17*(1), 521–549. DOI: 10.1146/annurev-clinpsy-081219-120307 PMID: 33534615

Moumne, S., Hall, N., Böke, B. N., Bastien, L., & Heath, N. (2021). Implicit theories of emotion, goals for emotion regulation, and cognitive responses to negative life events. *Psychological Reports*, *124*(4), 1588–1620. DOI: 10.1177/0033294120942110 PMID: 32674669

Nijhof, S. L., Vinkers, C. H., van Geelen, S. M., Duijff, S. N., Achterberg, E. J. M., van der Net, J., Veltkamp, R. C., Grootenhuis, M. A., van de Putte, E. M., Hillegers, M. H. J., van der Brug, A. W., Wierenga, C. J., Benders, M. J. N. L., Engels, R. C. M. E., Kors van der Ent, C., Vanderschuren, L. J. M. J., & Lesscher, H. M. B. (2018). Healthy play, better coping: The importance of play for the development of children in health and disease. *Neuroscience and Biobehavioral Reviews*, *95*, 421–429. Advance online publication. DOI: 10.1016/j.neubiorev.2018.09.024 PMID: 30273634

Pergantis, P., Bamicha, V., Doulou, A., Christou, A. I., Bardis, N., Skianis, C., & Drigas, A. (2025). Assistive and Emerging Technologies to Detect and Reduce Neurophysiological Stress and Anxiety in Children and Adolescents with Autism and Sensory Processing Disorders: A Systematic Review. *Technologies*, *13*(4), 144. DOI: 10.3390/technologies13040144

Pericas, C., Clotas, C., Espelt, A., López, M. J., Bosque-Prous, M., Juárez, O., & Bartroli, M. (2022). Effectiveness of school-based emotional education program: A cluster-randomized controlled trial. *Public Health, 210*, 142–148. DOI: 10.1016/j.puhe.2022.06.013 PMID: 35970016

Pinto, C. (2022). Neuropedagogy for multicultural classrooms: The neuromethodology for inclusion. *MLS Inclusion and Society Journal, 2*(2), 207–218. DOI: 10.56047/mlsisi.v2i2.1676

Poole, K. L., Santesso, D. L., Van Lieshout, R. J., & Schmidt, L. A. (2018). Trajectories of frontal brain activity and socio-emotional development in children. *Developmental Psychobiology, 60*(4), 353–363. DOI: 10.1002/dev.21620 PMID: 29457644

Popovic, D., Ruef, A., Dwyer, D. B., Antonucci, L. A., Eder, J., Sanfelici, R., Kambeitz-Ilankovic, L., Oztuerk, O. F., Dong, M. S., Paul, R., Paolini, M., Hedderich, D., Haidl, T., Kambeitz, J., Ruhrmann, S., Chisholm, K., Schultze-Lutter, F., & Falkai, P. (2020). Traces of trauma: A multivariate pattern analysis of childhood trauma, brain structure, and clinical phenotypes. *Biological Psychiatry, 88*(11), 829–842. DOI: 10.1016/j.biopsych.2020.05.020 PMID: 32782139

Ruba, A. L., & Pollak, S. D. (2020). The Development of Emotion Reasoning in Infancy and Early Childhood. *Annual Review of Developmental Psychology, 2*(1), 503–531. DOI: 10.1146/annurev-devpsych-060320-102556

Russell, J. D., & Herringa, R. J. (2021). Editorial: The Preschool Emotional Brain. *Journal of the American Academy of Child and Adolescent Psychiatry, 60*(1), 29–31. DOI: 10.1016/j.jaac.2020.08.012 PMID: 32890671

Seth, R. (2023). Children with cancer: Shared care and transition of care. *Indian Journal of Pediatrics, 90*(12), 1232–1236. DOI: 10.1007/s12098-023-04644-3 PMID: 37368222

Tabibnia, G. (2024). Neuroscience education as a tool for improving stress management and resilience. *Current Opinion in Behavioral Sciences, 59*, 101401. DOI: 10.1016/j.cobeha.2024.101401

Tan, P. Z., Oppenheimer, C. W., Ladouceur, C. D., Butterfield, R. D., & Silk, J. S. (2020). A review of associations between parental emotion socialization behaviors and the neural substrates of emotional reactivity and regulation in youth. *Developmental Psychology, 56*(3), 516–527. DOI: 10.1037/dev0000893 PMID: 32077721

Tillery, R., Howard Sharp, K. M., Okado, Y., Long, A., & Phipps, S. (2015). Profiles of Resilience and Growth in Youth With Cancer and Healthy Comparisons. *Journal of Pediatric Psychology*, *41*(3), 290–297. DOI: 10.1093/jpepsy/jsv091 PMID: 26423321

Voineskos, A. N. (2020). Mapping effects of childhood trauma onto brain systems and behavior. *Biological Psychiatry*, *88*(11), 810–811. DOI: 10.1016/j.biopsych.2020.08.009 PMID: 33153524

Wang, Y., Zhu, Z., Chen, B., & Fang, F. (2018). Perceptual learning and recognition confusion reveal the underlying relationships among the six basic emotions. *Cognition and Emotion*, •••, 1–14. DOI: 10.1080/02699931.2018.1491831 PMID: 29962270

Yu, C. (2019). (in Review). Endocrine consequences of childhood cancer therapy and transition considerations. *Pediatrics*, *48*(8), e326–e332. DOI: 10.3928/19382359-20190729-02 PMID: 31426101

Chapter 10

Neuropedagogical Impact of ABA Behavioral Interventions on Communication in Autism

Elmahdi Tejdid
https://orcid.org/0009-0005-5241-8147
The Faculty of Letters and Human Sciences Dhar El Mehraz, Sidi Mohamed Ben Abdellah University, Fez, Morocco

Mohamed El Himer
https://orcid.org/0009-0001-1665-3650
Sidi Mohamed Ben Abdellah University of Fès, Morocco

ABSTRACT

This article examines the effectiveness of a training program based on the Applied Behavior Analysis (ABA) method on improving and ameliorating the verbal communication skills of four autistic Moroccan children. This program monitors four children aged between 7 to 9 years while undergoing a teaching program of six different verbal Moroccan Arabic expressions and phrases. The results reveal significant improvement in spontaneous verbal expression production, with success rates ranging from 48% to 60%. Although post-monitoring follow-ups show persistence of the acquired skills, the participants cannot practice the last acquired skills clearly and spontaneously. These results indicate that ABA is an effective method for strengthening the verbal communication skills of autistic Moroccan children,

DOI: 10.4018/979-8-3373-3581-0.ch010

however, repetition and regular follow-ups to retain the acquired skills is of paramount importance. This paper contributes to the literature by providing empirical information on the adaptation of ABA in a Moroccan context.

INTRODUCTION

The American Psychiatric Association (2013) considers autism a neurodevelopmental disorder (NDD). It is characterized by persistent deficits in social communication and restricted, repetitive behaviors. Verbal communication is a challenge for children with autism. Therefore, the ability to clearly and adequately express needs, desires, and emotions is closely related to their social, cognitive, and emotional development. Applied behavior analysis (ABA) has been shown to be effective in the development of behaviors in individuals with this disorder. This treatment specifically aims to develop functional communication skills while reducing behaviors that may disrupt them.

ABA originated from the pioneering work of Lovaas and Sundberg. In recent years, according to Lovaas and Sundberg, autism educators and professionals have effectively used the ABA approach, achieving good results in developing the skills of autistic children (Lovaas, 1987; Sundberg, 2008). However, despite unprecedented success, ABA remains underexplored in cultural contexts other than the American context, as well as in the Moroccan context. It is in this context that the study aims to test the effectiveness of a demand-driven, ABA-based oral expression program with Moroccan children diagnosed with autism.

Although ABA has proven effective in developing social and language skills, the experimental team knows surprisingly little about its performance outside of Western contexts, particularly in countries like Morocco. Most studies do not take into account the specificities of each autistic child during their interventions. This is why it is crucial to adapt ABA methods to the Moroccan context, where specialized autism resources and professional training opportunities remain scarce.

In this sense, the experiment aims to explore how applied behavioral analysis (ABA) can develop the verbal expression of autistic children, in this case requests based on their individual needs and their Moroccan cultural specificities.

To answer these questions, the research focuses on several questions: Does the ABA-based training program improve the verbal communication skills of autistic children? What are the parameters that influence the effectiveness of ABA? At what point can the experimental team speak of generalization and maintenance of acquired verbal communication skills?

Two main hypotheses guide this research. First, the application of an ABA-based oral training program will lead to a significant improvement in verbal communication, measured by an increase in the spontaneous production of verbal expressions. Second, the acquired skills will persist after the intervention ends but will require regular follow-up to maintain them.

This research moves from theory to practice. Theoretically, it enriches the literature by evaluating the effectiveness of ABA in a Moroccan context. Practically, it offers concrete recommendations to Moroccan professionals and families. The study aims to evaluate the effectiveness of an ABA program to improve the verbal communication skills of Moroccan autistic children, by analyzing the changes before and after the intervention and identifying the factors influencing its success .

1. Verbal Communication Skills of Children with Autism and Applied Behavior Analysis (ABA)

1.1. Verbal Communication in Autism

According to the 2013 Diagnostic and Statistical Manual of Mental Disorders (DSM-5), children with autism spectrum disorder (ASD) experience ongoing challenges. These challenges involve social communication. They also exhibit restricted and repetitive behaviors. Verbal communication is a crucial skill among these challenges. It is essential for developing their independence. It is equally important for successful social integration. Many struggle to express their needs. They struggle to express their desires or emotions. This limitation significantly hinders their interactions with the world. Formulating requests is therefore fundamental. This skill allows them to express everyday needs. They can ask for help. They can signal when they are hungry. They can simply ask for a break.

These skills are vital. They aid participation in daily life. They reduce challenging behaviors. These behaviors often arise from inadequate communication.

Language learning is a challenge for many autistic children. Some don't speak. Others use words much later than neurotypical children. Still others learn to speak, but in a limited way. They may repeat the same words over and over again. This is called echolalia. They sometimes repeat phrases heard in other people's homes. They repeat television dialogue. But they don't always do this to express a personal thought. This complicates effective everyday communication.

Social language is often another challenge. The natural rhythm of conversations eludes them. They don't know when to speak. They don't know when to listen. Some only want to talk about their passions. Many avoid eye contact. They often interpret language very literally. A phrase like "Get out!" can throw them off. Sarcasm is often incomprehensible to them. Jokes also elude them because they require reading between the lines. All these obstacles make simple interactions overwhelming. They then become very anxious.

These communication barriers hinder bonding. They often play alone. They feel profoundly lonely, as conversations do not come naturally to them. Expressing a thought in words is so difficult that they require constant help. They need their parents. They need their teachers, even for the most basic needs. This dependence complicates the development of their independence. In addition, the inability to clearly express their feelings generates anxiety in social situations.

Finding alternative means of communication is therefore essential. Using images is one solution. Using gestures or specialized devices can make all the difference.

Appropriate support methods allow for gradual improvement. Their interactions with the world then become more effective.

Oral expression gives children real power over their environment. Saying "Help" in a difficult situation is a way of seeking support. This simple expression reduces frustration. For example, saying "I want water" helps meet a need. The child no longer depends entirely on others to make themselves understood. Another example is asking for a break. Saying "I need a break" helps them calm down before too much stress escalates. These simple requests make it easier to control daily activities.

An experimental team teaching verbal communication encounters a real obstacle. Children struggle to apply their skills elsewhere. Imagine a child saying "I want a drink" at home. The same child may remain silent at school or at the park. Why? Their minds associate these skills with specific contexts. The glass of water in the kitchen doesn't evoke the fountain at school. Sometimes they simply don't see the point of communicating in an unfamiliar place. Why ask for water without having experienced how words make things happen?

The experimental team, composed of adults, then intervenes. Without deliberate prompting from parents, teachers, and therapists, these expressions remain trapped in their original context. The magic works through patient repetition. They must be used everywhere: in the playground, at the grocery store. They must be shown that "I want to drink" also works at their grandmother's house.

Several strategies help overcome these difficulties. Visual aids, such as pictograms, aid in understanding key statements. Breaking skills into small steps makes structured approaches effective. ABA's Discrete Trial Teaching (DTT) is one example. It allows for step-by-step mastery with plenty of practice. Actively involving parents and caregivers is also essential. They help apply new learning in different contexts. If a child uses a new communication skill at home, at school, and in the community, they will be able to stabilize this skill.

The team uses positive reinforcement. They offer verbal rewards. They give a high five or a short explanation. These motivators stimulate the desire to communicate. They encourage children to interact with others in new ways.

Children with disabilities face many obstacles. Complex and impractical coping strategies make things difficult.

These communication skills are very useful. They help children feel independent. They help them feel safe and healthy in their environment. They allow them to maintain a stable emotional state.

Most ABA-based educational programs collaborate with other organizations. They provide effective materials for professionals, parents, and caregivers. This material is crucial for those who struggle to use these devices. The ultimate goal is always to improve children's quality of life.

1.2. What is the Application for the Analysis Application?

For competition specialists, the application of behavior analysis (ABA) is a fundamental approach to the principles of competition aimed at modifying the development of competition uses and adapting all problematic cells (Cooper, Heron and Heward, 2020). This method pays particular attention to social interactions, language, etc., through the techniques used in structures and adaptations for children. It is in this context that ABA is part of the fundamental idea that sports equipment comes into play and adapts to sports equipment that adapts to the best possible performance, from the simplest to the most complex competitions.

Moreover, as Granpeesheh says, research highlights that early and intensive ABA interventions produce significant improvements in communication skills in children with ASD (Granpeesheh et al., 2009). In fact, the experimental team can say that this is consistent with the study's emphasis on structured verbal training for Moroccan children aged 7 to 9 years.

Teaching children to make requests—one of the most basic forms of verbal communication—is typically a priority in ABA programs (Sundberg, 2008). By learning to make requests, children finally express their needs. This gives them newfound control over their environment. This ability fosters greater independence. It also reduces frustrations. These frustrations previously stemmed from their inability to communicate.

ABA relies on proven, evidence-based principles to carefully assess and shape behaviors. Fundamentally, this approach uses strategic reinforcement techniques, rewarding the child for desired behaviors. For example, when teaching a verbal request like "I want a drink": practitioners might start with hands-on coaching and then gradually reduce their coaching until the child can articulate the request completely independently.

The scientific value of ABA lies in its personalization. Professionals first conduct in-depth assessments. This helps them identify each learner's unique motivations. For a music-loving child, for example, they might suggest musical toys. This tailored approach precisely targets each child's needs.

These professionals intelligently integrate these preferences into their teaching strategies to stimulate engagement. By adapting both the context before behaviors appear and subsequent responses, ABA can induce behavioral changes based on the child's natural interests. This makes learning more effective.

Verbal requests, or " mands " in ABA, are essential. They allow children to express their needs concretely. A child learns to say "I'm hungry." They no longer cry. They no longer engage in inappropriate behavior. They now communicate in a way that those around them understand. Granting these requests reduces frustration. It also streamlines interactions with caregivers. A calm routine is then established for everyone.

It is in this context that ABA focuses not only on learning requests but also aims to cover a wide range of skills, from basic social skills like greeting or waiting one's turn, to more complex skills like holding a real conversation or solving everyday problems. ABA's effectiveness lies in the way it breaks these skills down into small, sequential, and progressive steps. Children are encouraged to master one small step before tackling the next, gradually building their confidence and ensuring lasting progress. In this case, ABA is similar to building a house brick by brick, rather than trying to build it all in one piece. ABA's effectiveness also lies in its flexibility and pragmatism. ABA aims to teach children practical ways to communicate by reinforcing their efforts to motivate and encourage them to repeat the same newly acquired verbal utterances. In this sense, this approach gives autistic children the verbal tools they need to gain independence. This naturally leads to fewer tantrums and challenging behaviors. The real magic happens when ABA is personalized to each child's specific situation and used thoughtfully throughout the program. Parents tell educators they see improvements in communicating requests.

1.3. Verbal Communication Requirements

In ABA, asking is called "manding." This may sound like a strange term, I admit. These requests are essential. They help children develop their communication skills. Being able to ask for what they want is crucial. Being able to express what's bothering them is just as important. This creates a vital link between their inner world and the outside world.

Skinner, in 1957, put forward a fundamental idea about verbal behavior. He suggested that requests arise naturally from a need. A child is hungry. He is uncomfortable. He longs for a toy. These inner urges drive him to use words. They drive him to use gestures to get what he needs. The original motivation is simple: "I want it, so I will ask for it." This triggers communication.

From birth, children instinctively express their needs. Long before they speak, babies cry. They point. They use facial expressions. They communicate their hunger, discomfort, or desire for attention. As they grow, these natural attempts evolve. First, they reach for objects. Then they produce specific sounds. Finally, they form words and sentences. This innate need for contact is the foundation of all language.

Even children with disabilities retain that fundamental desire to express themselves. They may simply require different tools. They may need alternative approaches to achieve this. The beauty of working with them lies in their perseverance. They always find ways to make us understand their needs.

A hungry child might say, "I want to eat." Overwhelmed by loud noises, they might ask, "I need a break." These phrases are called " mands " in ABA therapy. They take various forms depending on the needs:

* Some use words.
* Others prefer gestures or images.
* Others still cry, not having learned to communicate better.

Understanding these signs is essential to helping them grow. Teachers and professionals must be attentive to them. This vigilance allows for calmer responses. It often helps prevent difficult behaviors from escalating. Effective communication also helps autistic children. It allows them to gradually develop their social skills.

What makes these requests particularly important is that they are motivated by the child's current needs. Unlike simply naming objects or answering clear, direct questions, these moments reflect true, real emotions. A child who says "water" when thirsty isn't just using words; they're beginning to manage their emotions. Thus, communication becomes a tool for managing emotions and acting independently.

Through ABA therapy, children often manage to connect their thoughts to actions that produce results. Constant support helps them understand that expressing themselves, showing images, or using gestures is more effective than simply breaking down when they need something. This is also the case when some children have real children, who have had the opportunity to do so, because all the objects they have chosen are in the public domain, in a storage place, or the answer on the so-called car if they have a difficult face, if they start to find more expensive objects. Verbal outlets allow this activity to be initiated. This change encourages children to remove obstacles to learning new content. It is thanks to the presence of the family that they encounter more problems without difficulty and without adapting to them, which affects external activities related to the nature of the family and allows them to control their lives and create good relationships with their environment.

Before embarking on an ABA program, it's essential to understand how a child currently asks. This first step can tell you a lot about their communication style and what may be hindering it. By observing a child in their daily environment, whether at home or at school, you begin to identify patterns. Do they use words?

Do they point? Do they pressure adults to respond to their wishes? Or do they have meltdowns when they can't express themselves?

It's equally important to identify what truly motivates the child. Every child has their own interests that appeal to them, such as dinosaurs, music, or chocolate milk. These motivations are valuable for learning to communicate because they give children a reason to turn to others.

Consider a child who is motivated by food. Teaching them simple phrases like "want to snack" becomes very effective. They immediately see the value in communicating. Nothing teaches expression better than getting exactly what you want. I've observed children barely communicating. They would suddenly become impatient to practice. This impatience stemmed from a simple realization: certain words consistently brought them their favorite treats.

Observing what a child already knows is only the first step. The real work begins when ABA therapists develop an action plan to develop the required skills. Some children do better with highly structured practice sessions (this is the "discrete trial teaching" part), while others learn best by incorporating communication practice into everyday moments, such as snack time or trips to the park.

Here's how it usually goes: The therapist may hold the child's favorite toy car out of reach. This creates a natural opportunity for the child to communicate. At first, they may simply reach for it, and the therapist helps them say or sign "car" or "want car." With the child's slightest attempt, however imperfect, they immediately get the car and receive enthusiastic praise.

The magic happens over time. As the child learns to ask, the therapist gradually steps back. Perhaps they used to accept a simple "car," but now expect a "I want a car" or "I want the car, please." The support gradually fades until the child is asking for things confidently and on their own. I've seen this process transform frustrated children who couldn't express their needs into children who proudly use their words to get what they want.

Learning to ask isn't limited to therapy rooms. The main advantage of ABA is that children can use these skills everywhere. For example, an autistic child who can ask for water or say "I want a drink" during a session should do the same at school, in the park, or elsewhere, such as at their grandmother's house. This requires practice in different places and with different members of the family. The child can try new sentences with the same meaning, for example, by practicing with loved ones. This allows requests to be met without provoking aggression or anger. ABA therefore uses personalized, step-by-step techniques to help autistic children use these skills in the classroom, on the playground, and at recess. This generalization is gradually programmed, leading to appropriate behaviors.

The impact goes far beyond simply improving communication. When children master the request, they acquire fundamental skills that promote their social connections and language development, which in turn impacts their development.

Autistic children often struggle to express their needs. They struggle to express their feelings. This difficulty can hinder their autonomy. It can also hinder their social integration. Cognitive behavioral therapy (CBT) then intervenes. It uses behavioral techniques. It thus offers a clear path to the development of verbal skills.

Teaching them to make requests is essential. This skill is fundamental. They need it to interact with the world. The experimental team systematically rewards these positive behaviors. They use ABA therapy for this. Several benefits result from this:

* Children are less frustrated because they communicate better.
* They become more independent.
* Their general well-being improves.

It's impressive to see the power of these targeted interventions. They transform a child's challenges into practical skills. Skills they will use throughout their lives.

2. Methodology

2.1. The Method Adopted and Its Objective

Arrahma Children's Association "Spina Bifida" in Fez, Morocco, is not just a facility: it offers genuine support for autistic children aged 6 and over (once an official diagnosis has been made by a child psychiatrist). What makes this facility unique is that they don't just work directly with the children, but also take a whole-family approach. They monitor the children's academic performance while ensuring that the adults around them, whether healthcare professionals or parents, receive the necessary training. This includes workshops for beginners. These workshops cover the fundamentals and teach behavioral therapy techniques.

The holding of this trial in Arrahma is important. It demonstrates the mobilization of community organizations. They are thus filling critical gaps. These gaps concern the specialized care of these children.

This study focused on a rather practical goal: teaching four autistic children to say six common phrases in Moroccan Arabic. The experimental team members used simple but crucial phrases like "I want to drink" (/ na. ʃ.rɔb /), "I want to eat" (/ na. kɔl /), "I want to play" (/ na. laːb /), "I want to go to the bathroom" (/ twa. lɛ /), "I want to take a break" (/ safi /), and "Help me" (/ sɑ ːː dni ː/). The experimental team didn't choose these phrases at random: they cover basic needs that come up constantly throughout the day. The real impact is that once these children were able to use these phrases, they not only communicated better, but they became more independent and experienced much less frustration when trying to express their needs to others.

Given the structure of this study, they adopted a fairly straightforward experimental approach to determine whether ABA therapy actually helped autistic children communicate better. They clearly defined what they were measuring: the ABA program was the manipulated element (the independent variable) and the improvement in the children's oral skills was the dependent variable.

When selecting participants, they started with thirteen children and then narrowed their selection to just four for their test group. Their sample had an 80% confidence level with a 30% margin of error, which clearly illustrates the statistical framework used.

The researchers divided the children into two groups: the four who received specialized ABA therapy (experimental group) and the other nine who simply continued their usual programming (control group).

They didn't assign the children randomly. They carefully considered the composition of the groups. The children were similar on important factors. These factors included the severity of their autism. They also included their initial communication skills. Age and gender (boys or girls) were also taken into account.

This randomization step is crucial. It provides certainty: the observed improvements are indeed due to ABA therapy. They are not due to simple chance. Nor are they the result of a group composed of children who were initially less affected.

Examining their method reveals one overriding priority: the protection of these children. Their entire approach was based on a solid ethical foundation. They weren't just looking for results. Their underlying goal was to treat every child with dignity. This consideration was constant, present throughout the process.

The team made it a point to respect the children at every stage, demonstrate professional integrity, and use rewards wisely. In this regard, they didn't rely on generic incentives. They paid attention to what each child truly appreciated and valued, using praise and concrete rewards in ways that encouraged progress without making the children overly dependent on rewards for speaking up.

All educators demonstrated absolute seriousness and great confidentiality. The detailed observations of the autistic children's verbal behavior and other data collected during the session were not inventoried, but were kept confidential, in accordance with current ethical rules. This ethical and personalized attention demonstrated that these were not just subjects and objects of research, but vulnerable children with specific emotional needs who deserved special attention.

2.2. Measuring Instruments and WB-Mapp Guide

To monitor these children's language development, the experimental team members implemented a focused observation method that examined communication from three key perspectives. First, they identified what had actually prompted the child to speak. Then, they carefully analyzed their responses. Finally, they observed the adults' reactions to their communication attempts. By capturing this complete interaction cycle, the experimental team collected robust data that allowed us to understand each child's unique progress and provide appropriate support.

The experimental team created specific scenarios to help the children learn certain phrases. To teach “I want to drink,” the teachers showed them water or pretended to be thirsty. For “I want to play,” they brought out toys they liked or suggested fun games that excited them. The teachers didn’t limit themselves to artificial training sessions: they used real, everyday situations whenever possible. Mealtimes became natural opportunities for practice. They then worked on the phrase “I want to eat.” They also watched for signs of fatigue. This triggered training in saying “I want to take a break.” By connecting these phrases to real situations, the children began to understand. They grasped the meaning of the words. Above all, they learned when to use them. They learned how to use them in real life.

A dedicated team monitored these children's reactions in each situation; I worked with a social worker and a psychologist. They considered it a victory whenever a child used the right phrase at the right time, such as “I want to drink” when offered water. If they simply pointed or gestured instead of speaking, they didn't consider it a failure, but rather an opportunity to practice more in subsequent sessions. Thanks to this detailed monitoring, they could see precisely which phrases each child had mastered and identify specific areas where they still needed help.

The effectiveness of this approach lies in the provision of concrete, actionable information. For example, when they noticed that a child was regularly using gestures instead of speaking, they could immediately adapt their teaching strategy. They could then present that phrase more often throughout the day. They provided additional encouragement when they tried to use it. They also created additional practice situations. These situations were designed to require them to use those specific words. The ability to refine the methods was crucial. Real-time observations made this possible. This allowed them to constantly adapt the approach. This adaptation was made according to each child's stage of learning.

The systematic approach of analyzing the entire communication cycle—what triggers children to speak, their responses, and those of adults—created a truly effective framework for language development. The strength of this method lies in its combination of detailed observation and adaptable teaching techniques. This balanced strategy allowed us to offer personalized support throughout each child's communication journey, while maintaining clear ways to measure their progress. Ultimately, they developed a practical, evidence-based system that truly helped these children express their needs more effectively in everyday life.

The experimental team also made sure to track behavioral consequences in the observation grid. This simply means that they recorded the teacher's reaction after the child said or did not say the studied sentence. These responses varied from primary to secondary reinforcers, depending on each child's motivation.

The approach focused on six essential phrases. These phrases served daily communication. "I want to drink" and "I want to eat" expressed a need. "I want to play" formulated a request for activity. "Toilet" indicated a physiological need. "Help me" was a request for assistance. "I want to take a break" enabled emotional regulation.

Teaching occurred in natural contexts. It occurred in meaningful moments. This method created a direct connection. The connection linked the word to its concrete utility. The therapists watched for the precise moment. They observed the child's true desire. Their urge to play with a specific toy triggered the incentive. They prompted them to formulate the corresponding request. Only then did they fulfill it.

Each successful use triggered reinforcement. This reinforcement was carefully chosen. Rewards matched individual motivations. They were never left to chance. Social praise could be a reward. So could access to a coveted toy. A small treat worked, too. This instant gratification created a positive association. The association linked verbal expression to the satisfaction of the need. It encouraged future reuse.

The effectiveness lay in this synergy. The synergy united a natural context and personalized reinforcement. The children gradually understood. They learned to pronounce the words. Above all, they discovered when to use them. They understood why to use them. The approach transformed everyday situations. Meals became learning opportunities. So did signs of fatigue. The children experienced the power of communication in a concrete way. They learned to influence their environment.

The assessment scale developed for this study goes beyond simply monitoring progress. It offers a comprehensive view of these children's communication learning. Its analysis examines three fundamental elements: what precedes speech (antecedents), what the child actually says or does (behavior), and what immediately follows (consequences). This triadic method reveals the mechanisms of their communication development.

This three-pronged approach has several advantages. It allows for a clear visualization of progress made. It accurately identifies persistent weaknesses. Its effectiveness lies in its dual nature: structural and personalized. Professionals apply the fundamental principles of ABA. But they constantly adapt them to each child's unique situation. This flexibility ensures that interventions are relevant to each learner.

The end result is a highly effective intervention that actually helps these autistic children develop the verbal skills they need most.

The study tracked how often children said specific sentences they were taught. It measured how often children verbally used target phrases like “I want to drink” (/ na. ʃ.rɔb /), “I want to eat” (/ na . kɔl /), “I want to play” (/ na. laːb /), “Toilet” (/ twa . lɛt /), “Help me” (/sɑː.ʕid . niː/), and “I want to take a break” (/ safi /).

During each session, they noted three key things: what happened just before the child tried to communicate (what they called the antecedents), whether or not the child said the target sentence (their behavior), and how they responded to their attempt (the consequences), such as praising them or helping them correct their speech.

This careful monitoring allowed us to have a very clear vision of each child's progress in their verbal communication journey. Unlike more subjective approaches, this method allowed us to observe concrete progress over time.

They wanted unbiased observations. So they required at least a 90% agreement rate between observers. Myself, the social worker, and the psychologist had to agree. We all had to observe the same thing. Note whether the child had said the sentence or not. This agreement had to occur in at least nine cases out of ten. In the event of occasional disagreement about what they heard, they discussed it. They discussed it until they reached a consensus.

This high level of agreement was not a mere formality. It was absolutely crucial. It guaranteed the relevance of the data. Without this consistency between observers, the results lacked scientific value. They also lost reliability.

To identify children's preferred objects, they used the paired-trial method. This method determines the most effective reinforcers. It involves presenting the child with two stimuli—two toys, for example, or two foods. Then noting their choice. Each stimulus is presented once with another. This helps establish a clear hierarchy of preferences.

For example, a child systematically chooses a ball over a book. The ball will then be considered a more powerful reinforcer. It will better motivate the child to communicate. This method allows for systematic assessment. It is also objective. It can test a large number of stimuli. It offers a hierarchical view of preferences. This view is essential for adapting interventions and thus maximizes their effectiveness.

For example, a child prefers a musical toy to a puzzle. This toy will serve as a reward. It will encourage the child to produce verbal utterances.

This preference assessment should be conducted regularly. Ideally, before each teaching session. Autistic children frequently change their preferences. These changes stem from their interests. They also stem from their emotional state. Environmental factors also play a role.

The initial assessment of four participants used the VB-MAPP tool. This tool helped identify each child's preferences. It also revealed their emerging communication skills.

Participant 1 showed interest in certain toys. The horse and the spinning top particularly motivated him. Participant 2 preferred edible objects such as the lollipop or the cookie. He also liked specific toys: the soccer ball and the harmonica. Participant 3 was attracted to chocolate, cars, and puzzles. Participant 4 preferred candy, the motorcycle, and the ball. These individual preferences directly guided the choice of reinforcers. These motivators were essential during the pre-intervention sessions.

In terms of skills, each participant presented a unique profile. Participant 1 had difficulties with touch, hearing, and requesting. However, he was making progress in independent play and motor imitation. Participant 2 was weak in requesting and visual performance. However, he was developing social and sonographic skills. Participant 3 excelled in some aspects of tactile and visual autonomy. However, he experienced difficulties with requesting and sonographic performance. Participant 4 encountered obstacles with requesting and vocal performance. However, he distinguished himself by strong motor imitation.

These results highlight an absolute necessity: individualized interventions. We must strengthen deficient skills. We must also build on each child's strengths. Identifying each participant's preferences is therefore fundamental. Educators can then select truly effective reinforcers. This selection motivates children and facilitates their participation in learning activities.

Analyzing emerging skills and gaps is equally crucial. It allows us to target specific weaknesses and build on existing strengths. This individualized approach is based on accurate data. It is essential to optimize the effectiveness of interventions. It supports children's overall development in a targeted and adaptive manner.

2.3. The Individualized Educational Program

Following the assessment of the four children, priority objectives were defined. This definition was collaborative. The psychologist, educators, and parents participated. Given the short duration of the intervention, the focus was on a central objective: improving demand. This verbal operant is essential for appropriate communication.

The personalized project, or curriculum, addressed individual needs. It met five specific criteria: specificity, measurability, action, realism, and temporality. Spontaneous requests were chosen for their everyday usefulness. "I want to drink" is one example. "Help me" is another. These phrases have an important ability: to reduce problematic behaviors.

The selection of these phrases followed a simple principle: their relevance in everyday situations. They allow children to express their needs clearly. They do so in a functional way. For example, "I want to drink" is useful during meals. It is also useful in cases of thirst. "Help me" is useful in difficult situations.

These targeted skills were aimed at a crucial replacement. They were to replace problematic actions. Tantrums are one. Tearful fits are another. The ultimate goal was to provide more effective means. Children could then express their desires. They could express their needs.

experimental team members designed the program around clear, specific, measurable goals, such as “the child repeats five two-syllable words ” or “asks for help appropriately.” Each goal had a specific target, such as achieving 80% success after several attempts. They set deadlines for each step so they could track progress and adapt the approach if problems arose. Parents and guardians are actively involved. They participate in choosing priorities. They thus ensure the program's appropriateness. The program must meet the children's basic needs. Parents have clearly expressed their wishes. They want their children to make simple requests. “I want to eat” is a concrete example. “I want to drink” is another. These skills are aimed at daily independence.

This close collaboration allows for tailor-made programs. We develop personalized programs for each child. These programs meet their priority needs. They also respond to the expectations of families. This dual approach ensures the relevance of the interventions and their effectiveness.

The experimental team created tailor-made programs. These programs had a specific goal: to teach children how to ask. They used practical, everyday expressions. The approach adhered to strict criteria. It was specific and measurable. Pragmatic and realistic. It was also time-limited. This solid framework helped these autistic children. It improved their oral skills.

At the heart of this approach is an ABA structure. This structure is carefully designed. It supports children in their development. It leads them toward communicative success. Repetitive exercises are abandoned. Instead, they develop meaningful interactions. Language then becomes a powerful medium. It allows children to connect with others.

By observing AZ's (Participant 1) progress, for example in pronouncing “/ na.ʃ.rɔb /” (I want to drink), they can see the method in action. The professionals start by showing him how to do it by holding a cup and pronouncing the words clearly with an encouraging smile that makes him want to try. When AZ tries to say it, even if it's not perfect, they immediately respond with motivating praise or give him one of those colorful star-shaped stickers he loves.

The children's level improved during the experiment as they practiced the program statements in different situations.

They constantly repeated the expression “/na.kɔl/ ” (I want to eat) during academic sessions at the association, as well as in different contexts with their parents, for example, while preparing dinner at home, in a supermarket and in bakeries.

The SL educator noted that the AZ child in care was making remarkable progress in producing this statement in several formal and informal settings. What's great, she says, is that the AZ child sometimes expresses his natural need for food when he's hungry. This proves that ABA techniques are improving the child's communication skills. It remains to be seen whether he will produce the acquired statements in appropriate situations in the future.

"ZA" (Participant 2) in the experimental group shows an attraction to bubbles; their teacher uses them as a reward when they manage to say "toilet" or "I want to go to the toilet."

In the same context, the third child, "ML" (Participant 3), fascinated by electronic spinning tops, can play with them by saying "/ safi /" (pause), in order to be able to start playing after a reading session, for example. These rewards are not implemented randomly, but aim to help them understand the importance of producing verbal utterances at the appropriate moments of communication.

Successful moments are counted in the progress of the educational program based on ABA techniques; when the fourth child, K (Participant 4), says "/na.laːb/ " (I want to play) upon seeing his favorite ball, or when all four children at separate intervals say "/sɑː.ʕd.niː/ " to ask for help from teachers or other peers, this demonstrates the success of the program based on this approach.

Moreover, the use of children's oral language in the educational program promotes verbal understanding of the program's statements, as these children frequently encounter and use them in their daily lives, far from the association generally established with Standard Arabic in these school programs. Their everyday language helps them better express their basic needs, thus helping to reduce their frustration and difficult or inappropriate behaviors.

Mastering the program's statements, based on the ABA approach, allows children to interact with their environment. It is important to emphasize that the importance of the chosen verbal statements lies in their ability to meet the children's vital needs, thus meeting the expectations of parents and teachers. These statements aim to strengthen children's autonomy, communication skills, and quality of life.

It is in this context that the expressions "/ na. ʃ.rɔb /" (I want to drink), "/ na.kɔl /" (I want to eat), /toilette/ allow the child to truly express his thirst, his vital and emotional need. This can only develop his social, mental and physical abilities.

As for the expressions "/sɑː.ʕid.niː/ " (Help me) and "/ safi /" (Stop), they concretely strengthen social bonds by providing an appropriate way to ask for help and take a break from difficult situations. It is in this context that the integration of these expressions into a structured school curriculum can improve verbal skills, reduce moments of frustration and crisis, and promote the overall development of autistic children, while meeting the expectations of families and specialists regarding their effective inclusion.

Evidence shows that early intervention can provide children with the resources they need to thrive in a variety of everyday situations by ensuring that social connections improve in positive ways.

These statements constituting the educational program are linked to the motivational operations (MOs), key components of the VB-MAPP (Sundberg, 2017). Indeed, MOs represent the circumstances that promote the child's motivation to engage in learning tasks.

When a child, for example, expresses thirst, water becomes a valuable reward that can help them learn phrases such as "I want to drink." By harnessing these natural motivations, educators can gradually improve the productivity of teaching sessions.

In short, although the VB-MAPP does not specifically describe practical methods for combining MOs with each learning stage to better control learning, MO-related concepts are integrated into the sections on motivation, reinforcement, and instructional approaches.

Experiments reveal that combining these motivational strategies with the basic reward techniques of the ABA approach is very useful for the development of verbal behavior in autistic children.

Thus, the use of assessment tools such as the observation sheet and the VB-MAPP manual guide made it possible to concretely observe and assess new learning and, consequently, the interests of each child. This made it possible to develop a solid personalized learning plan and better monitor their progress. The adopted procedure laid the foundations for a structured intervention aimed at developing verbal language skills in order to ensure a progressive improvement in the quality of life of autistic children.

3. Structured Teaching Sessions, Analysis of Results, and Discussion

The objective of this session is to report on the implementation of the ABA-based educational program in order to gradually measure its impact on the verbal abilities of autistic children in the experimental group. To ensure a methodical approach, the experiment was validated by ABA trainees. In this context, the initial results of the evaluation demonstrated that, while the children did not produce these statements independently at first, they did so successfully with repetitive assistance. This section analyzes the changes observed, the difficulties encountered, and the practical significance of these results, while proposing alternatives to improve future interventions based, of course, on the ABA approach.

3.1. The Structured Teaching Program

The learning program for the four autistic children, the experimental group, was implemented using a structured and personalized ABA-based strategy. The experiment therefore included the use of assessment rubrics for each participating child to monitor their progress during rehearsals and school exercises introducing the verbal statements of the program, while remaining faithful to the VB-MAPP guidelines (Sundberg, 2008).

These grids allow each child's development to be precisely monitored by noting moments of success and failure to identify where experimentation should intensify repetition exercises if necessary.

To achieve this, the educators carefully selected items and reinforcers for the four children, based on the results of the preference assessments. The personalization of each program, adapted to the profile of each participating child, maximized their motivation through the use of stimuli that increased their involvement in the production of verbal utterances.

The program included a diversification of reinforcers, between tangible elements (toys, food) and social elements (encouragements such as "Well done"). These reinforcers were administered to participating children immediately after the achievement of a target skill, in accordance with the principles of the ABA approach. The intensity of reinforcement was measured and adapted according to the effort made by the children, as suggested by Cooper, Heron, and Heward (2020), in order to maintain a balance between motivation and the children's progress in producing the verbal utterances of the program.

Differentiated reinforcement has also been used to encourage correct responses and reduce errors. This technique involves combining social (such as verbal praise) and material (such as favorite toys or foods) reinforcers, depending on each child's preferences. For example, a child who successfully utters a target sentence such as "I want to drink" (/ na. ʃ.rɔb /) may receive a social reward ("Good job!") and access to their favorite toy. However, if an error is made, appropriate guidance is provided to help the child correct their response, without positive reinforcement.

The sessions were organized to alternate between maintenance instructions (skills already mastered) and target instructions (new skills to be acquired), in order to maintain a balance between consolidating acquired skills and learning new skills. For example, a child who has already mastered the request "I want to eat" (/na.kɔl/) can be encouraged to practice this skill while learning to say "Help" (/sɑː.ʕid.niː/) .

Finally, support was gradually implemented and adapted to each child. For example, to teach a new skill, verbal or physical support may be initially offered, then gradually reduced as the child gains independence. ABA aims to reduce margins of error and promotes learning without frustration or crisis.

The experience encourages teaching sessions to begin with association activities between the educator and the autistic child to establish a positive teacher-child relationship, using favorite objects to reinforce approach behaviors in a playful and natural setting.

The second step of each session is to give children simple instructions, such as “What do you want?”, to encourage cooperation.

Immediate verbal prompts were implemented to help children formulate requests such as “I want a drink” or “Help me,” thereby avoiding errors through errorless teaching (Cooper et al., 2020).

These incentives were gradually reduced to encourage the emergence of spontaneous responses. When a child expressed a request without assistance, a larger reinforcer was used to consolidate this successful behavior, in accordance with the principles of differentiated reinforcement (Sundberg, 2008).

The session aimed to alternate two teaching methods: discrete trial training (DTT) for structured sessions and naturalistic teaching (NET) to integrate learning into natural contexts, such as mealtimes or play (Cooper et al.). To better structure the intervention, experimental team members alternated between DTT and NET to achieve generalization, in accordance with Schreibman et al.'s (2015) recommendations on naturalistic strategies.

Given the structured trials, teaching 'I want to eat' (/na.kɔl/) during mealtimes helped children reproduce the utterance in different real-life contexts.

It is worth noting that each session began with posture instructions to reinforce acquired skills, followed by targeted instructions to teach new expressions, all in a natural way.

Discriminative stimuli (DS) were presented clearly, and an error-correction procedure was implemented if necessary. To facilitate learning, experimental team members used shaping techniques, rewarding successive approximations of the utterances (e.g., “na” then “ko” before reaching “ nakol ”) (Skinner, 1957).

Finally, the experimental team members regularly assessed the children's progress by adjusting the number of attempts and objectives according to their individual needs. This structured and flexible approach maximized the program's effectiveness, promoting children's autonomy and verbal communication while maintaining their motivation and engagement.

The difficulties we encountered at the beginning of the matching process concerned THE four children, WHO had tendency has direct their attention to THE games rather than towards us. During the period of educational monitoring, the children showed strong resistance to simple instructions. To adapt to these difficulties, we intensified the pairing sessions (person, places and activities) as well as the educational monitoring, in order to establish a relationship of trust with the children.

Faced with the disruptive behavior and lack of cooperation of two of the children, presenting varying degrees of difficulty during teaching sessions, We to have We opted to alternate between 80% easy objectives and 20% difficult objectives, while planning regular breaks during the sessions. All these adjustments produced positive and beneficial results for the educational process, benefiting, of course, from the advice and corrections of the supervisors.

3.2. Procedure

a. The Reference Level

The baseline of children's behaviors was established during three initial intervention sessions. These sessions included oral rehearsals of the target utterances, supported by iconic or audiovisual aids representing real-life situations. For example, pictures or videos showing a child drinking, eating, or playing were used to evoke the contexts in which utterances such as "I want to drink" (/ na. ʃ.rɔb /) or "I want to play" (/ na. la:b /) are relevant. These visual aids helped children understand the link between the utterances and real-life situations, while also providing a structured learning environment.

The next phase involved motivating children to produce these phrases by responding to their wants and needs. To help a child learn to say "I want to eat" (/na.kɔl/), the experimental team members created a simulated hunger situation in the presence of food. They used words and gestures to help the children form these sentences and gradually improve their pronunciation. When a child did not understand "I want to drink" well, they could guide them verbally ("Say /na.ʃ.rɔb/ ") and then show them the correct way to say it.

They didn't order the sentences by difficulty, but shuffled them around throughout the sessions. This kept the learning interesting and prevented the children from falling into a predictable order. A typical session alternated between sentences like "toilet" (/twa.lɛt/), "help me" (/sɑː.ʕid.niː/), and "I want to take a break" (/ safi /), depending on the situation and each child's motivations at the time.

They did not reward children for their speech efforts unless they needed help formulating their requests correctly. When needed, they guided them and offered social encouragement (such as a smile or a "Well done!") to encourage and motivate them to try again. This approach helped build positive bonds between children and their communication partners, while preventing them from becoming overly dependent on physical rewards.

b. Wheat Program Intervention and the Modality of the Quoting Tests

The program teaches children with autism to express themselves verbally in everyday situations, starting in the classroom, based on the principles of Applied Behavior Analysis (ABA) (Cooper, Heron, & Heward, 2020). Children first learn to identify program phrases and when to use them, and then to grasp their meaning. For example, they learn to associate the phrase "I want to drink" (/ na. ʃ.rɔb /) with the sight of a glass of water or the feeling of thirst. Experimental team members then create a consistent routine to encourage the use of these phrases, building on children's natural preference for repetition and predictable patterns (Sundberg, 2008, p. 60).

This routine is designed to be flexible, allowing it to adapt to the different stimuli encountered during daily interactions.

Initially, children practice repeating sentences in a controlled setting where the situations and expected responses are clearly defined. For example, during a structured activity, members of the experimental team might encourage a child to say "I want to eat" (/na.kɔl/) in the presence of food. Once this basic step is mastered, they work to have the child use these sentences independently to express specific needs, such as asking for help (/sɑː.ʕid.niː/) or signaling that they need a break (/ safi /).

To facilitate this process, contextual questions are used to guide children in identifying appropriate situations. For example, questions like "Is there any food?" or "Do you need help?" help children understand when and how to use affirmations. A correct answer results in positive reinforcement, such as verbal praise ("Well done!") or the awarding of tokens that can be exchanged for rewards (toys, favorite activities, etc.). The number of tokens required to obtain a reward gradually increases, thus strengthening children's autonomy and perseverance.

The expected success rate also evolves over the sessions, going from 50% in the first sessions to 90% in the last, according to the principle of differentiated reinforcement (Cooper et al., 2020). This gradual progression helps maintain children's motivation while adjusting expectations based on their progress. In the event of an error, a verbal and discreet reminder of the rule and advice are provided to help the child correct their answer without frustration.

The intervention includes 31 sessions organized from 9 a.m. to 1 p.m., integrating meals, leisure and academic activities to encourage the natural observation of progress.

Utterance proficiency is assessed by probing, meaning that a trial is successful if the child produces the target utterance unaided for three consecutive sessions, under the observation of at least two raters (Sundberg, 2008). For example, a child validates the utterance "I want to eat" after three successful probes. This method ensures solid acquisition and generalization of skills across diverse contexts.

c. Follow-Up and Post- Intervention

Two follow-ups were planned to assess the maintenance of acquired skills: the first, two weeks after the intervention, and the second, three weeks later. These follow-ups aimed to verify whether the children spontaneously used the learned statements. The verbal stimuli remained the same, but no reinforcement was provided, except in the case of failure, where the child repeated the statement without reward. Each follow-up consisted of two sessions over two days to cover all the statements in different contexts. These assessments took place between February and March, during the second school semester.

3.3. Analysis of Results, Discussion and Recommendations

a. Analysis of Results

During the February-March intervention, the experimental team members witnessed the remarkable progress of four exceptional children, each of whom discovered the power of language in their own way. Although they all worked with the same basic set of sentences, their learning paths perfectly reflected their individual personalities and needs. The following image presents the results of this first intervention period:

Figure 1. Participants' use of intervention expressions

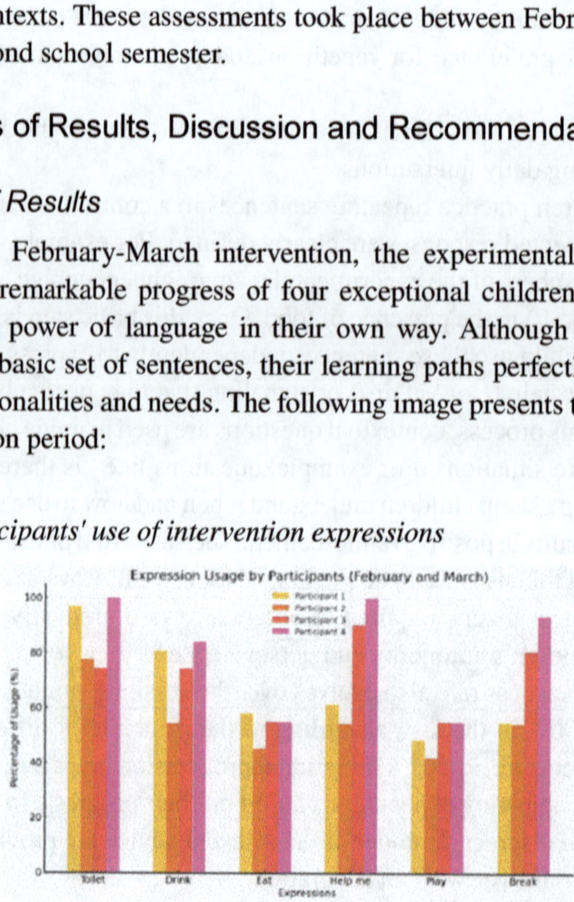

Participant 1's exceptional achievement—pronouncing the word "toilet" with 96.77% accuracy—brought a significant change to his daily life and a welcome relief to his family. His 80.65% accuracy for "drinking" was often accompanied by a gentle gesture: reaching for his favorite blue cup. Even more encouraging, his growing ability to ask for help (61.29%) in difficult times marked a significant milestone in his emotional development.

Participant 2 demonstrated a strong connection with the program's phrases, using "restroom" with a frequency accuracy of 77.42% after quickly understanding its purpose. His requests for " help" and "break" (approximately 54%) often appeared during sensory overloads, early signs of his ability to recognize and express his needs before becoming overwhelmed.

Participant 3 stood out for his impressive use of "help" (90.32%), clearly demonstrating his growing trust in others. This child often used "pause" (80.64%) when bored or struggling with slow schoolwork, while his spontaneous requests of "I want to drink" (74.19%) to fetch water demonstrated growing independence.

Participant 4, meanwhile, used "help" with perfect accuracy (100%), adapting his tone to the urgency of the situation. The same was true for "break," with a frequency of 93.54%. He therefore systematically received calming gestures, such as moving to a quiet place. Interestingly, follow-up data revealed that while concrete needs such as "toilet" and "help me" were well remembered by all participants, more emotional expressions such as "break" required more constant reinforcement.

This observation allows us to tailor future support to each child's developmental priorities. Beyond these statistics, the experience also noted embodied human moments, such as proud smiles when a word leads to success, or the feeling of reassurance when a need is met, as well as tender gestures during early attempts at communication. These human gestures remind us that true progress isn't just about percentages, but rather is manifested by each growing expression of confidence, independence, and connection, all expressed through attentiveness and patience.

The experience therefore has a broader vision, highlighting both learning and the ability to connect with the world as a human being, each in their own way and at their own pace.

As for the post-intervention phase, here are the data from the experiment, as presented in the following image representing the results of the post-intervention period:

Figure 2. Participants' use of post-intervention expressions

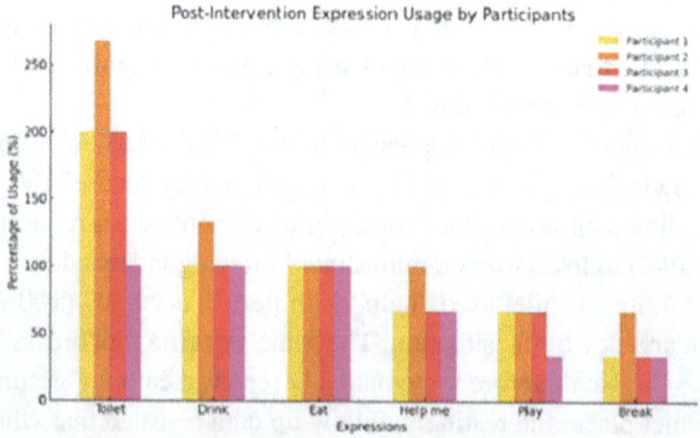

Participant 1 used "toilet" at 200%, and "drink" and "play" at 100%, while "break" remained at only 33.33%. Participant 2 excelled with "toilet" at 266.66% and "drink" at 133%, while "play" reached 66.67%. Participant 3 showed high use of "help me" (200%) and "drink" (100%), but "break" remained low at 33.33%. Participant 4 used almost all expressions at 100%, except for "play" (66.67%) and "break" (33.33%).

These results suggest that some phrases, particularly "pause," still require further reinforcement. Ongoing support, extended sessions, and regular follow-up will be essential to sustain these skills, avoid regression, and tailor interventions to each child's unique journey. Reflecting on the weeks following the intervention, there was much more to be seen than just data. It was a series of small victories, steady progress, and sincere reminders of areas where support is still needed. Participant 1's remarkable 200% use of "toilet" demonstrated how easily this phrase had become part of his daily life.

However, he rarely uses the word "break" (33.33%), which reveals that abstract learning can take time to acquire, unlike immediate needs such as "drink" or "play", which are easily acquired.

Participant 2's exclusive use of the term "toilet" (266.66%) demonstrated how well he had generalized this skill to different environments, from home to school to the playground. Furthermore, his use of the term "play" (66.67%) revealed that learning to ask for joy and pleasure is as important a process as expressing one's basic needs.

Participant 3's frequent use of "help me" (200%) demonstrates both growing confidence in seeking support and an ability to maintain attention, while the score for "break" remained at 33.33%, a reminder that emotional regulation develops slowly. It is important to note that emotional needs take time to express themselves and take shape in the child participant.

Participant 4's near-perfect use of most expressions revealed considerable progress, and his rather moderate results for “game” and “break” demonstrated a more general trend compared to the rest of the participants.

The experience concluded that children must be helped not only to express their needs, but also their joys and their need for space.

Each child's journey clearly showed that concrete needs integrate more quickly into their vocabulary, while emotional language requires more time, creativity, and patience. Each percentage gave us deeper insights, not only into progress, but also into how each child learns and communicates. Communication development is as unique as each child.

Moving forward, the experimental team will focus on naturally introducing more complex expressions throughout the day, increasing opportunities for spontaneous communication during play, and using visual tools to make abstract ideas more accessible. Perhaps the most significant result has been seeing these simple words come to life and transform into real messages that the children now confidently use in their daily lives.

Ultimately, these numbers represent much more than data: they are milestones in each child's personal journey toward discovering their voice. The paths may look different, but they all lead to the same beautiful destination: authentic self-expression and the deep connection that comes from true understanding.

b. Discussion

According to Virués -Ortega, meta-analyses confirm some of ABA's effects. These effects are moderate to significant on communication. However, most studies involve Western populations. Moroccan results show success rates of 48 to 60%. This effectiveness is comparable. It suggests that cultural adaptations could improve results. The use of Moroccan Arabic sentences is one example.

Verbal behavior training significantly improved communication. This approach is based on the principles of ABA. The children learned the target sentences. They continued to use them after the program. This persistence occurred even without immediate rewards. This suggests true integration of the skills. The children were not using them just to obtain rewards.

The team did, however, observe individual differences. Some specific difficulties persist. The persistence of acquired verbal behaviors is a positive indicator. It occurs after the cessation of systematic reinforcements. It demonstrates integration into the daily communication repertoire.

For example, phrases like “Toilet” or “Help me” continue to be used. This use in natural contexts indicates some generalization. This persistence was not uniform, however. The use of "Pause" decreased among some participants. This highlights a need: some phrases require more sustained reinforcement, especially those that are less frequent or less motivating.

A slight decrease in targeted behaviors was observed after one month. Less frequent utterances such as "Pause" were affected. A gradual recovery followed. The children retained some acquired skills. This recovery may come from procedural memory. Rehearsal in natural contexts also contributes to it.

This trend reveals a persistent fragility of certain statements. They require occasional reminders. Occasional reinforcement then becomes necessary. This prevents the risk of regression.

The involvement of parents and educators appears to be a key factor. It helps maintain the progress made. It also facilitates its generalization. The Moroccan context, however, presents a notable limitation. Involvement there was limited. This limitation stems from the lack of training available to families. It also stems from the absence of appropriate ABA resources.

Parents and educators, however, play an essential role. They ensure the generalization of skills at home. They also guarantee it at school. Without adequate support, this mission becomes difficult. Ensuring the continuity of progress in diverse contexts requires structured support. This limitation underscores an absolute necessity: collaboration between all stakeholders. Professionals, families, and educational institutions must work together. This synergy ensures the sustainability of interventions.

Existing verbal skills influenced effectiveness. Children who were already communicating assimilated the target sentences more easily. Children with intellectual difficulties require a different approach. So do those with severe communication problems. For example, they require additional visual aids. Pictures can help them. So can alternative systems like PECS. These tools facilitate comprehension. They aid in the practical use of sentences.

The experiment concludes that longer sessions are important. Additional sessions would be beneficial. They would allow these children to learn more thoroughly. They would memorize better. They would then apply the targeted skills in different contexts. Thus, children facing intellectual difficulties require personalized methods. Those with complex communication barriers also require personalized teaching methods. It is advisable to personalize teaching methods for them. Extending the duration of sessions often becomes necessary.

What works best is close collaboration. Therapists must work with educators. Parents and teachers must join them. Together, they create tailored approaches. These approaches address the specific challenges of each participant.

Experience has clearly demonstrated this necessity. Interventions must be individually tailored. Each program must be personalized. This personalization is based on each child's unique profile.

To achieve this, parents and teachers must be trained. They must be fully involved in the program. Training in ABA techniques is essential. It ensures consistency between structured sessions. These sessions are organized between the association and the school. Consistency with their daily lives must also be maintained.

Future research should target a broader group. This group should have common characteristics. A similar intellectual disability, for example. Significant communication difficulties as well.

c. Guidelines and Recommendations

Alnemary 's work in Saudi Arabia is noteworthy . This work demonstrated the success of ABA adapted to the Arab context. This successful adaptation is due to its cultural relevance. Therefore, training Moroccan parents in Darija seems promising. Using Moroccan Arabic to explain the ABA approach is crucial. Incorporating local reinforcers could improve assimilation. This would also promote better generalization.

To improve practices in Moroccan autism centers, ongoing professional training is essential. This training must be adapted to the sociocultural context. When parents master the basics of this approach, they become good caregivers. They can then collaborate effectively with teachers. This collaboration ensures a harmonious continuity of learning at home.

Children's needs are constantly evolving over time. This evolution makes ongoing assessment crucial. Regular follow-ups allow teams to measure progress and adjust approaches accordingly.

Strengthening networks between specialists is vital. ABA specialists must collaborate with educators. Psychologists and healthcare professionals must join them. This network would promote more comprehensive support. It would also ensure greater consistency.

By implementing these suggestions, specialized centers would become more efficient. They would improve the verbal skills of autistic children. This would strengthen the children's overall well-being. These measures would help better serve this community throughout Morocco.

CONCLUSION

The ABA study conducted with Moroccan autistic children yielded encouraging results. These results confirm the team's initial impressions. The ABA approach demonstrates real local effectiveness. The children's communication skills have improved. Their ability to speak spontaneously has progressed. Their expression of needs has developed. A clear link emerges between ABA work and this progress.

Caution remains necessary, however. The study involved only a few participants. Every autistic child is unique. Each situation presents specificities. Each need requires special attention. These results do not allow for generalization. Individual improvements are promising. But the small sample size requires caution. The diversity of autistic manifestations reinforces this need.

Responses vary from child to child. This variation underscores a fundamental requirement. ABA programs must be tailored to each individual. This personalization is essential to their effectiveness.

Despite these limitations, the study provides valuable insights. It sheds light on the specificities of verbal skills. It identifies key factors influencing ABA. Motivation is one of these factors. So is symptom severity. So is the quality of the intervention.

Methodological rigor strengthens the validity of the results. It provides a solid foundation for future research. The study provides empirical data. It offers practical recommendations. These elements help healthcare professionals. They assist educators. They support families.

The ultimate goal remains clear: to improve the quality of life of autistic children. Overcoming difficulties with verbal communication is crucial. This success promotes their social inclusion. Further studies will be necessary. They will need to include more participants and explore diverse cultural contexts. This research will deepen our understanding of the mechanisms of ABA and refine intervention strategies.

The study focused on verbal communication. However, nonverbal children could benefit from other systems. PECS is one example. Future Moroccan studies would be useful. They could explore PECS simultaneously with ABA. This combination would address broader communication needs.

THANKS

We express eternal gratitude. We particularly thank the psychologist Mr. Oussama Zentar . We also thank the association's psychologist, Mr. Mohammed Jabbad . His constructive comments accompanied each step of the program. We thank all the association's educators. A special mention for Mr. Mohammed Sahl . His contribution to this project was invaluable.

REFERENCES

Alnemary, F. M., Aldhalaan, H. M., Simon-Cereijido, G., & Alnemary, F. M. (2017). Services for children with autism in Saudi Arabia. *Autism, 21*(5), 592–602. DOI: 10.1177/1362361316664868 PMID: 28610540

American Psychiatric Association. (2013). *Diagnostic and Statistical Manual of Mental Disorders* (5th ed.)., DOI: 10.1176/appi.books.9780890425596

Boyd, B. A., Hume, K., McBee, M. T., Alessandri, M., Gutierrez, A., Johnson, L., Sperry, L., & Odom, S. L. (2014). Comparative effectiveness of LEAP, TEACCH, and model-nonspecific special education programs for preschool children with autism spectrum disorders. *Journal of Autism and Developmental Disorders, 44*(2), 366–380. DOI: 10.1007/s10803-013-1877-9 PMID: 23812661

Carr, M. E., Moore, D. W., & Anderson, A. (2014). Self-management interventions for students with autism: A meta-analysis of single-center research. *Exceptional Children, 81*(1), 28–44. DOI: 10.1177/0014402914532235

Cooper, J. O., Heron, T. E., & Heward, W. L. (2020). *Applied Behavior Analysis* (3rd ed.). Pearson.

Ganz, J. B., Davis, J. L., Lund, E. M., Goodwyn, F. D., & Simpson, R. L. (2012). Meta-analysis of PECS with individuals with ASD: An investigation of targeted and nontargeted outcomes, participant characteristics, and implementation phase. *Research in Developmental Disabilities, 33*(2), 406–418. DOI: 10.1016/j.ridd.2011.09.023 PMID: 22119688

Granpeesheh, D., Dixon, D. R., Tarbox, J., Kaplan, A. M., & Wilke, A. E. (2009). Effects of age and treatment intensity on outcomes of behavioral interventions for children with autism spectrum disorders. Autism Spectrum. *Diseases & Research, 3*(4), 1014–1022. DOI: 10.1016/j.rasd.2009.06.007

Kasari, C., Kaiser, A., Goods, K., Nietfeld, J., Mathy, P., Landa, R., Murphy, S., & Almirall, D. (2014). Communication interventions for minimally verbal children with autism: A sequential randomized multiple assignment trial. *Journal of the American Academy of Child and Adolescent Psychiatry*, *53*(6), 635–646. DOI: 10.1016/j.jaac.2014.01.019 PMID: 24839882

Koegel, L. K., Singh, A. K., & Koegel, R. L. (2010). Improving academic motivation in children with autism. *Journal of Autism and Developmental Disorders*, *40*(9), 1057–1066. DOI: 10.1007/s10803-010-0962-6 PMID: 20221791

Leaf, J. B., Leaf, R., McEachin, J., Taubman, M., Ala'i-Rosales, S., Ross, R. K., Smith, T., & Weiss, M. J. (2016). Applied behavior analysis is a science and, therefore, progressive. *Journal of Autism and Developmental Disorders*, *46*(2), 720–731. DOI: 10.1007/s10803-015-2591-6 PMID: 26373767

Lovaas, O. I. (1987). Behavioral treatment and normal educational and intellectual functioning in young children with autism. *Journal of Consulting and Clinical Psychology*, *55*(1), 3–9. DOI: 10.1037/0022-006X.55.1.3 PMID: 3571656

Makrygianni, M. K., Gena, A., Katoudi, S., & Galanis, P. (2018). Effectiveness of Applied Behavior Analysis Interventions for Children with Autism Spectrum Disorders: A Meta-Analysis. *Research in Autism Spectrum Disorders*, *51*, 18–31. DOI: 10.1016/j.rasd.2018.03.006

Peters-Scheffer, N., Didden, R., Korzilius, H., & Sturmey, P. (2011). A meta-analytic review of the effectiveness of comprehensive ABA-based early intervention programs for children with autism spectrum disorders. *Research in Autism Spectrum Disorders*, *5*(1), 60–69. DOI: 10.1016/j.rasd.2010.03.011

Reichow, B., Hume, K., Barton, E. E., & Boyd, B. A. (2018). Early Intensive Behavioral Intervention (EIBI) for young children with autism spectrum disorder (ASD). *Cochrane Database of Systematic Reviews*, *5*(10), CD009260. Advance online publication. DOI: 10.1002/14651858.CD009260.pub3 PMID: 29742275

Schreibman, L., Dawson, G., Stahmer, A. C., Landa, R., Rogers, S. J., McGee, G. G., & Halladay, A. (2015). Naturalistic developmental behavioral interventions: Empirically validated treatments for autism spectrum disorders. *Journal of Autism and Developmental Disorders*, *45*(8), 2411–2428. DOI: 10.1007/s10803-015-2407-8 PMID: 25737021

Skinner, B. F. (1957). *Behavior verbal*. Appleton-Century -Crofts. DOI: 10.1037/11256-000

Smith, T., & Iadarola, S. (2015). Evidence update on autism spectrum disorders. *Journal of Clinical Child and Adolescent Psychology, 44*(6), 897–922. DOI: 10.1080/15374416.2015.1077448 PMID: 26430947

Sundberg, M. L. (2008). *VB-MAPP: Verbal Behavior Milestone Assessment and Placement Program*. AVB Press.

Tincani, M. and Devis, K. (2011). Quantitative synthesis and analysis of the components of single-participant studies on the image exchange communication system. *Education specialized and specialized, 32* (6), 458-470. https://doi.org/DOI: 10.1177/0741932510362494

Virués-Ortega, J.Virués -Ortega. (2010). Behavior analytic intervention applied to autism in early childhood: Meta-analysis, meta-regression, and dose-response meta-analysis of multiple outcomes. *Clinical Psychology Review, 30*(4), 387–399. DOI: 10.1016/j.cpr.2010.01.008 PMID: 20223569

Chapter 11
Impact of Neuroeducation on Teaching Learning Process

Subharthi Das
https://orcid.org/0009-0004-8861-8477
Kazi Nazrul University, India

Santu Karmakar
https://orcid.org/0009-0007-6092-7974
Kazi Nazrul University, India

ABSTRACT

Neuroeducation is an evolving field, with interdisciplinary nature, which combines the knowledge of the neuroscience with classroom practice as a way to improve instruction and learning. We consider in this chapter the ways in which neuroeducation can enhance cognitive development and neuroplasticity, the formation of memory, and the management of their emotions by connecting the teaching strategies to brain functioning. Based on a systematic literature review, we speak about the effect of neuroeducation on the student outcomes, the impact of artificial intelligence and neurofeedback in individualized learning, and the formation of adaptive, brain-based pedagogies. The evidence indicates that neuroeducation-based strategies arouse the metacognition process, increase the involvement of the learner as well as elevating academic performance. In addition, the collaboration of neuroeducation with sustainable educational efforts creates inclusive, personalized, and future-rooted environments that enables both educators and learners.

DOI: 10.4018/979-8-3373-3581-0.ch011

INTRODUCTION

The concept of neuroeducation has emerged from an increasing recognition of the necessity to tailor educational approaches to meet the varied needs of learners (Pradeep et al., 2024). Today, the field of education has been going through many transformations propelled by the modern changes in the teaching approach and psychology. Neuroeducation is one of the most prevalent trends in contemporary education. It is an interdisciplinary field that synthesises neuroscience, psychology, and education (Jolles & Jolles, 2021). Neuroeducation aims to improve our understanding of how the brain learns and uses this information to improve teaching methods, curriculum development, and educational results (Pradeep et al., 2024). Exploring the cognitive and emotional functions of the brain, neuroeducation advocates important insights that challenge the conventional educational system and promote more effective and inclusive learning environments. Essentially, neuroeducation examines how neural processes, including memory, attention, and emotional control, affect learning (Gerdes et al., 2015). Evidence obtained in this field points to the value of coordinating teaching practices with the human brain's natural way of obtaining and storing information. The transition aids in education to shift away from non-rigid and non-uniform education methods. This is capable of recognising individual differences and expanding the natural plasticity of the brain. The ability to enhance instructional design is one of the most remarkable effects of neuroeducation (Fragkaki et al., 2022). Quality Teachers can create instruction that increases engagement, retention, and understanding by gaining an understanding of brain processing. In this regard, studies of memory integration have revealed that spaced repetition and active recall can also be used to facilitate the long-lasting storage of information (Squire et al., 2015). The application of these concepts in our modern-day classrooms will facilitate the learning not only of information but also the ability of students to be able to access and correspondingly use them (Abadzi, 2006). Additionally, neuroeducation makes a significant contribution to students with special learning needs.

Different neurological studies have contributed to the understanding of dyslexia, ADHD, and autism spectrum disorders, whose understanding permits the instructors to institute certain interventions that can address the issues (Stringer & Tommerdahl, 2015). Neuroeducation emphasises the connection between emotions and learning (Pradeep et al., 2024). The limbic system in the brain controls emotional reactions and determines motivation, reminiscence, and choice. It was shown that good feelings, like curiosity and feeling of achievement, can improve cognitive performance, whereas bad feelings, like fear and anxiety, can disrupt learning, on the other hand (García, 2024). This assists educators in creating safe and conducive conditions in which students feel important and inclined to pursue new ideas (Stassinopoulos,

2023). Social-emotional learning (SEL) programs are based on neuroeducation principles. They are becoming more and more widespread to assist students and develop their emotional intelligence and resilience, along with the ability to connect with others, all of which are necessary characteristics of success in academia and life (Schnitzer, 2019). Neuroeducation highlights the importance of fostering metacognition, which is the ability to think about one's thinking (Mefteh, 2024). When the students are urged to reflect on how they learn, make goals, and measure their development, this enables them to be in charge of their learning. Studies in neuroeducation indicate that metacognitive techniques stimulate the brain's prefrontal cortex, enhancing skills in problem-solving, critical thinking, and decision-making (Mefteh, 2024). The use of metacognition, which is incorporated into the curriculum, teaches students lifelong learning skills that extend beyond the school years. The rise of technology has expanded the influence and application of neuroeducation in contemporary education (Pradeep et al., 2024). Brain-imaging, eye tracking, and data analytics tools can be used to provide rich details about student learning and can make it possible to provide timely feedback and student-personalised learning. Educational technologies, such as adaptive learning platforms and gamified applications, apply neuroeducation principles to accommodate different learning speeds and styles (Shiwlani et al., 2024). The developments not only enhance academic performance but also provide better access to high-quality education, filling equity and opportunity gaps. However, effectively integrating neuroeducation into current education systems requires careful planning and collaboration (Bendriyanti et al., 2024). Lecturers, policymakers, and researchers need to collaborate and translate other complex neuroscience bodies of knowledge to transform them into strategies that can be deployed in the classroom. Professional development programs that provide teachers with knowledge and skills in neuroeducation are crucial for their successful implementation (Fragkaki et al., 2022).

REVIEW OF RELATED LITERATURE

Neuroeducation and Learning Outcomes

Research indicates that applying neuroeducation principles can significantly enhance learning outcomes. A systematic review done by Huangal-Scheineder et al. (2024) emphasises the fact that cognitive explanation enables the development of teaching strategies to synchronise with the mechanisms of the brain to learn and therefore show better academic results. What is more, the neuroscientific literacy of teachers is highlighted by a study by Howard-Jones (2014) to implement brain-based learning methods properly. This evidence indicates that the application of neuroscience in educational activities may become more productive in terms of the learning process. Neuroeducation provides insights into teaching by explaining how the brain processes and retains information. Approach to teaching reflecting on neural development discusses the topic in that Jolles and Jolles (2021) and Zadina (2015) emphasise connecting scientific research and the teaching practice to enrich the methods.

Teaching Strategies Improvement

Neuroeducation provides valuable insights into effective teaching strategies by elucidating how the brain processes and retains information. In a study conducted by Goswami (2004), the author discusses the development of the brain in understanding how a teacher can use this information to teach in a manner that contributes to the development of thinking. Moreover, an overview presented by Bruer (1997) discusses the use of neuroscience in education, pointing to the serious consequences of the existing gap between scientific research and education in schools. These studies underscore the potential of neuroeducation to inform and enhance teaching methodologies, leading to more effective educational practices. Applying neuroeducation principles enhances learning outcomes by aligning teaching methods with cognitive processes. Pradeep et al. (2024) identify the relationship between brain understanding and academic performance, whereas Caballero & Llorent (2022) note that educators need to become neuroscientific literate to support the brain-based approach.

Integration with Sustainable Education Practices

Integrating neuroeducation with sustainable education practices involves creating learning environments that support long-term cognitive and emotional development. Zull's (2002) paper is an analysis of how conceptualisation of the development of the brain can lead to curriculum design, which can facilitate lifelong learning. These findings are supported by another study conducted by Jensen (2005), which relates that the development of the brain and the resultant effect on learning may be influenced by some elements of the environment, including the classroom design and classroom methods of teaching. These insights suggest that incorporating neuroeducation principles into sustainable education practices can foster environments that support the holistic development of students. Integrating neuroeducation into sustainable education fosters cognitive and emotional development. Nievas & Del Pilar Gallardo-Montes (2023) also investigate its contribution to the design of the curriculum, and Pradeep et al. (2024) consider the impact of such factors as the classroom environment on brain development. These studies highlight neuroeducation's role in creating holistic learning environments.

Research Gap

Although neuroeducation is increasingly gaining momentum, the existing body of literature is disintegrated. Numerous experiments deal with individual elements like cognitive neuroscience, brain-based strategies, and educational technology, but do not take into consideration a comprehensive framework that ties the different components together. In addition, few studies have been done on how neuroeducation, artificial intelligence, neurofeedback, and sustainable learning practices relate to one another synergistically. The second gap is that of classroom practices of applying neuroeducation. Theoretical frameworks and neuroscience background are researched properly, but their interpretation into practical application is not clear to most teachers. It is also rare to find studies on how neuroeducation can reinforce the growth of metacognition, emotional self-management, and individualised learning specifically within the diverse or resource-limited learning contexts.

JUSTIFICATION OF THE STUDY

The study is imperative because it appears to integrate interdisciplinary studies of neuroeducation and its use in the present-day teaching-learning proceedings. The research will offer a critical understanding regarding the impact of neuroeducation on cognitive development, instructional design, incorporation of technology, as well as the sustainability of education by obtaining a systematic literature review on the topic. Its results will be of special value in guiding educators, policymakers, and curriculum developers in instituting evidence-based classroom approaches. Moreover, the research points to the emergence of the need to create individual and inclusive models of education that take into consideration the specifics of individual differences of learners, encourage their lifelong learning, and enhance educational equity. The research is topical and current due to the growing popularity of applying AI and neurofeedback in a classroom; it may provide some practical knowledge to make education more effective, adaptive, and far-sighted.

OBJECTIVES

1. To explore the role of neuroeducation in improving learning outcomes for students
2. To assess the impact of technology-driven neuroeducation tools, such as AI and neurofeedback, on individualised learning plans

3. To analyse the role of neuroeducation in enhancing teaching strategies for students
4. To investigate the role of Neuroeducation in Sustainable Learning Practices

METHODOLOGY

This paper uses a Systematic literature review (SLR) to critically review the impact of neuroeducation on the teaching-learning process. The SLR method was chosen because the synthesis of interdisciplinary research on neuroscience, psychology, and education needed to be conducted in a structured, transparent, and comprehensive way.

Search Strategy

The thorough search also ensued across academic databases such as Google Scholar, Scopus, Web of Science, and PubMed. The following keywords were used in different permutations: neuroeducation, brain-based learning, educational neuroscience, AI in education, neurofeedback, and sustainable learning.

Inclusion and Exclusion Criteria

Original articles were considered, in English, and published in peer-reviewed journals, book chapters, or conference proceedings. The criterion was that only those studies that directly address neuroeducation and its educational ramifications were chosen. Exclusions were used on non-academic sources, related studies, or papers that had no theoretical or empirical value.

Selection and Data Analysis

Figure 1 shows the selection process which followed the requirements of the PRISMA Flow Diagram. As part of this systematic review, we have closely followed the PRISMA 2020 (Preferred Reporting Items for Systematic Reviews and Meta-Analyses) framework to attain transparency, replicability and methodological rigour. An extensive search was undertaken in Scopus, Web of Science, Google Scholar, SpringerLink, and PubMed. A resulting set of 115 records was deduplicated, and 95 articles were used as primary screening through their titles and abstracts, which resulted in excluding 17 records that did not satisfy the relevance criteria. The entire content of the remaining 78 articles was then evaluated regarding eligibility; one of the studies was eliminated due to conceptual overlap with an article that was already included. As a result of this, a total of 77 studies were included in the final qualitative synthesis.

Figure 1. PRISMA 2020 flow diagram

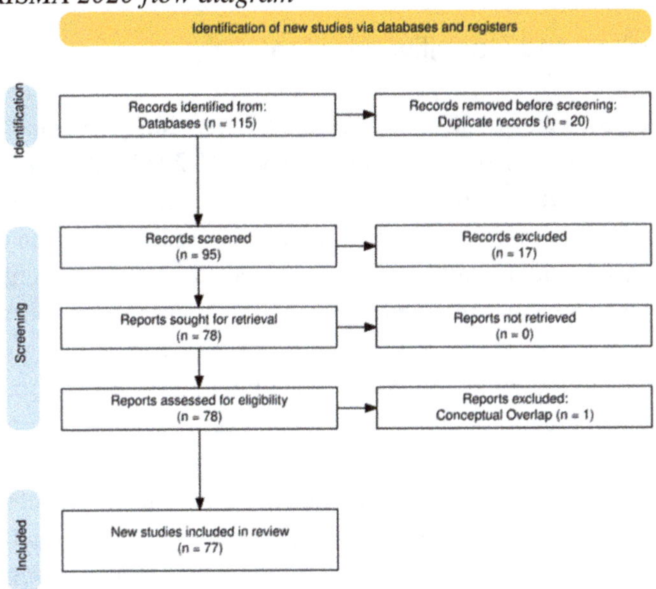

Generated using the PRISMA2020 R package (Haddaway et al., 2022)

FINDINGS

To Explore the Role of Neuroeducation in Improving Learning Outcomes for Students

Comprehending Neuroeducation and Its Core Principles

Neuroeducation is based on the idea that insights into how the brain learns can greatly enhance teaching methods (Pradeep et al., 2024). A fundamental principle of neuroeducation is neuroplasticity, which refers to the brain's capacity to reorganise itself by creating new neural connections throughout a person's life. This versatility emphasises the need to create interesting, challenging, and stimulating settings that will give students a challenging way of learning and focus on shaping their minds (Pradeep et al., 2024). The other area of concern is the importance of memory in the learning process. It has been proved that such methods as providing spaced repetition, active recalls, and learning in multi-sensory environments can enhance the retention and encoding process (Ghanbari et al., 2019). Incorporating these strategies in the teaching process, educators can create more effective learning experiences to comply with how the brain receives and retrieves information.

Neuroeducation and Cognitive Growth

One of the key benefits of neuroeducation is its ability to enhance cognitive development through specific interventions (AV & V, 2022). Studies have revealed that mindfulness practice and brain training are among the activities that could enhance the attention span, working memory, and executive function capacity that are crucial in academic attainment (Diéguez et al., 2024). Mindfulness has been reported to relieve stress and anxiety in students, creating a more favourable learning environment (Capiro, Gleason, & Powers, 2019). Neuroeducation also highlights the significance of emotional regulation in cognitive growth (Capiro, Gleason, & Powers, 2019). Emotional conditions may significantly influence learning because, under the impact of high stress, memory and decision-making processes may be hampered. The best thing educators can do is to teach their students self-control techniques and to provide them with a favourable emotional atmosphere so they can think clearly and find the strength to focus on their academic challenges.

Tailored Learning Through Neuroeducation

A particularly promising aspect of neuroeducation is its ability to customise learning experiences according to individual cognitive profiles (Doukakis & Vlamos, 2021). Studies have indicated that every student is different in the way he or she processes information because there exist differences in both the structure and the functioning of the brain. Neuroeducation supports the use of assessments and tools, such as neurofeedback and cognitive diagnostics, to identify each student's unique learning needs and strengths (García, 2024). Personalised learning plans based on neuroeducation can tackle specific issues, such as learning disabilities or attention deficits, while also capitalising on students' strengths (Vaninsky, 2017). As one example, neurofeedback procedures have been quite fruitful in improving attention and concentration in students with ADHD (Rahmani et al., 2022). Like, educators can apply insights from neuroeducation to create differentiated instruction that accommodates various learning styles, thereby optimising each student's potential.

Enhancing Instructional Practice

Neuroeducation offers a solid foundation for improving teaching methods by providing research-based insights into how students learn most effectively (Marshall & Bolt-Lee, 2022). The acknowledgement of the brain's preference for visual and spatial information has led to the use of common tools such as concept mapping and the use of visual aids in education. These strategies help the students to sort out and make sense of the complicated information in a more appropriate manner. Also, the significance of feedback in the learning process is another area where neuroeducation has greatly influenced teaching practices (Fragkaki et al., 2022). Neuroscience research highlights that prompt and positive feedback on the part of the learner can reinforce the neuronal pathways concerning learning. Teachers who provide concrete, prompt feedback allow pupils to internalise what has been taught and increase self-esteem. Lesson pacing is another important issue. Research in neuroeducation suggests that students are better at retaining information when lessons are divided into smaller, manageable segments, with regular breaks to allow the brain to process and consolidate what it has learned (Ghanbari et al., 2019).

Supporting Lifelong Learning Abilities

Neuroeducation is not only about enhancing academic achievements, as it also allows students to acquire some skills to be lifelong learners (Jolles & Jolles, 2021b). In a sense, by making metacognition emerge, a sense of how they have learned, they are students who are emboldened to be in control of their education. Metacognitive strategies, including goal setting, self-monitoring, and metacognitive thinking, also assist the student to be more autonomous and active in education (Paciarotti & Bertozzi, 2023). Neuroeducation, as well, emphasises the importance of developing a growth mindset that keeps students inspired enough to approach a challenge as an opportunity to develop, rather than as an obstacle. In my research, Yeager & Dweck (2012) found that a growth mindset was paired with a higher strength of motivation, resilience, and academic achievement.

To Assess the Impact of Technology-Driven Neuroeducation Tools, Such as AI and Neurofeedback, on Individualised Learning Plans

The Emergence of Technology in Neuroeducation

Neuroeducation uses the mechanisms of how the brain successfully learns and processes information, which has culminated in the appearance of technology-based tools of neuroeducation (Howard-Jones et al., 2014). These are the tools that are combined with neuroscience and sophisticated technological solutions to produce results in the form of the cognitive profile, learning tendencies, and strengths or weaknesses in the students. Technologies like adaptive learning systems powered by AI, neurofeedback or wearable solutions that allow measuring the activity of the brain (Aithal et al., 2024). Learning platforms equipped with AI and developed by companies like DreamBox and Smart Sparrow analyse data about their performance to adapt to their teaching material dynamically (Saputra et al., 2024). On the same note, neurofeedback systems also provide real-time data on brain activity, which allows students to develop self-control capabilities that can enhance focusing and attention span (Patel et al., 2021). The mentioned instruments are at the forefront of individual learning plans and help one to ensure the exact, data-driven information about the needs of a student.

Technology as a Means of Facilitating Personalisation

One of the main strengths of technology-based neuroeducation tools is the ability to foster personalised learning. The traditional learning methods are often a one-size-fits-all way of teaching, and this cannot support the variances that are experienced by the students. However, the neuroeducation tools use data analytics to personalise information. As an example, through analysing performance patterns, AI algorithms can help detect the gaps in understanding and change the curriculum based on them. Such individualisation will ensure that specific instruction is provided to the students based on their learning pace and pattern. According to the research published by Ziegler et al. (2022), the use of AI-powered learning platforms promotes high academic performance and engagement level among students about their colleagues attending classroom-based courses.

Mitigating Learning Challenges

Some of the neuroeducation tools that have been created by technology can be used to help students with a learning disability, either attention deficit hyperactivity disorder (ADHD), dyslexia, or autism spectrum disorder (ASD). Neurofeedback treatment techniques are effective in enhancing attention and reducing impulsiveness among ADHD students through training them to enhance their brainwave patterns (Thompson & Thompson, 1998). Another way in which AI-based tools can be of benefit to students with dyslexia is the ability to provide text-to-speech, visual support, and other assistive technologies to support the processing of the information (Barua et al., 2022). Such instruments also make it possible to identify learning challenges early enough, and thereby take proactive measures by educators.

Well-known platforms like CogniFit and Lumosity can offer a detailed report on the strengths and weaknesses of the individual in terms of cognitive capacity, making the teachers better prepared to come up with a specific strategy to challenge those aspects that they experience trouble with (Siricharoen, 2023).

Enhancing Student Autonomy

The neuroeducation tools that are enhanced with technology contribute to the active student engagement in their educational efforts (Howard-Jones et al., 2014). Such tools usually encompass the features to prompt self-assessment and goal-setting, thus prompting students to monitor their progress and make specific changes. Individual dashboards provide students with personal control over their achievements and the possibility to set their learning goals (Song et al., 2024). The examples of such applications are Khan Academy and others. Neurofeedback systems also lead to student independence by empowering the learners to have the skills associated with controlling their cognitive and emotional states (Mohammadi et al., 2023). By way of a concrete example, a student who uses a neurofeedback device to monitor the level of focus in the course of their studying can be taught to notice distractive factors and to correctly switch their attention. Such an autonomous system of learning makes the learner independent and resilient, which are key lifelong learning competencies.

Teacher Support and Professional Development

Even though it seems that the greatest number of benefits of neuroeducation tools driven by technology lead to students, it is also worth noting that they contribute to the strength of educators (Jolles & Jolles, 2021). These tools provide teachers with in-depth information about how students are doing, and this information will help the teachers identify trends so that they can adjust their teaching methods. AI-led systems will have the capability of generating in-depth reports to find out the strengths and weaknesses of the students, enabling teachers to make specific interventions. The process of professional development is also becoming more biased to the training of using the tools of neuroeducation (Jolles & Jolles, 2021; Pradeep et al., 2024). Teachers with such experience will have an upper hand when it comes to integrating technology in their classrooms, thus creating an overall instructor quality improvement.

To Analyse the Role of Neuroeducation in Enhancing Teaching Strategies for Students

Promoting a Student-Centred Learning Environment

The importance of neuroeducation is in the emphasis on acknowledging personal differences in studying (McFarland, 2017). The differences in cognitive abilities, processing speeds, and learning styles between students may be explained by the dissimilarity in their brain development and functioning (Lövdn et al., 2020). Educators will be able to adapt the topic of their instructions to suit the varied demands of the learners by applying the principles of neuroeducation (Bendriyanti et al., 2024). An example can be considered when some students may become good visual learners requiring diagrams and charts to teach effectively, and other students can be more effectively taught using auditory methods, e.g. lectures or discussions. Neuroeducation promotes the use of multimedia, multimodal teaching, which involves the incorporation of visual, auditory and kinaesthetic modules to deal with learners of varying preferences (Pashler et al., 2008).

Enhancing Memory Retention Through Evidence-Based Strategies

The ability to remember is one of the main elements of the learning process, and neuroeducation provides valuable information about the strategies that can be used to improve the memory of things (Dubinsky & Hamid, 2024). Neuroscience also supports the effectiveness of several interventions, including spaced repetition, active teens and storytelling, in enhancing memory retention (Kang, 2016). Spaced repetition involves rehashing concepts at regular intervals, which strengthens neuronal connections and promotes an ability to remember over a long period (Yuan, 2022). Active recall ensures that memory recall is encouraged instead of passive readings and hence increases memory consolidation (Roediger & Butler, 2010). Storytelling in a piece of educational content is helpful as the information it conveys is more contextual, which makes it easy to remember as it engages both brain hemispheres, as cognitive and emotional (Ginting et al., 2024).

Boosting Engagement Through Attention Mechanisms

Neuroeducation throws much light on the role of attention in the learning process because attention acts as a doorstep to memory and understanding (Ansari et al., 2011). A study of neuroscience shows that lessons with an emotional touch, as well as being personally relevant and new, show that the brain is more attentive (Goldberg, 2022). Teachers can use this insight to come up with carefully crafted methods that help them gain and maintain the attention of the learners (Hossen & Uddin, 2023). As an example, a provocative question, a surprise fact or a real-life application can be interesting to start a lesson, it draws the attention of students and makes them interested in the topic of study (Chin & Osborne, 2008). Also, it is recommended to organise changes of the activity frequently, including physical activity or gamified elements, to keep the mind engaged with long-term learning (Capatina et al., 2024).

Maintaining Emotional Regulation and a Favourable Learning Environment

Interaction between emotion and learning is another area where the understanding of neuroeducation contributes much to the improvement of teaching methods. Emotions may either support or impede the learning process; an example is that stress and anxiety may disrupt the cognitive processes, whereas a positive emotional state may lead to their improvement analogously through heightened creativity, problem-solving skills and information processing (Robinson et al., 2013). Teachers who receive neuroeducation grow well-prepared to develop a positive classroom atmosphere that allows emotional security and reduces pressure (Fitzgerald et al., 2022). Mindfulness exercises, growth mindset interventions, and positive reinforcements as techniques may help students to manage their emotions and learn with more confidence (Lindsay et al., 2018).

Metacognition Facilitation and Self-Regulated Learning Provision

A technological process called neuroeducation also emphasises the value of metacognition, i.e., thinking about own mental processes, in enhancing learning performance (Shekh-Abed, 2024). Teaching metacognitive skills to students, namely, self-monitoring, goal-setting, and reflection skills, helps educators enable learners to take charge of their learning tasks (Desautel, 2009). As an example, the activities can be devised by the teachers and they require students to gauge their understanding of a topic or their plans on progress on the assignments. These habits not only improve academic outcomes but also provide students with lifelong learning essential skills (Shloul et al., 2024).

To Investigate the Role of Neuroeducation in Sustainable Learning Practices

Supporting Long-Term Retention and Application

Neuroeducation focuses mainly on the methodologies that enhance memory storage and enable knowledge transfer, all of which are paramount to lasting learning outcomes (Pradeep et al., 2024). It has a neuroscience basis, envisioning the importance of using spaced repetition and active recall as a person can strengthen the neural connections, thus reinforcing the ability to recall the information over time (Dubinsky & Hamid, 2024). As an example, as opposed to conducting tedious study sessions that include cramming, teachers can adopt a plan of spreading out learning and reviewing fundamental ideas now and then (Carpenter et al., 2022). This approach encompasses the brain mechanism of consolidation of information in an idle state of sleep and rest, a process that contributes to the entrenchment of knowledge into long-term memory (Rasch & Born, 2013). Moreover, neuroeducation supports the construction of curricula that promote knowledge application in other situations (Jolles & Jolles, 2021). The given strategy aligns with the nature of brain connection and connection-making capabilities to find certain possibilities between ideas and helps students in making generalisations of their learning and transferring it to new experiences (Goldberg, 2022).

Developing Lifelong Learning Skills

The development of learning and lifelong education is all about providing people and students with skills and mindsets of continuous learning (Ben-Eliyahu, 2021). One of the most important elements that was emphasised by neuroeducation is metacognition, or the ability to think about oneself thinking (Stanton et al., 2021). In the process of developing metacognitive skills, students learn more about their own strong and weak sides as well as their favourite learning approaches (Hartman, 2001). As an illustration, setting goals, monitoring progress, and reflecting on educational experiences teach the students to be independent learners (Neo et al., 2022). The approach can encourage self-direction and adaptability and can thus help the learners to carry on with positive learning even when they get out of the formal educational setting (She et al., 2023). Moreover, neuroeducation promotes the growth mindset that is the belief in the ability to improve and develop skills and abilities with determination and hard work (Ng, 2018). Investigation by Carol Dweck and her associates has indicated that resilience and motivational abilities to pursue education as lifelong learners can be improved by having a growth mindset (Moser et al., 2011).

Integrating Emotional Regulation and Well-Being

Sustainable learning is not only an intellectual affairs problem; emotional health is also an influential factor (Moreira et al., 2021). Neuroeducation highlights the importance of emotion as a part of the learning process, which suggests that positive emotional experiences may promote memory performance, creativity, and problem-solving, the continued stress of which may inhibit such skills (Li et al., 2020). When mindfulness practice, stress management techniques, and the social-emotional learning (SEL) programs are integrated, educators can create the settings in which the students can feel safe, appreciated, and motivated (Schonert-Reichl et al., 2014). As an example, the mindfulness training has been found to become effective in increasing concentration and reducing anxiety, resulting in students being able to become more engaged in their studies. Not only do these methods promote academic performance, but they also allow the development of emotional resilience, which is a necessary skill when operating sustainably and effectively and overcoming life and work difficulties (Ross et al., 2023).

Promoting the Collaborative and Contextual Learning

Sustainability learning also tends to be social, which means that collaboration, communication, and the skills to work with various teams are involved (Van Mierlo & Beers, 2018). This is affirmed by the Neuroeducation that advocates the brain as being sensitive to social and contextual learning (Pradeep et al., 2024). All of the above-listed group activities, peer teaching and project-based learning methods are rooted in neuroeducation and encourage collaboration and critical thinking (Mutanga, 2024). Such methods stimulate several parts of the brain and make the process much more interesting and easier to memorise. Also, through placement in the context of the real world, educators will be able to increase the relevance and purposefulness of lessons, which will lead to the student discovering the importance of what he is learning and encouraging him to persevere (O'Neill & Short, 2023).

Aligning Learning Practices with Environmental and Societal Sustainability

A new topic of concern is the combination of neuroeducation and environmental sustainability in learning. Educators can also promote sustainable habits in the personal and professional life of students by inclusive into the curriculum lessons about how the brain works about decision-making, and behaviour (Goldberg, 2022). As an example, neuroeducation can guide the way of teaching students the psychology of habit-building and enable them to make sustainable choices. Also, knowing how the brain reacts under a social dilemma and ethical issues could lead to educators planning lessons that bring about empathy, world citizenship, and responsibility (Coumans & Wark, 2024).

EDUCATIONAL IMPLICATIONS

Based on the principles of neuroeducation, it is possible to draw several practical implications on how to enhance the teaching-learning practice in the modern classroom. By matching the natural learning processes in the brain to instructional design, the student engagement, retention of knowledge and cognitive development would be greatly improved. In addition, neuroeducation strategies that use technology facilitate inclusive learning and individualised learning of different learner profiles. Key implications include:

1. **Brain-Aligned Instructional Design.** The integration of neuroplasticity based, spaced repetitions, active recall and multisensory input-based strategies can enhance long-term retention and conceptual understanding in students.
2. **Increased Student motivation and involvement.** Techniques of neuroeducation that focus on curiosity, relevance, and emotional safety can reinforce attention, motivation, and academic perseverance.
3. **Individualised Learning Using Neuro-Technologies.** The adaptive learning frameworks supported by AI-based systems and neurofeedback applications can support students with diverse learning requirements, such as students with ADHD or dyslexia (as well as any other learning issues) with carefully tailored learning experiences.
4. **Metacognition and Lifelong Learning Skills Promotion.** The ability to monitor themselves, reflect, and set goals as a strategy to metacognition will enable students to have control over the learning process, which will make them gain independence even when they are outside of the school environment.
5. **Thoughts on Inclusion with Diverse Learners.** The neurocognitive insights make differentiated teaching and early intervention possible to make sure that students with different developmental and socio-emotional backgrounds have equal opportunities to receive learning.
6. **Development of Teacher Professional Competence.** The ongoing growth in neuroscience-based pedagogy is what allows educators to have access to new techniques to improve cognitive development, attention, and emotional regulation. This guarantees the successful transfer of scientific knowledge into the teaching process.

7. **Evidence based Educational Decision Making.** The combination of neuroeducation-based learning analytics allows educators and schools to track the progress of learners more precisely, detect the cognitive barriers at a earlier stage, and create specific intervention programs based on the objective data.
8. **Influencing Support of Emotionally Safe Learning Environments.** Neuroeducation focuses on the fact that moods and thinking are closely connected. Positive reinforcement, stress-reduction strategy and prioritisation of psychological safety can facilitate better memory consolidation and increased persistence of learning in schools.
9. **Greater Access and Equity to Learning.** Brain-based learning practices support differentiated teaching and assistive technologies that support neurodivergent children. This eliminates disparities in performance whereby students with different capabilities are given equal chances to learn.
10. **Future Ready Skills Development: Alignment.** Neuroeducation promotes the skills needed in 21st century jobs and lifelong personal growth by fostering executive functioning, problem-solving, adaptability, and creativity.

LIMITATIONS

1. **Language Limitation:** All articles covered in the review are restricted to those published in the English language; thus, we will miss important research done in other languages, which might impact the global nature and the viability of the results.
2. **Database Coverage:** Although massive scholarly resources, like Scopus, Web of Science, Google Scholar, and PubMed, were used, some relevant research in obscure or local journals could have been missed.
3. **Technological Limitations:** The argument of AI and neurofeedback devices is grounded on recent technological advancements, some of which are at experimental phases. The process of their widespread use and long-term effect remains poorly studied.

NEUROETHICS AND CLASSROOM NEUROTECHNOLOGY PRIVACY

Implementing neurotechnology into the learning process creates serious ethical and privacy concerns. EEG signals or signal readings of the neural stimulation indicate the areas of cognition, attention, and emotion that touch the inner world of the human mind. Since such information may incriminate mental privacy, identity, and even freedom of thought, it must be handled as special-category data that requires extra-protection, limited use, and explicit ethical management.

Data Classification and Sensitivity

Neural and affective information should be established as one of the most sensitive personal data. These cues are capable of revealing personal information about the internal condition of students, and therefore, they are particularly susceptible to being abused or misinterpreted. This means that schools and vendors need to implement the same level of protection that exists in biometric or health data, which includes high access control, encryption, and reduced collection and storage.

Consent and Agency

The use of any neural data in any case must be at least voluntary, founded on previously, without charge, informed, specific consent by parents or other people in charge, and appropriate student assent. Consent should be voluntary and never be taken by way of implication, and one should not be subjected to a penalty, either academic or social, due to refusal to consent. All the consent forms must be written in plain language to clarify what data are captured, how the data will be interpreted, by whom they will be accessed and how long they will be stored, and how they will be secured. The students must not be conditioned to feel that they cannot pause or stop the recording and continue without penalty, because that is respecting autonomy and comfort.

Privacy-by-Design Safeguards

The privacy-by-design approach should be the basis of any development and implementation process. Data minimization (only collecting the data that is necessarily needed to serve specific educational goals) should be applied, as much processing as possible should be performed on-device or at the edge to avoid unnecessary data transfer, and data transmission and storage should be encrypted. Role-based access control, authentication, and deep audit logs are required to ensure accountability. The vendors have to comply with clear contractual obligations on data-processing, restrict third-party disclosure, and accept liability on breach or abuse.

Purpose: Restriction and Ethical Application

A high-stakes decision cannot be made using neural data, like grading, disciplinary action, academic placement, or teacher appraisal. They should continue to be voluntary, well-being-based, and pedagogical and in accordance with community-agreed outcomes, like promoting self-regulation, engagement, or reflective teaching. The implementation of all use cases should be preceded by the documentation of all the use cases, which must be approved by a transparently governed process.

Government and Transparency

Institutions need to perform a Data Protection Impact Assessment (DPIA) to trace out data flow, risk assessment, re-identification, and misuse, being just a few examples, and document mitigation and remaining risk acceptance before any pilot or deployment. Findings of such tests ought to be presented in simple, easy-to-understand reports. Vendors, protocol approval, audit monitoring, and handling complaints and incident response should be vetted and handled by a governance committee consisting of educators, parents, students, and the data-protection officer. The incident response plan must have clear notification, containment, recovery, and remediation timelines that ensure there is clear communication with the families and regulators.

Openness and Data Rights

Families and students should be allowed to access, correct, and demand deletion of neural data. When feasible, outputs must be anonymized or pooled, and the shortest possible retention times and sunset provisions may be necessary so that data can be destroyed, particularly after the project. The transparency creates trust and ensures that it is in line with the privacy law and the ethical expectations.

Equity, Culture, and Inclusion

The ethical implementation should take into account culture and equity implications. The neural data interpretation and communication must be culturally responsive without being stigmatizing or deterministic concerning cognition. Low-cost or non-technological options should be offered in schools so that all can participate and digital gaps cannot be further widened.

Professional Ethics: Pedagogical

Neuroethics and neuroscientific literacy should be trained to teachers and facilitators to prevent over-interpretation or neuro-essentialist thinking that might end up perpetuating bias or dehumanizing students to neural value scales. Ethical awareness must be connected with professional development and practical application in the classroom, making the use of it responsible and informed.

Fairness and Oversight of Algorithms

Every analytic algorithm should be tested and audited against bias, accuracy, and reliability with regard to different groups of students. Frequent reviews of performance and an independent audit should also be done to promote fairness and validity. A perceived bias or degradation must initiate open remediation.

Conformity to Human Rights and Neurorights

Lastly, classroom neurotechnology must be consistent with the emerging human-rights-based practices and global discourse of neurorights - defending mental privacy, cognitive liberty, and freedom of thought, particularly in the case of children. Ethical innovation in the area should uphold the dignity and autonomy of the learner as the key principles of education.

RECOMMENDATIONS

1. **Teacher Training and Professional Development:** Postulates of neuroscience must be included in teacher training modules in educational institutions, both in pre-service and in-service. This will help the educators gain an understanding of how to use brain-based instructional strategies, including metacognitive scaffolding, emotional regulation methods and using differentiated instructions to meet the variance of cognitions.
2. **Combination of AI and neurofeedback software:** Artificial intelligence, neurofeedback equipment, and learning analytics based on data can be promoted in the classrooms to facilitate individual learning. Educators can use these tools to learn more about the cognitive patterns of each student to establish an adaptive learning environment that suits their requirements and encourages them to learn more.
3. **Operator Lesson Redesign Utilising Neuroeducation Principles:** Learning resources and techniques used in the curriculum should be redesigned to incorporate fundamental neuroeducation principles as neuroplasticity, spaced learning, active recall and growth mindset. Due focus must be set on multisensory, student-driven, and theoretically consistent content that is consistent with brain processing and storage patterns.

4. **Social-Emotional Learning (SEL) integration:** There is evidence showing emotions have an influence on the learning process, and thus, are integrated into the neuroeducation research. Emotional intelligence, resilience, mindfulness and positive learning environments that can facilitate cognitive growth and academic success should be promoted in these programs.
5. **Special Needs and Diverse Learners:** The use of neuroeducation in the field of learning disabilities sheds light on how to treat learning deficiencies, including ADHD, dyslexia and autism. These insights should be applied by educational settings in planning individual and focused interventions based on neurocognitive assessment and evidence-based practices.

CONCLUSION

Neuroeducation is a movement that is changing the modern-day learning environment and process due to the integration of neuroscience, psychology and pedagogical knowledge into the resulting educational experiences to enhance learning. This study shows how neuroeducation plays a more decisive role in improving student engagement, cognitive development, and teaching methods. Educators must use and improve the learning environments they create by using such concepts as neuroplasticity, memory retention techniques and emotional management techniques. Integration of neuroeducation tools based on technology, namely, artificial intelligence, and neurofeedback has further optimised learning experiences to address the individual cognitive needs. The innovations not only reinforce students with existing learning problems but also advance metacognitive skills essential to a life-time learning process. Moreover, the synergy between neuroeducation and sustainable teaching and learning promotes the holistic cognitive development as well as environmental awareness and social responsibility. Despite the vast range of opportunities that neuroeducation holds, it requires constant research, training in the field and policies to make it effective and successful. As a way of improving its applications, future studies ought to look into the long-term impact of neuroeducation in other learning settings. Finally, the implementation of neuroeducation can help to develop more adaptable and child-centred educational frameworks that will meet needs in academic and personal growth.

REFERENCES

Abadzi, H. (2006). *Efficient learning for the poor.* The World Bank eBooks. https://doi.org/DOI: 10.1596/978-0-8213-6688-2

Aithal, P. S., Prabhu, S., & Aithal, S. (2024). Future of higher education through technology prediction and forecasting. SSRN *Electronic Journal.* https://doi.org/DOI: 10.2139/ssrn.4901474

Ansari, D., De Smedt, B., & Grabner, R. H. (2011). Neuroeducation – a critical overview of an emerging field. *Neuroethics*, *5*(2), 105–117. DOI: 10.1007/s12152-011-9119-3

AV. B., & V, R. (2022). Implications of neuroscience/neuroeducation in the field of education to enhance the learning outcomes of the students. *Journal of Positive School Psychology, 6*, 6502–6510. https://www.journalppw.com/index.php/jpsp/article/view/8636

Barua, P. D., Vicnesh, J., Gururajan, R., Oh, S. L., Palmer, E., Azizan, M. M., Kadri, N. A., & Acharya, U. R. (2022). Artificial intelligence-enabled personalized assistive tools to enhance education of children with neurodevelopmental disorders—A review. *International Journal of Environmental Research and Public Health, 19*(3), 1192. DOI: 10.3390/ijerph19031192

Ben-Eliyahu, A. (2021). Sustainable learning in education. *Sustainability (Basel), 13*(8), 4250. DOI: 10.3390/su13084250

Bendriyanti, R. P., Setyawan, A., Kurniasih, N., & Citrawati, T. (2024). Integrating neuroeducation into educational management: A breakthrough for enhancing elementary education. *BIO Web of Conferences, 146*, 01098. https://doi.org/DOI: 10.1051/bioconf/202414601098

Bruer, J. T. (1997). Education and the brain: A bridge too far. *Educational Researcher, 26*(8), 4–16. DOI: 10.3102/0013189X026008004

Caballero, M., & Llorent, V. J. (2022). The effects of a teacher training program on neuroeducation in improving reading, mathematical, social, emotional, and moral competencies of secondary school students: A two-year quasi-experimental study. *Revista de Psicodidáctica (English Ed.), 27*(2), 158–167. https://doi.org/DOI: 10.1016/j.psicoe.2022.04.002

Capatina, A., Juarez-Varon, D., Micu, A., & Micu, A. E. (2024). Leveling up in corporate training: Unveiling the power of gamification to enhance knowledge retention, knowledge sharing, and job performance. *Journal of Innovation & Knowledge, 9*(3), 100530. DOI: 10.1016/j.jik.2024.100530

Capiro, N. M., Gleason, A. L., & Powers, S. (2019). *The impact of a neuroeducation-based wellness curriculum on Generation Z: Implementing mind-body connection* (Doctoral dissertation, Lynn University). SPIRAL. https://spiral.lynn.edu/etds/344

Carpenter, S. K., Pan, S. C., & Butler, A. C. (2022). The science of effective learning with spacing and retrieval practice. *Nature Reviews Psychology, 1*(9), 496–511. DOI: 10.1038/s44159-022-00089-1

Chin, C., & Osborne, J. (2008). Students' questions: A potential resource for teaching and learning science. *Studies in Science Education, 44*(1), 1–39. DOI: 10.1080/03057260701828101

Coumans, J. V. F., & Wark, S. (2024). Impact of problem-based learning coaching and neuroeducation in the development of 21st-century lifelong learners. *Mind, Brain and Education : the Official Journal of the International Mind, Brain, and Education Society, 18*(1), 35–42. DOI: 10.1111/mbe.12406

Desautel, D. (2009). Becoming a thinking thinker: Metacognition, self-reflection, and classroom practice. *Teachers College Record, 111*(8), 1997–2020. DOI: 10.1177/016146810911100803

Diéguez, M. P., García, M. C., Asencio, E. N., & Vergara-Moragues, E. (2024). Executive function training through a mindfulness-based neuroeducational program in elementary school students. *Mindfulness, 15*(11), 2739–2749. Advance online publication. DOI: 10.1007/s12671-024-02474-8

Doukakis, S., & Vlamos, P. (2021). Enhancement programming skills and transforming knowledge of programming through neuroeducation approaches. *arXiv (Cornell University).* https://doi.org//arxiv.2105.09779DOI: 10.48550

Dubinsky, J. M., & Hamid, A. A. (2024). The neuroscience of active learning and direct instruction. *Neuroscience and Biobehavioral Reviews, 163*, 105737. DOI: 10.1016/j.neubiorev.2024.105737

Fitzgerald, M. M., Shipman, K., Pauletic, M., Ellesworth, K., & Dymnicki, A. (2022). Promoting educator social emotional competence, well-being, and student–educator relationships: A pilot study. *Mental Health & Prevention, 26*, 200234. DOI: 10.1016/j.mhp.2022.200234

Fragkaki, M., Mystakidis, S., & Dimitropoulos, K. (2022). Higher education faculty perceptions and needs on neuroeducation in teaching and learning. *Education Sciences*, *12*(10), 707. DOI: 10.3390/educsci12100707

García, M. T. M. (2024). Bridging the gap: Leveraging neuroeducation to enhance teaching methodologies. *Korea TESOL Journal, 20*(2). https://koreatesol.org/sites/default/files/pdf_publications/20241227_%EC%A0%80%EB%84%90%2020_2_%ED%91%9C%EC%A7%80%ED%8F%AC%ED%95%A8.pdf#page=13

Gerdes, L., Tegeler, C. H., & Lee, S. W. (2015). A groundwork for allostatic neuroeducation. *Frontiers in Psychology*, *6*. Advance online publication. DOI: 10.3389/fpsyg.2015.01224

Ghanbari, S., Haghani, F., & Akbarfahimi, M. (2019). Practical points for brain-friendly medical and health sciences teaching. *Journal of Education and Health Promotion*, *8*(1), 198. DOI: 10.4103/jehp.jehp_135_19

Ginting, D., Woods, R. M., Barella, Y., Limanta, L. S., Madkur, A., & How, H. E. (2024). The effects of digital storytelling on the retention and transferability of student knowledge. *SAGE Open*, *14*(3), 21582440241271267. Advance online publication. DOI: 10.1177/21582440241271267

Goldberg, H. (2022). Growing brains, nurturing minds—Neuroscience as an educational tool to support students' development as life-long learners. *Brain Sciences*, *12*(12), 1622. DOI: 10.3390/brainsci12121622

Goswami, U. (2004). Neuroscience and education. *The British Journal of Educational Psychology*, *74*(1), 1–14. DOI: 10.1348/000709904322848798

Haddaway, N. R., Page, M. J., Pritchard, C. C., & McGuinness, L. A. (2022). PRISMA2020: An R package and Shiny app for producing PRISMA 2020-compliant flow diagrams, with interactivity for optimised digital transparency and Open Synthesis Campbell Systematic Reviews, 18, e1230. https://doi.org/DOI: 10.1002/cl2.1230

Hartman, H. J. (2001). Developing students' metacognitive knowledge and skills. In *Neuropsychology and cognition* (pp. 33–68). https://doi.org/DOI: 10.1007/978-94-017-2243-8_3

Hossen, M. K., & Uddin, M. S. (2023). Attention monitoring of students during online classes using XGBoost classifier. *Computers and Education: Artificial Intelligence*, *5*, 100191. DOI: 10.1016/j.caeai.2023.100191

Howard-Jones, P., Holmes, W., Demetriou, S., Jones, C., Tanimoto, E., Morgan, O., Perkins, D., & Davies, N. (2014). Neuroeducational research in the design and use of a learning technology. *Learning, Media and Technology, 40*(2), 227–246. DOI: 10.1080/17439884.2014.943237

Howard-Jones, P. A. (2014). Neuroscience and education: Myths and messages. *Nature Reviews. Neuroscience, 15*(12), 817–824. DOI: 10.1038/nrn3817

Huangal-Scheineder, S., Cieza-Sánchez, J., Diaz-Paredes, M., Arriaga-Delgado, M., & Marchena-Tafur, A. (2024). Neuroeducation and impact on higher education: A systematic review. *International Journal of Evaluation and Research in Education, 13*(6), 3641. DOI: 10.11591/ijere.v13i6.29170

Jensen, E. (2005). *Teaching with the brain in mind.* Association for Supervision and Curriculum Development. https://www.google.co.in/books/edition/Teaching_with_the_Brain_in_Mind/KP5QBAAAQBAJ?hl=en&gbpv=1

Jolles, J., & Jolles, D. D. (2021). On neuroeducation: Why and how to improve neuroscientific literacy in educational professionals. *Frontiers in Psychology, 12*, 752151. Advance online publication. DOI: 10.3389/fpsyg.2021.752151

Kang, S. H. K. (2016). Spaced repetition promotes efficient and effective learning. *Policy Insights from the Behavioral and Brain Sciences, 3*(1), 12–19. DOI: 10.1177/2372732215624708

Li, L., Gow, A. D. I., & Zhou, J. (2020). The role of positive emotions in education: A neuroscience perspective. *Mind, Brain and Education : the Official Journal of the International Mind, Brain, and Education Society, 14*(3), 220–234. DOI: 10.1111/mbe.12244

Lindsay, E. K., Chin, B., Greco, C. M., Young, S., Brown, K. W., Wright, A. G. C., Smyth, J. M., Burkett, D., & Creswell, J. D. (2018). How mindfulness training promotes positive emotions: Dismantling acceptance skills training in two randomized controlled trials. *Journal of Personality and Social Psychology, 115*(6), 944–973. DOI: 10.1037/pspa0000134

Marshall, L. L., & Bolt-Lee, C. E. (2022). A neuroeducation and cognitive learning-based strategy to develop active learning pedagogies for accounting education. *The Accounting Educators' Journal, 32*. https://www.aejournal.com/ojs/index.php/aej/article/view/689

McFarland, D. J. (2017). How neuroscience can inform the study of individual differences in cognitive abilities. *Reviews in the Neurosciences, 28*(4), 343–362. DOI: 10.1515/revneuro-2016-0073

Mefteh, K. C. (2024). *Active pedagogy and neuroeducation: In-depth reflections for innovative teaching*. IntechOpen eBooks. https://doi.org/DOI: 10.5772/intechopen.114368

Mohammadi, Y., Bozorgkhou, H., Hadavi, S. M., Shojaei, M., Khodadadi, F. R., Najafi, S., Karimi, Z., & Sarvestani, M. M. (2023). The effectiveness of neurofeedback on the management of academic performance in students with academic failure: Experimental research. *Annals of Medicine and Surgery (London)*, *85*(6), 2677–2682. DOI: 10.1097/MS9.0000000000000823

Moreira, P. A., Inman, R. A., Hanel, P. H., Faria, S., Araújo, M., Pedras, S., & Cunha, D. (2021). Engagement and disengagement with sustainable development: Further conceptualization and evidence of validity for the Engagement/Disengagement in Sustainable Development Inventory (EDiSDI). *Journal of Environmental Psychology*, *79*, 101729. DOI: 10.1016/j.jenvp.2021.101729

Moser, J. S., Schroder, H. S., Heeter, C., Moran, T. P., & Lee, Y. (2011). Mind your errors. *Psychological Science*, *22*(12), 1484–1489. DOI: 10.1177/0956797611419520

Mutanga, M. B. (2024). Students' perspectives and experiences in project-based learning: A qualitative study. *Trends in Higher Education*, *3*(4), 903–911. DOI: 10.3390/higheredu3040052

Neo, T., Amphawan, A., Hew, S., Neo, M., Hamidani, K., & Chang, Y. (2022). Inculcating student problem-solving skills through self-directed learning in a smart learning environment. *EDULEARN ... Proceedings*, *1*, 326–332. DOI: 10.21125/edulearn.2022.0100

Ng, B. (2018). The neuroscience of growth mindset and intrinsic motivation. *Brain Sciences*, *8*(2), 20. DOI: 10.3390/brainsci8020020

Nievas, P. P., & Del Pilar Gallardo-Montes, C. (2023). The neuroeducation training of students in the degrees of early childhood and primary education: A content analysis of public universities in Andalusia. *Education Sciences*, *13*(10), 1006. DOI: 10.3390/educsci13101006

O'Neill, G., & Short, A. (2023). Relevant, practical and connected to the real world: What higher education students say engages them in the curriculum. *Irish Educational Studies*, •••, 1–18. DOI: 10.1080/03323315.2023.2221663

Paciarotti, C., & Bertozzi, G. (2023). The impact of cross-cutting pedagogical features based on neuroeducation advances: Project-based learning vs. traditional lecturing in engineering education. *Journal of Engineering Education*, *37*(3), 17–32. DOI: 10.16920/jeet/2024/v37i3/24002

Pashler, H., McDaniel, M., Rohrer, D., & Bjork, R. (2008). Learning styles. *Psychological Science in the Public Interest*, *9*(3), 105–119. DOI: 10.1111/j.1539-6053.2009.01038.x

Patel, K., Katz, C. N., Kalia, S. K., Popovic, M. R., & Valiante, T. A. (2021). Volitional control of individual neurons in the human brain. *Brain*, *144*(12), 3651–3663. DOI: 10.1093/brain/awab370

Pradeep, K., Anbalagan, R. S., Thangavelu, A. P., Aswathy, S., Jisha, V. G., & Vaisakhi, V. S. (2024). Neuroeducation: Understanding neural dynamics in learning and teaching. *Frontiers in Education*, *9*, 1437418. Advance online publication. DOI: 10.3389/feduc.2024.1437418

Rahmani, E., Mahvelati, A., Alizadeh, A., Mokhayeri, Y., Rahmani, M., Zarabi, H., & Hassanvandi, S. (2022). Is neurofeedback effective in children with ADHD? A systematic review and meta-analysis. *Neurocase*, *28*(1), 84–95. DOI: 10.1080/13554794.2022.2027456

Rasch, B., & Born, J. (2013). About sleep's role in memory. *Physiological Reviews*, *93*(2), 681–766. DOI: 10.1152/physrev.00032.2012

Robinson, O. J., Vytal, K., Cornwell, B. R., & Grillon, C. (2013). The impact of anxiety upon cognition: Perspectives from human threat of shock studies. *Frontiers in Human Neuroscience*, *7*. Advance online publication. DOI: 10.3389/fnhum.2013.00203

Roediger, H. L.III, & Butler, A. C. (2010). The critical role of retrieval practice in long-term retention. *Trends in Cognitive Sciences*, *15*(1), 20–27. DOI: 10.1016/j.tics.2010.09.003

Ross, P. M., Scanes, E., & Locke, W. (2023). Stress adaptation and resilience of academics in higher education. *Asia Pacific Education Review*. Advance online publication. DOI: 10.1007/s12564-023-09829-1

Saputra, I., Kurniawan, A., Yanita, M., Putri, E. Y., & Mahniza, M. (2024). The evolution of educational assessment: How artificial intelligence is shaping the trends and future of learning evaluation. *Indonesian Journal of Computer Science*, *13*(6). Advance online publication. DOI: 10.33022/ijcs.v13i6.4465

Schnitzer, K. E. (2019). *Discovering the educational implications of neuropsychological research: Understanding the impact of neuroeducation instruction on fifth-grade students and their teachers* (Doctoral dissertation, San Diego State University). ProQuest Dissertations Publishing. https://www.proquest.com/openview/79fd118aa695afe8d9dcca55afdba70c/1?pq-origsite=gscholar&cbl=18750&diss=y

Schonert-Reichl, K. A., Oberle, E., Lawlor, M. S., Abbott, D., Thomson, K., Oberlander, T. F., & Diamond, A. (2014). Enhancing cognitive and social–emotional development through a simple-to-administer mindfulness-based school program for elementary school children: A randomized controlled trial. *Developmental Psychology*, *51*(1), 52–66. DOI: 10.1037/a0038454

She, C., Liag, Q., Jiang, W., & Xing, Q. (2023). Learning adaptability facilitates self-regulated learning at school: The chain mediating roles of academic motivation and self-management. *Frontiers in Psychology*, *14*, 1162072. Advance online publication. DOI: 10.3389/fpsyg.2023.1162072

Shekh-Abed, A. (2024). Metacognitive self-knowledge and cognitive skills in project-based learning of high school electronics students. *European Journal of Engineering Education*, •••, 1–16. DOI: 10.1080/03043797.2024.2374479

Shiwlani, A., Hasan, S. U., & Kumar, S. (2024). Artificial intelligence in neuroeducation: A systematic review of AI applications aligned with neuroscience principles for optimizing learning strategies. *Journal of Digital and Social Sciences.* https://doi.org/DOI: 10.47205/jdss.2024(5-IV)50

Shloul, T. A., Mazhar, T., Abbas, Q., Iqbal, M., Ghadi, Y. Y., Shahzad, T., Mallek, F., & Hamam, H. (2024). Role of activity-based learning and ChatGPT on students' performance in education. *Computers and Education Artificial Intelligence*, *6*, 100219. DOI: 10.1016/j.caeai.2024.100219

Siricharoen, N. (2023). Creative brain training apps and games can help improve memory, cognitive abilities, and promote good mental health for the elderly. *EAI Endorsed Transactions on Context-Aware Systems and Applications*, *9*(1). Advance online publication. DOI: 10.4108/eetcasa.v9i1.3524

Song, C., Shin, S., & Shin, K. (2024). Implementing the dynamic feedback-driven learning optimization framework: A machine learning approach to personalize educational pathways. *Applied Sciences (Basel, Switzerland)*, *14*(2), 916. DOI: 10.3390/app14020916

Squire, L. R., Genzel, L., Wixted, J. T., & Morris, R. G. (2015). Memory consolidation. *Cold Spring Harbor Perspectives in Biology*, *7*(8), a021766. DOI: 10.1101/cshperspect.a021766

Stanton, J. D., Sebesta, A. J., & Dunlosky, J. (2021). Fostering metacognition to support student learning and performance. *CBE Life Sciences Education*, *20*(2), fe3. DOI: 10.1187/cbe.20-12-0289

Stassinopoulos, R. L. (2023). *Cultivating student engagement and enhancing teaching self-efficacy in higher education STEM: A neuroeducation framework* (Doctoral dissertation, Johns Hopkins University). Johns Hopkins Institutional Repository. http://jhir.library.jhu.edu/handle/1774.2/68866

Stringer, S., & Tommerdahl, J. (2015). Building bridges between neuroscience, cognition and education with predictive modeling. *Mind, Brain and Education : the Official Journal of the International Mind, Brain, and Education Society, 9*(2), 121–126. DOI: 10.1111/mbe.12076

Thompson, L., & Thompson, M. (1998). Neurofeedback combined with training in metacognitive strategies: Effectiveness in students with ADD. *Applied Psychophysiology and Biofeedback, 23*(4), 243–263. DOI: 10.1023/A:1022213731956

Van Mierlo, B., & Beers, P. J. (2018). Understanding and governing learning in sustainability transitions: A review. *Environmental Innovation and Societal Transitions, 34*, 255–269. DOI: 10.1016/j.eist.2018.08.002

Vaninsky, A. (2017). Educational neuroscience, educational psychology, and classroom pedagogy as a system. *American Journal of Educational Research, 5*(4), 384–391. DOI: 10.12691/education-5-4-6

Yeager, D. S., & Dweck, C. S. (2012). Mindsets that promote resilience: When students believe that personal characteristics can be developed. *Educational Psychologist, 47*(4), 302–314. DOI: 10.1080/00461520.2012.722805

Yuan, X. (2022). Evidence of the spacing effect and influences on perceptions of learning and science curricula. *Cureus*. Advance online publication. DOI: 10.7759/cureus.21201

Zadina, J. N. (2015). The emerging role of educational neuroscience in education reform. *Psicologia Educativa, 21*(2), 71–77. DOI: 10.1016/j.pse.2015.08.005

Zull, J. E. (2002). *The art of changing the brain: Enriching the practice of teaching by exploring the biology of learning*. Stylus Publishing. https://moodle2.units.it/pluginfile.php/561006/mod_resource/content/1/el200409_zull.pdf

Chapter 12
Factors Affecting Learning From a Neuropedagogical Perspective

Didem Kılıç
https://orcid.org/0000-0002-2250-8580
Aksaray University, Turkey

Yasemin Taşkıner Şereflioğlu
https://orcid.org/0000-0002-7309-2589
Ministry of Education, Turkey

Necdet Sağlam
Hacettepe University, Turkey

ABSTRACT

Numerous neurophysiological and biochemical factors can either impede or facilitate the learning process by affecting the brain's structure and function. The findings of neuroscience research provide substantial scientific evidence suggesting that emotional states, such as motivation, attention, stress, and anxiety, have a direct impact on the process of learning. Neuropedagogy provides educators with insights to enhance their understanding of individual learners by approaching neurologically based expressions that directly affect learning from a neuroscientific perspective. This chapter clarifies the neurophysiological effects of emotional states, including motivation, attention, stress, and anxiety, on learning. Additionally, it will address the cognitive aspect of how these factors influence the learning process.

DOI: 10.4018/979-8-3373-3581-0.ch012

1. INTRODUCTION

From the beginning of the 19th century, a great number of scientific studies have been conducted with the purpose of explaining human behavior and gaining a deeper understanding of the phenomena of learning by attempting to answer the question, "How does learning occur?" Even though the fact that behavioral, cognitive, and social learning theories offer important explanations on human learning, the fact that learning is characterized by biological and physiological changes in the brain (Hebb, 1949) has become increasingly significant, particularly after the second half of the 20th century. In this context, educational sciences have evolved and started to connect the inquiry of "How does the brain learn?" with insights from psychology and pedagogy (Ansari, Coch, & De Smedt, 2011; Carew & Magsamen, 2010; Ferrari & McBride, 2011; Fischer, Goswami, & Geake, 2010; Sousa, 2011).

Learning is characterized as a neurophysiological and biochemical process occurring in the brain, wherein stimuli from the social environment, received through sensory organs, induce changes in the brain's structure and functioning (Caine & Caine, 1991; Hebb, 1949). Consequently, it is essential to clarify the structure and functioning of the brain to enhance the understanding of the learning process and to develop more effective educational approaches. Neuroscience, which uses diverse brain imaging techniques to understand the structure and function of the brain, contributes significant results to the scientific literature through multidisciplinary research. The impressive scientific findings of neuroscience research have also been reflected in the field of education, leading the way for a neurophysiological and biochemical viewpoint on the concept of learning.

The empirical evidence from studies on the brain and cognition, particularly through brain imaging techniques, has established neuroscience as a focal area of inquiry across a wide range of academic disciplines. Neuroscience has also become a significant phenomenon in educational sciences due to its remarkable insights into the concept of learning and the factors affecting it (Geake, 2004; Goswami, 2004). This connection between neuroscience and education initiated the advancement of neuropedagogy and highlighted the necessity of investigating brain structures in educational contexts (Ansari, De Smedt, & Grabner, 2012; Sigman, Peña, Goldin, & Ribeiro, 2014).

Neuropedagogy, which has evolved alongside advancements in brain imaging, not only offers significant insights into the concept of learning but also explains the reasons for learning differences between individuals by substantial neurophysiological and neurobiological evidence (Goswami, 2020; Thomas, Ansari, & Knowland, 2019). This field provides insightful information regarding the impact of internal and external factors on learning; hence, it contributes to the development of a wide range of pedagogical approaches through the integration of cognitive neuroscience, psychology, and educational research (Watagodakumbura, 2017; Sousa, 2011).

Neuropedagogy, with its relatively recent historical development, is advancing rapidly and represents a significant trend in the field of educational sciences. A growing body of neuropedagogical research is being conducted to elucidate the differences in learning processes of individuals with typical development by utilizing the structure and function of the brain; to base the developmental differences of individuals with atypical development, such as ADHD, autism, dyscalculia, and dyslexia, on neuroscience-based information; and to provide neurophysiological evidence for the measures that can be taken to better understand the individual learner and improve the quality of education (Byrnes, 2012). Furthermore, neuropedagogy research correlates factors such as attention, stress, and anxiety, which directly affect learning, with biological and physiological findings (Carew & Magsamen, 2010) and also emphasizes the significance of motivation, which is directly related to an individual's interest, ability, and well-being and seen as the main trigger of learning, supported by neurological evidence (Cleveland-Innes & Campbell, 2012; Leventon, Stevens, & Bauer, 2014; McGaugh, McIntyre, & Power, 2002). Research in this domain offers neurophysiological evidence regarding the structuring of learning environments (Geake, 2004; Howard-Jones, 2011; Watagodakumbura, 2017; Sousa, 2011), linking neuroplasticity and neurogenesis to the processes of learning and memory formation (Maguire, Frackowiak, & Frith, 1997; Maguire et al., 2003; Sarrasin et al., 2008; Woollett & Maguire, 2012) to present a neurophysiological and biochemical perspective on learning. The primary objective of neuropedagogical research is to establish a novel paradigm for understanding brain function and cognition in educational contexts, while also offering neurophysiological and biochemical evidence to support the education of individuals equipped with 21st-century competencies (Campbell, 2011; Carew & Magsamen, 2010; Fischer, Goswami, & Geake, 2010).

Neuropedagogy provides educators with research findings that offer the opportunity to gain a deeper understanding of the neurological foundations of the learning process. Recent research indicates that a thorough analysis of the brain's working principles is essential for understanding individual differences and enhancing the quality of teaching. When learning and the factors affecting learning are considered, sensory stimuli directly impact the activation of brain structures, the duration of information retention in memory, and the organization of knowledge through associations with other information. Designing learning environments and learning materials informed by neuropedagogical research, enabling the brain to regulate sensory input and facilitate targeted learning, will enhance educational quality. Developing educational methods that consider emotions, reduce stress and anxiety through enhanced attention, and stimulate motivation has become a crucial imperative in 21st-century educational paradigms.

In this chapter, firstly, how the brain structure and functioning affect learning will be explained under the "brain and learning" section. Next, neurologically based expressions that directly affect learning are presented from a neuroscience-informed educational perspective. In the 3rd section, fundamental affective and cognitive factors -motivation, attention, stress, and anxiety- treated in dedicated sections. Each section begins with the definition of the factor, is detailed with cognitive and behavioral impacts, and is based on a neurobiological basis. The section then continues with learning implications and concludes with suggestions for classroom practice. At the end of the chapter, there is a glossary of key words where some terms are briefly explained.

2. BRAIN AND LEARNING

During human interaction with the environment, the brain receives numerous sensory inputs, both consciously and unconsciously. The brain processes these stimuli within the neurological system, which ultimately leads to changes in the individual's cognitive, affective, or kinesthetic experiences. These changes, which are identifiable as learning, can be regarded as the work of neurophysiological pathways in the brain responding to perceived stimuli. From a neurophysiological perspective, learning involves the perception of sensory stimuli from internal or external environments by receptors, their transient incorporation into sensory memory, and their subsequent short- or long-term retention through alterations in the brain's structure and physiology via synaptic modifications. It is the capacity to consciously recognize the activations induced by sensory stimuli in the pertinent brain regions, to retain them in memory, and to connect them with prior information (Camina & Güell, 2017; Squire, 2004). The learning process is affected by numerous external and internal factors, although it is essentially influenced by the brain's biochemical composition and neurophysiological functioning.

The examination of cellular and molecular dimensions of learning reveals significant effects of neurogenesis and neuroplasticity on cognitive processes and memory formation. The brain structure, whose development is largely completed in the womb, can change itself in adulthood (Bruel-Jungerman, Laroche, & Rampon, 2005; Cameron, Tanapat, & Gould, 1998; Hill, Storandt, & Malley, 1993; Kempermann, Kuhn, & Gage, 1998; Zhao, Deng, & Gage, 2008). Research on neurogenesis, which elucidates the brain's ability to undergo self-modification, has significantly impacted the last century by demonstrating that new neurons or glial cells can develop in the adult human brain.

Neurogenesis is the process by which new neurons, dendrites, axons, or glial cells are formed. It is characterized by the proliferation and differentiation of neural stem cells, as well as the survival of neonatal neurons (Zhao, Deng, & Gage, 2008). Research demonstrates that physical activity (Ma et al., 2017; Morris, 1984; Nokia et al., 2016) and enriched environmental situations (Kempermann & Gage, 2002; Morris, 1984; Nilsson et al., 1999) stimulate neurogenesis through their impact on arousal, indicating that the brain is capable of self-modification in adulthood.

The adult brain can undergo neuronal modulation during learning and memory formation, particularly when subjected to physical exercise and enriched environmental situations (Bruel-Jungerman, Laroche, & Rampon, 2005; Cameron, Tanapat, & Gould, 1998; Hill, Storandt, & Malley, 1993; Kempermann, Kuhn, & Gage, 1998). The Morris swimming pool test (Morris, 1984), a significant study involving rats, demonstrates enhanced cognitive performance in a labyrinth during spatial learning tasks and highlights critical results related to neurogenesis. The positive correlation between physical exercise and enriched environments with neurogenesis offers significant evidence for neurogenesis by elucidating the enhanced cell division, differentiation, and survival of newly generated neurons in the dentate gyrus of the hippocampus, an essential region for memory formation (Kempermann & Gage, 2002; Morris, 1984).

Neuroplasticity is a further aspect that offers significant explanations for learning (Berlucchi & Buchtel, 2009; Stepanyants, Hof, & Chklovskii, 2002). Neuroplasticity is a neural mechanism that explains how all sensory inputs perceived by an individual throughout their lifespan create new connections in neural networks or correlate existing connections with new situations (Costandi, 2019; Turhan & Özbay, 2016). The concept of neuroplasticity, which explains substantial changes in the structure and function of the brain, refers to a person's ability to acquire appropriate behaviors in different situations through increasing their learning capacity (Galvan, 2010).

Research on neuroplasticity offers significant neurophysiological insights into learning through synaptic interactions, including the formation of new synapses, changes in connections among existing synapses, and increased dendritic branching (Buonomano & Merzenich, 1998). It demonstrates that from the moment of infancy to death, depending on age and experience, new synaptic connections can be formed while unused synaptic interactions can be pruned, so revealing the brain's capacity to modify its structure and physiology through learning (Kania, Wrońska, & Zięba, 2017).

Neuroplasticity, which offers important facts about memory formation and learning, is influenced by various factors. Factors like age (Kirov, Goddard, & Harris, 2004), activity (Butz, Wörgötter, & Ooyen, 2009), frequency of repetitions (Moritz-Gasser & Duffau, 2013), and gender (Kuo, Paulus, & Nitsche, 2006) influence neuroplasticity at different levels. Particularly, factors such as enhanced environmental stimulation, deviation from routine, and the diversity of sensory information utilized in the learning process significantly influence neuroplasticity. However, factors that negatively impact neuroplasticity, such as stress and anxiety, may induce undesirable structural or functional alterations in the brain (Vance, Roberson, McGuinness, & Fazeli, 2010).

Neurogenesis and neuroplasticity, which influence the brain's structure and physiology, offer important information regarding the learning process and the factors that impact learning. These neural processes explaining the development of knowledge and skills (Maguire, Frackowiak, & Frith, 1997; Maguire et al., 2003; Sarrasin et al., 2008; Woollett & Maguire, 2012) prove the brain's capacity for self-modification in reaction to new situations (Maino, 2009). Consequently, it is essential to account for aspects that promote neurogenesis and neuroplasticity, including repetition, physical exercise, deviation from routine, and enriched environmental stimuli, when planning instructional strategies for improving an individual's learning potential. Moreover, removing anxiety and stress, which negatively affect neural communication, in educational settings will enhance the quality of learning.

The brain's construction, capable of integrating sensory, affective, and cognitive behaviors through its modular connections, indicates that it regulates all cognitive functions, enabling learning. In 21st-century education, incorporating an understanding of brain structure and physiology in educational planning becomes crucial for improving the understanding of individual learners, analyzing the origins of learning differences, and enhancing teaching quality. In the next section, factors that affect learning positively or negatively by affecting the structure and functioning of the brain will be discussed.

3. NEUROPHYSIOLOGICAL AND BIOCHEMICAL EVIDENCE OF FACTORS AFFECTING LEARNING

Numerous neurophysiological and biochemical factors can either impede or facilitate the learning process by affecting the brain's structure and function. The findings of neuroscience research provide substantial scientific evidence suggesting that emotional states, such as motivation, attention, stress, and anxiety, have a direct impact on the process of learning. Neuropedagogy provides educators with insights to enhance their understanding of individual learners by approaching neurologically based expressions that directly affect learning from a neuroscientific perspective (Morett, Morett, Hawes, & Dommett, 2021; Willis, 2008). This chapter clarifies the neurophysiological effects of affective states, including motivation, attention, stress, and anxiety, on learning. Additionally, it will address the cognitive aspect of how these factors influence the learning process.

3.1. Emotions From a Neuropedagogical Perspective

Life experiences elicit varying emotions in response to specific moments. Any stimulus, regardless of its prior association with a specific event, provokes unique emotional responses in our brain. Different stimuli can elicit varying emotions in individuals, and similar stimuli may provoke distinct reactions among different people. The psychophysiological responses that humans exhibit to internal or external stimuli are known as emotions, and they are characterized as a complex state that combines thoughts and behaviors (Zhang, Yin, Chen, & Nichele, 2020). Emotional states, which significantly influence decision-making, perception, and communication, are shaped by subjective experiences and act as a mechanism for decision-making in the initiation of new actions, being affected by individuals' past experiences (Leventon, Stevens, & Bauer, 2014).

3.1.1. Cognitive and Behavioral Impact

Emotions, such as anger, fear, anxiety, stress, happiness, sadness, and jealousy, are influenced by the nature of stimuli, the duration of exposure, and prior experiences, and they directly affect the brain's structure and physiology. These emotional states significantly influence learning by directly impacting individual motivation, leading to either positive or negative outcomes in memory formation and recall (Leventon, Stevens, & Bauer, 2014; Oggiano, 2022).

Emotional states in response to stimuli significantly influence fundamental life experiences, including attention, motivation, interest, perception, self-regulation, decision-making, communication, and action (Leventon, Stevens, & Bauer, 2014; Pekrun, 2014). These emotional states, which also have an impact on the moment of learning, arise as a subjective outcome between the stimulus and the individual experiencing it. A situation linked to a positive or negative stimulus from an individual's past will influence their response to that stimulus in any new and specific context (Hamann, Ely, Grafton, & Kilts, 1999; Leventon, Stevens, & Bauer, 2014).

Researchers arguing that emotion and cognition should not be considered separately assert that cognitive emotional behaviors are related to neurophysiological processes in the brain (Damasio, 1994; Davis & Whalen, 2001; Dolan, 2002; Phelps, 2006). In this context, emotional arousals that influence learning processes, including attention, perception, motivation, memory formation, and recall, directly impact cognitive performance. A study examining the relationship between memory formation, recall processes, and emotional arousal found that emotional stimuli positively influence memory formation (Steinmetz, Addis, & Kensinger, 2010).

3.1.2. Neurobiological Basis

Emotional states, such as anger, fear, anxiety, stress, happiness, and sadness, linked to stimuli, elicit distinct neurophysiological responses in the brain. The neural circuits associated with these emotions in the brain are primarily linked to the amygdala, orbitofrontal cortex, and superior temporal sulcus (Adolphs, 2001; Gostolupce, Iordanova, & Lay, 2021; Sotres-Bayon & Quirk, 2010). The amygdala, known as the emotional brain, regulates cognitive functions like reward, motivation, attention during emotional events, and decision-making, significantly influencing the learning process, particularly memory formation (Gallagher, Graham, & Holland, 1990; Murray, 2007; Pessoa, 2008). The amygdala, central to emotional processing, interacts with the hippocampus, which is involved in memory formation, and the prefrontal cortex, which contributes to cognitive performance. Consequently, the activation of the amygdala is crucial for information processing, including attention during learning, as well as memory formation and recall (Gostolupce, Iordanova, & Lay, 2021; LaBar & Cabeza, 2006; Pessoa, 2008). The amygdala seems to influence the intensity of conscious memory for experiences based on their emotional significance, irrespective of whether the emotion is positive or negative (Hamann, Ely, Grafton, & Kilts, 1999; Yonelinas & Ritchey, 2015).

3.1.3. Learning Implications

Learning and memory formation processes should not be considered independent of the emotional factor, and educational planning that ignores the emotional factor in the learning environment and process, as well as educational innovations that do not take emotions into account, will be quite incomplete in achieving holistic educational goals (Brookfield, 2006; Lehman, 2006). Neglecting emotional factors and viewing the learner only as a mechanical data perceiver would result in overlooking a significant influence on education (Cleveland-Innes & Campbell, 2012). It is important to remember that the classroom has an atmosphere that is very open to emotional arousal. Students may be excited about learning, hope to succeed, feel proud of their achievements, be surprised when they discover a new solution, worry about failing exams, feel embarrassed about low grades, or be bored during class. They may also experience social emotions such as admiration, empathy, anger, contempt, or jealousy with peers and teachers (Pekrun, 2014).

The research results indicate a significant relationship between emotion and cognition, demonstrating that emotions directly influence cognitive performance. Consequently, the learning process must always incorporate emotional considerations in its planning (Brookfield, 2006; Lehman, 2006). Humans, as social beings, experience various emotions in the brain neurophysiology that are linked to different social relationships through stimuli. Additionally, all emotional arousal, which directly influences brain neurophysiology and regulates learning, is personal and unique, associated with the interaction between the stimulus and the individual. Therefore, learning is an individual process, so it is essential to plan instruction with consideration for individual differences. Since one of the determinants of the learning process is the individual's approach to learning, the next section will continue with the motivation factor.

3.2. Motivation From a Neuropedagogical Perspective

The initial prerequisite for the learning process to start or continue is for the individual to have a positive approach towards the process. This approach, characterized as motivation, serves as the primary catalyst for an individual to initiate or persist in any action (Ryan & Deci, 2000). Motivation, influenced by external or internal stimuli, is characterized as the willingness to attain a goal or the desire to realize one's potential, serving as the foundation for an individual's engagement in the process (Jovanovic & Matejevic, 2014). Extrinsic motivation refers to actions driven by external expectations, aimed at achieving specific outcomes rather than focusing on the behavior itself. Intrinsic motivation involves performing a task with passion and deriving satisfaction from the activity itself. Intrinsic motivation involves engaging in an activity for the inherent satisfaction it provides, while extrinsic motivation is driven by the anticipation of external rewards, such as material or verbal recognition (Eisenberger & Shanock, 2003; Ryan & Deci, 2000).

3.2.1. Cognitive and Behavioral Impact

The literature presents various perspectives on the intrinsic and extrinsic motivators that link the individual to the learning process. The behaviorist approach and social cognitive learning theories elucidate the foundations of extrinsic motivators and demonstrate the impact of reward and reinforcement on learning. These theories suggest that when the goals attained during the execution of a desired action are reinforced with suitable rewards, the frequency of the action's occurrence and repetition increases, thereby facilitating high-level learning (Morgan, 1977; Ormrod, 1990). Some scientists argue that external motivators, such as rewards, diminish or fail to enhance intrinsic motivation (Deci & Ryan, 1985; Jovanovic & Matejevic, 2014; Kohn, 1993). However, certain research findings suggest that, under specific conditions, external rewards may actually boost intrinsic motivation (Cameron & Pierce, 1994; Eisenberger & Cameron, 1996; Eisenberger, Pierce, & Cameron, 1999). These authors suggest that while autonomy may diminish with such rewards, the perception of competence may concurrently increase, potentially enhancing the individual's intrinsic motivation to engage in the process.

Significant scientific research and evidence exist about the neurophysiology of reward in the brain, which is believed to activate motivation (Berridge & Robinson, 1998; Bissonette & Roesch, 2015; Camara, Rodriguez-Fornells, & Münte, 2009). These studies indicate that neurophysiological and biochemical changes resulting from the stimulation of the brain's reward regions influence the frequency of learning and its repetition by eliciting a sensation of pleasure or impulse in the individual (Bissonette & Roesch, 2015).

Motivation, regulated by several impulses such as the gratification of success, self-validation, receipt of rewards, avoidance of punishment, intrinsic satisfaction, feelings of affection, and appreciation, underpins an individual's engagement and focus in the learning process. Motivation enhances learning and cognitive abilities, offers feedback for advanced skills, and contributes to the development of an individual's expertise (Eisenberger & Shanock, 2003). The knowledge and skills acquired from enhanced thinking and learning, driven by motivation, will positively influence the frequency of repetition in similar future actions (Sternberg, 1985). Scientific studies indicate that optimizing a highly motivated individual's negative thoughts regarding other variables in the learning process can enhance learning outcomes to the desired level (Bahlmann, Aarts, & D'Esposito, 2015; Holroyd & Nick, 2012; Ng, 2018; Ritonga, Ahmad, Rosniati, & Dasrizal, 2025).

3.2.2. Neurobiological Basis

Although learning is fundamentally a cognitive process, the regulation of social-emotional processes is crucial for effective learning to occur. In this context, important factors influencing learning include the necessity for internal or extrinsic motivation and the expectation of reward. The main neurotransmitter in the brain linked to the reward system is dopamine. Dopamine synthesized in the ventral tegmental area traverses the mesocorticolimbic pathway, which plays an important role in reward and motivation, to reach the prefrontal cortex or nucleus accumbens (Björklund & Dunnett, 2007; Horvitz, 2000; Kelley & Berridge, 2002). Activations in these areas demonstrate that motivated individuals exhibit higher levels of learning (Dubinsky & Hamid, 2024).

Research indicates that motivation significantly influences cognitive control, primarily through mechanisms involving the frontal cortex and dopamine. A study examined the correlation between dopamine, which significantly influences the brain's reward and motivation systems, and the frontal lobe, the foundation of cognitive control, by monitoring individuals' cognitive processes based on reward expectation. The study identified significant correlations between the medial frontal areas, associated with the motivational aspects of behavior, and the lateral frontal regions, which are primarily responsible for cognitive control, along with observed increases in activity (Bahlmann, Aarts, & D'Esposito, 2015). A neurophysiological study examining the relationship between learning and motivation revealed increased activation in the anterior cingulate cortex, a region associated with cognitive control, during goal-motivated learning processes (Holroyd & Nick, 2012). A study on emotion, motivation, and brain plasticity revealed that the amygdala, responsible for emotions, and the hippocampus, associated with memory, function collaboratively, demonstrating a positive correlation between the two structures (Ritonga, Ahmad, Rosniati, & Dasrizal, 2025).

3.2.3. Learning Implications

Various studies demonstrate the significant relationship between motivation and cognition, indicating that neural activations within fundamental brain structures during social interactions directly influence all stages of learning. Consequently, numerous factors directly influence learning, including the learner's motivation at the time of instruction, the alignment of the learning material with the individual's interests and capabilities, the person's psychological or physical health, the physical attributes of the learning environment, the physical, mental, or emotional traits of the instructor, the instructional techniques employed, the materials utilized, and the individuals in the environment with whom the learner interacts socially and their attitudes towards them. All of these factors are perceived by neurons through sensory stimuli, leading to activation in relevant brain regions that either facilitate or impede learning. Consequently, all variables influencing the learning process must be regulated at an optimal level to ensure the brain is receptive to learning and to stimulate individual motivation.

3.2.4. Classroom Applications

Getting out of routine can be effective in motivating students by attracting their attention. Getting out of routine significantly supports learning by creating important neurophysiological effects on brain plasticity.

By encouraging students' autonomy, intrinsic motivation will be achievable. Students' autonomy can be improved by providing chances for information discovery, offering options, and allowing students to take the initiative in guiding their own learning (Ryan & Deci, 2009).

One of the most effective strategies for motivating students is to attract their attention. The following part will discuss the effects of attention on learning. The impact of attention on learning will be discussed in the following section.

3.3. Attention From a Neuropedagogical Perspective

The human brain encounters numerous sensory stimuli continuously, even during stable periods. Many various inputs, such as sounds from different sources, light beams from different objects in the environment, smells, tastes, and tactile stimuli, are detected by neurons and activate the brain in a neurophysiological way. However, we can only perceive stimuli that we direct our attention to. At this phase, the fundamental components of attention are identified as focus, maintenance, and orientation (Baddeley, 1990; Nesic, Kostic, Cicevic, & Nesic, 2011). Focus involves the selection of stimuli from numerous sources and is associated with selective attention. Selective attention refers to the orientation and perception toward stimuli considered significant, depending on an individual's physiological needs or interests. The persistence of focus on a certain activity, object, or circumstance is explained by sustained attention (Baddeley, 1990 Furthermore, an individual has the ability to attend to multiple stimuli simultaneously. It is referred to in the literature as divided attention and implies the capacity to focus on at least two stimuli simultaneously (Anderson, 1995).

3.3.1. Cognitive and Behavioral Impact

Attention, a cognitive process that inhibits the perception of other stimuli by concentrating on a specific one, is influenced by the brain's neurophysiology and represents an individual's selection among perceived stimuli (Eysenck & Keane, 2000; LaBerge, 2001; LaBerge, 2002). Focusing on a specific stimulus in the context of physiological needs, interest, ability, and current motivation levels results in the neglect of other stimuli and enhances the sensory response to the attended stimulus (Colby, 1991).

The sensory stimuli we consciously perceive are associated with selective attention. Selective attention, influenced by individual interest, ability, and physiological needs, serves as the fundamental process for focusing on specific stimuli. The fact that we continue to pay attention to any stimulus we focus on is explained by the concept of sustained attention (Baddeley, 1990). Furthermore, while we can voluntarily perceive any stimulus, we can also involuntarily direct our attention. While stimuli such as ambient temperature and amount of light affect involuntary attention, a person's levels of interest, ability, and motivation are directly related to perceiving stimuli related to voluntary attention (Näätänena, Gaillard, & Mäntysalo, 1980). Given this information, voluntary and selective attention is crucial for accurately directing consciousness, perception, and motivation towards the intended stimuli essential for learning (Soysal, Yalçın, & Can, 2008).

Attention serves as the primary factor in both the initiation and continuation of learning processes, underpinning cognitive functions including consciousness, perception, reasoning, decision-making, memory formation, and recall. This process, despite its limited capacity, enables conscious perception and is the principal factor in the transfer of inputs from sensory records to short-term memory. Consciousness functions as a mechanism for processing information, utilizing attention to execute control functions (Nesic, Kostic, Cicevic, & Nesic, 2011). Therefore, this relationship between attention and consciousness is an important determinant in memory formation processes (Umilta, 1988a; Umilta, 1988b). Activation of attention, which facilitates conscious perception of stimuli, optimally enhances perception, memory formation, and cognitive quality. Consequently, the processes of learning and memory formation are initiated.

The stimuli on which we focus our attention create activation in the relevant brain areas, thus accelerating the transition from sensory recording to short-term memory. The transition of a perceived stimulus from sensory memory to short-term memory, as well as the duration the stimulus remains in sensory memory, is directly proportional to both selective attention and sustained attention directed towards the stimulus (Nesic, Kostic, Cicevic, & Nesic, 2011). Attention is regarded as a crucial factor in maintaining consciousness and facilitating memory formation (Umilta, 1988a; Umilta, 1988b). Consequently, directing selective attention towards the stimulus facilitates orientation towards the intended target and markedly influences the speed of perception and learning. Activities that are effective in maintaining attention have the potential to increase opportunities for student learning (Grammer, Xu, & Lenartowicz, 2021).

3.3.2. Neurobiological Basis

Attention, while often regarded as a singular process, is a neurophysiological phenomenon that involves various brain structures (Colby, 1991). Examining brain neurophysiology in the case of attention reveals the activation of various brain structures (Coull & Nobre, 1998). Various scientific research indicates that the cerebral cortex is especially engaged in the perception of sensations and the allocation of attention to stimuli (Mäki-Marttunen et al., 2014; Coull & Nobre, 1998). The cerebral cortex, the most active neuronal pathway in neuroanatomy concerning cognition and attention, facilitates the allocation of attention to various sensory stimuli through its distinct lobes. In particular, the frontal lobe, which controls working memory, is engaged in the formation of selective attention (Knight, Hillyard, Woods, & Neville, 1981); the ventromedial prefrontal cortex (anterior cingulate) is activated in the initiation and maintenance of attention (Ertuğrul & Rezaki, 2006); and the parietal lobe is activated during visual spatial attention (Mesulam, 1983). In addition, the amygdala, which establishes a relationship between emotions and attention, triggers motivation by increasing attention in emotional arousal (Murray, 2007).

A study on attention examined individuals who experienced difficulties in focusing on a specific stimulus. Neurophysiological evidence indicates that lesions in the parietal lobe, particularly in the right hemisphere, impair attention focus, leading to diagnoses of Attention Deficit Hyperactivity Disorder (ADHD) in affected individuals (Hynd et al., 1990; Rueckert & Grafman, 1996; Tamm, Menon, & Reiss, 2006). Research indicates that the frontal lobes of individuals with ADHD are smaller than those of typically developing individuals and that there is asymmetry between the right and left frontal lobes, with the right lobe being smaller than the left (Hynd et al., 1990).

3.3.3. Learning Implications

The studies on attention clearly demonstrate that sensory, affective, and cognitive behaviors are neurophysiologically interrelated. Consequently, the use of stimuli that increase attention in instructional environments, utilizing learning materials and subjects aligned with the individual's interests, abilities, gender, and age, and eliminating irrelevant distractions that may distract attention and are irrelevant to the subject matter are essential precautions that should be taken in the learning process.

3.3.4. Classroom Applications

Implementing activities that foster active engagement in the classroom will significantly enhance academic success by improving attention (Rapport, Kofler, Alderson, Timko, & DuPaul, 2009; Schwanz, Palm, & Brallier, 2007). Therefore, designing a learning process that enables individuals to focus their attention and developing appropriate teaching materials are crucial for accomplishing the learning. Ensuring active participation through different activities such as watching videos and using visual and audio materials will help extend the attention span. Natural settings and imagery profoundly influence attention and enhance cognitive focus during the learning process (Dettweiler, Gerchen, Mall, Simon, & Kirsch, 2022; Schertz, Meidenbauer, & Berman, 2021). Students' attention and active engagement are increased when they are shown videos with context-related natural stimuli (Ki, Kelly, & Parra, 2016).

Meditation, which enables the regulation of attention and awareness (Cahn & Polich, 2006), aims to focus better on cognitive processes (Kasala et al., 2014). Meditation and breathing exercises implemented during the learning process will establish essential conditions for effective learning by enhancing attention and focus.

Meditation and breathing exercises are also known to reduce stress. The subject of stress and how it affects learning will be covered in the following section.

3.4. Stress From a Neuropedagogical Perspective

Stress refers to the biochemical or neurophysiological responses of the body, which are nonspecific reactions to sensory stimuli (Selye, 1956), aimed at maintaining homeostatic balance (Kaptan & Üzüm, 2016). Stress, which can impact the body in several ways, is also a significant factor in cognitive processes, including learning, memory formation, and recall. Stress, influenced by subjective experiences in response to various stimuli, can provide diverse effects on individuals based on the source, duration (acute or chronic), and intensity of the stimulus (Dickerson & Kemeny, 2004; Gewirtz & Radke, 2010). Such effects can directly impact the functioning of all organs and lead to psychological, physiological, or sociological issues (Pehlivan, 1995).

3.4.1. Cognitive and Behavioral Impact

Reactions vary according to the subjective perceptions elicited by the stressor in the individual. During periods of stress, various physiological and psychological responses can occur, including increased pulse rate, heightened blood pressure, rapid breathing, altered perception, difficulties with attention and concentration, and diminished motivation (Becker et al., 2018; Domes, Heinrichs, Reichwald, & Hautzinger, 2002). Prolonged stress can lead to negative impacts on daily life, including sleep disorders, nutritional deficiencies, heightened anxiety, depression, fatigue, reluctance, and diminished self-confidence (Pehlivan, 1995). Furthermore, stress, which directly influences conscious perception, serves as a significant factor in the learning process (Cordero, Merino, & Sandi, 1998; Diamond, 2005).

Research on stress's effect on learning and memory formation shows that both the duration of stress and the timing of exposure to the stressor are important. Chronic stress adversely impacts memory performance (Bangasser & Shors, 2010; Lupien & McEwen, 1997; McEwen, 2006), although several studies indicate that acute stress may have either beneficial or detrimental effects on memory formation (Diamond et al., 2006; Domes, Heinrichs, Reichwald, & Hautzinger, 2002; Lindau, Almkvist, & Mohammed, 2016; Schwabe et al., 2012; Shields, Sazma, McCullough, & Yonelinas, 2017). Analysis of the studies revealed that prolonged stress leads to cell death, particularly in the CA3 region of the hippocampus, which adversely impacts memory performance due to chronic stress (Lupien & McEwen, 1997; McEwen, 2006). In acute stress situations, the impact on memory formation can differ based on the timing of stress exposure during the learning process (Schwabe et al.,

2012). Research indicates that stress experienced before or during memory encoding impedes memory formation (Diamond et al., 2006; Shields, Sazma, McCullough, & Yonelinas, 2017). However, acute stress can enhance memory formation when there is minimal temporal disparity between the stressor and memory encoding (Domes, Heinrichs, Reichwald, & Hautzinger, 2002; Shields, Sazma, McCullough, & Yonelinas, 2017). There is also evidence that memory performance is positively affected when the stressor and study material are in the same physical environment and when stress exposure occurs after encoding (Shields, Sazma, McCullough, & Yonelinas, 2017). According to these studies, stressful experiences may tend to enhance acquisition-related processes (Roozendaal, 2003). Relevant research results suggest that acute and tolerable stress can enhance memory performance (Lindau, Almkvist, & Mohammed, 2016). The evidence indicates that both the duration and timing of stress exposure have distinct effects on memory formation and retrieval processes.

3.4.2. Neurobiological Basis

Numerous brain regions are influenced by stress, particularly the neuroendocrine structures that impact the functioning of various areas, notably the cerebral cortex, limbic system (including the amygdala and hippocampus), thalamus, hypothalamus, and reticular activating system (Dedovic et al., 2009; Schloesser, Huang, Klein, & Manji, 2008). The most important neuroendocrine system that is activated in stressful situations and affects the structure and physiology of the brain is the hypothalamic-pituitary-adrenal (HPA) axis (Francis & Meaney, 1999). The HPA axis is activated during stress, usually when an organism's homeostasis is disrupted. In such instances, a series of hormones is released in response to a physical or psychological threat. Corticotropin-releasing factor (CRF) is initially released from the hypothalamus, which subsequently stimulates the release of adrenocorticotropic hormone (ACTH) from the pituitary gland into the bloodstream. ACTH ultimately promotes the secretion of glucocorticoids, specifically cortisol, from the adrenal cortex (Dedovic et al., 2009; Lupien et al., 2005). The release of cortisol directly influences various cognitive processes, particularly memory formation and recall (Schwabe & Wolf, 2010). An explicit example of such hormonal modulation is Cushing's syndrome. Individuals with this medical disorder experience challenges in learning and performance due to excessive secretion of cortisol (Starkman, Gebarski, Berent, & Schteingart, 1992). In healthy individuals, the secretion of stress hormones can influence learning processes, often resulting in a deficiency of certain signals. High concentrations of glucocorticoids and stressful manipulations lead to weakened reception of declarative information in healthy participants (Kirschbaum et al., 1996). Stress, which also has significant effects on neurogenesis and neuroplasticity (Kaptan & Üzüm, 2016), suppresses neurogenesis by preventing the formation of new neurons and inhibits new synapse formation by affecting long-term potentiation (LTP) (McEwen, 2006; Rocher, Spedding, Munoz, & Jay, 2004). The results indicate that stress directly impacts the brain's structure and physiology, influencing all bodily functions and significantly affecting learning processes. Consequently, implementing strategies to reduce stress in educational processes and environments will substantially enhance the quality of education.

3.4.3. Learning Implications

These stress-related neurophysiological consequences are crucial biological proof that stress should be managed in educational settings and throughout the learning process. When examining the elements that can lead to stress, we can list things like low self-esteem, mental and psychological issues, the teacher's reactions, the expected rewards to be earned during the teaching process, or the punishments to be meted out for reactions and failures, and the inadequate physical conditions of the learning environment. Assume the educator knows how these factors can cause stress and affect the individual neurophysiologically. In that case, he/she can make more accurate arrangements for the teaching process and employ more appropriate methods and techniques to improve the quality of learning.

3.4.4. Classroom Applications

Breathing exercises and mindfulness exercises will be useful in lowering stress because meditation has a favorable impact on a person's ability for managing stress.

Out-of-class learning activities and outdoor activities involve processes that allow students to be more independent and active. These activities can further improve the quality of learning by reducing factors like stress and anxiety. Findings that cortisol release is regulated in the brain in out-of-class learning environments confirm this information (Schertz, Meidenbauer, & Berman, 2021). Activities that are effective in reducing stress also help to alleviate anxiety. This section will then continue with another affective factor that affects learning: anxiety.

3.5. Anxiety From a Neuropedagogical Perspective

Anxiety is characterized as a feeling of worry and tension that occurs in reaction to threats, losses, or anticipated negative outcomes (Hyde, Ryan, & Waters, 2019). Anxiety influences the brain's neurophysiology and elicits undesirable biological, physiological, or psychological responses. It refers to irrational perceptions that predominantly arise before a perceived threat (Beck & Clark, 1997). Anxiety, frequently confused with fear, is distinct in that it lacks a specific source, is generally less intense, and persists for a longer duration than fear (Budak, 2000; Hyde, Ryan, & Waters, 2019; Manav, 2011).

3.5.1. Cognitive and Behavioral Impact

Anxiety problems represent a condition characterized by inner restlessness, which may arise from various factors, including stress, a sense of helplessness, perceived threats, or vulnerability to such danger (Şahin & Seven, 2020). Anxiety occurs through several responses to threats, including cognitive apprehension (verbal-subjective), avoidance (overt motor activities), or muscle tension (somato-visceral activity), resulting in physical symptoms such as sweating, trembling, heart palpitations, and nausea (Lang, 1968). Besides various negative reactions encountered during anxiety, distraction and focus problems can be regarded as fundamental challenges that may arise. Anxiety disorder, commonly known as "social anxiety disorder" in the literature, is known to impair attention control due to neurophysiological factors. Consequently, impairment in voluntary control of attention is considered a significant characteristic of anxiety disorders (Wieser, Pauli, & Mühlberger, 2009).

Research indicates that stimuli that can cause high levels of anxiety can reduce activity in the ventromedial prefrontal cortex, making it difficult to focus attention on the stimulus (Kim, Gee, Loucks, Davis, & Whalen, 2011). The effects of anxiety on attention are also explained by Attentional Control Theory (Eysenck, Derakshan, Santos, & Calvo, 2007). This theory explains that during anxiety, the inhibition and orientation processes of memory are directly affected. Whereas the inhibition process of memory explains the prevention of attention to non-task stimuli, the orienting process is explained as the continuation of selective attention to stimuli even when the focus of attention shifts. This theory, which explains the relationship between anxiety and cognition, suggests that anxiety not only impairs attentional control but also increases attention to threat-related stimuli, thereby hindering the individual's ability to concentrate on relevant issues (Eysenck, Derakshan, Santos, & Calvo, 2007).

There are also studies suggesting that keeping anxiety at an optimal level serves as a performance-enhancing stimulus. In this context, while anxiety is often associated with negative effects on processing efficiency, some scientific studies indicate that anxiety may not impair and can even enhance performance quality when it prompts the use of compensatory strategies, such as increased effort and greater utilization of processing resources (Eysenck, Derakshan, Santos, & Calvo, 2007).

3.5.2. Neurobiological Basis

The examination of neurophysiological effects of anxiety on the brain revealed a significant interaction among the limbic system, responsible for emotional regulation, the prefrontal cortex, which influences cognitive performance (Kenwood, Kalin, & Barbas, 2022), and the hippocampus, the center for memory (Roozendaal, McEwen, & Chattarji, 2009). Examination of the results of this interaction reveals that the amygdala, activated during situations of fear and anxiety, influences memory formation and retrieval processes (Bishop, Duncan, Brett, & Lawrence, 2004; Kenwood, Kalin, & Barbas, 2022; Murray, 2007; Roozendaal, McEwen, & Chattarji, 2009; Stein, Simmons, Feinstein, & Paulus, 2007). Furthermore, research indicates that high anxiety impacts the prefrontal cortex, which regulates attention in the learning process, leading to a reduction in both attention and motivation towards the desired stimulus (Kim, Gee, Loucks, Davis, & Whalen, 2011; Mogg & Bradley, 1998). Another critical event that anxiety affects in the brain is neurogenesis. Research indicates a correlation between adult hippocampal neurogenesis and anxiety, with evidence suggesting that high anxiety negatively impacts the production or survival of new neurons (Mirescu & Gould, 2016).

3.5.3. Learning Implications

Anxiety is a condition that negatively affects an individual's ability to engage with their environment or objectives. Higher levels of anxiety can result in significant psychological, physiological, or biological disorders. Extreme anxiety disorders not only impact attention and motivation but also lead to issues such as the creation of negative scenarios in response to perceived threats (Stuijfzand, Creswell, Field, Pearcey, & Dodd, 2018), lower self-esteem (Goldin et al., 2013), depression, and difficulties in social relationships (Kenwood, Kalin, & Barbas, 2022). Given these challenges, it is imperative to manage anxiety to enable kids to enhance their academic performance while also improving their physical, psychological, and social well-being, thereby fostering a sense of confidence. Consequently, factors including the identification of personal learning strategies, problem-solving abilities, elevated self-perception, self-esteem, psychological and physiological well-being—particularly during adolescence—adaptation of social acceptance expectations to personal desires, and attention control can be optimized through effective anxiety management, thereby enhancing learning outcomes (Zhang, Su, Peng, Yang, & Cheng, 2011).

3.5.4. Classroom Applications

Meditation, mindfulness and breathing exercises help minimize stress and anxiety by reducing activation in the amygdala region of the brain (Desbordes, et al., 2012).

Activities that can be effective in reducing anxiety, as well as stress reduction, are out-of-class learning environments and outdoor activities.

Subsequently is always important to remember that students' emotional states should be taken into account in classroom practices and that emotions should not be ignored from the learning process.

4. EDUCATIONAL TAKEAWAYS

Neuropedagogy enables educators to better understand the learner by examining learning and the factors that affect it from a neurophysiological and biochemical perspective. Additionally, it provides educators with crucial recommendations on issues like organizing learning environments, adopting appropriate methods and approaches for the teaching process, and improving educational programs specifically for the individual.

According to the results of educational neuroscience studies focusing on the neurophysiological and biochemical processes of learning, enriched environmental stimuli and sensory data diversity (Turhan & Özbay, 2016), physical exercise (Bruel-Jungerman, Laroche, & Rampon, 2005; Hill, Storandt, & Malley, 1993), activities that will trigger long-term consolidation (Butz Wörgötter, & Ooyen, 2009), getting out from routine (Stiles & Jernigan, 2010), repetitive stimuli (Moritz-Gasser & Duffau, 2013), learning processes that will minimize stress and anxiety by increasing attention and trigger neuroplasticity (Vance, Roberson, McGuinness, & Fazeli, 2010) not only support learning but also have significant effects on memory performance and positively affect the capacity to retain information in long-term memory. Teaching activities developed in light of these findings will enable a significant transformation in transferring theoretical knowledge in the field of educational neuroscience to practical applications.

Based on the scientific evidence, it can be asserted that incorporating emotional stimulation into the learning process results in effective outcomes by activating significant neurophysiological responses in the brain, enhancing interaction among cortical regions, and ultimately improving memory formation processes. This section of the book analyzes factors affecting learning, including motivation, attention, stress, and anxiety, through a neuropedagogical perspective. In this regard, it can be argued that effective management of these factors throughout the learning process will make substantial contributions to the improvement of learning quality.

REFERENCES

Adolphs, R. (2001). The neurobiology of social cognition. *Current Opinion in Neurobiology, 11*(2), 231–239. DOI: 10.1016/S0959-4388(00)00202-6

Anderson, J. R. (1995). *Cognitive psychology and its implications* (4th ed.). W. H. Freeman and Company.

Ansari, D., Coch, D., & De Smedt, B. (2011). Connecting education and cognitive neuroscience: Where will the journey take us? *Educational Philosophy and Theory, 43*(1), 37–42. DOI: 10.1111/j.1469-5812.2010.00705.x

Ansari, D., De Smedt, B., & Grabner, R. H. (2012). Neuroeducation – A Critical Overview of An Emerging Field. *Neuroethics, 5*(2), 105–117. DOI: 10.1007/s12152-011-9119-3

Baddeley, A. (1990). *Human Memory: Theory and Practice.* Allyn and Bacon.

Bahlmann, J., Aarts, E., & D'Esposito, M. (2015). Influence of motivation on control hierarchy in the human frontal cortex. *The Journal of Neuroscience : The Official Journal of the Society for Neuroscience, 35*(7), 3207–3217. DOI: 10.1523/JNEUROSCI.2389-14.2015

Bangasser, D. A., & Shors, T. (2010). Critical brain circuits at the intersection between stress and learning. *Neuroscience and Biobehavioral Reviews, 34*(8), 1223–1233. DOI: 10.1016/j.neubiorev.2010.02.002

Beck, A. T., & Clark, D. A. (1997). An information processing model of anxiety: Automatic and strategic processes. *Behaviour Research and Therapy, 35*(1), 49–58. DOI: 10.1016/S0005-7967(96)00069-1

Becker, S. P., Jarrett, M. A., Luebbe, A. M., Garner, A. A., Burns, G. L., & Kofler, M. J. (2018). Sleep in a large, multi-university sample of college students: Sleep problem prevalence, sex differences, and mental health correlates. *Sleep Health, 4*(2), 174–181. DOI: 10.1016/j.sleh.2018.01.001

Berlucchi, G., & Buchtel, H. (2009). Neuronal plasticity: Historical roots and evolution of meaning. *Experimental Brain Research, 197*(3), 307–319. DOI: 10.1007/s00221-008-1611-6

Berridge, K. C., & Robinson, T. (1998). What is the role of dopamine in reward: Hedonic impact, reward learning, or incentive salience? *Brain Research. Brain Research Reviews, 28*(3), 309–369. DOI: 10.1016/S0165-0173(98)00019-8

Bishop, S., Duncan, J., Brett, M., & Lawrence, A. D. (2004). Prefrontal cortical function and anxiety: Controlling attention to threat-related stimuli. *Nature Neuroscience*, *7*(2), 184–188. DOI: 10.1038/nn1173

Bissonette, G. B., & Roesch, M. (2015). Neurophysiology of reward-guided behavior: Correlates related to predictions, value, motivation, errors, attention, and action. *Current Topics in Behavioral Neurosciences*, *27*(1), 199–230. DOI: 10.1007/7854_2015_382

Björklund, A., & Dunnett, S. (2007). Dopamine neuron systems in the brain: An update. *Trends in Neurosciences*, *30*(5), 194–202. DOI: 10.1016/j.tins.2007.03.006

Brookfield, S. D. (2006). *The skillful teacher: On technique, trust and responsiveness in the classroom*. Jossey-Bass.

Bruel-Jungerman, E., Laroche, S., & Rampon, C. (2005). New neurons in the dentate gyrus are involved in the expression of enhanced long-term memory following environmental enrichment. *The European Journal of Neuroscience*, *21*(2), 513–521. DOI: 10.1111/j.1460-9568.2005.03875.x

Budak, S. (2000). *Psikoloji sözlüğü* (1. baskı b.). Ankara: Bilim ve Sanat Yayınları.

Buonomano, D. V., & Merzenich, M. (1998). Cortical plasticity: From synapses to maps. *Annual Review of Neuroscience*, *21*(1), 149–186. DOI: 10.1146/annurev.neuro.21.1.149

Butz, M., Wörgötter, F., & Ooyen, A. (2009). Activity-dependent structural plasticity. *Brain Research. Brain Research Reviews*, *60*(2), 287–305. DOI: 10.1016/j.brainresrev.2008.12.023

Byrnes, J. P. (2012). How neuroscience contributes to our understanding of learning and development in typically developing and special-needs students. In K. R. Harris, S. Graham, T. Urdan, C. B. McCormick, G. M. Sinatra, & J. Sweller, *Educational Psychology Handbook* (s. 561–595). American Psychological Association. DOI: 10.1037/13273-019

Cahn, B. R., & Polich, J. (2006). Meditation states and traits: EEG, ERP, and neuroimaging studies. *Psychological Bulletin*, *132*(2), 180–211. DOI: 10.1037/0033-2909.132.2.180

Caine, R. N., & Caine, G. (1991). *Making connections: Teaching and the human brain*. Association for Supervision and Curriculum Development.

Camara, E., Rodriguez-Fornells, A., & Münte, T. (2009). Functional connectivity of reward processing in the brain. *Frontiers in Human Neuroscience*, *2*(19), 1–14.

Cameron, H. A., Tanapat, P., & Gould, E. (1998). Adrenal steroids and N-methyl-d-aspartate receptor activation regulate neurogenesis in the dentate gyrus of adult rats through a common pathway. *Neuroscience, 82*(2), 349–354. DOI: 10.1016/S0306-4522(97)00303-5

Cameron, J., & Pierce, W. (1994). Reinforcement, reward, and intrinsic motivation: A meta-analysis. *Review of Educational Research, 64*(3), 363–423. DOI: 10.3102/00346543064003363

Camina, E., & Guell, F. (2017). The neuroanatomical, neurophysiological and psychological basis of memory: Current models and their origins. *Frontiers in Pharmacology, 8*(438), 1–16. DOI: 10.3389/fphar.2017.00438

Campbell, S. R. (2011). Educational neuroscience: Motivations, methodology, and implications. *Educational Philosophy and Theory, 43*(1), 7–16. DOI: 10.1111/j.1469-5812.2010.00701.x

Carew, T. J., & Magsamen, S. H. (2010). Neuroscience and education: An ideal partnership for producing evidence-based solutions to guide 21st century learning. *Neuron, 67*(5), 685–688. DOI: 10.1016/j.neuron.2010.08.028

Cleveland-Innes, M., & Campbell, P. (2012). Emotional presence, learning, and the online learning environment. *International Review of Research in Open and Distance Learning, 13*(4), 268–292. DOI: 10.19173/irrodl.v13i4.1234

Colby, C. L. (1991). The neuroanatomy and neurophysiology of attention. *Journal of Child Neurology, 6*(1).

Cordero, M. I., Merino, J., & Sandi, C. (1998). Correlational relationship between shock intensity and corticosterone secretion on the establishment and subsequent expression of contextual fear conditioning. *Behavioral Neuroscience, 112*(4), 885–891. DOI: 10.1037/0735-7044.112.4.885

Costandi, M. (2019). *Nöroplastisite (1. b.). (Ş. Taş, Çev.).* Pan Yayıncılık.

Coull, J. T., & Nobre, A. (1998). Where and when to pay attention: The neural systems for directing attention to spatial locations and to time intervals as revealed by both PET and fMRI. *The Journal of Neuroscience : The Official Journal of the Society for Neuroscience, 18*(18), 7426–7435. DOI: 10.1523/JNEUROSCI.18-18-07426.1998

Damasio, A. R. (1994). Descartes' error and the future of human life. *Scientific American, 271*(4), 144. DOI: 10.1038/scientificamerican1094-144

Davis, M., & Whalen, P. J. (2001). The amygdala: Vigilance and emotion. *Molecular Psychiatry*, *6*(1), 13–34. DOI: 10.1038/sj.mp.4000812

Deci, E. L., & Ryan, R. (1985). The general causality orientations scale: Self-determination in personality. *Journal of Research in Personality*, *19*(2), 109–134. DOI: 10.1016/0092-6566(85)90023-6

Dedovic, K., Duchesne, A., Andrews, J., Engert, V., & Pruessner, J. C. (2009). The brain and the stress axis: The neural correlates of cortisol regulation in response to stress. *NeuroImage*, *47*(3), 864–871. DOI: 10.1016/j.neuroimage.2009.05.074

Desbordes, G., Negi, L., Pace, T., Wallace, B., Raison, C., & Schwartz, E. (2012). Effects of mindful-attention and compassion meditation training on amygdala response to emotional stimuli in an ordinary, non-meditative state. *Frontiers in Human Neuroscience*, *6*, 1–15. DOI: 10.3389/fnhum.2012.00292

Dettweiler, U., Gerchen, M., Mall, C., Simon, P., & Kirsch, P. (2022). Choice matters: Pupils' stress regulation, brain development and brain function in an outdoor education project. *The British Journal of Educational Psychology*, •••, 1–22.

Diamond, D. M. (2005). Cognitive, endocrine and mechanistic perspectives. *Nonlinearity in Biology Toxicology and Medicine*, *3*(1), 1–7. DOI: 10.2201/nonlin.003.01.001

Diamond, D. M., Campbell, A. M., Park, C. R., Woodson, J. C., Conrad, C. D., Bachstetter, A. D., & Mervis, R. F. (2006). Influence of predator stress on the consolidation versus retrieval of long-term spatial memory and hippocampal spinogenesis. *Hippocampus*, *16*(7), 571–576. DOI: 10.1002/hipo.20188

Dickerson, S. S., & Kemeny, M. E. (2004). Acute stressors and cortisol responses: A theoretical integration and synthesis of laboratory research. *Psychological Bulletin*, *130*(3), 355–391. DOI: 10.1037/0033-2909.130.3.355

Dolan, R. J. (2002). Emotion, cognition, and behavior. *Science*, *298*(5596), 1191–1194. DOI: 10.1126/science.1076358

Domes, G., Heinrichs, M., Reichwald, U., & Hautzinger, M. (2002). Hypothalamic–pituitary–adrenal axis reactivity to psychological stress and memory in middle-aged women: High responders exhibit enhanced declarative memory performance. *Psychoneuroendocrinology*, *27*(7), 843–853. DOI: 10.1016/S0306-4530(01)00085-3

Dubinsky, J. M., & Hamid, A. A. (2024). The neuroscience of active learning and direct instruction. *Neuroscience and Biobehavioral Reviews*, *163*, 1–21. DOI: 10.1016/j.neubiorev.2024.105737

Eisenberger, R., & Cameron, J. (1996). Detrimental effects of reward: Reality or myth? *Journal of the American Psychoanalytic Association, 51*, 1153–1166.

Eisenberger, R., Pierce, W., & Cameron, J. (1999). Effects of reward on intrinsic motivation—negative, neutral, and positive: Comment on deci, koestner, and ryan. *Psychological Bulletin, 125*(6), 677–691. DOI: 10.1037/0033-2909.125.6.677

Eisenberger, R., & Shanock, L. (2003). Rewards, intrinsic motivation, and creativity: A case study of conceptual and methodological isolation. *Creativity Research Journal, 15*(2-3), 121–130. DOI: 10.1080/10400419.2003.9651404

Ertuğrul, A., & Rezaki, M. (2006). Prefrontal korteks ve şizofreni. *Klinik Psikofarmakoloji Bülteni, 16*(2), 118–127.

Eysenck, M. W., Derakshan, N., Santos, R., & Calvo, M. (2007). Anxiety and cognitive performance: Attentional control theory. *Emotion (Washington, D.C.), 7*(2), 336–353. DOI: 10.1037/1528-3542.7.2.336

Eysenck, M. W., & Keane, M. (2000). *Cognitive Psychology. A Student's Handbook* (4. baskı b.). London: Psychology Press.

Ferrari, M., & McBride, H. (2011). Mind, brain, and education: The birth of a new science. *LEARNing Landscapes, 5*(1), 85–100. DOI: 10.36510/learnland.v5i1.533

Fischer, K. W., Goswami, U., & Geake, J. (2010). The future of educational neuroscience. *Mind, Brain and Education : the Official Journal of the International Mind, Brain, and Education Society, 4*(2), 68–80. DOI: 10.1111/j.1751-228X.2010.01086.x

Francis, D. D., & Meaney, M. (1999). Maternal care and the development of stress responses. *Current Opinion in Neurobiology, 9*(1), 128–134. DOI: 10.1016/S0959-4388(99)80016-6

Gallagher, M., Graham, P. W., & Holland, P. C. (1990). The amygdala central nucleus and appetitive pavlovian conditioning: Lesions impair one class of conditioned behavior. *The Journal of Neuroscience : The Official Journal of the Society for Neuroscience, 10*(6), 1906–1911. DOI: 10.1523/JNEUROSCI.10-06-01906.1990

Galvan, A. (2010). Neural plasticity of development and learning. *Human Brain Mapping, 31*(6), 879–890. DOI: 10.1002/hbm.21029

Geake, J. (2004). Cognitive neuroscience and education: Two-way traffic or one-way street? *Westminster Studies in Education, 27*(1), 87–98. DOI: 10.1080/0140672040270107

Gewirtz, J. C., & Radke, A. K. (2010). Effects of stress on learning and memory. *Encyclopedia of Behavioral Neuroscience, 1*, 461-468.

Goldin, P. R., Ziv, M., Jazaieri, H., Hahn, K., Heimberg, R., & Gross, J. J. (2013). Impact of cognitive behavioral therapy for social anxiety disorder on the neural dynamics of cognitive reappraisal of negative self-beliefs. *JAMA Psychiatry*, *70*(10), 1048–1056. DOI: 10.1001/jamapsychiatry.2013.234

Gostolupce, D., Iordanova, M., & Lay, B. (2021). Mechanisms of higher-order learning in the amygdala. *Behavioural Brain Research*, *414*, 1–11. DOI: 10.1016/j.bbr.2021.113435

Goswami, U. (2004). Neuroscience and educatio. *The British Journal of Educational Psychology*, *74*(1), 1–14. DOI: 10.1348/000709904322848798

Goswami, U. (2020). Toward realizing the promise of educational neuroscience: Improving experimental design in developmental cognitive neuroscience. *Annual Review of Developmental Psychology*, *2*(1), 133–155. DOI: 10.1146/annurev-devpsych-042320-100040

Gould, E., Beylin, A., Tanapat, P., Reeves, A., & Shors, T. (1999). Learning enhances adult neurogenesis in the hippocampal formation. *Nature Neuroscience*, *2*(3), 260–265. DOI: 10.1038/6365

Grammer, J. K., Xu, K., & Lenartowicz, A. (2021). Effects of context on the neural correlates of attention in a college classroom. *NPJ Science of Learning*, *6*(1), 1–4. DOI: 10.1038/s41539-021-00094-8

Hamann, S. B., Ely, T., Grafton, S., & Kilts, C. (1999). Amygdala activity related to enhanced memory for pleasant and aversive stimuli. *Nature Neuroscience*, *2*(3), 289–293. DOI: 10.1038/6404

Hebb, D. O. (1949). *The organization of behavior; a neuropsychological theory*. Wiley.

Hill, R. D., Storandt, M., & Malley, M. (1993). The impact of long-term exercise training on psychological function in older adults. *Journal of Gerontology*, *48*(1), 12–17. DOI: 10.1093/geronj/48.1.P12

Holroyd, C. B., & Nick, Y. (2012). Motivation of extended behaviors by anterior cingulate cortex. *Trends in Cognitive Sciences*, *16*(2), 122–128. DOI: 10.1016/j.tics.2011.12.008

Horvitz, J. C. (2000). Mesolimbocortical and nigrostriatal dopamine responses to salient non-reward events. *Neuroscience*, *96*(4), 651–656. DOI: 10.1016/S0306-4522(00)00019-1

Howard-Jones, P. A. (2011). A multiperspective approach to neuroeducational research. *Educational Philosophy and Theory*, *43*(1), 24–30. DOI: 10.1111/j.1469-5812.2010.00703.x

Hyde, J., Ryan, K. M., & Waters, A. M. (2019). Psychophysiological markers of fear and anxiety. *Current Psychiatry Reports*, *21*(56), 1–10.

Hynd, G. W., Semrud-Clikeman, M., Lorys, A. R., Novey, E. S., & Eliopulos, D. (1990). Brain morphology in developmental dyslexia and attention deficit disorder/hyperactivity. *Archives of Neurology*, *47*(8), 919–926. DOI: 10.1001/archneur.1990.00530080107018

Jovanovic, D., & Matejevic, M. (2014). Relationship between rewards and intrinsic motivation for learning. *Procedia: Social and Behavioral Sciences*, *149*, 256–260. DOI: 10.1016/j.sbspro.2014.08.287

Kania, B. F., Wrońska, D., & Zięba, D. (2017). Introduction to neural plasticity mechanism. *Journal of Behavioral and Brain Science*, *7*(2), 41–49. DOI: 10.4236/jbbs.2017.72005

Kaptan, Z., & Üzüm, G. (2016). Erişkin hipokampal nörogenezin öğrenme ve hafıza fonksiyonlarındaki rolü. *Türk Nöroloji Dergisi = Turkish Journal of Neurology*, *22*, 149–155. DOI: 10.4274/tnd.68889

Kasala, E. R., Bodduluru, N., Maneti, Y., & Thipparaboina, R. (2014). Effect of meditation on neurophysiological changes in stress mediated depression. *Complementary Therapies in Clinical Practice*, *20*(1), 74–80. DOI: 10.1016/j.ctcp.2013.10.001

Kelley, A. E., & Berridge, K. (2002). The neuroscience of natural rewards: Relevance to addictive drugs. *The Journal of Neuroscience : The Official Journal of the Society for Neuroscience*, *22*(9), 3306–3311. DOI: 10.1523/JNEUROSCI.22-09-03306.2002

Kempermann, G., & Gage, F. (2002). Genetic determinants of adult hippocampal neurogenesis correlate with acquisition, but not probe trial performance, in the water maze task. *The European Journal of Neuroscience*, *16*(1), 129–136. DOI: 10.1046/j.1460-9568.2002.02042.x

Kempermann, G., Kuhn, H., & Gage, F. (1998). Experience-induced neurogenesis in the senescent dentate gyrus. *The Journal of Neuroscience : The Official Journal of the Society for Neuroscience*, *18*(9), 3206–3212. DOI: 10.1523/JNEUROSCI.18-09-03206.1998

Kenwood, M. M., Kalin, N. H., & Barbas, H. (2022). The prefrontal cortex, pathological anxiety, and anxiety disorders. *Neuropsychopharmacology : Official Publication of the American College of Neuropsychopharmacology*, *47*(1), 260–275. DOI: 10.1038/s41386-021-01109-z

Ki, J. J., Kelly, S., & Parra, L. (2016). Attention strongly modulates reliability of neural responses to naturalistic narrative stimuli. *The Journal of Neuroscience : The Official Journal of the Society for Neuroscience*, *36*(10), 3092–3101. DOI: 10.1523/JNEUROSCI.2942-15.2016

Kim, M. J., Gee, D., Loucks, R., Davis, F., & Whalen, P. (2011). Anxiety dissociates dorsal and ventral medial prefrontal cortex functional connectivity with the amygdala at rest. *Cerebral Cortex (New York, N.Y.)*, *21*(7), 1667–1673. DOI: 10.1093/cercor/bhq237

Kirov, S. A., Goddard, C., & Harris, K. (2004). Age-dependence in the homeostatic upregulation of hippocampal dendritic spine number during blocked synaptic transmission. *Neuropharmacology*, *47*(5), 640–648. DOI: 10.1016/j.neuropharm.2004.07.039

Kirschbaum, C., Wolf, O., May, M., Wippich, W., & Hellhammer, D. (1996). Stress- and treatment-induced elevations of cortisol levels associated with impaired declarative memory in healthy adults. *Life Sciences*, *58*(17), 1475–1483. DOI: 10.1016/0024-3205(96)00118-X

Knight, R. T., Hillyard, S. A., Woods, D. L., & Neville, H. J. (1981). The effects of frontal cortex lesions on event-related potentials during auditory selective attention. *Electroencephalography and Clinical Neurophysiology*, *52*(6), 571–582. DOI: 10.1016/0013-4694(81)91431-0

Kohn, A. (1993). *Punished by rewards: The trouble with gold stars, incentive plans, A's, praise, and other bribes*. Mifflin and Company.

Kuo, M.-F., Paulus, W., & Nitsche, M. (2006). Sex differences in cortical neuroplasticity in humans. *Neuroreport*, *17*(16), 1703–1707. DOI: 10.1097/01.wnr.0000239955.68319.c2

LaBar, K. S., & Cabeza, R. (2006). Cognitive neuroscience of emotional memory. *Nature Reviews. Neuroscience*, *7*(1), 54–64. DOI: 10.1038/nrn1825

LaBerge, D. (2001). Attention, consciousness, and electrical wave activity within the cortical column. *International Journal of Psychophysiology*, *43*(1), 5–24. DOI: 10.1016/S0167-8760(01)00176-3

LaBerge, D. (2002). Attentional control: Brief and prolonged. *Psychological Research*, *66*(4), 220–233. DOI: 10.1007/s00426-002-0097-2

Lang, P. J. (1968). *Fear reduction and fear behavior: Problems in treating a construct. J. Schlien içinde, Research in Psychotherapy.* American Psychiatric Press.

Lehman, R. (2006). The role of emotion in creating instructor and learner presence in the distance education experience. *Journal of Cognitive Affective Learning*, *2*(2), 12–26.

Leventon, J. S., Stevens, J., & Bauer, P. (2014). Development in the neurophysiology of emotion processing and memory in school-age children. *Developmental Cognitive Neuroscience*, *10*, 21–33. DOI: 10.1016/j.dcn.2014.07.007

Lindau, M., Almkvist, O., & Mohammed, A. (2016). Effects of stress on learning and memory. G. Fink (Dü.) içinde, *Stress: Concepts, cognition, emotion, and behavior* [). Academic Press.]. *Cilt*, *1*, 153–160.

Lupien, S. J., Fiocco, A., Wan, N., Maheu, F., Lord, C., Schramek, T., & Tu, M. (2005). Stress hormones and human memory function across the lifespan. *Psychoneuroendocrinology*, *30*(3), 225–242. DOI: 10.1016/j.psyneuen.2004.08.003

Lupien, S. J., & McEwen, B. (1997). The acute effects of corticosteroids on cognition: Integration of animal and human model studies. *Brain Research. Brain Research Reviews*, *24*(1), 1–27. DOI: 10.1016/S0165-0173(97)00004-0

Ma, C.-L., Ma, X.-T., Wang, J.-J., Liu, H., Chen, Y.-F., & Yang, Y. (2017). Physical exercise induces hippocampal neurogenesis and prevents cognitive decline. *Behavioural Brain Research*, *317*, 332–339. DOI: 10.1016/j.bbr.2016.09.067

Maguire, E. A., Frackowiak, R., & Frith, C. (1997). Recalling routes around london: Activation of the right hippocampus in taxi drivers. *The Journal of Neuroscience : The Official Journal of the Society for Neuroscience*, *17*(18), 7103–7110. DOI: 10.1523/JNEUROSCI.17-18-07103.1997

Maguire, E. A., Spiers, H., Good, C., Hartley, T., Frackowiak, R., & Burgess, N. (2003). Navigation expertise and the human hippocampus: A structural brain imaging analysis. *Hippocampus*, *13*(2), 250–259. DOI: 10.1002/hipo.10087

Maino, D. M. (2009). Neuroplasticity: Teaching an old brain new tricks. *Revista Optometra*.

Mäki-Marttunen, V., Pickard, N., Solbakk, A.-K., Ogawa, K., Knight, R., & Hartikainen, K. (2014). Low attentional engagement makes attention network activity susceptible to emotional interference. *Neuroreport*, *25*(13), 1038–1043. DOI: 10.1097/WNR.0000000000000223

Manav, F. (2011). Kaygı kavramı. *Toplum Bilimleri Dergisi*, *5*(9), 201–211.

McEwen, B. S. (2006). Protective and damaging effects of stress mediators: Central role of the brain. *Dialogues in Clinical Neuroscience*, *8*(4), 367–381. DOI: 10.31887/DCNS.2006.8.4/bmcewen

McGaugh, J. L., McIntyre, C., & Power, A. (2002). Amygdala modulation of memory consolidation: Interaction with other brain systems. *Neurobiology of Learning and Memory*, *78*(3), 539–552. DOI: 10.1006/nlme.2002.4082

Mesulam, M. M. (1983). The functional anatomy and hemispheric specialization for directed attention: The role of the parietal lobe and its connectivity. *Trends in Neurosciences*, *6*, 384–387. DOI: 10.1016/0166-2236(83)90171-6

Mirescu, C., & Gould, E. (2016). Stress and adult neurogenesis. *Hippocampus*, *16*(3), 233–238. DOI: 10.1002/hipo.20155

Mogg, K., & Bradley, B. P. (1998). A cognitive-motivational analysis of anxiety. *Behaviour Research and Therapy*, *36*(9), 809–848. DOI: 10.1016/S0005-7967(98)00063-1

Morett, L. M., Morett, L. M., Hawes, Z., & Dommett, E. J. (2021). Why educational neuroscience needs educational and school psychology to effectively translate neuroscience to educational practice. *Frontiers in Psychology*, *11*(618449), 1–7.

Morgan, C. T. (1977). *A Brief Introduction to Psychology*. McGraw-Hill, Inc.

Moritz-Gasser, S., & Duffau, H. (2013). The anatomo-functional connectivity of word repetition: Insights provided by awake brain tumor surgery. *Frontiers in Human Neuroscience*, *7*(405), 1–4. DOI: 10.3389/fnhum.2013.00405

Morris, R. (1984). Developments of a water-maze procedure for studying spatial learning in the rat. *Journal of Neuroscience Methods*, *11*(1), 47–60. DOI: 10.1016/0165-0270(84)90007-4

Murray, E. A. (2007). The amygdala, reward and emotion. *Trends in Cognitive Sciences*, *11*(11), 489–497. DOI: 10.1016/j.tics.2007.08.013

Näätänena, R., Gaillard, W. K., & Mäntysalo, S. (1980). Brain Potential Correlates of Voluntary and Involuntary Attention. *Progress in Brain Research*, *54*, 343–348. DOI: 10.1016/S0079-6123(08)61645-3

Nesic, M., Kostic, J., Cicevic, S., & Nesic, V. (2011). Neurofizioloske osnove paznje - Neurophysiology of attention. *Godisnjak za Psihologiju*, *8*(10), 7–25.

Ng, B. (2018). The neuroscience of growth mindset and intrinsic motivation. *Brain Sciences*, *8*(20), 1–10. DOI: 10.3390/brainsci8020020

Nilsson, M., Perfilieva, E., Johansson, U., Orwar, O., & Eriksson, P. S. (1999). Enriched environment increases neurogenesis in the adult rat dentate gyrus and improves spatial memory. *Journal of Neurobiology*, *39*(4), 569–578. DOI: 10.1002/(SICI)1097-4695(19990615)39:4<569::AID-NEU10>3.0.CO;2-F

Nokia, M. S., Lensu, S., Ahtiainen, J. P., Johansson, P. P., Koch, L. G., Britton, S. L., & Kainulainen, H. (2016). Physical exercise increases adult hippocampal neurogenesis in male rats provided it is aerobic and sustained. *The Journal of Physiology*, *594*(7), 1855–1873. DOI: 10.1113/JP271552

Oggiano, M. (2022). Neurophysiology of emotions. In *T. Heinbockel (Dü.), Neurophysiology - networks, plasticity, pathophysiology and behavior*. Intechopen. DOI: 10.5772/intechopen.106043

Ormrod, J. E. (1990). *Human learning: Principles, theories, and educational applications*. Merrill Publishing Co.

Pehlivan, İ. (1995). *Yönetimde stres kaynakları*. Pegem Yayınları.

Pekrun, R. (2014). Emotions and learning. *Educational Practices Series*, *24*, 1–31.

Pessoa, L. (2008). On the relationship between emotion and cognition. *Nature Reviews. Neuroscience*, *9*(2), 148–158. DOI: 10.1038/nrn2317

Phelps, E. A. (2006). Emotion and cognition: Insights from studies of the human amygdala. *Annual Review of Psychology*, *57*(1), 27–53. DOI: 10.1146/annurev.psych.56.091103.070234

Rapport, M. D., Kofler, M., Alderson, R., Timko, T.Jr, & DuPaul, G. (2009). Variability of attention processes in ADHD: Observations from the classroom. *Journal of Attention Disorders*, *12*(6), 563–573. DOI: 10.1177/1087054708322990

Ritonga, A. R., Ahmad, L., Rosniati, H., & Dasrizal, D. (2025). Optimizing learning environments through the lens of neuroscience: A study on the role of emotion, motivation, and brain plasticity. *Jurnal Pendidikan Islam*, *6*(1), 12–19.

Rocher, C. Spedding, M., Munoz, C., & Jay, T. (2004). Acute stress-induced changes in hippocampal/prefrontal circuits in rats: Effects of antidepressants. *Cerebral Cortex, 14*(2), 224-229.

Roozendaal, B. (2003). Systems mediating acute glucocorticoid effects on memory consolidation and retrieval. *Progress in Neuro-Psychopharmacology & Biological Psychiatry*, *27*(8), 1213–1223. DOI: 10.1016/j.pnpbp.2003.09.015

Roozendaal, B., McEwen, B. S., & Chattarji, S. (2009). Stress, memory and the amygdala. *Nature Reviews. Neuroscience*, *10*(6), 423–433. DOI: 10.1038/nrn2651

Rueckert, L., & Grafman, J. (1996). Sustained attention deficits in patients with right frontal lesions. *Neuropsychologia, 34*(10), 953–963. DOI: 10.1016/0028-3932(96)00016-4

Ryan, R. M., & Deci, E. (2000). Self-determination theory and the facilitation of intrinsic motivation, social development, and well-being. *The American Psychologist, 55*(1), 68–78. DOI: 10.1037/0003-066X.55.1.68

Ryan, R. M., & Deci, E. L. (2009). Promoting self-determined school engagement: Motivation, learning and well-being. In Wentzel, K. R., & Wigfield, A. (Eds.), *Handbook of motivastion at school* (pp. 171–195). Routledge.

Şahin, H., & Seven, S. (2020). *Erken çocuklukta kaygı. H. Uzun (Dü.) içinde, Recent advances in education and sport researches*. Gece Kitaplığı.

Sarrasin, J. B., Nenciovici, L., Brault Foisy, L.-M., Allaire-Duquette, G., Riopel, M., & Masson, S. (2008). Effects of teaching the concept of neuroplasticity to induce a growth mindset on motivation, achievement, and brain activity: A meta-analysis. *Trends in Neuroscience and Education, 12*, 22–31. DOI: 10.1016/j.tine.2018.07.003

Schertz, K. E., Meidenbauer, K., & Berman, M. (2021). Understanding the affective benefits of interacting with nature.In E. Brymer, M. Rogerson, & J. Barton, *Nature and health. Physical activity in nature* (s. 7-22). Routledge. DOI: 10.4324/9781003154419-2

Schloesser, R. J., Huang, J., Klein, P. S., & Manji, H. K. (2008). Cellular plasticity cascades in the pathophysiology and treatment of bipolar disorder. *Neuropsychopharmacology : Official Publication of the American College of Neuropsychopharmacology, 33*(1), 110–133. DOI: 10.1038/sj.npp.1301575

Schwabe, L., Joëls, M., Roozendaal, B., Wolf, O. T., & Oitzl, M. S. (2012). Stress effects on memory: An update and integration. *Neuroscience and Biobehavioral Reviews, 36*(7), 1740–1749. DOI: 10.1016/j.neubiorev.2011.07.002

Schwabe, L., & Wolf, O. T. (2010). Learning under stress impairs memory formation. *Neurobiology of Learning and Memory, 93*(2), 183–188. DOI: 10.1016/j.nlm.2009.09.009

Schwanz, K. A., Palm, L., & Brallier, S. (2007). Attention problems and hyperactivity as predictors of college grade point average. *Journal of Attention Disorders, 11*(3), 368–373. DOI: 10.1177/1087054707305155

Selye, H. (1956). *The stress of life*. McGraw-Hill.

Shields, G. S., Sazma, M. A., McCullough, A. M., & Yonelinas, A. P. (2017). The effects of acute stress on episodic memory: A meta-analysis and integrative review. *Psychological Bulletin, 143*(6), 636–675. DOI: 10.1037/bul0000100

Sigman, M., Peña, M., Goldin, A. P., & Ribeiro, S. (2014). Neuroscience and education: Prime time to build the bridge. *Nature Neuroscience, 17*(4), 497–502. DOI: 10.1038/nn.3672

Sotres-Bayon, F., & Quirk, G. (2010). Prefrontal control of fear: More than just extinction. *Current Opinion in Neurobiology, 20*(2), 231–234. DOI: 10.1016/j.conb.2010.02.005

Sousa, D. A. (2011). Mind, brain, and education: The ımpact of educational neuroscience on the science of teaching. *LEARNing Landscapes, 5*(1), 37–43. DOI: 10.36510/learnland.v5i1.529

Soysal, A. Ş., Yalçın, K., & Can, H. (2008). Bilişsel psikoloji kapsamında yer alan dikkat teorileri. *New Symposium Journal, 46*(1), 35-41.

Squire, L. R. (2004). Memory systems of the brain: A brief history and current perspective. *Neurobiology of Learning and Memory, 82*(3), 171–177. DOI: 10.1016/j.nlm.2004.06.005

Starkman, M. N., Gebarski, S., Berent, S., & Schteingart, D. (1992). Hippocampal formation volume, memory dysfunction, and cortisol levels in patients with Cushing's syndrome. *Biological Psychiatry, 32*(9), 756–765. DOI: 10.1016/0006-3223(92)90079-F

Stein, M. B., Simmons, A. N., Feinstein, J. S., & Paulus, M. P. (2007). Increased amygdala and insula activation during emotion processing in anxiety-prone subjects. *The American Journal of Psychiatry, 164*(2), 318–327. DOI: 10.1176/ajp.2007.164.2.318

Steinmetz, K. R., Addis, D., & Kensinger, E. (2010). The effect of arousal on the emotional memory network depends on valence. *NeuroImage, 53*(1), 318–324. DOI: 10.1016/j.neuroimage.2010.06.015

Stepanyants, A., Hof, P., & Chklovskii, D. (2002). Geometry and structural plasticity of synaptic connectivity. *Neuron, 34*(2), 275–288. DOI: 10.1016/S0896-6273(02)00652-9

Sternberg, R. J. (1985). *Beyond IQ: A triarchic theory of human intelligence*. Cambridge University Press.

Stiles, J., & Jernigan, T. (2010). The basics of brain development. *Neuropsychology Review, 20*(4), 327–348. DOI: 10.1007/s11065-010-9148-4

Stuijfzand, S., Creswell, C., Field, A. P., Pearcey, S., & Dodd, H. (2018). Research Review: Is anxiety associated with negative interpretations of ambiguity in children and adolescents? A systematic review and meta-analysis. *Journal of Child Psychology and Psychiatry, and Allied Disciplines, 59*(11), 1127–1142. DOI: 10.1111/jcpp.12822

Tamm, L., Menon, V., & Reiss, A. L. (2006). Parietal attentional system aberrations during target detection in adolescents with attention deficit hyperactivity disorder: Event-related fMRI evidence. *The American Journal of Psychiatry, 163*(6), 1033–1043. DOI: 10.1176/ajp.2006.163.6.1033

Thomas, M. S., Ansari, D., & Knowland, V. C. (2019). Annual research review: Educational neuroscience: Progress and prospects. *Journal of Child Psychology and Psychiatry, and Allied Disciplines, 60*(4), 477–492. DOI: 10.1111/jcpp.12973

Turhan, B., & Özbay, Y. (2016). Erken çocukluk eğitimi ve nöroplastisite. *Uluslararası Erken Çocukluk Eğitimi Çalışmaları Dergisi, 1*(2), 54–63.

Umilta, C. (1988a). *Orienting of Attention. F. Boller, & J. Grafman (Dü) içinde, Handbook of Neuropsychology*. Elsevier.

Umilta, C. (1988b). The control operations of consciousness. A. Marcel, & E. Bisiach (Dü) içinde, *Consciousness in contemporary science* (s. 334-356). Clarendon Press/Oxford University Press.

Vance, D. E., Roberson, A., McGuinness, T., & Fazeli, P. (2010). How neuroplasticity and cognitive. *Journal of Psychosocial Nursing and Mental Health Services, 48*(4), 23–30. DOI: 10.3928/02793695-20100302-01

Watagodakumbura, C. (2017). Principles of curriculum design and construction based on the concepts of educational neuroscience. *Journal of Education and Learning, 6*(3), 54–69. DOI: 10.5539/jel.v6n3p54

Wieser, M. J., Pauli, P., & Mühlberger, A. (2009). Probing the attentional control theory in social anxiety: An emotional saccade task. *Cognitive, Affective & Behavioral Neuroscience, 9*(3), 314–322. DOI: 10.3758/CABN.9.3.314

Willis, J. (2008). Building a bridge from neuroscience to the classroom. *Phi Delta Kappan, 89*(6), 424–427. DOI: 10.1177/003172170808900608

Woollett, K., & Maguire, E. A. (2012). Exploring anterograde associative memory in London taxi drivers. *Neuroreport, 23*(15), 885–888. DOI: 10.1097/WNR.0b013e328359317e

Yonelinas, A. P., & Ritchey, M. (2015). The slow forgetting of emotional episodic memories: An emotional binding account. *Trends in Cognitive Sciences, 19*(5), 259–267. DOI: 10.1016/j.tics.2015.02.009

Zhang, J., Yin, Z., Chen, P., & Nichele, S. (2020). Emotion recognition using multi-modal data and machine learning techniques: A tutorial and review. *Information Fusion, 59*, 103–126. DOI: 10.1016/j.inffus.2020.01.011

Zhang, Z., Su, H., Peng, Q., Yang, Q., & Cheng, X. (2011). Exam anxiety induces significant blood pressure and heart rate increase in college students. *Clinical and Experimental Hypertension (New York, N.Y.), 33*(5), 281–286. DOI: 10.3109/10641963.2010.531850

Zhao, C., Deng, W., & Gage, F. (2008). Mechanisms and functional implications of adult neurogenesis. *Cell, 132*(4), 645–660. DOI: 10.1016/j.cell.2008.01.033

KEY TERMS AND DEFINITIONS

Adrenocorticotropic hormone (ACTH): A hormone secreted by the anterior pituitary gland, particularly when a person experiences stress.

Amygdala: An almond-shaped structure in the temporal lobe that is a component of the limbic system. Through widespread connections with other brain areas has numerous viscerosensory and autonomic functions as well as an important role in memory, emotion, perception of threat, and fear learning.

Anterior cingulate cortex: A part of the brain's limbic system involved in emotional and cognitive processing, with implications for attention, autonomic functions, and emotional stability.

Cerebral cortex: The layer of gray matter that covers the outside of the cerebral hemispheres in the brain and is associated with higher cognitive functions, such as language, learning, perception, and planning.

Corticotropin-releasing factor (CRF): A neuropeptide produced by the hypothalamus that is important in the control of the hypothalamic–pituitary–adrenal response to stress.

Cortisol: A corticosteroid hormone whose glucocorticoid activity increases blood sugar levels.

Dentate girus: A simple cortical region that is an integral portion of the larger functional brain system called the hippocampal formation.

Dopamine: A neurotransmitter that has an important role in motor behavior and is implicated in numerous mental conditions and emotional states.

Frontal lobe: One of the four main lobes of each cerebral hemisphere of the brain, lying in front of the central sulcus. It is concerned with motor and higher order executive functions.

Glucocorticoids: Any corticosteroid hormone that acts chiefly on carbohydrate metabolism.

Hippocampus: A seahorse-shaped part of the forebrain, in the basal medial region of the temporal lobe, that is important for declarative memory and learning.

Hypothalamic-pituitary-adrenal (HPA) axis: A major mammalian system maintaining body homeostasis by regulating the neuroendocrine and sympathetic nervous systems as well as modulating immune function.

Hypothalamus: Part of the diencephalon of the brain, lying ventral to the thalamus, that contains nuclei with primary control of the autonomic (involuntary) functions of the body.

Limbic system: The limbic system is a group of interconnected brain structures that help regulate emotions and behavior.

Long-term potentiation (LTP): An enduring increase in synaptic strength induced by learning or experimentally by repetitive activity,

Mesocorticolimbic pathway: A neural pathway that transports dopamine from the ventral tegmental area (VTA) to the nucleus accumbens and amygdala, and is believed to play a role in reward, desire, and emotional processing,

Neurogenesis: The production of new neurons during early nervous system development and throughout the lifespan.

Neuroplasticity: The ability of the nervous system to change in response to experience or environmental stimulation.

Neurotransmitter: Any of a large number of chemicals that can be released by neurons to mediate transmission of nerve signals across the junctions (synapses) between neurons.

Nucleus accumbens: A structure located in the basal forebrain that plays a crucial role in the regulation of motivated behaviors and reward processing.

Orbitofrontal cortex: the cerebral cortex of the ventral part of each frontal lobe, critical to goal-directed behavior and learning,

Parietal lobe: One of the four main subdivisions of each cerebral hemisphere. Parts of the parietal lobe participate in somatosensory activities, visual activities, and auditory activities.

Prefrontal cortex: The most anterior (forward) part of the cerebral cortex of each frontal lobe in the brain.

Reticular activating system: A part of the reticular formation thought to be particularly involved in the regulation of arousal, alertness, and sleep–wake cycles.

Superior temporal sulcus: A region in the brain that is involved in various social processes, such as language perception and understanding the thoughts and intentions of others (theory of mind).

Thalamus: The thalamus is a mostly gray matter structure of the diencephalon that has many essential roles in human physiology

Ventral tegmental area (VTA): A heterogeneous brain structure that serves a central role in motivation and reward processing.

Chapter 13
Bridging Brain Science and Neural Pathways to Pedagogical Possibilities and Classroom Practice: Neuropedagogical Strategies for Effective Learning

Ashraf Alam
https://orcid.org/0000-0001-6178-1187
Alliance University, Bengaluru, India

ABSTRACT

This chapter explores the integration of neuroscience into educational practice through the lens of neuropedagogy, to enhance student engagement and learning outcomes. It presents foundational principles such as neuroplasticity, synaptic plasticity, and cognitive load theory, and connects them with practical strategies targeting attention, memory, executive function, and emotional regulation. Applications across early childhood, secondary, higher, and inclusive education are critically examined, with attention to cultural and developmental contexts. The chapter addresses infrastructural, ethical, and epistemic challenges, cautioning against neuromyths, technological overreach, and inequitable access. It concludes with forward-looking policy recommendations grounded in responsible innovation, critical teacher education, equity-oriented funding, and pluralistic research. Positioning neuropedagogy as a transformative and context-sensitive framework, the chapter emphasizes its potential to relook education as both brain-aligned and socially just.

DOI: 10.4018/979-8-3373-3581-0.ch013

1. INTRODUCTION

The advent of the twenty-first century has inaugurated a paradigmatic inflection point in the nexus between neurobiological research and pedagogical praxis (David et al., 2025; Shvarts-Serebro et al., 2024). Amid an intensifying imperative to recalibrate educational systems in response to increasingly heterogeneous cognitive, affective, and sociocultural learner profiles, neuropedagogy has emerged as a transdisciplinary field situated at the confluence of cognitive neuroscience, developmental psychology, educational theory, and epistemology (Sen, 2022; Bielenia-Grajewska, 2014; Hernández Fernández, 2022; Mácajová, 2013). It departs from the historically dominant paradigms of behaviorism and sociocultural constructivism not by displacing them, but by extending their scope through biologically plausible frameworks of learning acquisition, memory consolidation, and executive regulation (Boboxolovna, 2022; Arum, 2025). At its core, neuropedagogy interrogates the neural substrates of learning and reframes instruction not merely as the transference of knowledge, but as the intentional modulation of synaptic connectivity and neurocognitive engagement (Glińska-Lachowicz, 2017; Alkhassawneh & Al Sharif, 2025; Chojak, 2018; Fernández, 2022). The exigency of this epistemic realignment is emphasised by empirical indicators of systemic educational failure. The Global Education Monitoring Report that came out in 2023 highlights that over 260 million children worldwide are functionally excluded from foundational literacy and numeracy competencies, despite expanded enrolment metrics. In India, the ASER report of 2022 assessment revealed that a mere one-fifth of Grade 3 government school students could perform at a Grade 1 reading level, while the National Assessment of Educational Progress of 2022 in the United States documented unprecedented regression in core academic domains, particularly among historically marginalized student populations. These deficits are not adequately explicable through resource constraints alone; rather, they signal an epistemological incongruence between how learning is neurologically mediated and how it is institutionally operationalized.

Prevailing instructional architectures, predicated on didactic delivery, rote repetition, and high-stakes evaluative schemas, frequently ignore the neuropsychological correlates of cognition, such as attentional regulation, affective modulation, and working memory capacity (Schlaggar, 2007; Temirbekova, 2025). Despite a proliferation of reformist rhetoric, the structural inertia of content-heavy curricula persists in many national systems, often resulting in cognitive overload and attenuated long-term retention (Lakhmotova et al., 2024; Savchenko et al., 2023). The scientific literature is unequivocal, stating that sustained cognitive engagement is predicated on the strategic distribution of cognitive load, affective safety, and opportunities for meaningful elaboration (Mamaniyazovna, 2025; Torres Martín, 2024). Yet, classroom ecologies in many contexts remain cognitively dysregulated, particularly for students exposed to chronic adversity, whose neurobiological capacity for learning is compromised by toxic stress, hypervigilance, or executive dysfunction (Nurmakhanova et al., 2021; Allaberdieva, 2019). Against this backdrop, neuropedagogy posits a science-informed alternative, grounded in empirical advancements in neuroplasticity, synaptic potentiation, and the interface between cognitive load theory and attentional gating (Kaplinskiy et al., 2022; Lohvynenko et al., 2023). The notion of neuroplasticity, i.e., the brain's capacity for structural and functional reconfiguration in response to environmental stimuli, problematizes essentialist conceptions of intelligence and introduces pedagogical possibilities for adaptive scaffolding across the lifespan (Matveev, 2024; Rashwan, 2024). Likewise, synaptic plasticity elucidates the Hebbian mechanisms through which repeated activation patterns strengthen neuronal networks, highlighting the pedagogical salience of spaced retrieval, multimodal encoding, and contextualized rehearsal (Barros & Fernández, 2022; Oliveira, 2024). Concurrently, cognitive load theory, originally formulated by Sweller, delineates the working memory constraints that delimit effective instruction and reinforces the imperative to sequence, simplify, and scaffold content delivery to facilitate schema automation.

Moreover, affective neuroscience foregrounds the role of emotion as a modulator of cognition. Elevated cortisol levels, that is common among learners experiencing social marginalization or institutional exclusion, impair hippocampal function and attenuate neurogenesis. Conversely, positive emotional states such as curiosity, belonging, and self-efficacy enhance synaptic transmission and neurochemical receptivity. In this view, the affective atmosphere of the classroom is not ancillary but constitutive of cognitive accessibility (Kuznietsov & Kostiukevych, 2024; Cavadas et al., 2019). Thus, pedagogical design must engage the whole brain, i.e., cognitive, emotional, and social, if it is to be authentically transformative (Pervushina, 2019; Silva, 2021). Yet the translational application of neuroscience to education is replete with epistemic and practical challenges. The proliferation of so-called "*brain-based*" pedagogies has often been accompanied by the dissemination of scientifically unfounded myths, or "*neuromyths*," including reductive dichotomies (e.g., left-brain vs. right-brain dominance) and learning style taxonomies unsupported by empirical evidence (Téllez et al., 2018; Yermakova et al., 2023). As Howard-Jones in 2014 and others have noted, these misconceptions arise not solely from miscommunication but from a structural disarticulation between neuroscientific epistemologies and pedagogical enactments. Neuropedagogy must therefore differentiate itself from popularized neuro-enthusiasm by committing to translational integrity, i.e., the rigorous, interdisciplinary negotiation between laboratory findings and the ecologies of classroom implementation (Herrera et al., 2023; Mystakidis et al., 2023).

Furthermore, a robust neuropedagogy must resist the ontological fallacy of neuro-essentialism, i.e., the presumption that educational phenomena can be wholly explained via neural correlates (Friedman et al., 2019; Fontalvo, 2019). Human cognition is not reducible to neural circuitry; it is embedded in sociohistorical structures, linguistic repertoires, and relational ontogenies (Macias et al., 2024; Díaz & Granda, 2022). The development of executive functions, for example, is co-constructed within cultural matrices that privilege either individual agency or collective responsibility, which in turn shape cognitive strategies and learning dispositions (Bożena, 2020; Mamaniyozovna, 2025). Sociocultural theorists such as Vygotsky, as well as contemporary proponents of embodied and enactive cognition, emphasize the situatedness of learning, i.e., the ways in which sensorimotor experience, symbolic mediation, and social interaction coalesce to constitute cognitive development. Thus, neuropedagogy must be inherently interdisciplinary, integrating insights from cognitive science, critical pedagogy, medical anthropology, and developmental ethics. While neuropedagogy has achieved discursive traction in some educational systems, such as Finland's post-2016 curricular reforms and Singapore's Ministry-led neurocognitive studies, its institutional adoption remains sporadic and geographically skewed. Educational systems in sub-Saharan Africa, Latin America, and much of South and Southeast Asia often lack the fiscal bandwidth, digital infrastructure, or professional development ecosystems to mainstream such innovations. Moreover, even in resource-rich settings, uptake tends to be uneven, driven by individual educator initiative rather than systemic mandates. This fragmentation highlights the need for multiscalar policy interventions, from national curriculum design and teacher education reforms to local school-level innovations and international research consortia.

Simultaneously, the technologization of education, especially in the wake of the COVID-19 pandemic, has intensified both the potential and the precarity of neuro-informed learning tools. The deployment of AI-driven adaptive learning systems, neurofeedback wearables, and biometric engagement monitors offers novel affordances for personalization and formative assessment (Vargas Angulo et al., 2022; Melnyk et al., 2022). However, these same technologies raise serious ethical and epistemological concerns around algorithmic bias, datafication of learners, and the commodification of cognitive metrics (Pretorius, 2025; Contreras et al., 2025). If left unregulated, such tools risk exacerbating existing educational inequities, reinforcing surveillance logics, and displacing human pedagogical judgment. A critically grounded neuropedagogy must therefore attend to both the affordances and limitations of emerging technologies (Shiwlani et al., 2024; Antoniuk et al., 2022). It must interrogate not only the efficacy of digital interventions but also their governance, i.e., Who has access to them? Who designs and controls the algorithms? Whose knowledge paradigms are encoded in the software? And who is held accountable when such tools perpetuate harm? The field must adopt an anticipatory ethics that is proactive rather than reactive, ensuring that technological integration aligns with principles of transparency, justice, and learner autonomy. This chapter is animated by three interlocking imperatives. First, it seeks to address the structural disjuncture between advances in neurocognitive science and entrenched educational practices. Second, it proposes a conceptual and practical framework for the systemic implementation of neuropedagogical strategies, grounded in both empirical evidence and contextual responsiveness. Third, it advocates for an ethically reflexive approach to brain-based education, i.e., one that is attentive to power, plurality, and the sociomaterial conditions of learning.

To this end, the chapter proceeds in six sections. Section 2 explicates the foundational constructs of neuropedagogy, including neuroplasticity, synaptic consolidation, and cognitive load theory, and interrogates their pedagogical implications. Section 3 operationalizes these principles through evidence-informed strategies such as spaced repetition, dual coding, and emotional regulation, elucidating their neurocognitive mechanisms and instructional affordances. Section 4 examines their differentiated applications across educational stages, from early childhood to higher education to inclusive and neurodiverse classrooms, highlighting cultural adaptations and institutional requirements. Section 5 engages with the practical and ethical challenges of implementation, including inequitable access, pedagogical misapplication, digital surveillance, and cultural misalignment. Section 6 articulates a forward-facing agenda, outlining research priorities, policy levers, and ethical safeguards to guide the future of neuropedagogy in a rapidly evolving educational and technological landscape. The objective of this chapter is not to advocate neuropedagogy as a universal cure-all, but to advance it as a dynamic, critical, and context-sensitive paradigm for reimagining the future of education. It insists on the necessity of cognitive justice alongside scientific precision, and on the value of integrating brain-based insights into pedagogical frameworks that are inclusive, emancipatory, and globally relevant. In a world grappling with epistemic volatility, structural inequity, and the automation of cognition, aligning education with the neurobiological and sociocultural conditions of learning is not merely desirable, but is imperative.

2. FOUNDATIONAL PRINCIPLES OF NEUROPEDAGOGY

Neuropedagogy articulates a convergent epistemology that integrates the ontogeny of neural development with pedagogical theory, yielding a biologically plausible and culturally contingent framework for instructional design (Marrero & de las Mercedes, 2023; Lupu & Jurchescu, 2020). Unlike traditional didactic paradigms which often operate within a compartmentalized view of cognition, neuropedagogy reconfigures learning as a neurobiological, affective, and socioculturally situated process (Silva-López et al., 2015; de Oliveira et al., 2009). Its foundational architecture is scaffolded by interrelated constructs such as *neuroplasticity*, *synaptic plasticity*, and *cognitive load theory*, each offering a distinct yet interdependent lens through which educators can conceptualize and operationalize effective learning ecologies (Riccardi, 2023; Huseinova et al., 2024). These constructs are not isolated explanatory tools; rather, they constitute a dynamic triad that reveals how neural malleability, synaptic modulation, and cognitive resource management interact to influence knowledge acquisition, memory consolidation, and epistemic engagement (Shalom & Luria, 2022; Elouafi et al., 2021).

2.1 Neuroplasticity and Synaptic Plasticity

Neuroplasticity represents the brain's intrinsic capacity to undergo structural and functional reorganization in response to environmental input, experiential novelty, and task-specific engagement (Gasanova et al., 2022; Nikulochkina et al., 2022). It disrupts static models of intelligence and learning capacity by positing that synaptogenesis, dendritic arborization, and neurochemical modulation can occur well into adulthood, contingent on context-sensitive stimulation (Rasskazova et al., 2023; Borisovna & Valeryanovna, 2018). This principle has catalyzed a shift from essentialist paradigms, wherein learners are sorted and evaluated according to presumed fixed cognitive endowments, to constructivist neuroeducational paradigms that affirm learning as an emergent, dynamic, and reparative process (Fragkaki et al., 2022; Vorotyntseva et al., 2022). At the neural microarchitecture level, *synaptic plasticity*, the capacity for long-term potentiation (LTP) and long-term depression (LTD) of synaptic strength, provides the physiological basis for learning and memory. Hebbian theory, encapsulated in the dictum "*neurons that fire together wire together*," elucidates how repeated, contextually salient activation of specific neural networks enhances synaptic efficiency, thereby increasing the probability of future activation and retrieval. This phenomenon substantiates pedagogical strategies such as *spaced repetition, multisensory encoding*, and *cross-modal integration*, which are designed to stimulate co-activation across distributed neural substrates.

In practical terms, instructional designs that employ *interleaved learning, dual coding*, and *constructivist sequencing* capitalize on this principle. For instance, integrating visuospatial representations with linguistic narration in teaching physics not only recruits the visuospatial sketchpad and phonological loop of Baddeley's working memory model but also promotes cross-hemispheric interaction, resulting in deeper encoding and long-term consolidation. The inclusion of *affective salience*, through narrative coherence, ethical dilemma, or personal relevance, further modulates synaptic receptivity via dopaminergic and noradrenergic pathways, reinforcing memory trace formation (Marievych et al., 2023; Zambrano & Mieles, 2023). However, the same neuroplastic mechanisms that enable learning can also reinforce maladaptive schemas. Repeated exposure to *epistemically shallow content*, culturally dislocated curricula, or emotionally dysregulating classroom environments can entrench ineffective cognitive heuristics and exacerbate learning inequalities (Yánez et al., 2025; Shulha et al., 2021). This highlights the ethical imperative of *pedagogical intentionality*, where repetition is not merely mechanical but embedded within *emotionally resonant, cognitively scaffolded, and socially anchored* learning contexts (Barba Tellez et al., 2018; Barros, 2022). Effective neuroeducation must therefore transcend content delivery and architect experiences that encode relational meaning and epistemic agency.

Moreover, *neuroplastic responsiveness is not uniformly distributed*. It is modulated by age, neurodevelopmental stage, sleep hygiene, nutritional status, and sociocultural capital (Supriatna et al., 2019; Pinzón Blanco & Téllez Sánchez, 2016). For example, during sensitive periods such as early childhood and adolescence, synaptic pruning and myelination are accelerated, making these windows particularly amenable to educational intervention (Yepes Landinez et al., 2024; Markiv et al., 2025). Simultaneously, chronic stressors, whether biological (e.g., inflammation), psychosocial (e.g., trauma), or environmental (e.g., poverty), elevate glucocorticoid levels, disrupt hippocampal neurogenesis, and compromise prefrontal cortex functionality. Hence, *psychosocial context is not peripheral* but fundamentally constitutive of neurocognitive outcomes. Pedagogical environments that are psychologically safe, socially inclusive, and culturally responsive activate the parasympathetic nervous system, downregulate stress responses, and facilitate the release of neurotrophic factors such as BDNF (Brain-Derived Neurotrophic Factor), which promotes synaptic growth. Therefore, *neuropedagogical fidelity* demands a dual emphasis on cognitive challenge and affective attunement, designing curricula that are not only intellectually rigorous but also emotionally sustainable.

2.2 Cognitive Load Theory

Cognitive Load Theory (CLT), rooted in information-processing models of cognition, provides a metacognitive apparatus for understanding the limitations of working memory in the context of instructional design. It posits that the efficacy of learning is inversely proportional to the overload of finite cognitive resources, primarily within the *visuospatial sketchpad and phonological loop*, which act as the primary holding structures for novel information prior to its integration into long-term memory. CLT distinguishes between *intrinsic, extraneous*, and *germane* cognitive load. Intrinsic load is governed by the inherent complexity of the material and the degree of interactivity between its constituent elements. Extraneous load arises from suboptimal instructional presentation, i.e., poor sequencing, cognitive dissonance, or irrelevant stimuli, which competes for neural resources. Germane load pertains to the mental effort expended in forming, refining, and automating schemas, the structured representations of knowledge in long-term memory. Effective neuropedagogical strategies aim to *minimize extraneous load, optimize intrinsic load* through strategic scaffolding, and *maximize germane load* by cultivating cognitive elaboration. For instance, introducing the concept of entropy in thermodynamics through progressively complex simulations, metaphors grounded in everyday experiences, and student-generated analogies can sequentially distribute cognitive load and reinforce schematic integration. Neuroimaging evidence supports this approach, e.g., fMRI and fNIRS studies reveal that excessive extraneous load activates the anterior cingulate cortex and dorsolateral prefrontal cortex, i.e., regions associated with error monitoring and executive overload, whereas optimized instruction correlates with more efficient fronto-parietal activation and higher retention rates.

However, interpreting CLT solely through the lens of neurocognitive efficiency can inadvertently perpetuate *pedagogical instrumentalism.* Learning, particularly in socio-culturally diverse and affectively complex environments, often involves *productive dissonance, strategic ambiguity, and epistemic disequilibrium* (Syrotkina et al., 2022; Pávová & Valent, 2020). Indigenous pedagogical frameworks, for example, emphasize communal observation, ritualized delay in formal instruction, and apprenticeship-based learning, all of which resist linear models of cognitive efficiency. Such practices, while seemingly at odds with CLT metrics, develop and nurture *intergenerational epistemologies*, *embodied cognition*, and *relational knowledge construction.* Thus, neuropedagogy must resist equating cognitive minimalism with pedagogical quality and instead embrace *contextual and epistemological pluralism* (Maidaniuk et al., 2023; Nefedchenko et al., 2023). Moreover, working memory is not a culturally neutral or affectively autonomous mechanism. *Stereotype threat*, *linguistic dissonance*, and *socioeconomic precarity* exert substantial influence on cognitive availability. Learners from marginalized backgrounds may enter classrooms with elevated baseline cognitive load, not due to poor design, but due to the *psychosocial taxations* of systemic inequity. This reframes CLT not merely as an instructional heuristic but as a *structural diagnostic*, a lens through which to interrogate the broader ecologies that modulate learning capacity.

CLT must therefore be integrated with trauma-informed and culturally sustaining pedagogies. This includes validating students' funds of knowledge, integrating mother-tongue instruction, and designing learning experiences that reflect the semiotics, ethics, and epistemologies of their communities. By aligning schematic construction with *narrative resonance and cultural legibility*, educators can shift germane load from a site of abstract cognitive effort to one of *meaningful intellectual engagement.* Affective neuroscience further reveals that emotional states act as filters for cognitive load. Positive affect, mediated through neurotransmitters like dopamine and serotonin, enhances attentional flexibility, promotes risk tolerance, and facilitates divergent thinking. Conversely, negative emotional valence contracts attentional focus, inhibits memory formation, and narrows exploratory behavior. Instructional practices that activate *curiosity, humor, aesthetic pleasure*, or *moral engagement* not only enhance motivation but also optimize the neural circuitry involved in *learning-to-learn.* The foundational tenets of neuropedagogy, i.e., neuroplasticity, synaptic modulation, and cognitive load calibration, do not operate in a vacuum. They must be *contextualized within culturally situated, emotionally responsive, and ethically reflexive* learning paradigms. Pedagogy, in this framework, is neither reductionist nor mechanistic; it is an embodied, dialogic, and transformational endeavor that requires educators to be both *scientifically literate* and *culturally fluent* (Corona et al., 2012; Marchak et al., 2021). The promise of neuropedagogy lies not in prescribing universal solutions but in constructing flexible, justice-oriented blueprints for learning, ones that honor both the neurobiological infrastructure of cognition and the lived realities of diverse learners (Slavikivna et al., 2023; Lyndina et al., 2023).

3. NEUROPEDAGOGICAL STRATEGIES FOR ENHANCING COGNITIVE FUNCTIONS

Contemporary neuropedagogical praxis advances a paradigm shift from monolithic models of instruction to neurobiologically optimized, affectively attuned, and contextually grounded learning environments (Lenska et al., 2022; Marrero, 2023). It draws upon the integrated functions of the central nervous system, namely attentional regulation, memory consolidation, executive processing, and emotional modulation, not as isolated domains of brain activity but as interdependent systems that scaffold intellectual development and self-directed learning (Wulan & Jamaris, 2023; Rakhmetova et al., 2024). This section operationalizes these domains into pedagogical strategies that are empirically substantiated, developmentally responsive, and culturally and structurally sensitive. It recognizes that cognition is neither apolitical nor acultural; rather, it is shaped by neurobiological predispositions, ecological constraints, and social imaginaries.

3.1 Attention, Memory, and Executive Function

Attention functions as the primary gating mechanism for learning, determining which stimuli are prioritized for encoding and which are filtered out as irrelevant noise. Neuroanatomically, attentional modulation involves intricate coordination between the prefrontal cortex, posterior parietal cortex, and the anterior cingulate cortex. Functional neuroimaging reveals that *phasic dopamine release*, particularly in the ventral tegmental area (VTA), is closely tied to the orienting response, thereby reinforcing the salience of novel or reward-predictive stimuli. Pedagogically, this underlines the value of *novelty infusion, predictive questioning,* and *multimodal attentional cues* in stimulating learner engagement. Yet the indiscriminate use of novelty can devolve into performativity rather than pedagogy. Empirical data from event-related potential (ERP) studies highlight that novelty must be *semantically anchored* to pre-existing knowledge schemas to produce sustained activation in the hippocampus and medial temporal lobe, i.e., regions associated with long-term encoding. Thus, instructional novelty must be cognitively coherent, culturally congruent, and strategically distributed to avoid habituation or distraction. Educators should use *anticipatory schema activation* through inquiry-based prompts, counterintuitive dilemmas, and real-world case simulations that simultaneously stimulate curiosity and epistemic uncertainty.

Memory formation, particularly the consolidation of explicit declarative memory, depends on repeated activation of hippocampal-neocortical networks. Strategies such as *spaced retrieval, interleaved practice, and dual coding* exploit neurobiological mechanisms like synaptic consolidation and reconsolidation windows. Spaced repetition, supported by robust empirical meta-analyses, optimizes the synaptic strengthening process by aligning review intervals with the forgetting curve, thereby promoting durable encoding. However, institutional pressures toward *syllabic acceleration* and *content coverage* frequently inhibit its effective implementation. Curricular realignment to accommodate *distributed learning cycles* must therefore be prioritized at the policy level. Interleaving, which involves alternating between conceptually related but procedurally distinct tasks, enhances *discriminative learning* and *far transfer* by activating multiple retrieval pathways and reducing cognitive fixation. Neurocognitively, this practice recruits the *dorsolateral prefrontal cortex* and *posterior parietal cortex*, enhancing cognitive flexibility. Yet interleaving is often perceived by learners as inefficient or confusing due to its non-linear structure. This necessitates *metacognitive scaffolding*, explicit instruction about learning processes, to normalize the productive discomfort of *desirable difficulty*.

The *dual coding hypothesis*, first articulated by Paivio and subsequently corroborated by neuroimaging studies, posits that concurrent activation of *verbal-linguistic* and *visuospatial* systems, mediated by the left temporal lobe and right parietal lobe respectively, enhances memory trace redundancy and retrieval accuracy. In practice, this entails pairing textual content with labeled diagrams, narrated animations, or schematic maps. However, *cognitive alignment* is paramount; extraneous visuals activate irrelevant neural pathways, increasing cognitive load and disrupting working memory efficiency. Effective dual coding must adhere to *principles of visual clarity, semantic congruence, and processing efficiency*, particularly for neurodivergent learners with atypical visual processing profiles. *Executive functions*, comprising inhibitory control, cognitive flexibility, and working memory, are orchestrated predominantly by the *prefrontal cortex*, with modulatory input from the anterior cingulate gyrus and basal ganglia. These functions underpin self-regulated learning, adaptive problem-solving, and goal-directed behavior. Pedagogical strategies that cultivate executive function include *structured goal-setting, task chunking, reflective journaling, and self-monitoring dashboards*. For example, the "*Plan-Do-Review*" model scaffolds temporal sequencing, performance monitoring, and error correction, i.e., the functions that are essential for metacognitive growth.

Digital platforms that incorporate *real-time feedback loops, visual progress trackers*, and *interactive scaffolds* have demonstrated efficacy in enhancing executive control, particularly in blended and online modalities. Nevertheless, their effectiveness is moderated by *technological access, digital literacy, and home support systems*, resources that remain unequally distributed across geographies and socio-economic strata. Hence, reliance on digital interventions without addressing infrastructural inequity risks exacerbating the *digital divide*. *Working memory*, the neural substrate for conscious manipulation of information, is particularly susceptible to *cognitive overload* and *environmental interference*. Neuropsychological studies demonstrate that working memory bandwidth is compromised under conditions of *stereotype threat, emotional dysregulation, and auditory or visual distraction*. Instructional design must therefore minimize *split attention, information redundancy, and format fragmentation*. For instance, integrating text explanations directly into diagrams rather than presenting them separately aligns with *cognitive load theory*, optimizing neural coherence and processing fluency. Importantly, what is often pathologized as a *cognitive deficit* may in fact reflect an affective or ecological constraint. Learners contending with *housing insecurity, familial trauma, or linguistic marginalization* exhibit reduced working memory performance not due to intrinsic deficits but due to *extraneous cognitive taxation*. Thus, designing for working memory efficiency must be reframed as a *structural and ethical endeavor*, encompassing emotional safety, identity affirmation, and epistemic inclusion.

3.2 Emotional Regulation and Affective Engagement

Far from being ancillary, emotion constitutes a core modulator of cognitive functioning. The *limbic system*, particularly the *amygdala* and *hippocampus*, mediates the encoding and retrieval of emotionally salient experiences. Neuroaffective research indicates that *positive affective states*, such as joy, curiosity, and hope, enhance *dopaminergic activity*, bolster *synaptic plasticity*, and promote *prefrontal-limbic connectivity*, thereby increasing attentional breadth, working memory span, and motivation. Pedagogically, cultivating emotional regulation involves both *intrinsic strategies* (e.g., mindfulness, cognitive reappraisal) and *extrinsic strategies* (e.g., relationship building, environmental design) (Patten, 2011; Chorab, 2017).

Mindfulness-based interventions (MBIs), including breath regulation, guided imagery, and proprioceptive awareness, have demonstrated efficacy in reducing cortisol levels, improving sustained attention, and enhancing self-regulatory capacity. However, the *cultural generalizability* of MBIs is limited; in some sociocultural contexts, such practices may conflict with normative expressions of spirituality, silence, or trauma responses. Alternatives such as *movement-based ritual, art therapy, or community storytelling* may serve as culturally congruent modalities for emotion modulation.

Cognitive reappraisal, a core strategy in emotion regulation, involves reframing a stimulus or event to alter its emotional impact. Functional MRI studies show increased activation in the *dorsomedial prefrontal cortex* and reduced amygdala reactivity during successful reappraisal. Educationally, reappraisal can be embedded in reflective writing prompts, dialogic inquiry, or personalized feedback. Yet its success presupposes *psychological safety, affective vocabulary, and relational trust*, conditions that may be absent in punitive or hierarchical educational systems. Thus, relational pedagogy must precede cognitive strategy. *Social-Emotional Learning* (SEL) frameworks offer a systemic approach to cultivating affective competencies, encompassing self-awareness, empathy, relational skills, and ethical decision-making. Meta-analytic evidence links SEL with improved academic achievement, reduced behavioral issues, and enhanced life trajectories. Nevertheless, SEL has drawn criticism for its potential *normative assimilation*, particularly when decoupled from community-based knowledge systems. Effective SEL must be *culturally sustaining, linguistically inclusive, and trauma-informed*, embedding localized practices of resilience and intergenerational wisdom. Equally critical is the *affective labor of educators*. Teachers function as emotional co-regulators, and their demeanor, responsiveness, and vulnerability shape classroom climate. Oxytocinergic responses associated with trust and belonging are facilitated by *authentic teacher-student relationships*, which in turn modulate neural pathways associated with motivation and persistence (Denha et al., 2023; Soichuk et al., 2022). Pedagogical content knowledge must thus be complemented by *emotional intelligence and attunement.*

The interface between cognition and emotion is *bidirectional and synergistic*. Learners who experience emotional containment are more likely to engage in cognitive risk-taking, while mastery experiences increase emotional resilience (Karasievych et al., 2021; Kuznietsov, 2024). Instructional strategies such as *collaborative inquiry, peer mentoring, and formative self-assessment* activate this reciprocal dynamic, fostering both epistemic agency and socio-emotional fluency. Neuropedagogical strategies that target attention, memory, executive control, and emotional regulation must be seen not as mechanistic protocols but as part of an *ecosystemic design for human flourishing* (de Barros Camargo & Fernández, 2025; Naumenko et al., 2024). Their implementation requires *neuroscientific literacy, pedagogical adaptability*, and *institutional commitment to equity and inclusion* (Houdé, 2007; Varga & Szécsi,

2018). When coherently synthesized, these strategies enable classrooms to function as *neurocognitive sanctuaries*, nurturing the embodied, emotional, and intellectual potential of all learners.

4. EDUCATIONAL APPLICATIONS OF NEUROPEDAGOGY ACROSS CONTEXTS

The operationalization of neuropedagogical principles across educational ecologies demands a meticulous attunement to the ontogenetic, sociocultural, and institutional heterogeneities of learners (Solano Orellana, 2025; Medvedieva et al., 2023). While the neurocognitive substrates of learning, such as neuroplasticity, synaptic potentiation, attentional control, and executive regulation, exhibit universal physiological underpinnings, their pedagogical translation is necessarily contingent upon developmental trajectories, socio-political constraints, curricular architectures, and cultural semiotics (Karamat, 2024; Silva-López et al., 2015). This section delineates how brain-informed pedagogical strategies can be dynamically contextualized across four distinctive domains: early childhood education, secondary schooling, tertiary education, and inclusive education for neurodivergent learners.

4.1 Early Childhood Education

The early developmental epoch, particularly the prenatal to age-five window, constitutes a neurobiological critical period characterized by exponential synaptogenesis, myelination, and synaptic pruning within the sensory-motor cortex, prefrontal regions, and limbic circuitry. During this phase, the neurodevelopmental plasticity of the child is at its zenith, rendering the brain exquisitely responsive to environmental stimuli, relational contingencies, and pedagogical affordances. Educational praxis at this stage must be undergirded by *sensorimotor integration*, as per Piagetian and Vygotskian developmental frameworks, but reframed through the lens of contemporary neuroscience. Multisensory engagements, i.e., combining auditory, kinesthetic, visual, and proprioceptive modalities, activate distributed cortical and subcortical networks, promoting inter-hemispheric communication via the corpus callosum and enhancing thalamocortical synchrony. For instance, pedagogical activities such as rhythmic chanting paired with gestural mirroring or tactile object manipulation during narrative construction reinforce Hebbian learning through cross-modal stimulation, optimizing the development of symbolic and prelinguistic schemas.

Sociodramatic play, an essential conduit for neural and social maturation, engages the prefrontal cortex, mirror neuron systems, and default mode network, thereby cultivating cognitive empathy, inhibitory control, and affective reasoning.

Empirical findings from longitudinal studies in Nordic early education systems and African community-based preschools affirm that structured play, when scaffolded by emotionally attuned adults, enhances working memory, affective regulation, and prosocial behavior. Importantly, play is not epistemologically frivolous but neurodevelopmentally foundational. Yet, the pedagogical landscape of early education is often distorted by premature academic acceleration driven by standardized readiness assessments and neoliberal performativity metrics. Such misalignment disregards the *developmentally sequenced neurocognitive readiness* of young learners and may precipitate dysregulation of the hypothalamic-pituitary-adrenal (HPA) axis, elevating cortisol levels and impairing executive maturation. Therefore, neuropedagogical fidelity in early childhood necessitates a radical reorientation toward *developmental appropriateness*, prioritizing rhythm, sensory exploration, secure attachment, and emergent meaning-making over curricular standardization.

4.2 Secondary Education

The adolescent phase marks a neurodevelopmental inflection point characterized by *synaptic refinement, dopaminergic modulation*, and heightened plasticity within the prefrontal cortex and mesolimbic pathways. These neurobiological transformations manifest in increased capacities for abstraction, self-reflection, and moral cognition, coupled with amplified emotional volatility and peer orientation. Instructional modalities such as *inquiry-based learning* (IBL) and *project-based learning* (PBL) are particularly congruent with the adolescent neurocognitive profile. IBL activates the dorsolateral prefrontal cortex and anterior cingulate cortex, areas responsible for hypothesis generation, metacognitive monitoring, and error detection. PBL, with its emphasis on collaborative epistemic construction, iterative problem-solving, and real-world application, recruits multiple executive networks and reinforces neuroplastic adaptability through sustained goal-directed behavior. Neuroimaging studies conducted in urban and rural secondary schools across South America and Southeast Asia show enhanced theta-gamma coupling in students engaged in high-autonomy, interdisciplinary projects, indicating deep attentional engagement and episodic memory encoding. However, successful deployment of such models necessitates *scaffolded cognitive architecture*, particularly for learners from under-resourced contexts or with interrupted educational trajectories (Fernandes & da Motta, 2019; Kichuk et al., 2024). Pedagogical design must ensure cognitive incrementality, emotional safety, and socio-cultural resonance.

Adolescents' heightened affective sensitivity, mediated by a temporarily asynchronous maturation of the limbic system relative to the prefrontal cortex, necessitates targeted *emotional regulation scaffolds*. Techniques such as guided journaling, restorative justice circles, and contemplative practice (e.g., breathwork or visualization) recalibrate the amygdala-prefrontal circuitry, promoting reflective awareness and impulse modulation. In post-conflict educational contexts, trauma-informed neuropedagogy that incorporates somatic regulation and attachment-sensitive teaching has yielded significant gains in both academic engagement and affective resilience. Moreover, the *sociopolitical valences of identity* during adolescence, particularly in relation to gender, caste, race, and socioeconomic stratification, interact dynamically with neurocognitive load. Phenomena such as stereotype threat and identity incongruence are shown to dysregulate working memory and suppress attentional bandwidth, especially among students from marginalized backgrounds. Thus, intersectionally aware neuropedagogy must integrate *critical pedagogy, inclusive curricula, and narrative co-construction*, ensuring that all learners encounter mirrors of their lived realities and epistemic agency within the learning environment.

4.3 Higher Education

Although the neuroplasticity of the adult brain diminishes relative to earlier life stages, it remains sufficiently robust, particularly in the hippocampus, anterior cingulate cortex, and prefrontal systems, to benefit from pedagogical environments that are intellectually provocative, emotionally validating, and metacognitively demanding (Gorozhankina et al., 2023; Tarasenko et al., 2020). The demands of tertiary education, i.e., synthesis, abstraction, and disciplinary transfer, necessitate *cognitive efficiency, self-regulation*, and epistemic curiosity. *Adaptive learning technologies*, underpinned by machine learning algorithms and cognitive diagnostics, represent a frontier in personalized pedagogy. These systems adjust content complexity, feedback latency, and pacing based on learner analytics, optimizing the zone of proximal development and minimizing extraneous load. Implementations across higher education institutions in the European Union, East Asia, and Latin America show promising reductions in academic attrition and improved engagement in foundational STEM and language courses. *Flipped classroom models*, wherein content acquisition is externalized and class time is reserved for dialogic engagement and collaborative synthesis, are congruent with adult learners' need for autonomy and application. When paired with synchronous deliberation and problem-solving, flipped models enhance retrieval strength, cross-domain transfer, and higher-order cognitive engagement. However, their efficacy is modulated by learners' metacognitive maturity and digital access, warranting equity-sensitive instructional design.

The cultivation of *metacognitive intelligence*, i.e., the ability to monitor, evaluate, and recalibrate one's learning processes, should be explicitly embedded in course architecture. Reflection protocols, strategic self-assessments, and formative feedback loops strengthen neural circuits associated with self-directed learning (Szécsi, Varga, & Mák, 2018; Mudryk et al., 2022). For adult learners navigating complex life roles—such as caregiving, employment, or migratory precarity, these strategies enhance both cognitive agency and academic persistence. Crucially, the neuropsychological sequelae of *academic anxiety, imposter syndrome, and institutional alienation*, manifested as prefrontal suppression, cortisol dysregulation, and attentional narrowing, demand structural interventions. Campus-wide wellness infrastructures, peer mentorship programs, inclusive pedagogy workshops, and universal design frameworks mitigate these neuroaffective barriers and democratize access to intellectual participation.

4.4 Inclusive and Neurodivergent Education

Perhaps the most ethically urgent application of neuropedagogy lies in its capacity to reconfigure education for learners with neurodevelopmental and cognitive divergences (Vynogradova et al., 2021; Hnoievska et al., 2021). Far from being neuropathological anomalies, conditions such as autism spectrum disorder (ASD), attention deficit hyperactivity disorder (ADHD), dyslexia, and dyspraxia represent *neurocognitive pluralism*, variations in information processing, attentional distribution, sensory perception, and affective communication. In the context of *autism education*, neuroimaging and eye-tracking studies underscore the necessity of *structured routines, visual supports, and predictable transitions*. Visual schedules, social stories, and low-stimulation classroom environments reduce sensory overload and facilitate prefrontal-limbic regulation. Augmentative and alternative communication (AAC) tools, ranging from PECS boards to speech-generating applications, enhance expressive capacity and socio-communicative fluency. For learners with *ADHD*, instructional modalities must be tailored to accommodate frontal-striatal circuitry differences that affect impulse regulation and sustained attention. Interventions such as *task chunking, kinesthetic movement breaks, and immediate reinforcement schedules* align with attentional profiles and reduce distractibility. Neurofeedback and executive coaching, though still emergent in accessibility, show promise in augmenting dopaminergic self-regulation.

In *dyslexic learning*, functional MRI studies reveal underactivation in the left temporoparietal region during phonological decoding tasks. Structured literacy approaches—such as the Orton-Gillingham method, employ *multisensory phonics, repetition, and kinesthetic coding* to strengthen orthographic mapping. Policy-driven implementation across national education systems in Iceland, India, and Canada illustrates that early neurodiagnosis coupled with structured intervention can dramatically equalize reading outcomes. Inclusive neuropedagogy transcends mere accommodations; it mandates a paradigm shift toward *design justice, ecological adaptability*, and co-constructed agency. Universal Design for Learning (UDL), co-teaching models, personalized learning plans, and caregiver-educator partnerships operationalize this ethos. The objective is not assimilation but *epistemic dignity*, the right of all learners to meaningfully participate in knowledge production according to their cognitive particularities. Neuropedagogy's translational efficacy hinges not merely on neurobiological insight but on its ethical deployment across complex educational terrains (Tafuri et al., 2024; Honcharuk et al., 2023). From sensorimotor play in early childhood to AI-enhanced personalization in higher education, and from adolescent inquiry to inclusive architectures for neurodivergent learners, the brain-aware educator must be simultaneously *scientifically literate, culturally competent, and politically conscious*. Only then can neuropedagogy transcend its diagnostic origins to become a transformative praxis for equitable, responsive, and humanizing education.

5. CHALLENGES AND ETHICAL CONSIDERATIONS IN IMPLEMENTATION

The operationalization of neuropedagogical paradigms within educational ecologies presents an intricate confluence of promise and peril (Balashova, Sofronova, & Stroganov, 2025; Kernas et al., 2024). While the alignment of instructional modalities with neurocognitive and affective architectures offers the prospect of pedagogical optimization, the translational fidelity from neurobiological insight to classroom practice is circumscribed by infrastructural disparities, epistemological asymmetries, and ethical indeterminacies. Implementation is fraught with tensions that emerge at the interstices of scientific validity, cultural legibility, institutional feasibility, and sociopolitical accountability (Barabanova & Kazlauskiene, 2020; Ahmedova & Narmetova, 2022). This section interrogates the multi-scalar impediments and normative quandaries embedded in the deployment of neuropedagogical strategies, advocating for reflexive, contextually nuanced, and ethically defensible praxis.

5.1 Infrastructural Constraints and Systemic Inequalities

The deployment of neuroscience-informed pedagogy is deeply conditioned by the material substrata and policy architectures of education systems (Kaplinskyi et al., 2024; Povoroznyuk et al., 2024). In affluent jurisdictions, educators may access neuroadaptive platforms, biometric feedback mechanisms, and interdisciplinary professional development, whereas under-resourced contexts, particularly in postcolonial peripheries, are typified by infrastructural fragility, pedagogical overburden, and epistemic dispossession. These asymmetries engender implementation bifurcations. High-leverage cognitive strategies, such as spaced retrieval, multimodal encoding, and differentiated executive function scaffolds, are often precluded by logistical exigencies, including inflexible timetables, overcrowded classrooms, and curricular hyperstandardization. Instructional fidelity is further undermined by performativity metrics tied to high-stakes assessment regimes, disincentivizing pedagogical innovation. In such milieus, the neurocognitive optimization of instruction risks devolving into a technocratic ideal, unmoored from the granular constraints of real-world praxis (Elouafi, Lotfi, & Talbi, 2023; Bilyk et al., 2022). Moreover, neoliberal audit cultures and datafication imperatives disproportionately encumber marginalized institutions, constraining epistemic agency and pedagogical discretion. Without structural recalibrations in resource distribution, workload rationalization, and curricular governance, neuropedagogy remains a discursive artifact rather than an operational reality (Bakhmat et al., 2023).

5.2 Misapplication, Oversimplification, and the Persistence of Neuromyths

The entrenchment of neuromythologies within public and professional consciousness constitutes a major epistemic hazard. Reductionist constructs, such as hemispheric learning dichotomies, cognitive capacity percentages, or rigid sensory modality classifications, persist despite their empirical refutation. These conceptual distortions proliferate via commodified professional development ecosystems that prioritize marketability over methodological rigor. The pedagogical acceptance of pseudoscientific frameworks dilutes the epistemic credibility of legitimate cognitive neuroscience, undermining both instructional efficacy and learner trust. For instance, typological learning styles not only lack neuroscientific substantiation but may also engender epistemic foreclosure, curtailing students' engagement with diverse cognitive pathways and modalities. Counteracting this epistemic erosion necessitates robust translational infrastructures that preserve the complexity of scientific findings while rendering them pedagogically actionable. Collaborative epistemic brokerage, facilitated through interdisciplinary consortia, open-access repositories, and educator-neuroscientist co-production frameworks, can mediate between theoretical sophistication and classroom applicability. Absent such scaffolds, the field is vulnerable to instrumentalization and epistemic drift.

5.3 Gaps in Professional Development and Epistemic Accessibility

The scalability of neuropedagogical praxis is contingent upon the cognitive readiness and epistemological fluency of educators (Zhurat et al., 2021; Koval et al., 2025). Yet in most educational systems, preservice and in-service training remain cognitively impoverished, temporally fragmented, and ideologically constrained.

The neurocognitive foundations of learning are often relegated to ancillary modules, depriving educators of the theoretical substrates necessary for interpretive engagement with neuroscientific literature. Epistemic inaccessibility further compounds this deficit. The semiotic density, disciplinary jargon, and paywalled publication of neuroscientific outputs render them inscrutable to practitioners lacking advanced training in cognitive neurobiology or psycholinguistics. Moreover, the epistemic hegemonies that prioritize Anglophone, Eurocentric, and neurotypical norms marginalize contextually salient knowledges. Bridging this chasm necessitates the development of translational epistemologies that are linguistically inclusive, culturally reflexive, and pedagogically situated. Intermediary professionals, epistemic translators with dual fluency in neuroscience and education, must be institutionalized as boundary actors within school systems. Concurrently, professional learning communities (PLCs) should be reconfigured as recursive, inquiry-based ecosystems that privilege critical reflection, peer mentorship, and context-responsive experimentation over top-down compliance.

5.4 Ethical Use of Educational Technologies and Cognitive Data

The convergence of educational neuroscience and algorithmic technology engenders a new epistemological regime in which the learner is constituted as a data-generating entity subject to biopolitical governance. Neurotechnologies, ranging from EEG-based attentional monitors to emotion-sensing wearables and AI-driven adaptive platforms, purport to optimize learning by interfacing directly with students' cognitive and affective states. Yet this techno-scientific aspiration is fraught with ethical volatility. The aggregation and algorithmic processing of biometric data raise critical questions around informed consent, data sovereignty, algorithmic opacity, and the encroachment of surveillance rationalities into pedagogical spaces. In many contexts, datafication proceeds with limited transparency, rendering students legible to systems but opaque to themselves. Predictive analytics may reify deficit framings, reinforcing structural inequities through automated sorting, differential access, or performance-based interventions lacking human interpretive nuance. A robust data ethics framework is therefore imperative—one that foregrounds privacy by design, participatory consent architectures, algorithmic explainability, and the pedagogical subordination of technology to human flourishing. Institutional procurement protocols must include independent ethical audits, while governance regimes should be aligned with international rights-based instruments. The goal is not to eschew neurotechnology, but to embed it within a normative scaffold that centers learner autonomy and epistemic justice.

5.5 Cultural Blind Spots and the Risk of Neurocentrism

An uncritical valorization of neurobiological determinism risks epistemological monism, wherein diverse modes of learning and knowing are subordinated to cerebral metrics. Such neurocentrism occludes the sociocultural, historical, and linguistic matrices that co-constitute educational experience. By pathologizing deviation from normative cognitive profiles, it may inadvertently reinscribe deficit discourses and marginalize non-Western epistemologies. Educational cognition is not merely a function of neural circuitry but an emergent phenomenon shaped by ontological orientation, cultural symbolism, and intersubjective resonance. For instance, communal modes of narration, embodied apprenticeship, and rhythmic mnemonic devices, prevalent in many Indigenous pedagogies, may elude neuroscientific validation yet possess profound educational efficacy. Neuropedagogy must thus engage in epistemic pluralism, embracing culturally sustaining pedagogies that recognize diverse knowledge ecologies (Patten, 2008; Bilier et al., 2023). Neuroimaging studies on storytelling, rhythm, and multimodal affect can serve to validate rather than supplant such traditions, facilitating a dialogical synthesis between scientific insight and cultural praxis. The neuroethical imperative is not to homogenize cognition, but to scaffold inclusive learning environments that honor the heterogeneity of neurodevelopmental and cultural trajectories.

5.6 Equity and the Unequal Distribution of Neuropedagogical Benefits

The diffusion of neuropedagogical innovation is patterned along lines of socioeconomic stratification (Solano & Vega, 2024; Pervushina, 2018). Elite educational institutions often function as testbeds for emergent cognitive strategies, while underfunded systems remain ensnared in outdated didacticism. This cognitive capital asymmetry threatens to calcify educational inequities, producing epistemic bifurcation wherein only privileged learners benefit from neuroaligned instruction. Addressing this imbalance necessitates redistributive logics and solidarity-based implementation frameworks. Public-private partnerships must be recalibrated to serve equity goals, while philanthropic and governmental investments should prioritize capacity-building in marginalized contexts. Open-source neuroeducation tools, localized knowledge translation centers, and community-based teacher training initiatives can democratize access to cognitive science innovations. Crucially, equity in neuropedagogy is not merely about resource parity but about contextual resonance (Tsymbal-Slatvinska et al., 2022; Moss-Zobel, 2024). Strategies must be indigenized, co-designed with community stakeholders, and attuned to learners' lived realities. Only then can neuroscience cease to be an elite epistemic enterprise and become a catalyst for educational justice.

6. FUTURE DIRECTIONS AND POLICY RECOMMENDATIONS

As neuropedagogy transitions from a heuristic construct to an emergent field of praxis situated at the confluence of cognitive neuroscience, educational philosophy, and sociotechnical systems, its trajectory will be determined not merely by neurobiological discovery but by the capacity of institutions to scaffold equitable, epistemically pluralistic, and ethically sound implementations (Elouafi, Lotfi, & Talbi, 2021; Williamson, Pykett, & Kotouza, 2025). The translation of brain-based insights into pedagogical architectures must transcend reductionist technocentrism, avoid commodified instrumentalism, and instead center contextual responsiveness, civic accountability, and pedagogical intentionality. This section articulates forward-looking strategies and policy imperatives to guide the maturation of neuropedagogy in ways that preserve its transformative potential while resisting epistemic capture and systemic exclusion (Vasilieva et al., 2023; Rusydiana, 2023).

6.1 Research Priorities, Laboratory Precision, and Ecological Validity

The epistemic legitimacy of neuropedagogy hinges on its methodological pivot from experimental reductionism to ecological resonance (Nykyporets et al., 2023; Ribtsun et al., 2023). Traditional paradigms in educational neuroscience, often delimited by small-N designs, neurotypical homogeneity, and culturally myopic samples, yield findings of limited translatability. Future research must foreground *situated cognition*, recognizing that neural processes are mediated by sociocultural practices, affective environments, and historical contingencies. A recalibration of research agendas toward *ethnographically enriched neuroscientific inquiry, design-based implementation research* (DBIR), and *participatory neuroethics* is imperative. Longitudinal, multi-site studies incorporating learners from neurodivergent, multilingual, and socioeconomically marginalized populations will enrich the fidelity and applicability of findings. Integrative models drawing from *cultural neuroscience, developmental systems theory*, and *critical pedagogy* can uncover how neural plasticity intersects with structural violence, linguistic hybridity, and educational precarity. Importantly, the epistemological scaffolding must also evolve. Rather than presuming universality in cognitive architecture, researchers should engage in *context-sensitive mapping of neurocognitive variability*. Recognizing the epistemic authority of neurodivergent individuals, Indigenous communities, and non-Western knowledge systems is not only ethically requisite but intellectually generative. Such repositioning would challenge the ontological hierarchies embedded in normative developmental psychology and engender pluralistic ontologies of learning.

6.2 Cognitive-Technical Ecosystem and Responsible Innovation in Neurotechnology

The neurotechnological frontier, encompassing *BCIs, EEG-integrated platforms, affective computing, and AI-mediated scaffolds*, offers unprecedented affordances for personalized learning trajectories, real-time feedback loops, and neural state monitoring. Yet the entanglement of such apparatuses with pedagogical infrastructures demands a rigorous *technopolitical critique*. Responsible innovation must supplant the uncritical valorization of novelty. This entails the *prefigurative design* of tools that embed inclusivity, data minimization, and user sovereignty into their architecture. Open-source protocols, explainable AI (XAI), and *federated learning models* can disrupt the proprietary asymmetries that currently monopolize the ed-tech landscape. *Consent-centric design* must accommodate varying capacities for assent, particularly among minors, and embed adaptive consent mechanisms over time. Moreover, pedagogical intentionality must guide technology adoption. The use of *neurofeedback* to support self-regulation should not devolve into behavioral compliance systems. Rather, it should be relationally embedded within dialogic pedagogy, emotional scaffolding, and critical reflection. The litmus test must remain: does the intervention expand learner agency, foster epistemic curiosity, and deepen relationality? Technologies devoid of narrative, culture, and co-construction risk reifying cognition as mechanistic rather than lived.

6.3 Teacher Formation, Epistemic Agency, and Translational Fluency

The epistemic agency of educators is the linchpin of any sustainable neuropedagogical ecosystem. Teachers are not conduits for neuroscientific orthodoxy; they are *interpretive agents, situated knowers, and pedagogical cartographers* who mediate between theory and context (Barros Camargo & Hernández Fernández, 2024; Gvozdii et al., 2022). Thus, teacher education must transcend content transmission and invest in *metacognitive capacity building, translational literacy, and critical epistemological reflexivity*. Pre-service programs must integrate neuroscience as an interdisciplinary anchor across curriculum design, differentiated instruction, and assessment theory. Pedagogical epistemology should include not only canonical texts but also critiques from *neurodiversity studies, feminist epistemology, and critical disability studies*, allowing future educators to navigate scientific complexity with nuance and justice sensitivity. In-service models must pivot from episodic workshops to *collaborative professional learning communities* (PLCs) sustained over time. These "*neuropedagogy circles*" should be protected epistemic spaces for collective inquiry, iterative experimentation, and context-specific adaptation. Digital knowledge commons, curated open-access repositories, and peer-reviewed implementation toolkits can democratize access, particularly for educators operating in resource-constrained environments. The institutional ecosystem must also support this epistemic labor. Policy levers, such as time allowances, reflective supervision, and microcredentialing, can incentivize engagement and signal its systemic value.

6.4 Systemic Alignment, Policy Patchwork, and Structural Enablers

Isolated innovation without structural alignment often succumbs to attrition. For neuropedagogy to scale meaningfully, macro-level levers must synchronize with meso-level initiatives and micro-level practices (Camargo & Fernández, 2024; Piddubna et al., 2023). This entails systemic reengineering across curricular, assessment, infrastructural, and regulatory domains. Curriculum policy must transcend behavioral objectives and embed *cognitive developmental milestones, affective scaffolds, and neurodivergence-sensitive frameworks*. National curricular documents should reflect *cognitive load theory, spacing and retrieval practice, and executive function development*, operationalized through exemplar pedagogical designs. Assessment policy must transition from norm-referenced, summative models to *formative, process-oriented evaluation* that captures *metacognition, transfer*, and *self-regulation*. Infrastructure investments must be equity-weighted. Budgetary allocations should support *sensory-friendly classroom design, assistive neurotechnologies, and teacher-learner ratios* conducive to personalized cognition-aligned pedagogy. Procurement guidelines must privilege *ethically certified edtech providers*, with enforceable benchmarks on *data privacy, pedagogical congruence*, and *universal design for learning* (UDL). Accountability regimes should evolve toward *learning health systems* that use disaggregated, anonymized data for iterative improvement. Key performance indicators must include *cognitive growth metrics, learner engagement indices, and psychosocial wellbeing markers*, displacing the myopic primacy of high-stakes standardized scores.

6.5 Institutionalizing Ethical Infrastructure and Global Governance

As educational systems become entangled with cognitive surveillance and algorithmic mediation, the need for *multi-level ethical governance* becomes imperative. At national levels, *independent ethics councils*, comprising educators, neuroscientists, ethicists, learners, and civil society, must be established to appraise neuroscience-related initiatives against criteria of justice, consent, and psychosocial harm mitigation. Institutional Review Boards (IRBs) must be epistemologically diversified to evaluate the neurodevelopmental appropriateness and cultural legibility of research protocols. Consent frameworks must be adaptive, context-sensitive, and embedded in *relational ethics* rather than bureaucratic formalism. At supranational levels, intergovernmental organizations must broker *normative compacts.* A Global Charter on Educational Neuroethics, co-developed by the Global South and Global North, can delineate baseline standards and facilitate mutual accountability. Platforms such as *South-South knowledge exchanges, global innovation hubs*, and *open-science consortia* must be prioritized to dismantle epistemic asymmetries and incubate locally resonant models.

6.6 Deterministic Drift and Technocratic Capture

To responsibly chart the future, the field must anticipate and inoculate against epistemic and ethical distortions. Foremost among these is *cognitive essentialism*, i.e., the reduction of learner potential to fixed neural correlates. Such frameworks elide the dynamic, socially mediated nature of learning and risk reintroducing eugenicist tropes under neuroscientific veneer. The technocratic capture of pedagogy, wherein algorithmic control supersedes relational pedagogy, must be staunchly resisted. If tools designed to enhance attention or monitor emotion are deployed without learner consent, cultural attunement, or pedagogical reciprocity, they morph into *cognitive panopticons* rather than emancipatory supports. Equally problematic is the *overpromising of scientific translationality*. Neuroscience, while revelatory, remains a developing science with contested boundaries. Policymakers, educators, and funders must cultivate *epistemic humility*, resisting premature extrapolation and instead embracing iterative, co-constructed, and contextually validated implementations. The guiding ethos must remain humanistic. Neuropedagogy must not aspire to engineer optimal learners for knowledge economies but to *nurture flourishing human beings*, that are cognitively attuned, emotionally resilient, and socially grounded.

REFERENCES

Ahmedova, M. T., & Narmetova, Y. K. (2022). Neuropedagogy and neyropsychology how developing New Nauka. *Society and innovations Special*, (02), 2181-1415.

Alkhassawneh, S., & Al Sharif, H. (2025). Perspectives Of Brain Research (Educational Neuroscience) on the Design and Implementation of Teaching Strategies in Educational Technology. *Journal of Neuroeducation*, *5*(2), 14–24. DOI: 10.1344/joned.v5i2.47695

Allaberdieva, K. (2019). The Main Neuropedagogic Possibilities Of Formation At Children Of Senior Preschool Age Of Creative Activity. *European Journal Of Research And Reflection In Educational Sciences*, *7*, 12.

Antoniuk, L., Olena, S. O. I. A., Kosovets, O., Klimishyna, A., Kovtoniuk, M., & Tryfonova, O. (2022). Ensuring the innovativeness of vocational education: Neuropedagogical aspect. *BRAIN. Broad Research in Artificial Intelligence and Neuroscience*, *13*(4), 242–263. DOI: 10.18662/brain/13.4/386

Arum, Y. P. (2025, July). Implementing Silence Pedagogy in English Language Teaching through a Neuropedagogical Approach in Indonesia. In *Proceedings of the World Conference on Foreign Language Education* (Vol. 2, No. 1, pp. 5-5).

Bakhmat, N., Dzhyhun, L., Mishchenko, M., Polishchuk, O., Savytska, O., & Dorofey, S. (2023). The Neuropedagogical Aspects of Mental and Cognitive Activity in Younger School-Age Children. *BRAIN. Broad Research in Artificial Intelligence and Neuroscience*, *14*(3), 182–193. DOI: 10.18662/brain/14.3/469

Balashova, E. S., Sofronova, L. V., & Stroganov, D. A. (2025). Legal and Regulatory Support of Neuropedagogy in the Russian Federation. *Russian Studies in Law and Politics*, *9*(1), 29–50. DOI: 10.12731/2576-9634-2025-9-1-216

Barabanova, I., & Kazlauskiene, A. (2020). Neuropedagogy: preconditions for application of neuroscience results in the education process while providing feedback. In *Technium: Romanian journal of applied sciences and technology: Proceedings of the 5th Technium conference 2020 (18.07. 2020, Romania).* (Vol. 2, No. 5, pp. 112-122). Technium Press.

Barba Tellez, M. N., Sotomayor, C. R., & Tobar, A. P. (2018). The Management of Neuropedagogical Processes of Learning and the Need for a Teacher Connected with Neuropedagogy. *Opuntia Brava*, *10*, 648.

Barros, C. D. (2022). Neuromethodology and neuroimaging for a teacher training. *Texto Livre*, *15*, e40454. DOI: 10.35699/1983-3652.2022.40454

Barros, C. D., & Fernández, A. H. (2022). Neuroscience, neuroeducation, neurodidactics and technology. *Texto livre, 15*, e41235.

Barros Camargo, C. D., & Hernández Fernández, A. (2024). Neuropedagogy and neuroimaging of artificial intelligence and deep learning.

Bielenia-Grajewska, M. (2014). Neuroscience and learning. In *Encyclopedia of science education* (pp. 1–7). Springer.

Bilier, O., Reshetniak, V., Vasko, O., Drokina, A., Klanichka, Y., & Barda, S. (2023). Innovative learning technologies for future elementary school teachers in the context of neuropedagogy. *BRAIN. Broad Research in Artificial Intelligence and Neuroscience, 14*(4), 66–81. DOI: 10.18662/brain/14.4/492

Bilyk, V., Bashtovenko, O., Biriukova, T., Osipov, V., Kriukova, M., & Tomich, L. (2022). Principles of Realization of Physical Therapy for Students: Modern Views of Neuropedagogy and Neuropsychology. *BRAIN. Broad Research in Artificial Intelligence and Neuroscience, 13*(1), 132–144. DOI: 10.18662/brain/13.1/272

Boboxolovna, X. S. (2022). From Pedagogical Technologies Based on Neuropedagogy in the Educational Process Use. *European Journal of Research Development and Sustainability, 3*(5), 58–61.

Borisovna, Z. M., & Valeryanovna, D. T. (2018). Conflict behavior of younger school children: neuropsychological and neuropedagogical optics. *Turkish Online Journal of Design, Art & Communication, 8*.

Bożena, P. (2020). Brain, mind and education–we have found the way, whether we are wandering along the wilderness? *Człowiek-Niepełnosprawność-Społeczeństwo, 48*(2), 59–68.

Camargo, C. D. B., & Fernández, A. H. (2024). Neuropedagogy and Neuroimaging of Artificial Intelligence and Deep Learning. *Educational Process: International Journal, 13*(3), 97–115. DOI: 10.22521/edupij.2024.133.6

Cavadas, A., Fernandes, R. M., Motta, C., Marques, C., & Oliveira, C. (2019, November). Estratégia neuropedagógica computacional para promover o desenvolvimento de jovens em áreas de risco e vulnerabilidade social. In *Workshop de Informática na Escola (WIE)* (pp. 773-782). SBC. DOI: 10.5753/cbie.wie.2019.773

Chojak, M. (2018). Neuropedagogy as a scientific discipline: Interdisciplinary description of the theoretical basis for the development of a research field. *International Journal of Educational and Pedagogical Sciences, 12*(8), 1084–1087.

Chorab, G. (2017). The neuropedagogical character of Howard Gardner's theory of five minds. *General and Professional Education, 2017*(3), 7–10.

Contreras, O. J. T., Vargas, S. F. P., & Mora, R. J. F. (2025). Aprendizaje del concepto de acto motor: Estrategia neuro pedagógica para estudiantes de pregrado en el área de neurorrehabilitación. *Educere: Revista Venezolana de Educación*, (92), 23–43.

Corona, F., Di Tore, S., & Cozzarelli, C. (2012). Implied neuropedagogy and symbolic interactionism: An interpretative system for the gesture language. *Continental Journal of Medical Research, 6*(2), 11.

David, L. E. T., Tabares, E. T., & Tabares, N. T. (2025). Neuropedagogía en la Educación Artística: Un Enfoque desde la Universidad del Atlántico-Colombia. *Ciencia y Reflexión, 4*(1), 1839–1853. DOI: 10.70747/cr.v4i1.194

de Barros Camargo, C., & Fernández, A. H. (2025). Profesionalización Docente en la Era Global: Reflexiones desde la Neuropedagogía y la Neuroimagen. *Revista Española de Educación Comparada*, (47), 511–527. DOI: 10.5944/reec.47.2025.44074

de Oliveira, C. E. T., Marques, C. V. M., Weber, C., Prata, P., & Souza, M. (2009). An Architectural Platform to Provide Integral Care for Cognitive Impaired Children through Neuropedagogical Metacognition. In *HEALTHINF* (pp. 466-473).

Denha, N., Hudyma, U., Krupskyi, Y., Dumanska, T., Heseleva, K., & Povidaichyk, M. (2023). Blended learning as a means of forming mathematical competence of future teachers of the new Ukrainian school: Neuropedagogical aspects. *BRAIN. Broad Research in Artificial Intelligence and Neuroscience, 14*(4), 82–94. DOI: 10.18662/brain/14.4/493

Díaz, Y. R., & Granda, M. K. V. (2022). La neuropedagogía lúdica como estrategia para reforzar la capacidad de cálculo numérico en el proceso de enseñanza y aprendizaje de la matemática. *Serie Científica de la Universidad de las Ciencias Informáticas, 15*(6), 220–230.

Elouafi, L., Lotfi, S., & Talbi, M. (2021). Progress report in neuroscience and education: Experiment of four neuropedagogical methods. *Education Sciences, 11*(8), 373. DOI: 10.3390/educsci11080373

Elouafi, L., Lotfi, S., & Talbi, M. (2021). Progress Report in Neuroscience and Education: Experiment of Four Neuropedagogical Methods. *Education Sciences, 2021*(11), 373. DOI: 10.3390/educsci11080373

Elouafi, L., Lotfi, S., & Talbi, M. (2023). Experimentation Using Neuropedagogical Methods. *Journal of Hunan University Natural Sciences, 50*(2).

Fernandes, R. M. M., & da Motta, C. L. R. (2019). Contributions of Computational Neuropedagogy for Teaching the Narrative Genre. In *INTED2019 Proceedings* (pp. 7333-7339). IATED.

Fernández, A. H. (2022). Neuropedagogy and neuroimaging. *Texto Livre*, *15*, e40453. DOI: 10.35699/1983-3652.2022.40453

Fontalvo, I. D. J. L. (2019). El clima escolar como estrategia neuropedagógica para la gestión de conocimiento. *Gestión Competitividad e Innovación*, *7*(1), 49–58.

Fragkaki, M., Mystakidis, S., & Dimitropoulos, K. (2022). Higher education faculty perceptions and needs on neuroeducation in teaching and learning. *Education Sciences*, *12*(10), 707. DOI: 10.3390/educsci12100707

Friedman, I. A., Grobgeld, E., & Teichman-Weinberg, A. (2019). Imbuing education with brain research can improve teaching and enhance productive learning. *Psychology (Irvine, Calif.)*, *10*(02), 122–311. DOI: 10.4236/psych.2019.102010

Gasanova, R. R., Setyaeva, N. N., Khoteeva, R. I., & Arpentieva, M. R. (2022). Socio-psychological and spiritual-moral problems of neurodidactics in inclusive practice. *Психопедагогика в правоохранительных органах, 27*(1 (88)), 79-86.

Glińska-Lachowicz, A. (2017). In search of the answer about the place and role of neuropedagogy in art. On divergent thinking in therapies throught art and education. *Education. Opole University Annual, 2*.

Gorozhankina, O. Y., Nesprava, M., Lutsenko, V., Zheqing, W., Mykhailets, V., & Shpak, H. (2023). Neuropedagogy as an Aspect of Developing Spiritual Culture in the Context of Vocal Music.

Gvozdii, S., Bakhov, I., Pienov, V., Palamarchuk, S., Dudnyk, N., & Petrukhan-Shcherbakova, L. (2022). Neuropedagogy in contemporary formal and non-formal education. *BRAIN. Broad Research in Artificial Intelligence and Neuroscience*, *13*(4), 264–279. DOI: 10.18662/brain/13.4/387

Hernández Fernández, A. (2022). Neuropedagogy and neuroimaging. *Texto Livre/ Texto Livre: Linguagem e Tecnologia, 15*.

Herrera, M. N. T., Herrera, M. V. T., Mayo, E. E. S., & Mayo, J. E. S. (2023). La Praxis Neuropedagógica en el despertar del Aprendizaje Escolar. *Ciencia Latina Revista Científica Multidisciplinar*, *7*(2), 6475–6490. DOI: 10.37811/cl_rcm.v7i2.5800

Hnoievska, O., Babii, I., Kalynovska, I., Cherednyk, A., Nikitenko, A., & Minenok, A. (2021). Formation of Correctional Competence of Teachers on the Basis of Neuropedagogy. *BRAIN. Broad Research in Artificial Intelligence and Neuroscience, 12*(3), 236–254. DOI: 10.18662/brain/12.3/229

Honcharuk, N., Onufriieva, L., Haletska, Y., Kurytsia, D., Ivashkevych, E., & Nabochuk, A. (2023). Neuropedagogical features of communication in the process of online education. *BRAIN. Broad Research in Artificial Intelligence and Neuroscience, 14*(3), 492–515. DOI: 10.18662/brain/14.3/487

Houdé, O. (2007). First insights on "neuropedagogy of reasoning". *Thinking & Reasoning, 13*(2), 81–89. DOI: 10.1080/13546780500450599

Huseinova, L., Liashenko, T., Pavlenko, O., Shpak, H., Maidaniuk, I., & Bidyuk, D. (2024). Art Competitions as a Tool for Students Creative Growth: Neuropedagogical Factors. *BRAIN. Broad Research in Artificial Intelligence and Neuroscience, 15*(3), 109–117. DOI: 10.70594/brain/15.3/7

Kaplinskiy, V., Voloshyn, S., Stakhiv, L., Oleksyuk, O., Ruskulis, L., & Haidaienko, I. (2022). Educational Needs of Society: Neuropedagogy as One of the Main Aspects of Motivation in Learning within Formal and Non-Formal Education. *BRAIN. Broad Research in Artificial Intelligence and Neuroscience, 13*(3), 225–235. DOI: 10.18662/brain/13.3/364

Kaplinskyi, V., Stoliarenko, O., Stoliarenko, O., Berezyuk, O., Chumak, M., & Hatezh, N. (2024). Developing Future Teachers' Creativity as a Crucial Element of Systemic Work in the Neuropedagogical Environment. *Revista romaneasca pentru educatie multidimensionala, 16*(3), 375-385.

Karamat, K. (2024). The Integration Between Neuropedagogy and Creativity in Higher Education. *American Journal of Technology and Applied Sciences, 20*, 67–71.

Karasievych, S., Halaidiuk, M., Kovalchuk, A., Oliinyk, M., Vykhrushch, V., Marionda, I., & Maksymchuk, I. (2021). Training future physical education teachers for physical and sports activities: Neuropedagogical approach. *BRAIN. Broad Research in Artificial Intelligence and Neuroscience, 12*(4), 543–564. DOI: 10.18662/brain/12.4/264

Kernas, A., Kotlomanitova, G., Kozyr, M., Myronenko, N., Sokolovska, S., & Stepanchenko, N. (2024). Professionalization of pedagogical activity of future teachers, formation of communicative competence as an aspect of neuropedagogy. *BRAIN. Broad Research in Artificial Intelligence and Neuroscience, 15*(1), 77–88. DOI: 10.18662/brain/15.1/537

Kichuk, Y., Gurevych, R., Bohush, O., Zasypkina, L., Shvets, O., & Bevz, O. (2024). The Role of Pedagogical Reflexology in Fostering Teacher's Professional Reflection in Neuropedagogy. *BRAIN. Broad Research in Artificial Intelligence and Neuroscience, 15*(4), 104–119. DOI: 10.70594/brain/15.4/8

Koval, V., Prytulyk, N., Sharan, O., Streletska, N., Dudnyk, N., & Koltok, L. (2025). Neuropedagogical Technologies for Training Future Primary School Teachers. *BRAIN. Broad Research in Artificial Intelligence and Neuroscience, 16*(1 Sup1), 27-40.

Kuznietsov, Y. (2024). *Innovative models of vocational education: A symbiosis of artificial intelligence, neuropedagogy, and the competency-based approach.* ПРОФЕСІЙНА ОСВІТА.

Kuznietsov, Y., & Kostiukevych, O. (2024). The influence of the integration of neuropedagogy, trend-watching, gamification, robotics, and immersive technologies on the development of pedagogical skills. *Scientia et societus, 1*(3), 92-103.

Lakhmotova, Y., Sadovets, O., Orlovska, O., Martynyuk, O., Myroshnychenko, V., & Lebedieva, L. (2024). Distance Learning of a Foreign Language in the Context of Neuropedagogical Factors. *BRAIN. Broad Research in Artificial Intelligence and Neuroscience, 15*(1), 105–121. DOI: 10.18662/brain/15.1/539

Lenska, S., Naumovska, N., Rudakova, N., Naumovska, O., Marchii-Dmytrash, T., & Sova, A. (2022). Neuropedagogical and Psychological Aspects of Play. *BRAIN. Broad Research in Artificial Intelligence and Neuroscience, 13*(4), 104–121. DOI: 10.18662/brain/13.4/378

Lohvynenko, T., Drozd, L., Marieieva, T., Hryntsiv, M., Prymakova, V., & Hrynyk, I. (2023). Neuropedagogical Principles as a Factor of Inclusive Education in the Context of Managerial Activity: European Experience. *BRAIN. Broad Research in Artificial Intelligence and Neuroscience, 14*(4), 212–227. DOI: 10.18662/brain/14.4/501

Lupu, C., & Jurchescu, D. (2020). Neuropedagogia. Metoda de cunoa tere i cercetare a creierului de către copii. *Journal for Neurology & Psychiatry of Child & Adolescent in Romania, 26*(2).

Lyndina, Y., Martynyuk, Z., Tovstohan, V., Babichenko, A., Mytsyk, H., & Samoilenko, I. (2023). Psychological and pedagogical technologies in working with children with special educational needs: Neuropedagogical aspect. *BRAIN. Broad Research in Artificial Intelligence and Neuroscience, 14*(1), 302–318. DOI: 10.18662/brain/14.1/421

Mácajová, M. (2013). Neuropedagogy and brain compatible learning--ideas for education in the 21st century. *Technologia Vzdelavania, 21*(3).

Macias, L. D. C., Montoya, L. M. S., & Hernández, R. G. (2024). La neuropedagogía y sus herramientas educativas para mejorar la enseñanza en la educación técnica profesional en el área de contabilidad. *RECIMUNDO, 8*(1), 385–399. DOI: 10.26820/recimundo/8.(1).ene.2024.385-399

Maidaniuk, I., Kavun, V., Tverdokhlib, N., Biryukova, L., Doroshenko, T., & Mashtaler, I. (2023). A Creative Approach to Preparing Inclusive Music Lessons: The Role of Neuropedagogy in Inclusive Music Education. *BRAIN. Broad Research in Artificial Intelligence and Neuroscience, 14*(4), 242–253. DOI: 10.18662/brain/14.4/503

Mamaniyazovna, X. S. (2025). Ethical viewpoint formation through effective neuropedagogical methods and technologies. *International Journal of Pedagogics, 5*(02), 211–215. DOI: 10.37547/ijp/Volume05Issue02-57

Mamaniyozovna, K. S. (2025). Neuropedagogical Technologies That Develop Analysis, Critical and Creative Thinking. *CURRENT RESEARCH JOURNAL OF PEDAGOGICS, 6*(02), 42–47. DOI: 10.37547/pedagogics-crjp-06-02-09

Marchak, D., Shvarts-Serebro, I., & Blonder, R. (2021). Crafting molecular geometries: Implications of neuro-pedagogy for teaching chemical content. *Journal of Chemical Education, 98*(4), 1321–1327. DOI: 10.1021/acs.jchemed.0c00306

Marievych, N., Oksana, K. R. U. S., Martyniv, L., Komarovska, O., & Kryzhanovska, T. (2023). Music and Game Activity of Elementary School Students as an Aspect of Neuropedagogy. *BRAIN. Broad Research in Artificial Intelligence and Neuroscience, 14*(1), 269–284. DOI: 10.18662/brain/14.1/419

Markiv, O., Zarivna, O., Khymai, N., Shalova, N., Shemet, V., Markiv, I., ... & Tymkiv, O. (2025). Mentoring as a Neuro-Pedagogical Tool of Motivation for Health Culture Formation Among the Students During Periods of War and Global Challenges. BRAIN. Broad Research in Artificial Intelligence and Neuroscience, 16(1 Sup1), 165-178.

Marrero, N. D. L. M. P. (2023). Dinámica de formación neurodidáctica de docentes desde la neuropedagogía: Neuro-didactic Dynamics Training Teachers from Neuropedagogy. *Papeles, 15*(29).

Marrero, P., & de las Mercedes, N. (2023). Dinámica de formación neurodidáctica de docentes desde la neuropedagogía. *Papeles: Revista de la Facultad de Educación Universidad Antonio Nariño, 15*(29).

Matveev, M. (2024). Digital neuropedagogy: harnessing cognitive science and technology for educational efficiency. *Journal of Teaching English for Specific and Academic Purposes*, 693-712.

Medvedieva, S. O., Stepanova, I. S., Nykyporets, S. S., & Ibrahimova, L. V. (2023). The application of a neuropedagogical approach while teaching English to students of higher educational establishments. *Перспективи та інновації науки.Nº 8: 13-24.*

Melnyk, O., Petryk, O., Lysohor, L., Pavlyk, O., Boiaryn, L., & Tykhonova, S. (2022). Current approaches to organizing the educational process in primary school: A neuroscientific approach. *BRAIN. Broad Research in Artificial Intelligence and Neuroscience. Vol. 13,Nº 1, Sup. 1: 01-21.*

Moss-Zobel, A. (2024, July). Neuropedagogy in Higher Education. In *ARPHA Conference Abstracts* (Vol. 7, p. e129736). Pensoft Publishers. DOI: 10.3897/aca.7.e129736

Mudryk, O., Ivakhnenko, A., Odynchenko, L., Dmytriieva, I., Ivanenko, A., & Shelever, O. (2022). Mental and Pedagogical Techniques in Teaching Children with Special Educational Needs: Neuropedagogical Aspect. *BRAIN. Broad Research in Artificial Intelligence and Neuroscience, 13*(4), 292–305. DOI: 10.18662/brain/13.4/389

Mystakidis, S., Christopoulos, A., Fragkaki, M., & Dimitropoulos, K. (2023). Online professional development on educational neuroscience in higher education based on design thinking. *Information (Basel), 14*(7), 382. DOI: 10.3390/info14070382

Naumenko, N., Kozlov, A., Palevych, S., Denysenko, A., Tverdokhlib, T., & Bashkir, O. (2024). Advancing the Career Development for Future Primary School Teachers in Ukraine: New Neuropedagogical Challenges. *Revista Romaneasca Pentru Educatie Multidimensionala, 16*(4), 29–51. DOI: 10.18662/rrem/16.4/906

Nefedchenko, V., Ostapenko, E., Bokhonko, Y., Gurevych, R., Shanaieva-Tsymbal, L., & Rud, O. (2023). Features of Information and Communication Technologies in the Educational Process: Neuroscience in Education.

Nikulochkina, O., Teslenko, T., Kokhanko, O., Sevastiuk, M., Yankovska, I., & Teletska, L. (2022). Neuro-pedagogical aspects of forming the professional competence of elementary school teachers and their interaction with students. *Revista Romaneasca Pentru Educatie Multidimensionala, 14*(4 Sup. 1), 128-154.

Nurmakhanova, D. E., Rakhmetova, A. K., Kassymbekova, D. A., Meiirova, G., & Rakhimzhanova, G. M. (2021). Neuropedagogy for improving the educational process in universities.

Nykyporets, S. S., Melnyk, O. D., Hadaichuk, N. M., Derun, V. H., & Chopliak, V. V. (2023). Neuropedagogical approach enhancing foreign language acquisition in non-linguistic higher education institutions. *Актуальні питання у сучасній науці.Nº 5: 341–355.*

Oliveira, J. E. (2024). Neuropedagogia e neurodidática na identificação precoce de transtornos no desenvolvimento cognitivo de crianças e adolescentes. *RECIMA21-Revista Científica Multidisciplinar-ISSN 2675-6218, 5*(2), e524886-e524886.

Patten, K. E. (2008). Toward a neuropedagogy of emotion.

Patten, K. E. (2011). The somatic appraisal model of affect: Paradigm for educational neuroscience and neuropedagogy. *Educational Philosophy and Theory, 43*(1), 87–97. DOI: 10.1111/j.1469-5812.2010.00712.x

Pávová, A., & Valent, M. (2020). Neuropedagogical knowledge in further education and counselling for teachers. In *10th International Adult Education Conference. Univerzita Karlova Pedagogická Fakulta, Prague.*

Pervushina, N. A. (2018). Neuropedagogy And Bioethics Symbolism: Place In Knowledge Management. *European Proceedings of Social and Behavioural Sciences.*

Pervushina, N. A. (2019). A semiotic diagnostics of study kits in the era of neuropedagogy. *ΠΡΑΞΗΜΑ. Problemy vizual'noy semiotiki–ΠΡΑΞΗΜΑ. Journal of Visual Semiotics, 4*, 194–205.

Piddubna, O., Maksymchuk, A., Lytvychenko, D., Revutska, O., Moskalenko, M., & Sopina, O. (2023). Implementing neuropedagogical innovation in schools: From theory to practice. *BRAIN. Broad Research in Artificial Intelligence and Neuroscience, 14*(2), 37–58. DOI: 10.18662/brain/14.2/443

Pinzón Blanco, D. M., & Téllez Sánchez, F. J. (2016). Neuropedagogical Tools: An Alternative to Improving Problem Solution Skills in Mathematics.

Povoroznyuk, R., Pocheniuk, I., Gaidash, A., Rybakova, K., Ostropalchenko, Y., & Saifutdinova, O. (2024). Neuropedagogical guidelines for translation studies: Perceiving the linguistic-cultural markers of the other (foreign) in translation. *Revista Romaneasca pentru Educatie Multidimensionala, 16*(4), 185-209.

Pretorius, L. (2025). An active learning intervention for in-service teachers: Self-determination theory, heutagogy, neuroeducation and the (altered) flipped classroom in practice. *Curriculum Perspectives, 45*(2), 1–14. DOI: 10.1007/s41297-024-00299-y

Rakhmetova, A. K., Meiirova, G., Balpanova, D. T., Baidullayeva, A. K., & Nurmakhanova, D. E. (2024). The Use of Elements of Neuropedagogy in the Creation of Virtual Simulators for In-Depth Study of Chemistry in Higher Education. *Journal of Technology and Science Education, 14*(2), 473–483. DOI: 10.3926/jotse.2532

Rashwan, H. K. A. (2024). *Bridging the Gap between Neuroscience and Education: What are Teachers' Perceptions of Applying "Neuropedagogy" to High School Classrooms?* (Master's thesis, The American University in Cairo (Egypt)).

Rasskazova, O., Anholenko, V., Pecherytsia, N., Hryhorenko, V. A., Tsybulina, I., Andreieva, M., & Yefimtseva, H. (2023). An Overview of the Principles of an Inclusive Approach in Education in Ukraine in the First Decade of the 21st Century as a Neuroscientific Factor. *BRAIN. Broad Research in Artificial Intelligence and Neuroscience, 14*(4), 373–387. DOI: 10.18662/brain/14.4/511

Ribtsun, Y., Bielova, O., Korolenko, V., Bolotnykova, T., Govorun, O., & Myttseva, O. (2023). Personality development in the paradigm of current neuropedagogy. *BRAIN. Broad Research in Artificial Intelligence and Neuroscience, 14*(4), 388–403. DOI: 10.18662/brain/14.4/512

Riccardi, M. (2023). How neuroscience and brain-based learning theory can enhance skill development of students in higher education. *Journal of Homeland Security Education, 16*, 1–6.

Rusydiana, I. (2023). Enhancing Learning Outcomes Through Neuropedagogy-Based Quantum Teaching. *Journal of Education and Religious Studies, 3*(03), 76–83.

Savchenko, O., Prystai, H., Hulych, M., Sobol, L., & Stupnytska, H. (2023). Neuropedagogy of Communication-Imitation. Opportunities for the Ukrainian English Teacher. *BRAIN. Broad Research in Artificial Intelligence and Neuroscience, 14*(3), 164–181. DOI: 10.18662/brain/14.3/468

Schlaggar, B. L. (2007). Are We Ready for a Neuropedagogy?.

Sen, A. (2022). Revisiting Brain-Based Learning: Strategies And Implications In The Higher Education Scenario. In *INTED2022 Proceedings* (pp. 10084-10090). IATED.

Shalom, M., & Luria, E. (2022). Neuro-pedagogy Course-Breaching the Borders Between Neuroscience and Education. *World Studies in Education, 23*(2), 51–67. DOI: 10.7459/wse/22.2.04

Shiwlani, A., Hasan, S. U., & Kumar, S. (2024). Artificial Intelligence in Neuroeducation: A Systematic Review of AI Applications Aligned with Neuroscience Principles for Optimizing Learning Strategies. *Journal of Development and Social Sciences, 5*(4), 578–593.

Shulha, L., Hnizdilova, O., Matishak, M., Marchii-Dmytrash, T., Yaroslavtseva, M., & Chorna, H. (2021). Developing Creative Abilities in Preschoolers in Painting Classes via the Principles of Neuropedagogy and Psychology of Creativity in Ukraine. *Revista Romaneasca Pentru Educatie Multidimensionala*, *13*(4), 614–632. DOI: 10.18662/rrem/13.4/501

Shvarts-Serebro, I., Ben-Yehudah, G., Elgavi-Hershler, O., Grobgeld, E., Katzof, A., Luzzatto, E., Shalom, M., & Zohar-Harel, T. (2024, June). Agents of change: Integration of neuropedagogy in pre-service teacher education. [). Frontiers Media SA.]. *Frontiers in Education*, *9*, 1369394. DOI: 10.3389/feduc.2024.1369394

SILVA, D. F. D. (2021). A neuropedagogia no processo de ensino e aprendizagem: uma abordagem da neurociência aplicada à educação no ensino fundamental I.

Silva-López, R. B., Fallad, J., Reyes-Ortiz, J. A., Bravo, M., & Rodriguez, J. (2015, December). Techno neuro pedagogy system: An instructional design methodology for customized online courses (virtual customized environment learning). In *2015 International Conference on Computational Science and Computational Intelligence (CSCI)* (pp. 281-286). IEEE. DOI: 10.1109/CSCI.2015.166

Silva-López, R. B., Reyes-Ortiz, J. A., Bravo, M., Federal, D., Fallad, J., de la Costa Sur, C. U., & Rodriguez, J. (2015). Techno Neuro Pedagogy System: an instructional design methodology for customized online courses. In *International Conference on Computational Science and Computational Intelligence*.

Slavikivna, B. O., Viktor, R., Oleksandrivna, V. O., Alina, D., Yurii, K., & Svitlana, B. (2023). Innovative Learning Technologies for Future Elementary School Teachers in the Context of Neuropedagogy.

Soichuk, R., Khrypun, D., Sydoruk, I., Serheieva, V., Shevchenko, V., & Shevchenko, S. (2022). Problems of organization of education of children with special educational needs in the conditions of contemporary primary school (in the context of neuropedagogy). *BRAIN. Broad Research in Artificial Intelligence and Neuroscience*, *13*(4), 383–397. DOI: 10.18662/brain/13.4/394

Solano, G., & Vega, M. (2024). Exploring Innovative Neuropedagogical Implications in English as a Foreign Language Teaching. *RUNAS. Journal of Education & Culture*, *5*(10), 12.

Solano Orellana, G. P. (2025). Exploring innovative neuropedagogical implications in english as a forign language teaching.

Supriatna, N., Fauzi, W. I., & Holilah, M. (2019). Social Studies Comic: Application of Neuropedagogy Approach To Social Studies Text Book of Smp Kelas Vii. *International Journal Pedagogy of Social Studies, 4*(2).

Syrotkina, Z., Bankul, L., Bukhniieva, O., Boychev, I., Gunko, N., & Chekhunina, A. (2022). The Arts as a Means of Developing Emotional Intelligence in the Context of Neuropedagogy. *BRAIN. Broad Research in Artificial Intelligence and Neuroscience, 13*(4), 306–320. DOI: 10.18662/brain/13.4/390

Szécsi, T., Varga, L., & Mák, V. (2018). Current trends, dilemmas and future directions in neuropedagogy in the field of early childhood. *Képzés és Gyakorlat: Neveléstudományi folyóirat, 16*(3), 51-58.

Tafuri, G., Scala, G., Di Lorenzo, G., & Gravino, G. (2024). Theoretical Review on inclusive education for children with special educational needs: From the main teaching techniques to the innovative aspects of neuropedagogy. *Journal of Inclusive Methodology and Technology in Learning and Teaching*, *4*(2).

Tarasenko, H., Zhurat, Y., Lipshyts, L., Soter, M., Chumak, L., Valchuk-Orkusha, O., & Melnyk, I. (2020). Developing Professional Subjectivity in Future Primary School Teachers in the Context of a Neuropedagogical Approach.

Téllez, M. N. B., Sotomayor, C. R., & Tobar, A. P. (2018). La gestión de los procesos neuropedagógicos del aprendizaje y la necesidad de un docente conectado con la neuropedagogía. *Opuntia Brava, 10*(2), 310–321.

Temirbekova, A. (2025). Neuropedagogical foundations of linguistics: Programming theory and practice. *International Journal of Pedagogics, 5*(03), 203–205. DOI: 10.37547/ijp/Volume05Issue03-58

Torres Martín, C. (2024). Neurodidáctica y transferencia del conocimiento a través del aprendizaje activo por competencias.

Tsymbal-Slatvinska, S., Maksymchuk, B., Saienko, V., Babii, I., Behas, L., Lemeshchuk, M., Chepka, O., Dychok, T., & Maksymchuk, I. (2022). Psycho-pedagogical experience of intellectual education in the views of Ukrainian and foreign pedagogues as the basis of modern neuropedagogy. *BRAIN. Broad Research in Artificial Intelligence and Neuroscience, 13*(4), 321–346. DOI: 10.18662/brain/13.4/391

Varga, L., & Szécsi, T. (2018). Neuropedagogy in Early Childhood in Hungary: Foundations and Micro-investigation. *Képzés És Gyakorlat: Training And Practice, 16*(3), 67–74. DOI: 10.17165/TP.2018.3.8

Vargas Angulo, L. E., Manuel SellanIcasa, V., Escobar Torres, A. F., & Ramos Fuentes, L. F. (2022). Neuropedagogía, sugerencias metodológicas para su aplicación en la enseñanza superior. *Roca: Revista Científico-Educacional de la Provincia de Granma, 18*(1).

Vasilieva, S. A., Reipolska, O. D., Podoliuk, S., Sadova, I., Danyliak, R., & Lozenko, A. (2023). The relationship between neuropedagogic approaches and the formation of skills of primary school students. *Revista Romaneasca Pentru Educatie Multidimensionala, 1*(15), 352–365. DOI: 10.18662/rrem/15.1/700

Vorotyntseva, O., Pozniak, O., Voitenko, A., Lopatina, H., Huz, I., & Husieva, T. (2022). The Preparation of Specialists for the Realization of Individual Education Path of Children with Special Educational Needs: Neuropedagogical Aspects. *BRAIN. Broad Research in Artificial Intelligence and Neuroscience, 13*(2), 97–112. DOI: 10.18662/brain/13.2/334

Vynogradova, O., Zdanevych, L., Sivak, N., Melnychuk, S., Polianovska, O., & Motoziuk, L. (2021). The system of modern social work with children with disabilities in the context of neuropedagogy: Traditions and Innovations. BRAIN. *Broad Research in Artificial Intelligence and Neuroscience, 12*(3), 287–302. DOI: 10.18662/brain/12.3/232

Williamson, B., Pykett, J., & Kotouza, D. (2025). Learning brains: Educational neuroscience, neurotechnology and neuropedagogy. *Pedagogy, Culture & Society*, •••, 1–21. DOI: 10.1080/14681366.2025.2521458

Wulan, S., & Jamaris, M. (2023). Increasing Children's Character Overt Behaviours by Neuro Pedagogy-Based Play. *Jurnal Pendidikan Usia Dini, 17*(2), 363–377. DOI: 10.21009/JPUD.172.12

Yánez, L. Y. C., Paredes, R. R. P., Guamarica, S. M. P., Naranjo, V. M. G., & Andrade, R. E. A. (2025). Abordando los retos de la educación del siglo XXI: perspectivas de la neuropedagogía para el aprendizaje y el desarrollo cognitivo integral.: Addressing the challenges of XXI st century education: perspectives of neuro pedagogy for comprehensive learning and cognitive development. *Revista Científica Multidisciplinar G-Nerando, 6*(1), ág-255.

Yepes Landinez, Y. A., Barón Peña, J. D., Campuzano Rojas, D., Barrera Sepulveda, C. Y., Cantor Herrera, A., González Giraldo, C. S., ... & Embus Alzate, V. (2024). Overview of Neuroeducation Basic Principles.

Yermakova, S., Ivanova, O., Horytska, O., Polishchuk, V., Polukhtovych, T., & Vivcharenko, T. (2023). Influence of the Neuro-Educational Environment on One's Socialization under Total Digitalization. *BRAIN. Broad Research in Artificial Intelligence and Neuroscience*, *14*(4), 593–611.

Zambrano, I. G. V., & Mieles, J. E. C. (2023). Neuropedagogical strategies for the attention of simple language delay in infants. *Revista San Gregorio*, *1*, 56–71.

Zhurat, Y., Lipshyts, L., Soter, M., Chumak, L., Tarasenko, H., Valchuk-Orkusha, O., & Melnyk, I. (2021). Developing professional subjectivity in future primary school teachers in the context of a neuropedagogical approach. *BRAIN. Broad Research in Artificial Intelligence and Neuroscience, 11*(2Sup1), 64-81.

Chapter 14
Brain-Based Learning From a Neuropedagogical Perspective in the Preschool Period

Nazan Kaytez
Faculty of Health Sciences, Department of Child Development, Çankırı Karatekin University, Turkey

ABSTRACT

Neuropedagogy relates children's psychological and cognitive development to neurophysiology. This provides the necessary information for creating scientifically based learning environments. Brain-based learning utilizes this knowledge and applies it in the classroom. It offers children a rich, stimulating environment, particularly during the preschool period when brain development is rapid. The primary goal of brain-based learning is to unlock children's learning potential by paying attention to individual differences and providing the right stimuli to create an effective learning environment. Teachers play the most crucial role in this regard. They must be thoroughly familiar with the principles of brain-based learning and be able to effectively guide children.

INTRODUCTION

The preschool period is a critical period when brain development is at its fastest. During this period, providing children with a rich and stimulating environment supports the formation of neural connections in the brain and enhances their learning potential (Perry, 2002). Learning occurs through the formation of new connections

DOI: 10.4018/979-8-3373-3581-0.ch014

between neurons in the brain and the strengthening of existing connections. This process is called neuroplasticity. Neuroplasticity is the brain's ability to reorganize itself in response to environmental stimuli, experiences, and learning activities (Doidge, 2007). This flexibility is particularly pronounced during the preschool years, meaning that experiences gained at an early age significantly influence a child's lifelong learning capacity (Goswami, 2004).

Neuropedagogy is a concept formed by combining the words neuroscience and pedagogy. This concept aims to optimize the learning experience. Neuropedagogy focuses on understanding the functions of the brain to implement education effectively. It also investigates how emotions affect learning and the conditions necessary for learning to be permanent. Neuropedagogy plays an essential role in supporting learning processes during the preschool period, when brain development is rapid (Ansari & Coch, 2006; Ansari et al., 2012). Certain neuropedagogical principles must be taken into consideration to support brain development during the preschool period. For example, providing children with a rich learning environment and sensory experiences is essential for brain development. Gross motor activities such as running, climbing, and balance games, as well as sensory experiences such as touching, smelling, and tasting, support children's brain development and learning. Similarly, different materials, toys, books, interactive activities, and safe and supportive social relationships are essential for brain development. Neuropedagogy guides teachers in this regard. Therefore, a teacher who is knowledgeable in neuropedagogy is aware of neurodevelopmental differences in children and understands that each child learns through different techniques and methods. One of these techniques and methods is brain-based learning (Özkan & Önder, 2021; Stevens Smith, 2020).

Brain-based learning emphasizes that learning is not solely composed of cognitive processes; emotional, social, and physiological factors also play an essential role in learning. It argues that learning is directly related to the structure and functioning of the brain. Therefore, it emphasizes the importance of brain development to make children's learning processes more effective. The brain-based learning approach emphasizes interactive and experiential learning. It also pays close attention to children's physiological processes (Jensen, 2005). It has a child-centered approach. It is opposed to rote learning. According to brain-based learning, new information should be taught by relating it to old information, and information should be related to examples from everyday life. Teachers should take into account the cognitive and emotional states of children and pay attention to individual differences among children (Sousa, 2011). In brain-based learning, the understanding that "*every brain is* unique" prevails. For example, some children are more inclined to auditory learning, while others are more inclined to visual learning. Therefore, teachers should not use the same approach to educate every child. Brain-based learning in the preschool period refers to a learning approach that is appropriate for the early stages of brain development. It offers various strategies to ensure that children learn by using their brain functions most efficiently. While neuropedagogy provides more theoretical knowledge about the brain, brain-based learning offers more concrete examples of application and methods (Değirmenci, 2021; Duman, 2015).

During the preschool period, the brain develops rapidly thanks to the connections established between neurons and synaptic plasticity. During this period, environmental stimuli and experiences contribute to the strengthening of connections in the brain. Therefore, the education and environmental stimuli that children receive in early childhood affect their learning capacity in the long term. During the preschool period, children generally need visual and auditory stimuli to explore the world (Caine & Caine, 2002; Tanrıdağ, 2018). Therefore, it is essential to provide children with the right stimuli. According to the brain-based learning approach, education delivered through games and activities makes learning more effective.

Additionally, teachers creating a safe and supportive atmosphere in the classroom facilitates the learning process. Brain-based learning also aims to develop children's creative thinking and problem-solving skills. It provides a learning environment that enhances children's mental flexibility and encourages them to explore and be curious (Duman, 2015). During the preschool period, children learn through social interaction. Brain-based learning supports children's social skills. Group games, cooperative games, and joint activities contribute to children's learning processes. Brain-based learning also emphasizes the importance of reinforcing and regularly reviewing the information learned. In the preschool period, children reinforce their learning processes through games, songs, and repetitive activities. This ensures that the information learned is retained (Özkan, 2015; Özkan & Önder, 2021). In this section, the neuropedagogical approach is discussed, focusing on brain development in the preschool period and how these characteristics interact with learning processes. Information is provided on brain-based learning principles and their implications for preschool education practices.

NEUROPEDAGOGICAL APPROACH

The neuropedagogical approach is an interdisciplinary approach that takes into account the brain development of children in the learning process. It encompasses the fields of education, neuroscience, and psychology. Neuropedagogy examines the structure of the brain, including structures related to learning such as the prefrontal cortex, limbic system, and mirror neurons. Emotional intelligence, motivation, and behavioral responses, which are essential topics in psychology, are also important topics in neuropedagogy (Ensari et al. 2021). Neuropedagogy, which relates children's psychological and cognitive development to neurophysiology, focuses on how children perceive the world, how they respond to stimuli in their environment, and how they learn, thereby developing teaching methods and creating scientifically based learning environments. Thus, it aims to facilitate children's learning both in and out of school and guides teachers and parents (Bissonette et al., 2015).

According to neuropedagogy, every child's brain structure, learning style, and educational needs are different. Therefore, when providing education, individual differences between children must be taken into account, and teaching methods should be developed accordingly. Children's emotional states also play an essential role in learning. Positive emotional states facilitate a child's learning, while negative emotional states, such as fear and anxiety, hinder learning. Again, an environment where the child feels safe and motivated is also crucial from a neuropedagogical perspective. Because, according to neuropedagogy, learning encompasses both cognitive and sensory, emotional, and social processes (Bendriyanti et al., 2024; Halmotov & Halmotov, 2022).

From a neuropedagogical perspective, the most essential feature of learning environments is that they support children's sensory development. According to the neuropedagogical approach, rich environments that stimulate all of a child's senses activate different parts of the brain and facilitate learning. Therefore, it is essential to have materials that develop children's senses in educational environments. However, these materials must be compatible with the age and developmental characteristics of the children. Physical movement and play are also important factors that facilitate children's learning. Children learn more easily through play. Active games, in particular, are of critical importance for children's brain development. This is because when children move, the brain releases proteins that facilitate learning, which in turn supports children's cognitive development (García, 2024; Gerdes, 2015). Active games support not only children's cognitive development but also their physical and emotional development. Therefore, learning environments must provide children with opportunities for physical movement. Again, the learning environment should reveal the child's curiosity and encourage active, hands-on, and experiential learning. Role modeling and imitation are also essential in learning. This is because modeling and imitation activate mirror neurons. Therefore, children must also be provided with environments where they can establish social relationships. From a neuropedagogical perspective, the learning environment should support all areas of the child's development, stimulate their senses, arouse curiosity, and make them feel emotionally secure. A child can only learn and unlock their potential in such an environment (Caballero & Llorent, 2022; Halmotov & Halmotov, 2022).

BRAIN DEVELOPMENT IN THE PRESCHOOL PERIOD

The brain is an organ that performs functions such as motor movements, organ functioning, learning, thinking, and remembering, and can perform many tasks simultaneously. It is surrounded by a membrane called the cortex and weighs approximately 1.25 kg in adults. Neurons consist of a cell body, dendrites, and axons. Learning occurs through the movements of nerve cells. These movements are facilitated by neurons, dendrites, and axons (Bonoma, 2017). The connection between nerve cells formed as a result of the interaction between dendrites and axons is called a synaptic connection. The more frequently the synaptic connections in the brain are used, the stronger the brain's development and learning. Therefore, an increase in synaptic connections is directly proportional to brain development. Brain development is a process that includes the formation of synaptic connections and their pruning (Güven, 2021; Sousa, 2011).

In the center of the brain, there is *the corpus callosum*, which connects the two hemispheres and facilitates the easy transfer of information from one hemisphere to the other. The outermost part of the brain hemispheres is called the cerebral cortex. The cerebral cortex is the starting point for inputs and outputs in the brain and also controls cerebellar movements. The part of the brain that extends downward inside the skull is called the brain stem. It is responsible for functions such as eye and facial movements, hearing, balance, and the functioning of the heart and respiratory muscles. Behind the skull and brain stem is the cerebellum (Gerdes et al., 2013; Stevens Smith, 2020). The cerebellum is the body's balance center and ensures coordination. The thalamus is the part that receives information from the sensory organs and sends it to the relevant areas. Another part of the brain is the hypothalamus. The hypothalamus is located below the thalamus and is responsible for functions such as body temperature, blood pressure, hunger, sleep, and thirst. Between the cerebellum, the forebrain, and the spinal cord is a section called *the pons*. The pons is where information is transmitted. It facilitates information transmission between the brain, spinal cord, and cerebellum (Oakes, 2017; Tanrıdağ, 2018).

Brain development begins at conception and continues until the end of adolescence. The early childhood years, also known as the preschool period, are a critical period for brain development. During this period, neural connections in the brain form and develop rapidly (Caine & Caine, 2002). When a baby is born, the brain weighs about one-fourth of the adult brain weight, which is approximately 350 grams. During the first six months, the child's brain weight reaches 50% of the adult brain, and during the first two years, it reaches 75%. In the following years, the brain's growth rate slows down. By the age of five, the brain weight is 90% of the adult brain weight, and by the age of ten, it is 95%. Brain development, which begins before birth, consists of stages such as the formation of neurons, the formation of axons and dendrites that connect neurons, the formation of synapses, the maturation of synapses, and the formation of tissues that surround the brain and enable effective communication (Doğan, 2021; Farmer-Dougan, & Alferink, 2013; Gerdes et al., 2013; Özkan, 2015).

When a baby is born, there are approximately 100 billion neurons in their brain, but most of these neurons are not connected. Connections between neurons are formed between the ages of 0 and 3 through the presentation of stimuli to the child. As the baby interacts with its environment, neurons connect and strengthen. Therefore, it is essential to establish effective communication with the baby from birth and provide stimuli that support sensory development. The first three years of life are particularly critical for brain development (Güven, 2021). When the right stimuli are provided to children during this period, the number of synapses at around 2-3 years of age is higher than in adults. Again, during this period, plasticity, i.e., the brain's capacity to reshape itself based on learning and experience, and frontal lobe development are very rapid. The prefrontal cortex is associated with skills such as attention, impulse control, problem-solving, and planning. In subsequent years, the connections in the child's brain become stronger, leading to further development of attention skills (Köksal, 2024; Tanrıdağ, 2018).

Brain and Learning

The brain, as the organ where learning takes place, has long been the subject of interest for researchers studying the relationship between the brain and learning. Many factors influence learning. In general, learning is defined as the perception of internal and external stimuli through the senses and their transmission to the brain. Connections related to learning occur in the middle and lower parts of the brain. For learning to occur, stimuli must first be sent to the brain through the sensory organs, and the brain must interpret these stimuli (Caine et al., 2016; Sharma, 2024). When stimuli are sent to the brain, the information received is transferred from sensory memory to short-term memory. Thus, the attention process necessary for learning begins. Information in short-term memory is stored for as long as the person pays attention to it (Alpar & Topan, 2016). When the person shifts their attention elsewhere, the information in short-term memory is erased. The part of the brain responsible for attention, memory, and recall is the hippocampus. Located in the middle of the brain, the hippocampus decides whether information will be sent to long-term memory. It processes information and helps us remember what we need. The hippocampus processes information based on curiosity, interest, and importance, which is why educators must design activities that positively influence the hippocampus (Camina

& Güell, 2017; Madi, 2014). This is because for learning to occur, the brain must perceive the stimuli as essential and send them to long-term memory.

The brain consists of two parts: the right and left hemispheres. The corpus callosum connects the two hemispheres and enables information to pass from one hemisphere to the other (Ansari, 2011; Barbey et al., 2013). The left hemisphere is responsible for logical and analytical thinking, verbal skills, language learning, mathematical calculation, decision-making, and problem-solving. In contrast, the right hemisphere is responsible for creativity, intuitive thinking, aesthetics, imagination, abstract thinking, three-dimensional thinking, and art-related functions. Although both hemispheres are responsible for different functions, they influence each other through neural connections while performing these functions, thereby enabling learning. The stronger the connection between the two hemispheres, the stronger the learning process. When the right and left hemispheres work in harmony, individuals can unlock their full potential. For this reason, it is crucial to provide children with an education that supports both hemispheres of the brain (Güven, 2021; Jensen, 2005).

Brain-Based Learning

Caine and Caine developed brain-based learning, which is a learning method related to neuroscience and cognitive psychology. The anatomy, structure, and function of the brain are the same in all humans, but perception, thinking, and learning techniques differ. This is because each individual reacts differently to an event, interprets it differently, and makes sense of it differently. Brain-based learning emerged as a result of research into the relationship between the brain's learning process and these individual differences. It is a learning approach based on the brain's natural operating principles (Caine & Caine, 2002; Caine et al., 2016).

Brain-based learning investigates how the brain works and uses this knowledge to achieve learning outcomes. Education and training are planned in line with the brain's operating mechanisms, to improve children's learning skills. In brain-based learning, information is not given directly to the child; instead, the aim is to stimulate the child's interest and curiosity and encourage them to use their brain actively. This approach is child-centered. In traditional education, the brain's natural learning process is not taken into account, and education is mainly based on memorization. In brain-based education, children are not expected to memorize, but to think and discover (Köksal, 2024; Maryati et al., 2020). In brain-based learning, children learn to ask questions, make sense of information, and establish cause-and-effect relationships. Concrete experiences are presented to children during the learning process. Children are encouraged to use strategies to structure and categorize information, thereby achieving meaningful learning. Additionally, information about the brain's functioning and structure is learned and internalized. The brain-based learning process consists of three stages: relaxed alertness, deep immersion, and active processing (Özkan & Önder, 2021).

- *Relaxed alertness*: During this process, the child does not experience stress and feels safe. There must be no stress or anxiety in the learning environment. Children learn more easily when they are not stressed or anxious. In such an environment, internal motivation is high. When children feel negative emotions such as inadequacy and helplessness, the brain perceives this as a threat, and learning does not take place. Therefore, when teaching a child something new, the teacher should relax the child. Only in this way can the child learn new information. It is imperative to approach children through play during the preschool period. Educators play a vital role in providing a relaxed and alert environment. The teacher must be knowledgeable about the subject and approach the child sincerely. The teacher can relax children through breathing exercises and imagination exercises. They should be knowledgeable in this area. When evaluating children, they should make sure that the environment is not stressful, i.e., that the children do not feel anxious (Can, 2025).
- *Deep immersion:* In this stage, children are presented with rich experiences. They are asked to focus on the content and visualize it mentally. In other words, information is not given to children directly; they relate the clues to real life and visualize them cognitively in their minds. As a result of the experiences they gain, changes occur in the structure and function of the brain, and new synaptic connections are established between nerve cells. Again, in this stage, attitudes, behaviors, and concepts that require knowledge and skills are integrated, and stories, examples, case studies, and scenarios related to them are used. Children are provided with a rich learning environment. The learning environment challenges the child, but this challenge is at a level that the child can achieve (Soyalp, 2022).
- *Active processing:* Children combine what they have learned in a way that is both personal and conceptual and internalize it. This creates a meaningful structure in the learning process. Children ask themselves questions such as "*What did I learn? Why did I learn it? What does it mean?*" This indicates that the child is actively processing. The goal at this stage is for the child to internalize the information through higher-level thinking activities. Thus, the child is aware of how they learned. The child can control their learning. With the active processing stage, it is possible to check what the child has learned and whether the targeted gains have been achieved (Özkan & Önder, 2021).

There are certain principles of brain-based learning. These principles are listed as follows (Caine & Caine, 2016).

- *The brain is a parallel processor:* The brain can perform many functions, such as thinking, imagining, and sensing, simultaneously. For example, when a person crosses the street, multiple areas of the brain (vision, hearing, speed, shape, etc.) can work at the same time.
- *Learning involves the entire physiology:* Emotions such as stress, anxiety, and fear negatively affect the brain. Therefore, educational programs should also cover such issues as coping with negative emotions, nutrition, and exercise.
- *The search for meaning is internal:* The brain perceives and records stimuli even during sleep. Meaning-making and acting accordingly are essential needs of the brain.
- *The search for meaning is formed through pattern recognition*: The brain rejects meaningless patterns. Pattern recognition is the meaningful organization and classification of information. Meaningless patterns are information that does not convey meaning.
- *Emotions are essential in pattern recognition:* Emotions and cognition influence each other. Positive emotions such as self-esteem are crucial to the internalization of information. Information must be internalized so that it can be recalled when needed.
- *The brain perceives parts and the whole simultaneously:* Both hemispheres of the brain interact with each other. The brain can divide information into parts or perceive parts as a whole (Özkan & Önder, 2021).
- *Learning requires both focused attention and environmental perception:* The brain focuses on a piece of information, but also assimilates information outside of that focus. It consciously carefully selects information.
- *Learning always involves conscious and unconscious processes:* Not everything we know is consciously perceived. Many environmental stimuli are recorded in the subconscious without our awareness and later emerge or influence the decisions we make. Thus, our experiences are formed. The brain remembers not only what is said but also experiences.
- *There are two types of memory:* The brain stores some things in memory without the need for repetition. In other words, we have a spatial memory system that allows information to remain in our long-term memory. For example, we don't need to think hard to remember where we were yesterday morning. This information is automatically stored in our spatial memory.
- *We understand and remember facts and skills best when they are structured in natural spatial memory.* Internal processes and social interaction shape

language. Language is learned through multifaceted interaction, i.e., experiences (Soyalp, 2022).

- *Learning is enriched by challenge but hindered by threat:* When the brain is challenged at an appropriate level, it can exert effort to learn, i.e., learn better, but when there are negative emotions such as intense anxiety or fear, the brain's perception process is negatively affected.
- *Every brain is unique:* Even though different people are exposed to the same stimuli, everyone's brain perceives them differently. Therefore, even though all humans have the same brain anatomy, the perception and learning systems in their brain structures are different. Brain-based learning emphasizes the importance of understanding how the brain works and planning instruction accordingly. It also liberates children and encourages them to explore. Brain-based learning relates learning to the principles of how the brain works and emphasizes that improving brain performance has a positive effect on learning (Özkan, 2015).

According to Jensen and McConchie (2020), there are five basic elements in the brain-based learning process. These are listed as (1) context, (2) triggers, (3) processes, (4) systems, and (5) structures.

- *Context:* There are internal and external factors that influence the learning process. These factors can positively or negatively affect the learning process. For effective learning, internal (motivation) and external (classroom temperature, lighting, and ventilation) conditions must be provided (Jensen and McConchie, 2020).
- *Triggers:* These are internal or external stimuli that initiate the learning process. Internal triggers originate from mental processes such as memory, while external triggers include hearing a sound, asking a question in class, or listening to music (Ritchey et al., 2016).
- *Processes:* involve the activation of specific mechanisms in the brain. Learning is the process of forming new connections between neurons (Oakes, 2017).
- *Systems:* The learning process occurs through the coordinated work of multiple systems. For example, the digestive and nervous systems can work together. Teachers need to be familiar with these processes and guide children accordingly (Anderson et al., 2018).
- *Structures:* The brain is composed of structures that perform a variety of functions. Multiple systems and structures interact within the brain and body.

Brain-based learning has been of interest for many years, particularly in the field of neuroscience. Many educators and researchers have investigated the benefits of brain-based learning. Brain-based learning is child-centered. Children are individuals who think about, investigate, and critique how and why they learn. In the brain-based learning process, children establish connections between what they have just learned and what they have learned previously, and share their knowledge, experiences, and life stories. They learn to collaborate in groups and fulfill their responsibilities (Murniati, et. al., 2023). They prepare questions about topics that interest them and conduct research while seeking answers to these questions, thus learning by asking questions. They enjoy researching issues they are interested in in depth and share their research findings with the class. They learn to control their emotions and share their feelings. They produce metaphors related to the topics they research. Their self-assessment skills develop, enabling them to take responsibility for their learning (Morett et. al. 2021).

The Application of Brain-Based Learning in Educational Environments from a Neuropedagogical Perspective

Brain-based learning is different from traditional education. The educational program, classroom environment, classroom management and organization, techniques and methods used by teachers, assessment processes, and the role of the child in the learning process are different from traditional education (Caine and Caine, 2002). Its most important feature is that it is child-centered. In brain-based learning, children learn to work both individually and in groups. In this approach, factors such as adequate nutrition and water intake, movement, and clean air are also important. Children must be adequately and balanced in their nutrition, drink water frequently, and classrooms must be well ventilated. Water and oxygen are the most important factors for learning. This is because when the water content in the blood decreases, the salt content increases, which leads to high blood pressure and stress. Similarly, low levels of oxygen and glucose in the blood cause fatigue and sleepiness, making effective learning impossible. Breitenstein et. al (2021) emphasised the important role of sleep in cognitive development processes such as memory, attention, synaptic pruning and emotional regulation. Wang et al. (2024) found that physical activity positively affects children's mental health and cognitive performance.

Another factor that is effective in learning is movement (Shabatat & Al-Tarawneh, 2016). According to Jensen (2005), movement motivates children and facilitates learning. Therefore, children need to engage in activities such as walking, stretching, and relaxing before an activity. Music and drama activities are recommended, especially when working with younger age groups. Children should also be allowed to move around during activities. In their research, Pacherero et al. (2025) examined the impact of physical activity on the cognitive development of pre-school children, concluding that movement is crucial for the development of executive functions, attention and memory.

Environmental factors play an essential role in brain-based learning. The classroom environment, temperature, lighting, colors, and materials used in the environment should be planned to impact the learning process positively. Classroom walls should be painted in colors that stimulate the mind, and visual stimuli (pictures, posters, graphics, etc.) and objects should be designed, without any distracting materials (Özkan, 2015). Teachers should make the classroom environment suitable for children both emotionally and physically. The classroom environment must be prepared in a way that is suitable for the way the brain works. Children must also be able to move around comfortably in the classroom.

Another critical point is that children must be able to see each other. Negative behaviors such as threats and bullying should never be allowed in the classroom. A brain-based classroom environment that facilitates learning was stated by Afshari (2025) to be effective in his research conducted in Iran. The classroom environment needs to be safe and peaceful. This is because when children feel tense, their adrenal glands release cortisol, which makes learning difficult. High cortisol levels hurt brain cells. At the same time, stress also lowers serotonin levels. Known as the happiness hormone, serotonin directly affects a person's mood, memory, and sleep patterns. Therefore, low serotonin is undesirable in terms of learning. It is also essential for teachers to understand children's emotions and provide education accordingly in brain-based learning. Therefore, teachers should plan learning activities that include relaxation exercises to reduce stress in situations that may cause anxiety, such as exams, and teach children to control their emotions. They should also prevent situations that may cause stress. For example, trying to force a child to do something they do not want to do (Duman, 2028; Özkan & Önder, 2021).

In brain-based learning, teacher activities should be planned according to the age and developmental characteristics of children. Again, when determining the duration of activities, children's developmental characteristics should be taken into account. Planned activities should support children's sensory development. The more senses an activity appeals to, the more information is processed in the brain. Teachers should help children individualize the information they are given. Children should be able to relate the information they are provided to their own experiences (Olofin & Olojo, 2022). Activities should allow children sufficient time and should incorporate holistic teaching. They should plan activities that support multiple intelligences and guide children in presentation and design. Teachers should not ask, *"What can I teach?"* but rather, *"How does the brain learn best?"* It is also essential for teachers to adopt brain-based learning and possess creative thinking skills (Soyalp, 2022). Değirmenci (2021) found a significant relationship between preschool teachers' creative thinking tendencies and their attitudes towards brain-based learning.

Music, drama, and mind mapping are some of the practical techniques used in brain-based learning. It is a well-known fact that music is an essential educational tool. Music affects not only children's emotional state but also their cognitive learning. Therefore, it should be used frequently, especially in the preschool period. Music causes several changes in brain functions. When children engage with music, they relax mentally, and their neurons and synapses become active. Music helps children develop their attention skills and enables them to see, hear, and act more quickly (Başdüvenci Kahya, 2023). Lu et al. (2025) found that music education positively affects inhibitory control, working memory and cognitive flexibility in three- to six-year-old preschool children.

Although brain-based learning is widely recognised as important in education, the widespread use of digital tools today creates some limitations (Çakmak et.al 2022). The abundance of moving images and sounds in these tools distracts children and hinders their learning (Cadena et. al.2020). According to Hutton et al. (2020), excessive use of digital tools during the preschool period negatively affects children's social, emotional and cognitive development, preventing them from reaping the benefits of these tools.

Celemete-Suarez et al. (2024) stated in their research that, while digital media can offer innovative learning experiences, excessive consumption can have negative effects on physical health, cognitive abilities and language development. The researchers also emphasised the importance of parent-child interaction in mitigating the impact of digital devices on children's cognitive and psychological development.

Brain-Based Learning and Assessment

The overall purpose of assessment is to determine the level of learning. Assessment in brain-based learning differs from traditional assessment methods. Children need to apply what they have learned in their daily lives. At the end of the learning process, both the child and the teacher conduct an assessment. In particular, children are encouraged to assess themselves and perceive their situation. The tools used in assessment should encourage children to think. (Soyalp, 2022). Assessment tools such as forms, portfolios, scoring guidelines, and development files that allow children to conduct group and peer assessments should also be used. Observation forms, portfolios, and development files are more commonly used in the preschool period. Verbal assessment is also preferred in brain-based learning. In a verbal assessment, the child's level of learning is determined by asking them questions. In addition to individual assessments, collaborative learning is also assessed (Can, 2025).

In assessment, children are not expected to give direct answers but to think and find the answers themselves. For example, asking children to draw a picture of a heart is not as effective as asking them to make a heart out of Play-Doh. Teachers should not make children feel that they are being assessed. In this situation, the child may become stressed, and the teacher may not be able to make an accurate assessment (Noureen, 2017; Polat, 2014). Teachers should be well aware of each child's learning style and take individual differences into account when making assessments. Again, they should not forget that every child's emotional development is different. The goal should always be to bring out the strengths of children. Children should be given feedback promptly, and they should also be allowed to provide feedback to each other. Play must be included in the learning and assessment process, and children should be assessed holistically (Özkan & Önder, 2021).

For an accurate assessment to be made, children must be taught correctly. It is essential to have an appropriate learning environment and to learn at the right time. Children's attention spans should be taken into account, and more difficult topics should be taught in the first hours. Fun techniques and methods should be used in the teaching process, and children should be allowed to move around between activities. Repetitions should be included after activities (Doğanay & Tok, 2012; Strickland, 2003).

The effectiveness of brain-based neuropedagogical interventions is generally evaluated using measurement approaches that encompass behavioural, cognitive, emotional, and neurophysiological dimensions of learning (Llana et. al., 2022). A child's cognitive processes, such as working memory, executive functions, attention, and problem-solving skills, are assessed using neuropsychological tests and standardised cognitive assessment scales (Frei-Landau et.al., 2023; Stang, 2022). Learning and academic performance are evaluated using behavioural measurements, and the impact of emotions on learning is assessed through attitude and self-efficacy questionnaires, as well as anxiety, motivation, and stress level measurements. The effect of the intervention on brain activity and neural processes is examined using brain-based measurements such as electroencephalography (EEG) and autonomic nervous system markers. Furthermore, evaluations can be conducted through structured classroom observations, teacher and child interviews, and case studies (Caine & Caine, 2002; Özkan, Önder, 2021; Volpicelli & Miniaci, 2024).

Brain-Based Learning in Preschool Education

The stimuli provided to children in the preschool period are significant for their brain development. In particular, children in this period need to have adequate and balanced nutrition and appropriate environmental conditions. Many children do not have regular eating habits at this age. However, in brain-based learning, it is recommended that healthy eating habits be instilled in children from an early age. It is also emphasized that children should drink water regularly, exercise, and have a regular sleep schedule. According to the brain-based learning approach, preschool education institutions should offer breakfast with a healthy menu. Children should be encouraged to drink water frequently, and classrooms should be ventilated (Polat, Akay & Aydın, 2021).

When planning activities for preschool children, their characteristics must be taken into account, and activities should be planned to support brain development. The more senses are stimulated during activities, the more information the brain processes. Therefore, children should be encouraged to explore and have their curiosity aroused. Information should be conveyed to children by relating it to real-life experiences. For example, if information about birds is being provided, children should also be allowed to observe birds. Outdoor trips and walks are essential for both the physical and mental development of children. Therefore, outdoor activities should be prioritized. In addition, children should be able to use the information they learn in real life (Aydın et al., 2012; Duman, 2018).

During activities, children should be encouraged to ask questions. They should find the answers themselves by asking questions. But most importantly, they should feel safe in the classroom environment. In a learning environment free of stress and anxiety, children participate in activities with enthusiasm and enjoyment and are more comfortable asking questions. Play is the most effective tool for preschool children. Brain-based activities should be combined with play when planning activities. Other techniques such as music, drama, stories, and tales should also be used. Materials that support the development of multiple senses should be available in the classroom. Children should discover the materials themselves, and the materials should be explained to them when needed. The temperature, lighting, and color scheme of the classroom should also be suitable for children (Özkan, 2015; Schiller and Willis, 2008).

Brain-based learning is also the most critical task of the teacher. Teachers should be well aware of the principles of brain-based learning. They should be mindful of each child's learning style. They should also guide children to find their learning styles. Activities should be planned and organized in a structured manner. The teacher should never use direct instruction but instead employ techniques such as mind maps, drama, music, storytelling, videos, question-and-answer sessions, and science and nature activities (Başdüvenci Kahya, 2023). For example, a picture can be shown to introduce the topic, thereby sparking the children's curiosity. Again, real-life examples can be used, and group work involving steps such as designing, finding, and explaining can be carried out. After the work, children should present what they have learned to their friends and share their opinions. Finally, they should end the day on a positive note. For example, activities such as dancing to music or playing games outdoors. Therefore, the most important thing in brain-based learning is the teacher's knowledge, attitude, and behavior. A teacher who gives positive feedback to children, understands their feelings, and can guide them correctly is very important (Duman, 2018; Sözer Çapan, 2014).

Brain-based learning plays a significant role in education. However, it can sometimes be misinterpreted, resulting in neuromyths. These are beliefs about the brain that are not based on scientific evidence. They arise from the incorrect or incomplete interpretation of scientific research results without thorough testing (Ching et. al., 2020). Definitive statements about the functioning of the right and left hemispheres of the brain, such as the claim that children interested in art are 'right-brained' or those who like mathematics are 'left-brained', are examples of neuromyths. However, both sides of the brain work together during the learning process (Torrijos et. al., 2020). Therefore, neuromyths that limit brain function can lead to misunderstandings about brain-based learning. Examples of such beliefs include the idea that the brain develops more quickly if it is stimulated in early childhood and that learning styles (visual, auditory, etc.) are fixed and unchanging

However, rather than overstimulating the brain, the correct approach is to provide high-quality stimuli. Furthermore, learning styles are not fixed or immutable (Garcia & Thompson, 2022; Gola et. al., 2022). The brain learns more easily when multiple senses (sight, hearing, touch and movement) are engaged. Therefore, teachers should plan activities that engage the senses and use more than one learning style. For example, they could use movement, music, and drama together in storytelling. Consequently, neuromyths can lead to incorrect practices and misguided approaches in education. Teachers therefore need to be aware of this issue (Boon, 2024; Herzberg, 2023).

Advantages and Limitations of Brain-based Learning from a Neuropedagogical Perspective in the Preschool Period

The preschool period is a critical time when the brain's ability to adapt to the environment and restructure itself is at its highest. During this period, children are highly sensitive to environmental stimuli (Papanastasiou et.al., 2017). While brain-based learning in the preschool period offers significant advantages in terms of a child's neuropedagogical development, it also brings some limitations and disadvantages. Brain-based learning supports neuroplasticity, enabling the formation of more and stronger synaptic connections in the child's brain. It also enhances higher-order thinking skills and improves learning retention. It supports children's development in multiple ways, ensuring simultaneous advancement of motor skills, social-emotional development and cognitive abilities. Children can apply the knowledge they gain during the learning process to their daily lives (Jolles & Jolles, 2021; Nievas & Montes, 2023). It lays the groundwork for a high-quality learning environment by increasing intrinsic motivation and focusing on individual differences. However, it also has some limitations alongside its advantages. For brain-based learning to be effectively implemented, teachers need to have a detailed knowledge of neuroscience and brain physiology. Teachers may struggle with issues such as adapting materials and the classroom atmosphere to reflect brain function, and may also experience difficulties in planning and implementing extracurricular activities. The need to constantly consider the individual physiological condition, interests, and needs of each child also increases the teachers' observation and evaluation burden. Brain-based learning requires a flexible program, which can make integration into existing education systems difficult. Furthermore, planning activities is time-consuming, leading to delays in covering all topics. This can cause even greater problems in classrooms with large student numbers (Boon, 2024 ; Holmes & Porayska-Pomsta, 2022).

CONCLUSION

The first years of life are of great importance because they form the foundation of an individual's development, and basic knowledge and skills are acquired during this period. One of the areas of development that shows rapid progress during this period is brain development. The brain is a fundamental organ that controls all organs in the body and directs learning processes, emotions, and thoughts. Technological advances have enabled the use of different imaging techniques to study brain development and have contributed significantly to scientific research. In this context, studies have revealed that the cognitive abilities and maturity of children in different age groups are related to brain development. It is stated that a baby's brain contains 100 billion brain cells (neurons) at birth, 10-15% of which are nerve cells (neurons) that enable learning and thinking. At the same time, the rest are auxiliary cells called glia that perform cleaning and nutrition functions. It is stated that brain development is rapid before and after birth, that this rapid growth and development is called the brain's growth spurt, and that the brain's growth spurt continues until the age of four. For the brain to develop and for the network of connections between neurons to form, children need environmental stimuli and experiences. In this context, as children interact with their environment and form secure bonds with their parents or caregivers, connections between neurons are formed, and brain development is positively supported. The number of connections between brain cells is closely related to the stimuli the child receives from the environment and environmental conditions. In this context, the brain development of children who are neglected and do not receive sufficient stimuli is negatively affected. This is because a child's brain development occurs through the presentation and repetition of new stimuli. Therefore, brain development plays a key role in a child's development. During specific periods of life, learning processes, in which thinking patterns, research, and discovery are important, take place in different ways. In this context, differences are seen in learning, information processing, and thinking patterns in infancy, childhood, and adulthood. The comprehensive structure of neuropedagogy explains all these situations. Neuropedagogy is a multidisciplinary field that takes into account the brain development of children in the learning process. The reason for its interdisciplinary nature is that it focuses on the holistic development of the individual by integrating the fields of psychology, neuroscience, and education. Neuropedagogy studies different areas of the brain, such as mirror neurons, the limbic system, and the prefrontal cortex. Emotional intelligence, motivation, and behavioral responses, which are among the most important areas of psychology, are also among the most critical areas of interest in neuropedagogy. Unlike traditional teaching models, neuropedagogy focuses on the individual's learning style, educational needs, and ability to progress at their own pace, thereby contributing to the maximum utilization of their potential. From this perspective, neuropedagogy takes learning out of the realm of a mere state and focuses on the psychological and physiological issues that support or hinder learning. In this context, neuropedagogy studies how the brain works to create an effective educational environment for children both in and out of school. It investigates the relationship between brain development and education. Brain-based learning, on the other hand, aims to create an effective learning process by studying how the brain works. Therefore, neuropedagogy is a broader concept than brain-based learning. Neuropedagogy provides the necessary information for scientifically based learning environments by relating children's psychological and cognitive development to neurophysiology. Brain-based learning, on the other hand, transfers this information to the classroom environment. However, the most crucial role in this regard falls on teachers. Teachers must have a thorough understanding of the principles of brain-based learning and be able to guide children accordingly.

REFERENCES

Afshari, A. (2025). The effectiveness of brain-compatible learning on academic self-concept and academic self-efficacy. *Avicenna Journal of Neuropsychophysiology, 11*(4), 146–152. DOI: 10.32592/ajnpp.2024.11.4.146

Alpar, M., & Topan, R. (2016). *Brain-based learning in foreign language instruction for children.* Gazi Publishing House.

Anderson, A. A., Parsa, K., Geiger, S., Zaragoza, R., Kermanian, R., Miguel, H., & Gandjbakhche, A. H. (2018). Exploring the role of task performance and learning style on prefrontal hemodynamics during a working memory task. *PLoS One, 13*(6), 1–16. DOI: 10.1371/journal.pone.0198257 PMID: 29870536

Ansari, D., & Coch, D. (2006). Bridges over troubled waters: Education and cognitive neuroscience. *Trends in Cognitive Sciences, 10*(4), 146–151. DOI: 10.1016/j.tics.2006.02.007 PMID: 16530462

Ansari, D., Coch, D., & De Smedt, B. (2011). Connecting education and cognitive neuroscience: Where will the journey take us? *Educational Philosophy and Theory,* Ansari, D., De Smedt, B., & *Grabner, R. H. (2012).* Neuroeducation - A Critical overview of an emerging field. *Neuroethics, 5*(2), 105–117. DOI: 10.1007/s12152-011-9119-3

Aydın, O., Madi, B., & Alpanda, S., & Sazcı, A. (2012). Neurodevelopmental evaluation of the MEB Preschool Education Program from a Neurodevelopmental Perspective. *M. Ü. Atatürk Faculty of Education Faculty of Educational Sciences Journal, 36*, 69–93.

Barbey, A. K., Koenigs, M., & Grafman, J. (2013). Dorsolateral prefrontal contributions to human working memory. *Cortex, 49*(5), 1195–1205. DOI: 10.1016/j.cortex.2012.05.022 PMID: 22789779

Başdüvenci Kahya, İ. (2023). *Music teachers' awareness levels regarding brain-based learning approaches and their reflection in music teaching practices.* Master's thesis. Marmara University.

Bendriyanti, R. P., Setyawan, A., Kurniasih, N., & Citrawati, T. (2024). Integrating neuroeducation into educational management: A breakthrough for enhancing elementary education. *BIO Web of Conferences,* 146, 01098. https://doi.org/DOI: 10.1051/bioconf/202414601098

Bissonette, G. B., & Roesch, M. (2015). Neurophysiology of reward-guided behavior: Correlates related to predictions, value, motivation, errors, attention, and action. *Current Topics in Behavioral Neurosciences*, *27*(1), 199–230. DOI: 10.1007/7854_2015_382 PMID: 26276036

Bonoma, V. (2017). Brain-based learning theory. *Journal of Education and Human Development.*, *6*(1), 27–43.

Boon, S. (2024). Brain-based learning: understanding how the brain shapes education. *Int. J. School Cognit. Psychol.* 11-380. doi: DOI: 10.35248/2469-9837.24.11.380

Breitenstein, R. S., Hoyniak, C. P., McQuillan, M. E., & Bates, J. E. (2021). Sleep and self- regulation in early childhood. *Advances in Child Development and Behavior*, *60*, 111–137. DOI: 10.1016/bs.acdb.2020.08.007 PMID: 33641790

Caballero, M., & Llorent, V. J. (2022). The effects of a teacher training program on neuroeducation in improving reading, mathematical, social, emotional, and moral competencies of secondary school students: A two-year quasi-experimental study. *Revista de Psicodidáctica (English Ed.),* 27(2), 158–167. https://doi.org/DOI: 10.1016/j.psicoe.2022.04.002

Cadena, K. A. Á., Alvarado, K. G. M., Asacata, D. E. P., & Chong, M. K. (2020). Tiempo en pantalla (televisión, computadora, celular, tabletas) en las relaciones interpersonales entre niños de 8 a 12 años. *Horiz. Rev. Investig. En Cienc. Educ.*, *4*, 258–266.

Caine, R. & Caine, G. (2002). *Brain-based learning*. Trans. G. Ülgen. Nobel Publishing

Caine, R. N., Caine, R. N., McClintic, C., & Klimek, K. J. (2016). 12 Brain/ Mind Learning Principles in Action. https://doi.org/. Access URL: https://sk .sagepub.com/book/mono/12-brain-mind-learning-principles-in-action-3e/tocDOI: 10.4135/9781483394275

Çakmak, Z., Akgün, İ. H., & Salur, M. (2022). Beyin temelli öğrenme ile ilgili akademik çalışmalarin incelenmesi. *Uluslararası Türkçe Edebiyat Kültür Eğitim (TEKE). Dergisi*, *11*(4), 1766–1784.

Camina, E., & Guell, F. (2017). The neuroanatomical, neurophysiological, and psychological basis of memory: Current models and their origins. *Frontiers in Pharmacology*, *8*(438), 1–16. DOI: 10.3389/fphar.2017.00438 PMID: 28713278

Can, S. (2025). *Development of a brain-based learning-oriented second-grade teaching program for physical education and games.* Master's thesis. Mugla Sıçkı Koçman University.

Ching, F. N. Y., So, W. W. M., Lo, S. K., & Wong, S. W. H. (2020). Preservice teachers' neuroscience literacy and perceptions of neuroscience in education: Implications for teacher education. *Trends in Neuroscience and Education, 21*, 1–9. DOI: 10.1016/j.tine.2020.100144 PMID: 33303109

Değirmenci, B. S. (2021). *The relationship between preschool teachers' creative thinking tendencies and brain-based learning.* Master's thesis. Uskudar University.

Doğan, H. (2021). Brain and sensory development in children. In *Neuropedagogy, Children, and the Brain* (pp. 40-55). Ed. (G. Güven, M. N. Tuğluk, B. Özkan). Hedef Publishing.

Doğanay, A., & Tok, G. (2012). *Principles and Methods of Teaching.* In A. Doğanay (Ed.), Brain Learning. A. Doğanay (Ed.), Brain-Based Learning (pp. 304-317). Ankara: Pegem.

Doidge, N. (2007). *The brain that changes itself: Stories of personal triumph from the Frontiers of Brain Science.* Penguin.

Duman, A. (2018). *The effect of cognitive activities included in the preschool education program based on brain-based learning on in a preschool education program in terms of their impact on readiness for elementary school.* Master's Master's thesis. Selçuk University.

Duman, B. (2015). *Why Brain-Based Learning?* Pegem Publishing.

Farmer-Dougan, V., & Alferink, L. A. (2013). Brain development, early childhood, and brain-based education: a critical analysis. In Wasserman, L. H., & Zambo, D. (Eds.), *Educating the Young Child 7: Early Childhood and Neuroscience—Links to Development and Learning* (pp. 55–76). Springer. DOI: 10.1007/978-94-007-6671-6_5

Frei-Landau, R., Grobgeld, E., & Guberman, R. (2023). Implementing digital neuroscience in special-needs-teacher education: Exploring student-teachers' multifaceted learning outcomes related to teaching children with neurodevelopmental disorders. *Frontiers in Psychology, 14*, 1232315. DOI: 10.3389/fpsyg.2023.1232315 PMID: 37599772

Garcia, M., & Thompson, R. (2022). Neuroeducation: Bridging neuroscience and education for effective teaching practices. *Educ. Neurosci. Rev., 10*, 115–130. DOI: 10.1080/1234567890123456

García, M. T. M. (2024). Bridging the gap: Leveraging neuroeducation to enhance teaching methodologies. *Korea TESOL Journal, 20*(2). https://koreatesol.org/sites/default/files/pdf_publications/20241227_%EC%A0%80%EB%84%90%2020_2_%ED%91%9C%EC%A7%80%ED%8F%AC%ED%95%A8.pdf#page=13

Gerdes, J., Durden, T. R., & Poppe, L. M. (2013). *Brain development and learning in the primary years.* G2198. Faculty Publications from CYFS. 77.

Gerdes, L., Tegeler, C. H., & Lee, S. W. (2015). A groundwork for allostatic neuro-education. *Frontiers in Psychology*, *6*. Advance online publication. DOI: 10.3389/fpsyg.2015.01224 PMID: 26347688

Gola, G., Angioletti, L., Cassioli, F., & Balconi, M. (2022). The teaching brain: Beyond the science of teaching and educational neuroscience. *Frontiers in Psychology*, *13*, 823832. DOI: 10.3389/fpsyg.2022.823832 PMID: 35356321

Goswami, U. (2004). Neuroscience and education. *The British Journal of Educational Psychology*, *74*(1), 1–14. DOI: 10.1348/000709904322848798 PMID: 15096296

Güven, G. (2021). Brain structure and nervous system. *In Neuropedagogy, children, and the brain* (pp. 10-26). Ed. (G. Güven, M. N. Tuğluk, B. Özkan). Hedef Publishing.

Halmotov, S., & Halmotov, M. (2022). *Neuropedagogy in working with children: A neuropedagogical support program. Pegem Publishing*. Pegem Publishing.

Holmes, W., & Porayska-Pomsta, K. (2022). Advances in educational neuroscience: How AI and neuroimaging inform personalized learning. *J. Educ. Neurosci.*, *14*, 1–15. DOI: 10.1177/153574002211414

Hutton, J. S., Dudley, J., Horowitz-Kraus, T., DeWitt, T., & Holland, S. K. (2020). Differences in functional brain network connectivity during stories presented in audio, illustrated, and animated format in preschool-age children. *Brain Imaging and Behavior*, *14*(1), 130–141. DOI: 10.1007/s11682-018-9985-y PMID: 30377932

Jensen, E. (2005). *Teaching with the brain in mind.* ASCD.

Jensen, E., & McConchie, L. (2020). *Brain-based learning: Teaching the way students learn.* SAGE Publications Ltd.

Jolles, J., & Jolles, D. (2021). On neuroeducation: Why and how to improve neuroscientific literacy in educational professionals. *Frontiers in Psychology*, *12*, 752151. DOI: 10.3389/fpsyg.2021.752151 PMID: 34925156

Köksal, N. (2024). *Brain-Based Learning.* Ed. Ö. Demirel. *New Directions in Education. Directions in education* (pp. 113-123). Pegem Publishing.

Llana, T., Fernandez-Baizan, C., Mendez-Lopez, M., Fidalgo, C., & Mendez, M. (2022). Functional near-infrared spectroscopy in the neuropsychological assessment of spatial memory: A systematic review. *Acta Psychologica, 224*, 103525. https://doi.org/, Y., Shi, L., & Musib, A.F. (2025) Effects of music training on executive functions in preschool children aged 3–6 years: systematic review and meta-analysis. *Front. Psychol.* 15:1522962. https://doi.org/DOI: 10.1016/j.actpsy.2022.103525Lu

Madi, B. (2014). *How does learning occur in the brain?* Efil Publishing.

Maryati, S. S., Purwanti, I., & Mubarika, M. P. (2020). The effect of brain-based learning on improving students' critical thinking ability and self-regulation. *Indonesian Journal of Integrated Science Education*, *2*(2), 162–171. DOI: 10.29300/ijisedu.v2i2.3333

Morett, L.M., Morett, L.M., & Hawes, Z., & Dommett, E.J. (2021). Educational neuroscience needs educational and school psychology to translate neuroscience into educational practice effectively. *Frontiers in Psychology, 11*(618449), 1–7. PMID: 33519642

Murniati, N., Susilo, H., & Listyorini, D. (2023). Retention achievement in brain-based whole learning is supported by students' scientific literacy and concept mastery. *Pegem Journal of Education and Instruction, 13*(3), 294–303. DOI: 10.47750/pegegog.13.03.30

Nievas, F., & Montes, M. (2023). Adapting pedagogical strategies through interdisciplinary neuroeducation: Meeting individual learning needs. *J. Educ. Psychol.*, *115*, 304–317. DOI: 10.1037/edu0000586

Noureen, G., Awan, R. N., & Fatima, H. (2017). Effect of brain-based learning on academic achievement of seventh graders in mathematics. *Journal of Elementary Education*, *27*(2), 85–97.

Oakes, L. M. (2017). Plasticity may change inputs as well as processes, structures, and responses. *Cognitive Development*, *42*, 4–14. DOI: 10.1016/j.cogdev.2017.02.012 PMID: 28993717

Olofin, S. O., & Olojo, O. J. (2022). Effect of brain-based strategy on senior secondary school students' performance in mathematics in Ekiti State. *International Journal of Education, Learning and Development*, *10*(2), 1–15. DOI: 10.37745/ijeld.13/vol10no2pp.1-15

Özkan, B. (2015). *Development of a scientific process skills scale for children aged 60-72 months and the effect of a brain-based learning science program on scientific process skills.* Master's thesis. Marmara University.

Özkan, B., & Önder, A. (2021). Brain-based learning in children. *Neuropedagogy in Children and the Brain* (pp. 148-155). Ed. (G. Güven, M. N. Tuğluk, B. Özkan). Hedef Publishing.

Papanastasiou, G. P., Drigas, A. S., & Skianis, C. (2017). Serious games in preschool and primary education: Benefits and impacts on curriculum course syllabus. *International Journal of Emerging Technologies in Learning, 12*(1), 44. Advance online publication. DOI: 10.3991/ijet.v12i01.6065

Perry, B. D. (2002). Childhood experience and the expression of genetic potential: What childhood neglect tells us about nature and nurture. *Brain and Mind, 3*(1), 79–100. DOI: 10.1023/A:1016557824657

Polat, Ö., Akay, D., & Aydın, E. (2021). Examination of the Ministry of National Education's 2013 preschool education program from the perspective of brain-based learning. Brain-based learning approach. *National Education Journal, 50*(229), 419–444.

Ritchey, M., Murty, V. P., & Dunsmoor, J. E. (2016). Adaptive memory systems for remembering the salient and the seemingly mundane. *Behavioral and Brain Sciences, 39*, 1–75. DOI: 10.1017/S0140525X15001922 PMID: 28347387

Shabatat, K., & Al-Tarawneh, M. (2016). The impact of a teaching-learning program based on a brain-based learning program on the achievement of female students in 9th grade in chemistry. *Higher Education Studies, 6*(2), 162–173. DOI: 10.5539/hes.v6n2p162

Sharma, A. (2024). Effectiveness of brain-based learning strategy using blended mode of teaching elementary school science students. *Educational Administration: Theory and Practice, 30*(4), 7294–7296. DOI: 10.53555/kuey.v30i4.2556

Sousa, D. A. (2011). *How the brain learns*. Corwin Press. DOI: 10.4135/9781452219684

Soyalp, T. (2022). *The effect of brain-based learning theory on the achievement and attitudes of 8th-grade students in science education. Master's thesis. Gazi University.* Master's thesis. Gazi University.

Sözer Çapan, A. (2014). *An investigation of the effect of an education program prepared according to the brain-based learning approach on the creativity skills of 5-year- old children*. Doctoral thesis. Marmara University.

Stang, K. (2022). *Brain-based learning methods and student achievement*. Master's thesis. Bethel University.

Stevens Smith, D. A. (2020). Brain-based teaching: Differentiation in teaching, learning, and motor skills. *Journal of Physical Education, Recreation & Dance, 91*(7), 34–42. DOI: 10.1080/07303084.2020.1781717

Strickland, K. (2003). *Brain-compatible learning in a high school classroom.* Master's thesis, Royal Roads University, British Columbia. Thesis, Royal Roads University, British Columbia.

Tanrıdağ, O. (2018). *The development of the child's brain.* Üsküdar University Publications.

Volpicelli, F., & Miniaci, M. C. (2024). Dopaminergic pathways and their impact on learning and motivation in educational contexts. *Biomedicines, 15*, 210–230. DOI: 10.1038/nrn1406

Wang, J., Yang, Y., Li, L., Yang, X., Guo, X., Yuan, X., Xie, T., Yang, K., & Zhuang, J. (2024). Comparative efficacy of physical activity types on executive functions in children and adolescents: A network meta-analysis of randomized controlled trials. *Journal of Science and Medicine in Sport, 27*(3), 187–196. DOI: 10.1016/j.jsams.2023.11.006 PMID: 38042755

Compilation of References

Abadzi, H. (2006). *Efficient learning for the poor.* The World Bank eBooks. https://doi.org/DOI: 10.1596/978-0-8213-6688-2

Abdul-Fattah, H. M. (2010). Semantic extension of loanwords in Jordanian Arabic. *SKASE Journal of Theoretical Linguistics*, *7*(1), 14–26.

Aboo Backer, M. B., & Manoharan, P. (2022). The Wayang and its enchanting little puppeteers: Exploring cognitive abilities of cerebral palsy children through performance. *Jurnal Gendang Alam (GA)*, *12*(1), 83–100. DOI: 10.51200/ga.v12i1.1930

Abu-Ras, W., Al-Kubaisi, A., Idris, L. B., & Aboul-Enein, B. H. (2025). The Role of Puppetry in Mental Health Promotion: A Scoping Review of its Efficacy and Applications. *The Arts in Psychotherapy*, *92*, 102251. Advance online publication. DOI: 10.1016/j.aip.2025.102251

AÇEV. (2018). *Faaliyet raporu 2018.* Anne Çocuk Eğitim Vakfı.

AÇEV. (2021). *Erken çocukluk programları etki analizi raporu.* Anne Çocuk Eğitim Vakfı.

AÇEV. (2023). *Faaliyet raporu 2023.* Anne Çocuk Eğitim Vakfı.

Adolphs, R. (2001). The neurobiology of social cognition. *Current Opinion in Neurobiology*, *11*(2), 231–239. DOI: 10.1016/S0959-4388(00)00202-6

Afshari, A. (2025). The effectiveness of brain-compatible learning on academic self-concept and academic self-efficacy. *Avicenna Journal of Neuropsychophysiology*, *11*(4), 146–152. DOI: 10.32592/ajnpp.2024.11.4.146

Ahmedova, M. T., & Narmetova, Y. K. (2022). Neuropedagogy and neyropsychology how developing New Nauka. *Society and innovations Special*, (02), 2181-1415.

Ahr, E. (2016). La lecture et le fonctionnement du cerveau pour une « neuropédagogie » de la lecture. *Administration & Éducation, 152*(4), 17–23. DOI: 10.3917/admed.152.0017

Ai, H., & Hu, J. (2014). Psychological resilience moderates the impact of social support on loneliness of "left-behind" children. *Journal of Health Psychology, 21*(6), 1066–1073. DOI: 10.1177/1359105314544992 PMID: 25139895

Aithal, P. S., Prabhu, S., & Aithal, S. (2024). Future of higher education through technology prediction and forecasting. SSRN *Electronic Journal.* https://doi.org/ DOI: 10.2139/ssrn.4901474

Aksu, G., Güzeller, C. O., & Eser, M. T.AKSU. (2019). The Effect of the Normalization Method Used in Different Sample Sizes on the Success of Artificial Neural Network Model. *International Journal of Assessment Tools in Education, 6*(2), 170–192. DOI: 10.21449/ijate.479404

Al-Azawei, A., Serenelli, F., & Lundqvist, K. (2016). Universal design for learning (UDL): A content analysis of peer-reviewed journal papers from 2012 to 2015. *The Journal of Scholarship of Teaching and Learning, 16*(3), 39–56. DOI: 10.14434/josotl.v16i3.19295

Al-Balhan, E. M., Khabbache, H., Watfa, A., Re, T. S., Zerbetto, R., & Bragazzi, N. L. (2018). Psychometric evaluation of the arabic version of the nomophobia questionnaire: Confirmatory and exploratory factor analysis – Implications from a pilot study in Kuwait among university students. *Psychology Research and Behavior Management, 11*, 471–482. DOI: 10.2147/PRBM.S169918 PMID: 30425594

Al-Batal, M. (1992). Diglossia proficiency: The need for an alternative approach to teaching. In *Georgetown University Round Table on Languages and Linguistics* (pp. 284–303). Georgetown University Press.

Albert, M. L., & Davies, M. (2018). Media use and brain development during adolescence. *Journal of the American Academy of Child & Adolescent Psychiatry.* https://pubmed.ncbi.nlm.nih.gov/29467362/

Aldred, C., & Green, J. (2019). The Preschool Autism Communication Therapy – an Evidence-Based Approach to Enhancing Early Autistic Development and Empowering Families. *Enfance, 1*(1), 119–131. DOI: 10.3917/enf2.191.0119

Alhassan, A. M. (2016). The impact of English loanwords on Arabic: A cognitive linguistic perspective. *International Journal of Linguistics, 8*(5), 15–30. DOI: 10.5296/ijl.v8i5.10028

Al-Hroub, A., & Al-Hroub, R. (2024). Empowering the Vulnerable: The Impact of SEL on Traumatized Children's Academic and Social Outcomes in Crises. *Current Psychiatry Reports*, *26*(12), 777–781. DOI: 10.1007/s11920-024-01555-8 PMID: 39523250

Alkhassawneh, S., & Al Sharif, H. (2025). Perspectives Of Brain Research (Educational Neuroscience) on the Design and Implementation of Teaching Strategies in Educational Technology. *Journal of Neuroeducation*, *5*(2), 14–24. DOI: 10.1344/joned.v5i2.47695

Al-Khatib, M. A., & Sabbah, E. S. (2008). Language choice in mobile text messages among Jordanian university students. *SKASE Journal of Theoretical Linguistics*, *5*(1), 28–42.

Allaberdieva, K. (2019). The Main Neuropedagogic Possibilities Of Formation At Children Of Senior Preschool Age Of Creative Activity. *European Journal Of Research And Reflection In Educational Sciences*, *7*, 12.

Allard, I. ABA en IME, Neuropsychiatrie de l'Enfance et de l'Adolescence, Volume 61, Issue 5,2013,Pages 295-301,ISSN 0222-9617, DOI: 10.1016/j.neurenf.2013.04.008

Alloway, T. P., & Alloway, R. G. (2013). Working memory across the lifespan: A cross-sectional approach. *Journal of Cognitive Psychology*, *25*(1), 84–93. DOI: 10.1080/20445911.2012.748027

Al-Mughirah, H. A. M., Al-Basala, A. S., & Al-Rumahi, H. M. (2025). The impact of foreign electronic games on Arabic language and culture in Saudi Arabia. *Arts for Linguistic & Literary Studies*, *7*(3), 68–87. DOI: 10.53286/arts.v7i3.2715

Alnemary, F. M., Aldhalaan, H. M., Simon-Cereijido, G., & Alnemary, F. M. (2017). Services for children with autism in Saudi Arabia. *Autism*, *21*(5), 592–602. DOI: 10.1177/1362361316664868 PMID: 28610540

Alotaibi, A., & Alzahrani, K. (2021). The effect of working memory on reading skills among middle school students. *The Journal of Educational Research*, *12*(2), 78–95.

Alpar, M., & Topan, R. (2016). *Brain-based learning in foreign language instruction for children*. Gazi Publishing House.

Al-Saqqaf, A. H. (2006). The linguistics of loanwords in Hadhrami Arabic. *International Journal of Bilingual Education and Bilingualism*, *9*(1), 75–93. DOI: 10.1080/13670050608668631

Althobaiti, A. A. T. (2024). *The Spread of English in Saudi Arabia: A Study of University Students' Attitudes and Language Use* (Doctoral dissertation, UNSW Sydney).

American Psychiatric Association. (2013). *Diagnostic and Statistical Manual of Mental Disorders* (5th ed.)., DOI: 10.1176/appi.books.9780890425596

Amrani, F., & Belyazid, S. (2021). Dyslexia and bilingualism: Challenges for Arabic-French learners in Morocco. *Journal of Language and Education*, *7*(3), 112–125.

An, J. (2025). Lexical borrowing as A Cultural Expectation in the Context of Globalization: A Case Study of Chinese President Xi Jinping's 2025 New Year Message. *International Journal of English Language Studies, 7*(1), 08-16.

Anderson, A. A., Parsa, K., Geiger, S., Zaragoza, R., Kermanian, R., Miguel, H., & Gandjbakhche, A. H. (2018). Exploring the role of task performance and learning style on prefrontal hemodynamics during a working memory task. *PLoS One*, *13*(6), 1–16. DOI: 10.1371/journal.pone.0198257 PMID: 29870536

Anderson, J. R. (1995). *Cognitive psychology and its implications* (4th ed.). W. H. Freeman and Company.

An, G. (2024). Domestication and Foreignisation in Translation Studies: A Bibliometric Analysis of WoS Core Journal Articles. *Journal of Intercultural Communication*, *24*(4), 13–22. DOI: 10.36923/jicc.v24i4.933

Ansari, D. (2012). Culture and education: New frontiers in brain plasticity. *Trends in Cognitive Sciences*, *16*(2), 93–95. DOI: 10.1016/j.tics.2011.11.016 PMID: 22206752

Ansari, D., & Coch, D. (2006). Bridges over troubled waters: Education and cognitive neuroscience. *Trends in Cognitive Sciences*, *10*(4), 146–151. DOI: 10.1016/j.tics.2006.02.007 PMID: 16530462

Ansari, D., Coch, D., & De Smedt, B. (2011). Connecting education and cognitive neuroscience: Where will the journey take us? *Educational Philosophy and Theory*, *43*(1), 37–42. DOI: 10.1111/j.1469-5812.2010.00705.x

Ansari, D., De Smedt, B., & Grabner, R. H. (2011). Neuroeducation – a critical overview of an emerging field. *Neuroethics*, *5*(2), 105–117. DOI: 10.1007/s12152-011-9119-3

Antoniuk, L., Olena, S. O. I. A., Kosovets, O., Klimishyna, A., Kovtoniuk, M., & Tryfonova, O. (2022). Ensuring the innovativeness of vocational education: Neuropedagogical aspect. *BRAIN. Broad Research in Artificial Intelligence and Neuroscience*, *13*(4), 242–263. DOI: 10.18662/brain/13.4/386

Arda, T. B., & Ocak, S. (2012). Social Competence and Promoting Alternative Thinking Strategies—PATHS Preschool Curriculum. *Educational Sciences: Theory & Practice*, *12*(4), 2691–2698.

Arens, A. K., Becker, M., & Möller, J. (2017). Social and dimensional comparisons in math and verbal test anxiety: Within- and cross-domain relations with achievement and the mediating role of academic self-concept. *Contemporary Educational Psychology*, *51*(August), 240–252. DOI: 10.1016/j.cedpsych.2017.08.005

Armstrong, R. A. (2019). Should Pearson's correlation coefficient be avoided? *Ophthalmic & Physiological Optics*, *39*(5), 316–327. DOI: 10.1111/opo.12636 PMID: 31423624

Arum, Y. P. (2025, July). Implementing Silence Pedagogy in English Language Teaching through a Neuropedagogical Approach in Indonesia. In *Proceedings of the World Conference on Foreign Language Education* (Vol. 2, No. 1, pp. 5-5).

Atkinson, R. C., & Shiffrin, R. M. (1968). Human memory: A proposed system and its control processes. In Spence, K. W., & Spence, J. T. (Eds.), *The psychology of learning and motivation: Advances in research and theory* (Vol. 2, pp. 89–195). Academic Press., DOI: 10.1016/S0079-7421(08)60422-3

Auer, P. (1998). *Code-switching in conversation: Language, interaction and identity*. Routledge.

Auliya, A., Aljanah, D. S., Sagala, R., Hijriyah, U., & Ghazi, F. (2025). The Digital Revolution in Arabic Language Learning: An Analysis of Trends, Results, and the Future of Language Education in the Digital Age. *RADEN INTAN: Proceedings on Family and Humanity*, *2*(1), 194–203. DOI: 10.47352/3032-503x.69

AV. B., & V, R. (2022). Implications of neuroscience/neuroeducation in the field of education to enhance the learning outcomes of the students. *Journal of Positive School Psychology, 6*, 6502–6510. https://www.journalppw.com/index.php/jpsp/article/view/8636

Aydın, A., & Ceylan, Ş. (2024, October). Navigating the digital world: Ethical implications of AI in early childhood education. In *VI Congreso Mundial con Infancia y Adolescencia: Educar para la felicidad* (pp. 1570–1579). Cáceres, Spain.

Aydın, O., Madi, B., & Alpanda, S., & Sazcı, A. (2012). Neurodevelopmental evaluation of the MEB Preschool Education Program from a Neurodevelopmental Perspective. *M. Ü. Atatürk Faculty of Education Faculty of Educational Sciences Journal*, *36*, 69–93.

Baarendse, P. J., Counotte, D. S., O'donnell, P., & Vanderschuren, L. J. (2013). Early social experience is critical for the development of cognitive control and dopamine modulation of prefrontal cortex function. *Neuropsychopharmacology : Official Publication of the American College of Neuropsychopharmacology, 38*(8), 1485–1494. DOI: 10.1038/npp.2013.47

Baddeley, A. (1990). *Human Memory: Theory and Practice*. Allyn and Bacon.

Baddeley, A. (2010). Working memory. *Current Biology, 20*(4), R136–R140. DOI: 10.1016/j.cub.2009.12.014

Baddeley, A. D. (1996). Exploring the central executive. *The Quarterly Journal of Experimental Psychology. A, Human Experimental Psychology, 49*(1), 5–28. DOI: 10.1080/713755608

Baddeley, A. D. (2000). The episodic buffer: A new component of working memory? *Trends in Cognitive Sciences, 4*(11), 417–423. DOI: 10.1016/S1364-6613(00)01538-2

Baddeley, A. D., & Hitch, G. J. (1974). Working memory. In Bower, G. A. (Ed.), *Recent advances in learning and motivation* (Vol. 8, pp. 47–89). Academic Press., DOI: 10.1016/S0079-7421(08)60452-1

Baddeley, A. D., & Logie, R. H. (1999). Working memory: The multiple-component model. In Miyake, A., & Shah, P. (Eds.), *Models of working memory: Mechanisms of active maintenance and executive control* (pp. 28–61). Cambridge University Press., DOI: 10.1017/CBO9781139174909.005

Bahlmann, J., Aarts, E., & D'Esposito, M. (2015). Influence of motivation on control hierarchy in the human frontal cortex. *The Journal of Neuroscience : The Official Journal of the Society for Neuroscience, 35*(7), 3207–3217. DOI: 10.1523/JNEUROSCI.2389-14.2015

Bahumaid, Showqi (2015). "Lexical Borrowing: The Case of English Loanwords in Hadhrami Arabic", *International Journal of Language and Linguistics*. Vol. 2, No. 6; December 2015

Bakhmat, N., Dzhyhun, L., Mishchenko, M., Polishchuk, O., Savytska, O., & Dorofey, S. (2023). The Neuropedagogical Aspects of Mental and Cognitive Activity in Younger School-Age Children. *BRAIN. Broad Research in Artificial Intelligence and Neuroscience, 14*(3), 182–193. DOI: 10.18662/brain/14.3/469

Balashova, E. S., Sofronova, L. V., & Stroganov, D. A. (2025). Legal and Regulatory Support of Neuropedagogy in the Russian Federation. *Russian Studies in Law and Politics, 9*(1), 29–50. DOI: 10.12731/2576-9634-2025-9-1-216

Balonyi Candal, D., & Brandão de Ávila, C. (2025). Phonological working memory and linguistic processing speed in inferential reading comprehension. *Psicologia: Reflexão e Crítica : Revista Semestral do Departamento de Psicologia da UFRGS, 38*(20), 2–16. DOI: 10.1186/s41155-025-00356-z

Bandura, A. (1977). *Social Learning Theory*. Prentice Hall.

Bang, D., Chen, J., Lapointe, R., & Naqi, S. (2012). Mind, brain, and education. *Cognitive Neuroscience*. https://etec512cognitiveneuroscience.wordpress.com/5-mind-brain-and-education/

Bangasser, D. A., & Shors, T. (2010). Critical brain circuits at the intersection between stress and learning. *Neuroscience and Biobehavioral Reviews, 34*(8), 1223–1233. DOI: 10.1016/j.neubiorev.2010.02.002

Barabanova, I., & Kazlauskiene, A. (2020). Neuropedagogy: preconditions for application of neuroscience results in the education process while providing feedback. In *Technium: Romanian journal of applied sciences and technology: Proceedings of the 5th Technium conference 2020 (18.07. 2020, Romania)*. (Vol. 2, No. 5, pp. 112-122). Technium Press.

Barba Tellez, M. N., Sotomayor, C. R., & Tobar, A. P. (2018). The Management of Neuropedagogical Processes of Learning and the Need for a Teacher Connected with Neuropedagogy. *Opuntia Brava, 10*, 648.

Barbey, A. K., Koenigs, M., & Grafman, J. (2013). Dorsolateral prefrontal contributions to human working memory. *Cortex, 49*(5), 1195–1205. DOI: 10.1016/j.cortex.2012.05.022 PMID: 22789779

Barnett, W. S., Jung, K., Yarosz, D. J., Thomas, J., Hornbeck, A., Stechuk, R., & Burns, S. (2008). Educational effects of the Tools of the Mind curriculum: A randomized trial. *Early Childhood Research Quarterly, 23*(3), 299–313. DOI: 10.1016/j.ecresq.2008.03.001

Barrim, M. (2025). The Role of memory in language processing in learner: Phonological memory and semantic memory as a model. *Atae Journal for Studies and Research, 18*, 65–81.

Barros Camargo, C. D., & Hernández Fernández, A. (2024). Neuropedagogy and neuroimaging of artificial intelligence and deep learning.

Barros, C. D., & Fernández, A. H. (2022). Neuroscience, neuroeducation, neurodidactics and technology. *Texto livre, 15*, e41235.

Barros, C. D. (2022). Neuromethodology and neuroimaging for a teacher training. *Texto Livre*, *15*, e40454. DOI: 10.35699/1983-3652.2022.40454

Barsalou, L. W. (2008). Grounded cognition. *Annual Review of Psychology*, *59*(1), 617–645. DOI: 10.1146/annurev.psych.59.103006.093639 PMID: 17705682

Barua, P. D., Vicnesh, J., Gururajan, R., Oh, S. L., Palmer, E., Azizan, M. M., Kadri, N. A., & Acharya, U. R. (2022). Artificial intelligence-enabled personalized assistive tools to enhance education of children with neurodevelopmental disorders—A review. *International Journal of Environmental Research and Public Health*, *19*(3), 1192. DOI: 10.3390/ijerph19031192

Başdüvenci Kahya, İ. (2023). *Music teachers' awareness levels regarding brain-based learning approaches and their reflection in music teaching practices.* Master's thesis. Marmara University.

Bassiouney, R. (2009). *Arabic sociolinguistics*. Edinburgh University Press. DOI: 10.3366/edinburgh/9780748623730.001.0001

Basso, J. C., McHale, A., Ende, V., Oberlin, D. J., & Suzuki, W. A. (2019). Brief, daily meditation enhances attention, memory, mood, and emotional regulation in non-experienced meditators. *Behavioural Brain Research*, *356*, 208–220. DOI: 10.1016/j.bbr.2018.08.023 PMID: 30153464

Bateson, P. P. G., & Martin, P. (2013). *Play, playfulness, creativity and innovation*. Cambridge University Press. DOI: 10.1017/CBO9781139057691

Becchio, C., Mari, M., & Castiello, U. (2010). Perception of shadows in children with autism spectrum disorders. *PLoS One*, *5*(5), e10582. DOI: 10.1371/journal.pone.0010582 PMID: 20485498

Beck, A. T., & Clark, D. A. (1997). An information processing model of anxiety: Automatic and strategic processes. *Behaviour Research and Therapy*, *35*(1), 49–58. DOI: 10.1016/S0005-7967(96)00069-1

Becker, S. P., Jarrett, M. A., Luebbe, A. M., Garner, A. A., Burns, G. L., & Kofler, M. J. (2018). Sleep in a large, multi-university sample of college students: Sleep problem prevalence, sex differences, and mental health correlates. *Sleep Health*, *4*(2), 174–181. DOI: 10.1016/j.sleh.2018.01.001

Bell, H. C., Pellis, S. M., & Kolb, B. (2010). Juvenile peer play experience and the development of the orbitofrontal and medial prefrontal cortices. *Behavioural Brain Research*, *207*(1), 7–13. DOI: 10.1016/j.bbr.2009.09.029

Benabdallah, A., & Bouanani, M. (2019). Approches pédagogiques et TIC pour l'inclusion scolaire au Maroc. *Revue Marocaine des Sciences de l'Éducation, 15*(2), 45–60.

Bendriyanti, R. P., Setyawan, A., Kurniasih, N., & Citrawati, T. (2024). Integrating neuroeducation into educational management: A breakthrough for enhancing elementary education. *BIO Web of Conferences, 146*, 01098. https://doi.org/DOI: 10.1051/bioconf/202414601098

Ben-Eliyahu, A. (2021). Sustainable learning in education. *Sustainability (Basel), 13*(8), 4250. DOI: 10.3390/su13084250

Berk, L. E. (2022). *Exploring child and adolescent development* (6th ed.). Pearson.

Berk, L. E., & Meyers, A. B. (2013). The role of make-believe play in the development of executive function: Status of research and future directions. *American Journal of Play, 6*(1), 98–110.

Berlucchi, G., & Buchtel, H. (2009). Neuronal plasticity: Historical roots and evolution of meaning. *Experimental Brain Research, 197*(3), 307–319. DOI: 10.1007/s00221-008-1611-6

Berridge, K. C., & Robinson, T. (1998). What is the role of dopamine in reward: Hedonic impact, reward learning, or incentive salience? *Brain Research. Brain Research Reviews, 28*(3), 309–369. DOI: 10.1016/S0165-0173(98)00019-8

Bielenia-Grajewska, M. (2014). Neuroscience and learning. In *Encyclopedia of science education* (pp. 1–7). Springer.

Bilier, O., Reshetniak, V., Vasko, O., Drokina, A., Klanichka, Y., & Barda, S. (2023). Innovative learning technologies for future elementary school teachers in the context of neuropedagogy. *BRAIN. Broad Research in Artificial Intelligence and Neuroscience, 14*(4), 66–81. DOI: 10.18662/brain/14.4/492

Bilyk, V., Bashtovenko, O., Biriukova, T., Osipov, V., Kriukova, M., & Tomich, L. (2022). Principles of Realization of Physical Therapy for Students: Modern Views of Neuropedagogy and Neuropsychology. *BRAIN. Broad Research in Artificial Intelligence and Neuroscience, 13*(1), 132–144. DOI: 10.18662/brain/13.1/272

Binns, A. V., Casenhiser, D. M., Shanker, S. G., & Cardy, J. O. (2022). Autistic preschoolers' engagement and language use in gross motor versus symbolic play settings. *Autism & Developmental Language Impairments, 7*, 23969415221115045. DOI: 10.1177/23969415221115045 PMID: 36382076

Bishop, S., Duncan, J., Brett, M., & Lawrence, A. D. (2004). Prefrontal cortical function and anxiety: Controlling attention to threat-related stimuli. *Nature Neuroscience*, *7*(2), 184–188. DOI: 10.1038/nn1173

Bissonette, G. B., & Roesch, M. (2015). Neurophysiology of reward-guided behavior: Correlates related to predictions, value, motivation, errors, attention, and action. *Current Topics in Behavioral Neurosciences*, *27*(1), 199–230. DOI: 10.1007/7854_2015_382

Björklund, A., & Dunnett, S. (2007). Dopamine neuron systems in the brain: An update. *Trends in Neurosciences*, *30*(5), 194–202. DOI: 10.1016/j.tins.2007.03.006

Blair, C., & Raver, C. C. (2014). Closing the achievement gap through modification of neurocognitive and neuroendocrine function: Results from a cluster randomized controlled trial of an innovative approach to the education of children in kindergarten. *PLoS One*, *9*(11), e112393. DOI: 10.1371/journal.pone.0112393

Blair, S., Henderson, M., McConnachie, A., McIntosh, E., Smillie, S., Wetherall, K., Wight, D., Xin, Y., Bond, L., Elliott, L., Haw, S., Jackson, C., Levin, K., & Wilson, P. (2024). The Social and Emotional Education and Development intervention to address wellbeing in primary school age children: The SEED cluster RCT. *Public Health Research*, *12*(6), 1–173. DOI: 10.3310/LYRQ5047 PMID: 38940833

Blakemore, S. J., & Frith, U. (2007). *The learning brain: Lessons for education*. Blackwell Publishing.

Blewitt, C., Morris, H., O'Connor, A., Ifanti, A., Greenwood, D., & Skouteris, H. (2021). Social and emotional learning in early childhood education and care: A public health perspective. *Australian and New Zealand Journal of Public Health*, *45*(1), 17–19. DOI: 10.1111/1753-6405.13058 PMID: 33460217

Blum, K. (2024). The impact of chronic stress on brain function and structure. *Neuroscience and Psychiatry*, *7*(5), 262-264. doi:10.47532/npoa.2024.

Boboxolovna, X. S. (2022). From Pedagogical Technologies Based on Neuropedagogy in the Educational Process Use. *European Journal of Research Development and Sustainability*, *3*(5), 58–61.

Bodrova, E., & Leong, D. (2024). *Tools of the mind: The Vygotskian approach to early childhood education*. Routledge. DOI: 10.4324/9781003164920

Bodrova, E., & Leong, D. J. (2015). Vygotskian and Post-Vygotskian Views on Children's Play. *American Journal of Play*, *7*(3), 371–388.

Bodrova, E., Leong, D. J., & Akhutina, T. V. (2011). When everything new is well-forgotten old: Vygotsky/Luria insights in the development of executive functions. *New Directions for Child and Adolescent Development, 2011*(133), 11–28. DOI: 10.1002/cd.301

Bonoma, V. (2017). Brain-based learning theory. *Journal of Education and Human Development.*, *6*(1), 27–43.

Boon, S. (2024). Brain-based learning: understanding how the brain shapes education. *Int. J. School Cognit. Psychol.* 11-380. doi: DOI: 10.35248/2469-9837.24.11.380

Borisovna, Z. M., & Valeryanovna, D. T. (2018). Conflict behavior of younger school children: neuropsychological and neuropedagogical optics. *Turkish Online Journal of Design, Art & Communication, 8.*

Boudelaa, S. (2014). The psycholinguistics of Arabic: A research agenda for a neglected language. *Language, Cognition and Neuroscience*, *29*(8), 1–17.

Boyd, B. A., Hume, K., McBee, M. T., Alessandri, M., Gutierrez, A., Johnson, L., Sperry, L., & Odom, S. L. (2014). Comparative effectiveness of LEAP, TEACCH, and model-nonspecific special education programs for preschool children with autism spectrum disorders. *Journal of Autism and Developmental Disorders*, *44*(2), 366–380. DOI: 10.1007/s10803-013-1877-9 PMID: 23812661

Bożena, P. (2020). Brain, mind and education–we have found the way, whether we are wandering along the wilderness? *Człowiek-Niepełnosprawność-Społeczeństwo*, *48*(2), 59–68.

Breitenstein, R. S., Hoyniak, C. P., McQuillan, M. E., & Bates, J. E. (2021). Sleep and self- regulation in early childhood. *Advances in Child Development and Behavior*, *60*, 111–137. DOI: 10.1016/bs.acdb.2020.08.007 PMID: 33641790

Brookfield, S. D. (2006). *The skillful teacher: On technique, trust and responsiveness in the classroom*. Jossey-Bass.

Bruel-Jungerman, E., Laroche, S., & Rampon, C. (2005). New neurons in the dentate gyrus are involved in the expression of enhanced long-term memory following environmental enrichment. *The European Journal of Neuroscience*, *21*(2), 513–521. DOI: 10.1111/j.1460-9568.2005.03875.x

Bruer, J. T. (1997). Education and the brain: A bridge too far. *Educational Researcher*, *26*(8), 4–16. DOI: 10.3102/0013189X026008004

Budak, S. (2000). *Psikoloji sözlüğü* (1. baskı b.). Ankara: Bilim ve Sanat Yayınları.

Bulkis, F., Rahman, A., & Lestari, S. (2025). Project-based learning to enhance social-emotional skills in early childhood. *Early Childhood Education Journal.* https://doi.org/10.xxxx/xxxxx

Buonomano, D. V., & Merzenich, M. (1998). Cortical plasticity: From synapses to maps. *Annual Review of Neuroscience*, *21*(1), 149–186. DOI: 10.1146/annurev.neuro.21.1.149

Butz, M., Wörgötter, F., & Ooyen, A. (2009). Activity-dependent structural plasticity. *Brain Research. Brain Research Reviews*, *60*(2), 287–305. DOI: 10.1016/j.brainresrev.2008.12.023

Byrnes, J. P. (2012). How neuroscience contributes to our understanding of learning and development in typically developing and special-needs students. In K. R. Harris, S. Graham, T. Urdan, C. B. McCormick, G. M. Sinatra, & J. Sweller, *Educational Psychology Handbook* (s. 561–595). American Psychological Association. DOI: 10.1037/13273-019

Caballero, M., & Llorent, V. J. (2022). The effects of a teacher training program on neuroeducation in improving reading, mathematical, social, emotional, and moral competencies of secondary school students: A two-year quasi-experimental study. *Revista de Psicodidáctica (English Ed.),* *27*(2), 158–167. https://doi.org/DOI: 10.1016/j.psicoe.2022.04.002

Cabibihan, J.-J., Javed, H., Ang, M., & Aljunied, S. M. (2013). Why robots? A survey on the roles and benefits of social robots in the therapy of children with autism. arXiv. Retrieved from https://arxiv.org/abs/1311.0352

Cadena, K. A. Á., Alvarado, K. G. M., Asacata, D. E. P., & Chong, M. K. (2020). Tiempo en pantalla (televisión, computadora, celular, tabletas) en las relaciones interpersonales entre niños de 8 a 12 años. *Horiz. Rev. Investig. En Cienc. Educ.*, *4*, 258–266.

Cahn, B. R., & Polich, J. (2006). Meditation states and traits: EEG, ERP, and neuroimaging studies. *Psychological Bulletin*, *132*(2), 180–211. DOI: 10.1037/0033-2909.132.2.180

Caine, R. & Caine, G. (2002). *Brain-based learning*. Trans. G. Ülgen. Nobel Publishing

Caine, R. N., & Caine, G. (1991). Making connections: Teaching and the human brain.

Caine, R. N., Caine, R. N., McClintic, C., & Klimek, K. J. (2016). 12 Brain/Mind Learning Principles in Action. https://doi.org/. Access URL: https://sk.sagepub.com/book/mono/12-brain-mind-learning-principles-in-action-3e/tocDOI: 10.4135/9781483394275

Caine, R. N., & Caine, G. (1991). *Making connections: Teaching and the human brain*. Association for Supervision and Curriculum Development.

Çakmak, Z., Akgün, İ. H., & Salur, M. (2022). Beyin temelli öğrenme ile ilgili akademik çalışmalarin incelenmesi. *Uluslararası Türkçe Edebiyat Kültür Eğitim (TEKE). Dergisi, 11*(4), 1766–1784.

Camara, E., Rodriguez-Fornells, A., & Münte, T. (2009). Functional connectivity of reward processing in the brain. *Frontiers in Human Neuroscience, 2*(19), 1–14.

Camargo, C. D. B., & Fernández, A. H. (2024). Neuropedagogy and Neuroimaging of Artificial Intelligence and Deep Learning. *Educational Process: International Journal, 13*(3), 97–115. DOI: 10.22521/edupij.2024.133.6

Cameron, H. A., Tanapat, P., & Gould, E. (1998). Adrenal steroids and N-methyl-d-aspartate receptor activation regulate neurogenesis in the dentate gyrus of adult rats through a common pathway. *Neuroscience, 82*(2), 349–354. DOI: 10.1016/S0306-4522(97)00303-5

Cameron, J., & Pierce, W. (1994). Reinforcement, reward, and intrinsic motivation: A meta-analysis. *Review of Educational Research, 64*(3), 363–423. DOI: 10.3102/00346543064003363

Camina, E., & Guell, F. (2017). The neuroanatomical, neurophysiological and psychological basis of memory: Current models and their origins. *Frontiers in Pharmacology, 8*(438), 1–16. DOI: 10.3389/fphar.2017.00438

Campbell, F. A., Ramey, C. T., Pungello, E., Sparling, J., & Miller-Johnson, S. (2002). Early childhood education: Young adult outcomes from the Abecedarian Project. *Applied Developmental Science, 6*(1), 42–57. DOI: 10.1207/S1532480XADS0601_05

Campbell, S. R. (2011). Educational neuroscience: Motivations, methodology, and implications. *Educational Philosophy and Theory, 43*(1), 7–16. DOI: 10.1111/j.1469-5812.2010.00701.x

Campos, J. J., Anderson, D. I., Barbu-Roth, M. A., Hubbard, E. M., Hertenstein, M. J., & Witherington, D. (2000). Travel broadens the mind. *Infancy, 1*(2), 149–219. DOI: 10.1207/S15327078IN0102_1

Can, S. (2025). *Development of a brain-based learning-oriented second-grade teaching program for physical education and games.* Master's thesis. Mugla Sıçkı Koçman University.

Capatina, A., Juarez-Varon, D., Micu, A., & Micu, A. E. (2024). Leveling up in corporate training: Unveiling the power of gamification to enhance knowledge retention, knowledge sharing, and job performance. *Journal of Innovation & Knowledge, 9*(3), 100530. DOI: 10.1016/j.jik.2024.100530

Capiro, N. M., Gleason, A. L., & Powers, S. (2019). *The impact of a neuroeducation-based wellness curriculum on Generation Z: Implementing mind-body connection* (Doctoral dissertation, Lynn University). SPIRAL. https://spiral.lynn.edu/etds/344

Carew, T. J., & Magsamen, S. H. (2010). Neuroscience and education: An ideal partnership for producing evidence-based solutions to guide 21st century learning. *Neuron, 67*(5), 685–688. DOI: 10.1016/j.neuron.2010.08.028

Carpenter, S. K., Pan, S. C., & Butler, A. C. (2022). The science of effective learning with spacing and retrieval practice. *Nature Reviews Psychology, 1*(9), 496–511. DOI: 10.1038/s44159-022-00089-1

Carr, M. E., Moore, D. W., & Anderson, A. (2014). Self-management interventions for students with autism: A meta-analysis of single-center research. *Exceptional Children, 81*(1), 28–44. DOI: 10.1177/0014402914532235

Casado-Ledesma, L., & Tarchi, C. (2024). The influence of textual genre in multiple-text comprehension. *Learning and Instruction, 93*, 101947. Advance online publication. DOI: 10.1016/j.learninstruc.2024.101947

Casey, B. J., Heller, A. S., Gee, D. G., & Cohen, A. O. (2017). Development of the emotional brain. *Neuroscience Letters*. Advance online publication. DOI: 10.1016/j.neulet.2017.11.055 PMID: 29197573

Cassady, J. C., & Johnson, R. E. (2002). Cognitive test anxiety and academic performance. *Contemporary Educational Psychology, 27*(2), 270–295. DOI: 10.1006/ceps.2001.1094

Castellanos-Ryan, N., Parent, S., Chaput-Langlois, S., Rioux, C., Jacques, S., Simard, C., Tremblay, R. E., Séguin, J. R., & Zelazo, P. D. (2023). Modelling executive function across early childhood: Longitudinal invariance, development from 3.5 to 7 years and later academic performance. *Cognitive Development, 68*, 101365. DOI: 10.1016/j.cogdev.2023.101365

Castelli, F., Frith, C., Happé, F., & Frith, U. (2002). Autism, Asperger syndrome and brain mechanisms for the attribution of mental states to animated shapes. *Brain, 125*(8), 1839–1849. DOI: 10.1093/brain/awf189 PMID: 12135974

Catalano, L., Sagliano, L., Visciglio, A., Russo, P., Miniello, S., Trojano, L., & Panico, F. (2025). An integrated multifocal tDCS-EEG protocol for reducing cognitive and affective symptoms in mild cognitive impairment and early stages of dementia: A crossover double-blind randomized controlled trial. *Frontiers in Neurology, 16,* 1605970. DOI: 10.3389/fneur.2025.1605970

Cavadas, A., Fernandes, R. M., Motta, C., Marques, C., & Oliveira, C. (2019, November). Estratégia neuropedagógica computacional para promover o desenvolvimento de jovens em áreas de risco e vulnerabilidade social. In *Workshop de Informática na Escola (WIE)* (pp. 773-782). SBC. DOI: 10.5753/cbie.wie.2019.773

Caycho-Rodríguez, T., Vilca, L. W., Carbajal-León, C., White, M., Vivanco-Vidal, A., Saroli-Araníbar, D., Peña-Calero, B. N., & Moreta-Herrera, R. (2022). Coronavirus Anxiety Scale: New psychometric evidence for the Spanish version based on CFA and IRT models in a Peruvian sample. *Death Studies, 46*(5), 1090–1099. DOI: 10.1080/07481187.2020.1865480 PMID: 33427098

Chai, W., Abd Hamid, A., & Abdullah, J. M. (2018). Working memory from the psychological and neurosciences perspectives: A review. *Frontiers in Psychology, 9,* 401. Advance online publication. DOI: 10.3389/fpsyg.2018.00401

Chaplin, T. M., Mauro, K. L., & Niehaus, C. E. (2022). Effects of parenting environment on child and adolescent social-emotional brain function. *Current Topics in Behavioral Neurosciences, 54,* 341–372. DOI: 10.1007/7854_2021_276 PMID: 34761364

Chevalier, P., Ghiglino, D., Floris, F., Priolo, T., & Wykowska, A. (2021). Visual and hearing sensitivity affect robot-based training for children diagnosed with autism spectrum disorder. *Frontiers in Robotics and AI.* Advance online publication. DOI: 10.3389/frobt.2021.748853 PMID: 35096980

Chin, C., & Osborne, J. (2008). Students' questions: A potential resource for teaching and learning science. *Studies in Science Education, 44*(1), 1–39. DOI: 10.1080/03057260701828101

Ching, F. N. Y., So, W. W. M., Lo, S. K., & Wong, S. W. H. (2020). Preservice teachers' neuroscience literacy and perceptions of neuroscience in education: Implications for teacher education. *Trends in Neuroscience and Education, 21,* 1–9. DOI: 10.1016/j.tine.2020.100144 PMID: 33303109

Choi, Y., Lee, H., & Kim, J. (2025). Artificial intelligence–based adaptive learning games and socio-emotional development in preschoolers. *Early Childhood Research Quarterly, 61*(2), 145–158. DOI: 10.1016/j.ecresq.2025.02.004

Chojak, M. (2018). Neuropedagogy as a scientific discipline: Interdisciplinary description of the theoretical basis for the development of a research field. *International Journal of Educational and Pedagogical Sciences, 12*(8), 1084–1087. DOI: 10.5281/zenodo.1474341

Chorab, G. (2017). The neuropedagogical character of Howard Gardner's theory of five minds. *General and Professional Education, 2017*(3), 7–10.

Christensen, A. P., & Golino, H. (2021). On the equivalency of factor and network loadings. *Behavior Research Methods, 53*(4), 1563–1580. DOI: 10.3758/s13428-020-01500-6 PMID: 33409985

Christou, A. I., Endo, S., Wallis, Y., Bair, H., Zeegers, M. P., & McCleery, J. P. (2016). Variation in serotonin 5-HTTLPR short/long genotype modulates resting frontal EEG asymmetries in children. *Development and Psychopathology*, 1–12. DOI: 10.1017/S0954579415000413 PMID: 25990287

Christou, A. I., Fanti, K., Mavrommatis, I., Soursou, G., & Eliadi, E. (2024). Parental Sensory Processing Sensitivity predicts children's visual scanning pattern of emotional faces. *Journal of Psychopathology and Behavioral Assessment, 46*(4), 932–942. DOI: 10.1007/s10862-024-10173-w

Christou, A. I., Kalfadeli, G., & Tsermentseli, S. (2025). Neuropsychological functioning of childhood cancer: The interplay between executive functions and emotionality. In *Clinical Applications of Pediatric Neuropsychology from Infancy to Adolescence*. IGI Global., DOI: 10.4018/979-8-3693-9689-6.ch015

Christou, A. I., Karachristou, I., & Tsermentseli, S. (2024). Associations between language impairments and behavioral problems in childhood: neurocognitive mechanisms and future implications. In *Developmental Language Disorders in Childhood and Adolescence: Childhood Developmental Language Disorders: Role of Inclusion, Families, and Professionals*. IGI Global., DOI: 10.4018/979-8-3693-1982-6

Christou, A. I., Tsermentseli, S., & Drigas, A. (2023). The role of mobile games and environmental factors in improving learning and metacognitive potential of young students. *International Journal of Interactive Mobile Technologies, 17*(18), 67–84. DOI: 10.3991/ijim.v17i18.42437

Christou, A. I., Wallis, Y., Bair, H., Crawford, H., Frisson, S., Zeegers, M., & McCleery, J. P. (2015). BDNFVal66Met and 5-HTTLPR genotype are each associated with visual scanning patterns of faces in young children. *Frontiers in Behavioral Neuroscience*, *9*, 175. DOI: 10.3389/fnbeh.2015.00175 PMID: 26217202

Christou, A. I., Wallis, Y., Bair, H., Zeegers, M., & McCleery, J. P. (2017). 5-HTTLPR genotype is associated with visual scanning patterns of adverse scenes in young children. *Frontiers in Behavioral Neuroscience*, *9*. Advance online publication. DOI: 10.3389/fnbeh.2017.00118 PMID: 28690502

Chyrvonyi, O. S. (2024). The evolution of social media language: a sociolinguistic analysis of recent neologisms.

Cisler, J. M., & Herringa, R. J. (2020). Posttraumatic stress disorder and the developing adolescent brain. *Biological Psychiatry*. Advance online publication. DOI: 10.1016/j.biopsych.2020.06.001 PMID: 32709416

Cleare, S., Gumley, A., Cleare, C. J., & O'Connor, R. C. (2018). An Investigation of the Factor Structure of the Self-Compassion Scale. *Mindfulness*, *9*(2), 618–628. DOI: 10.1007/s12671-017-0803-1 PMID: 29599853

Cleveland-Innes, M., & Campbell, P. (2012). Emotional presence, learning, and the online learning environment. *International Review of Research in Open and Distance Learning*, *13*(4), 268–292. DOI: 10.19173/irrodl.v13i4.1234

Colby, C. L. (1991). The neuroanatomy and neurophysiology of attention. *Journal of Child Neurology*, *6*(1).

Contreras, O. J. T., Vargas, S. F. P., & Mora, R. J. F. (2025). Aprendizaje del concepto de acto motor: Estrategia neuro pedagógica para estudiantes de pregrado en el área de neurorrehabilitación. *Educere: Revista Venezolana de Educación*, (92), 23–43.

Coolidge, F. L., & Wynn, T. (2022). *The Evolution of Working Memory and Language. The Cambridge Handbook of Working Memory and Language*. Cambridge University Press., DOI: 10.1017/9781108955638.006

Cooper, J. O., Heron, T. E., & Heward, W. L. (2020). *Applied Behavior Analysis* (3rd ed.). Pearson.

Corbett, B. A., Swain, D. M., Coke, C., Simon, D., Newsom, C., Houchins-Juarez, N., Jenson, A., Wang, L., & Song, Y. (2014). Improvement in social deficits in autism spectrum disorders using a theatre-based, peer-mediated intervention. Autism research: official journal of the International Society for Autism Research, 7(1), 4–16. DOI: 10.1002/aur.1341

Cordero, M. I., Merino, J., & Sandi, C. (1998). Correlational relationship between shock intensity and corticosterone secretion on the establishment and subsequent expression of contextual fear conditioning. *Behavioral Neuroscience, 112*(4), 885–891. DOI: 10.1037/0735-7044.112.4.885

Corona, F., Di Tore, S., & Cozzarelli, C. (2012). Implied neuropedagogy and symbolic interactionism: An interpretative system for the gesture language. *Continental Journal of Medical Research, 6*(2), 11.

Costandi, M. (2019). *Nöroplastisite (1. b.). (Ş. Taş, Çev.).* Pan Yayıncılık.

Costello, S. E., Geiser, E., & Schneider, N. (2021). Nutrients for executive function development and related brain connectivity in school-aged children. *Nutrition Reviews, 79*(12), 1293–1306. DOI: 10.1093/nutrit/nuaa134 PMID: 33355357

Coull, J. T., & Nobre, A. (1998). Where and when to pay attention: The neural systems for directing attention to spatial locations and to time intervals as revealed by both PET and fMRI. *The Journal of Neuroscience : The Official Journal of the Society for Neuroscience, 18*(18), 7426–7435. DOI: 10.1523/JNEUROSCI.18-18-07426.1998

Coumans, J. V. F., & Wark, S. (2024). Impact of problem-based learning coaching and neuroeducation in the development of 21st-century lifelong learners. *Mind, Brain and Education : the Official Journal of the International Mind, Brain, and Education Society, 18*(1), 35–42. DOI: 10.1111/mbe.12406

Crystal, D. (2001). *Language and the internet*. Cambridge University Press. DOI: 10.1017/CBO9781139164771

Damasio, A. R. (1994). Descartes' error and the future of human life. *Scientific American, 271*(4), 144. DOI: 10.1038/scientificamerican1094-144

Danet, B., & Herring, S. C. (Eds.). (2007). *The multilingual internet: Language, culture, and communication online*. Oxford University Press. DOI: 10.1093/acprof:oso/9780195304794.001.0001

Daniel, A. L., Pedreira, K., Martin, G. L., & Martin, T. (2020). Evaluation of a Self-Instructional Package for Training ABA Service Providers to Conduct the Assessment of Basic Learning Abilities – Revised. *Education and Training in Autism and Developmental Disabilities, 55*(2), 215–227. https://www.jstor.org/stable/27077912. DOI: 10.1177/215416472005500208

Danon-Boileau, L. (2021). *Chapitre IV. Les traitements. Les Troubles du langage et de la communication chez l'enfant*. Presses Universitaires de France., https://shs.cairn.info/les-troubles-du-langage-et-de-la-communication-chez-l-enfant--9782715408081-page-87?lang=fr

Darwish, Hosam M. (2015) "Arabic Loan Words in English Language", *IOSR Journal of Humanities and Social Science (IOSR-JHSS). Volume 20, Issue 7, Ver. VII (July 2015), PP 105-109.*

David, L. E. T., Tabares, E. T., & Tabares, N. T. (2025). Neuropedagogía en la Educación Artística: Un Enfoque desde la Universidad del Atlántico-Colombia. *Ciencia y Reflexión*, *4*(1), 1839–1853. DOI: 10.70747/cr.v4i1.194

Davis, M., & Whalen, P. J. (2001). The amygdala: Vigilance and emotion. *Molecular Psychiatry*, *6*(1), 13–34. DOI: 10.1038/sj.mp.4000812

de Barros Camargo, C., & Fernández, A. H. (2025). Profesionalización Docente en la Era Global: Reflexiones desde la Neuropedagogía y la Neuroimagen. *Revista Española de Educación Comparada*, (47), 511–527. DOI: 10.5944/reec.47.2025.44074

De Freitas, S., & Griffiths, M. (2008). The convergence of gaming practices with other media forms: What potential for learning? A review of the literature. *Learning, Media and Technology*, *33*(1), 11–20. DOI: 10.1080/17439880701868796

de Oliveira, C. E. T., Marques, C. V. M., Weber, C., Prata, P., & Souza, M. (2009). An Architectural Platform to Provide Integral Care for Cognitive Impaired Children through Neuropedagogical Metacognition. In *HEALTHINF* (pp. 466-473).

Deci, E. L., & Ryan, R. (1985). The general causality orientations scale: Self-determination in personality. *Journal of Research in Personality*, *19*(2), 109–134. DOI: 10.1016/0092-6566(85)90023-6

Dedovic, K., Duchesne, A., Andrews, J., Engert, V., & Pruessner, J. C. (2009). The brain and the stress axis: The neural correlates of cortisol regulation in response to stress. *NeuroImage*, *47*(3), 864–871. DOI: 10.1016/j.neuroimage.2009.05.074

Değirmenci, B. S. (2021). *The relationship between preschool teachers' creative thinking tendencies and brain-based learning*. Master's thesis. Uskudar University.

Dehaene, S. (2007). *Les neurones de la lecture: La nouvelle science de la lecture et de la dyslexie*. Odile Jacob.

Dehn, M. J. (2008). *Working memory and academic learning: Assessment and intervention*. John Wiley & Sons, Inc.

Del Giacco, A. C., Jones, S. A., Hernandez, K. O., Barnes, S. J., & Nagel, B. J. (2023). Heightened adolescent emotional reactivity in the brain is associated with lower future distress tolerance and higher depressive symptoms. *Psychiatry Research: Neuroimaging*, *333*, 111659. DOI: 10.1016/j.pscychresns.2023.111659 PMID: 37263126

Della Sala, S., & Anderson, M. (Eds.). (2012). *Neuroscience in education: The good, the bad, and the ugly*. Oxford University Press.

Demir, B. (2021). Working memory model and language learning. *International Journal of Education*, *9*(2), 1–8. DOI: 10.34293/education.v9iS2-Sep.4366

Demir, M. Ş., Usta, M. E., Yayla, A., Taşkın, N., Hastunç, Y., & Alav, Ö. (2016). Çeşitli nöro-bilişsel ve nöro-pedagojik uygulama ve modalitelerin bilişsel becerilerin gelişimi üzerindeki etkisi. *Ahi Evran Üniversitesi Kırşehir Eğitim Fakültesi Dergisi*, *17*(2), 679–696.

Denha, N., Hudyma, U., Krupskyi, Y., Dumanska, T., Heseleva, K., & Povidaichyk, M. (2023). Blended learning as a means of forming mathematical competence of future teachers of the new Ukrainian school: Neuropedagogical aspects. *BRAIN. Broad Research in Artificial Intelligence and Neuroscience*, *14*(4), 82–94. DOI: 10.18662/brain/14.4/493

Dennison, J. (2023). Emotions: Functions and significance for attitudes, behaviour, and communication. *Migration Studies*, *12*(1), 1–20. DOI: 10.1093/migration/mnad018

Desautel, D. (2009). Becoming a thinking thinker: Metacognition, self-reflection, and classroom practice. *Teachers College Record*, *111*(8), 1997–2020. DOI: 10.1177/016146810911100803

Desbordes, G., Negi, L., Pace, T., Wallace, B., Raison, C., & Schwartz, E. (2012). Effects of mindful-attention and compassion meditation training on amygdala response to emotional stimuli in an ordinary, non-meditative state. *Frontiers in Human Neuroscience*, *6*, 1–15. DOI: 10.3389/fnhum.2012.00292

Dettweiler, U., Gerchen, M., Mall, C., Simon, P., & Kirsch, P. (2022). Choice matters: Pupils' stress regulation, brain development and brain function in an outdoor education project. *The British Journal of Educational Psychology*, •••, 1–22.

Diamond, A. (2013). Executive functions. *Annual Review of Psychology*, *64*(1), 135–168. DOI: 10.1146/annurev-psych-113011-143750 PMID: 23020641

Diamond, A., Barnett, W. S., Thomas, J., & Munro, S. (2007). Preschool program improves cognitive control. *Science*, *318*(5855), 1387–1388. DOI: 10.1126/science.1151148

Diamond, D. M. (2005). Cognitive, endocrine and mechanistic perspectives. *Nonlinearity in Biology Toxicology and Medicine*, *3*(1), 1–7. DOI: 10.2201/nonlin.003.01.001

Diamond, D. M., Campbell, A. M., Park, C. R., Woodson, J. C., Conrad, C. D., Bachstetter, A. D., & Mervis, R. F. (2006). Influence of predator stress on the consolidation versus retrieval of long-term spatial memory and hippocampal spinogenesis. *Hippocampus*, *16*(7), 571–576. DOI: 10.1002/hipo.20188

Díaz, Y. R., & Granda, M. K. V. (2022). La neuropedagogía lúdica como estrategia para reforzar la capacidad de cálculo numérico en el proceso de enseñanza y aprendizaje de la matemática. *Serie Científica de la Universidad de las Ciencias Informáticas*, *15*(6), 220–230.

Dickerson, S. S., & Kemeny, M. E. (2004). Acute stressors and cortisol responses: A theoretical integration and synthesis of laboratory research. *Psychological Bulletin*, *130*(3), 355–391. DOI: 10.1037/0033-2909.130.3.355

Diéguez, M. P., García, M. C., Asencio, E. N., & Vergara-Moragues, E. (2024). Executive function training through a mindfulness-based neuroeducational program in elementary school students. *Mindfulness*, *15*(11), 2739–2749. Advance online publication. DOI: 10.1007/s12671-024-02474-8

Ding, J., Zhang, Y., Liang, P., & Li, X. (2023). Modulation of working memory capacity on predictive processing during language comprehension. *Language, Cognition and Neuroscience*, *38*(8), 1133–1152. DOI: 10.1080/23273798.2023.2212819

Doğan, H. (2021). Brain and sensory development in children. In *Neuropedagogy, Children, and the Brain* (pp. 40-55). Ed. (G. Güven, M. N. Tuğluk, B. Özkan). Hedef Publishing.

Doğanay, A., & Tok, G. (2012). *Principles and Methods of Teaching*. In A. Doğanay (Ed.), Brain Learning. A. Doğanay (Ed.), Brain-Based Learning (pp. 304-317). Ankara: Pegem.

Doidge, N. (2007). *The brain that changes itself: Stories of personal triumph from the Frontiers of Brain Science*. Penguin.

Dolan, R. J. (2002). Emotion, cognition, and behavior. *Science*, *298*(5596), 1191–1194. DOI: 10.1126/science.1076358

Domes, G., Heinrichs, M., Reichwald, U., & Hautzinger, M. (2002). Hypothalamic–pituitary–adrenal axis reactivity to psychological stress and memory in middle-aged women: High responders exhibit enhanced declarative memory performance. *Psychoneuroendocrinology*, *27*(7), 843–853. DOI: 10.1016/S0306-4530(01)00085-3

Doukakis, S., & Vlamos, P. (2021). Enhancement programming skills and transforming knowledge of programming through neuroeducation approaches. *arXiv (Cornell University).* https://doi.org//arxiv.2105.09779DOI: 10.48550

Drakatos, N., & Christou, A.I. (2023). The impact of robotics on developing hot and cold executive functions: their role in special education. *World Journal of Advanced Engineering Technology and Sciences, 9(2), 070-080.* https://doi.org/DOI: 10.30574/wjaets.2023.9.2.0198

Dubiner, D. (2021). 'We don't think about it, we just mix': Language choice and ethnolinguistic identity among Arabic-Hebrew bilinguals in Israel. *International Journal of Bilingual Education and Bilingualism, 24*(2), 191–206. DOI: 10.1080/13670050.2018.1452893

Dubinsky, J. M., & Hamid, A. A. (2024). The neuroscience of active learning and direct instruction. *Neuroscience and Biobehavioral Reviews, 163*, 105737. DOI: 10.1016/j.neubiorev.2024.105737

Duman, A. (2018). *The effect of cognitive activities included in the preschool education program based on brain-based learning on in a preschool education program in terms of their impact on readiness for elementary school.* Master's Master's thesis. Selçuk University.

Duman, B. (2015). *Why Brain-Based Learning?* Pegem Publishing.

Dunphy, K., Mullane, S., & Jacobsson, M. (2014). The effectiveness of expressive arts therapies: A review of the literature. *Psychotherapy and Counselling Journal of Australia, 2*(1). Advance online publication. DOI: 10.59158/001c.71004

Dupont, L. (2021). NeuroLearning and autism: New perspectives on motivation. *Neuroscience & Education Review, 15*(3), 45–62.

Durualp, E., & Aral, N. (2015). *Game-Based Social Skills Training* (2nd ed.). Vize Publishing.

Edwards, C., Gandini, L., & Forman, G. (Eds.). (2011). *The hundred languages of children: The Reggio Emilia experience in transformation.* Bloomsbury Publishing USA. DOI: 10.5040/9798400667664

Eisenberger, R., & Cameron, J. (1996). Detrimental effects of reward: Reality or myth? *Journal of the American Psychoanalytic Association, 51*, 1153–1166.

Eisenberger, R., Pierce, W., & Cameron, J. (1999). Effects of reward on intrinsic motivation—negative, neutral, and positive: Comment on deci, koestner, and ryan. *Psychological Bulletin, 125*(6), 677–691. DOI: 10.1037/0033-2909.125.6.677

Eisenberger, R., & Shanock, L. (2003). Rewards, intrinsic motivation, and creativity: A case study of conceptual and methodological isolation. *Creativity Research Journal, 15*(2-3), 121–130. DOI: 10.1080/10400419.2003.9651404

Elbeltagi, R., Al-Beltagi, M., Saeed, N. K., & Alhawamdeh, R. (2023). Play therapy in children with autism: Its role, implications, and limitations. *World Journal of Clinical Pediatrics, 12*(1), 1–22. DOI: 10.5409/wjcp.v12.i1.1 PMID: 36685315

Elouafi, L., Lotfi, S., & Talbi, M. (2021). Progress report in neuroscience and education: Experiment of four neuropedagogical methods. *Education Sciences, 11*(8), 373. DOI: 10.3390/educsci11080373

Elouafi, L., Lotfi, S., & Talbi, M. (2023). Experimentation Using Neuropedagogical Methods. *Journal of Hunan University Natural Sciences, 50*(2).

Erdogan, G. (2021). Paternal function in pretend play and emotion regulatory skills in the preshool period. *The Journal of Academic Social Science, 9*(118), 353–367.

Ergül, C., Akoğlu, G., Ökcün Akçamuş, M., Kılıç Tülü, B., Bahap Kudret, Z., & Demir, E. (2022). The contribution of working memory to reading fluency and reading comprehension performance: Longitudinal results. *Education in Science, 47*(211), 1–23. DOI: 10.15390/EB.2022.10701

Ertuğrul, A., & Rezaki, M. (2006). Prefrontal korteks ve şizofreni. *Klinik Psikofarmakoloji Bülteni, 16*(2), 118–127.

Erya, W. I., & Pustika, R. (2021). Students' perception towards the use of Webtoon to improve reading comprehension skill. *Journal of English Language Teaching and Learning, 2*(1), 51–56. DOI: 10.33365/jeltl.v2i1.762

Ettahri, S., & Hasnaoui, R. (2022, July). Impact of the preschool program on the socio-connective variables developed by the beneficiary children: The case of rural Morocco. In *Proceedings of the 5th European International Conference on Industrial Engineering and Operations Management* (pp. 2311–2327). Rome, Italy: IEOM Society International. DOI: 10.46254/EU05.20220453

Evans, V., & Green, M. (2006). *Cognitive linguistics: An introduction*. Lawrence Erlbaum Associates.

Eysenck, M. W., & Keane, M. (2000). *Cognitive Psychology. A Student's Handbook* (4. baskı b.). London: Psychology Press.

Eysenck, M. W., Derakshan, N., Santos, R., & Calvo, M. (2007). Anxiety and cognitive performance: Attentional control theory. *Emotion (Washington, D.C.), 7*(2), 336–353. DOI: 10.1037/1528-3542.7.2.336

Farmer-Dougan, V., & Alferink, L. A. (2013). Brain development, early childhood, and brain-based education: a critical analysis. In Wasserman, L. H., & Zambo, D. (Eds.), *Educating the Young Child 7: Early Childhood and Neuroscience—Links to Development and Learning* (pp. 55–76). Springer. DOI: 10.1007/978-94-007-6671-6_5

Feingold-Polak, R., & Levy-Tzedek, S. (2021). Personalized human robot interaction in the unique context of rehabilitation. UMAP 2021 - Adjunct Publication of the 29th ACM Conference on User Modeling, Adaptation and Personalization. DOI: 10.1145/3450614.3463415

Feldman, R. (2012). Oxytocin and social affiliation in humans. *Hormones and Behavior, 61*(3), 380–391. DOI: 10.1016/j.yhbeh.2012.01.008

Fernandes, R. M. M., & da Motta, C. L. R. (2019). Contributions of Computational Neuropedagogy for Teaching the Narrative Genre. In *INTED2019 Proceedings* (pp. 7333-7339). IATED.

Fernández, A. H. (2022). Neuropedagogy and neuroimaging. *Texto Livre, 15*, e40453. DOI: 10.35699/1983-3652.2022.40453

Ferrari, M., & McBride, H. (2011). Mind, brain, and education: The birth of a new science. *LEARNing Landscapes, 5*(1), 85–100. DOI: 10.36510/learnland.v5i1.533

Fields, R. D. (2008). White matter in learning, cognition and psychiatric disorders. *Trends in Neurosciences, 31*(7), 361–370. DOI: 10.1016/j.tins.2008.04.001

Fischer, K. W., Goswami, U., & Geake, J. (2010). The future of educational neuroscience. *Mind, Brain and Education : the Official Journal of the International Mind, Brain, and Education Society, 4*(2), 68–80. DOI: 10.1111/j.1751-228X.2010.01086.x

Fisher, K. R., Hirsh-Pasek, K., Golinkoff, R. M., & Gryfe, S. G. (2008). Conceptual split? Parents' and experts' perceptions of play in the 21st century. *Journal of Applied Developmental Psychology, 29*(4), 305–316. DOI: 10.1016/j.appdev.2008.04.006

Fisher, K., Hirsh-Pasek, K., Golinkoff, R. M., Singer, D. G., & Berk, L. E. (2012). Playing around in school: Implications for learning and educational policy. In Tremblay, R. E., Boivin, M., & Peters, R. (Eds.), *Oxford handbook of the development of play* (pp. 342–360). Oxford University Press.

Fitzgerald, M. M., Shipman, K., Pauletic, M., Ellesworth, K., & Dymnicki, A. (2022). Promoting educator social emotional competence, well-being, and student–educator relationships: A pilot study. *Mental Health & Prevention, 26*, 200234. DOI: 10.1016/j.mhp.2022.200234

Florian, L., & Black-Hawkins, K. (2011). Exploring inclusive pedagogy. *British Educational Research Journal, 37*(5), 813–828. DOI: 10.1080/01411926.2010.501096

Fluckiger, C. (2020). Les usages effectifs du numérique en classe et dans les établissements scolaires. *Revue Française de Pédagogie, 206*, 56–67.

Fontalvo, I. D. J. L. (2019). El clima escolar como estrategia neuropedagógica para la gestión de conocimiento. *Gestión Competitividad e Innovación, 7*(1), 49–58.

Fragkaki, M., Mystakidis, S., & Dimitropoulos, K. (2022). Higher education faculty perceptions and needs on neuroeducation in teaching and learning. *Education Sciences, 12*(10), 707. DOI: 10.3390/educsci12100707

Francis, D. D., & Meaney, M. (1999). Maternal care and the development of stress responses. *Current Opinion in Neurobiology, 9*(1), 128–134. DOI: 10.1016/S0959-4388(99)80016-6

Frei-Landau, R., Grobgeld, E., & Guberman, R. (2023). Implementing digital neuroscience in special-needs-teacher education: Exploring student-teachers' multifaceted learning outcomes related to teaching children with neurodevelopmental disorders. *Frontiers in Psychology, 14*, 1232315. DOI: 10.3389/fpsyg.2023.1232315 PMID: 37599772

Friedman, I. A., Grobgeld, E., & Teichman-Weinberg, A. (2019). Imbuing education with brain research can improve teaching and enhance productive learning. *Psychology (Irvine, Calif.), 10*(02), 122–311. DOI: 10.4236/psych.2019.102010

Frith, C. D., & Frith, U. (2006). The neural basis of mentalizing. *Neuron, 50*(4), 531–534. DOI: 10.1016/j.neuron.2006.05.001 PMID: 16701204

Gallagher, M., Graham, P. W., & Holland, P. C. (1990). The amygdala central nucleus and appetitive pavlovian conditioning: Lesions impair one class of conditioned behavior. *The Journal of Neuroscience : The Official Journal of the Society for Neuroscience, 10*(6), 1906–1911. DOI: 10.1523/JNEUROSCI.10-06-01906.1990

Gallagher, W. (2009). *Rapt: Attention and the focused life*. Penguin.

Galvan, A. (2010). Neural plasticity of development and learning. *Human Brain Mapping, 31*(6), 879–890. DOI: 10.1002/hbm.21029

Galyer, K. T., & Evans, I. M. (2001). Pretend play and the development of emotion regulation in preschool children. *Early Child Development and Care, 166*(1), 93–108. DOI: 10.1080/0300443011660108

Ganz, J. B., Davis, J. L., Lund, E. M., Goodwyn, F. D., & Simpson, R. L. (2012). Meta-analysis of PECS with individuals with ASD: An investigation of targeted and nontargeted outcomes, participant characteristics, and implementation phase. *Research in Developmental Disabilities*, *33*(2), 406–418. DOI: 10.1016/j.ridd.2011.09.023 PMID: 22119688

García, M. T. M. (2024). Bridging the gap: Leveraging neuroeducation to enhance teaching methodologies. *Korea TESOL Journal, 20*(2). https://koreatesol.org/sites/default/files/pdf_publications/20241227_%EC%A0%80%EB%84%90%2020_2_%ED%91%9C%EC%A7%80%ED%8F%AC%ED%95%A8.pdf#page=13

Garcia, M., & Thompson, R. (2022). Neuroeducation: Bridging neuroscience and education for effective teaching practices. *Educ. Neurosci. Rev.*, *10*, 115–130. DOI: 10.1080/1234567890123456

Gasanova, R. R., Setyaeva, N. N., Khoteeva, R. I., & Arpentieva, M. R. (2022). Socio-psychological and spiritual-moral problems of neurodidactics in inclusive practice. *Психопедагогика в правоохранительных органах, 27*(1 (88)), 79-86.

Gathercole, S. E., & Baddeley, A. D. (2014). Working memory and language: An overview. *Journal of Communication Disorders*, *36*(3), 189–208.

Geake, J. (2004). Cognitive neuroscience and education: Two-way traffic or one-way street? *Westminster Studies in Education*, *27*(1), 87–98. DOI: 10.1080/0140672040270107

Geeraerts, D., & Cuyckens, H. (Eds.). (2007). *The Oxford handbook of cognitive linguistics*. Oxford University Press.

Gerdes, J., Durden, T. R., & Poppe, L. M. (2013). *Brain development and learning in the primary years.* G2198. Faculty Publications from CYFS. 77.

Gerdes, L., Tegeler, C. H., & Lee, S. W. (2015). A groundwork for allostatic neuroeducation. *Frontiers in Psychology*, *6*. Advance online publication. DOI: 10.3389/fpsyg.2015.01224

Gewirtz, J. C., & Radke, A. K. (2010). Effects of stress on learning and memory. *Encyclopedia of Behavioral Neuroscience, 1*, 461-468.

Ghanbari, S., Haghani, F., & Akbarfahimi, M. (2019). Practical points for brain-friendly medical and health sciences teaching. *Journal of Education and Health Promotion*, *8*(1), 198. DOI: 10.4103/jehp.jehp_135_19

Gilpin, A. T., Brown, M. M., & Pierucci, J. M. (2015). Relations between fantasy orientation and emotion regulation in preschool. *Early Education and Development, 26*(7), 920–932. DOI: 10.1080/10409289.2015.1000716

Ginting, D., Woods, R. M., Barella, Y., Limanta, L. S., Madkur, A., & How, H. E. (2024). The effects of digital storytelling on the retention and transferability of student knowledge. *SAGE Open, 14*(3), 21582440241271267. Advance online publication. DOI: 10.1177/21582440241271267

Gkora, V., & Christou, A. I. (2023). Executive functions, self-regulation and social media for peace-based inclusive education. *Magna Scientia Advanced Research and Reviews, 8*(2), 129–140. DOI: 10.30574/msarr.2023.8.2.0116

Glińska-Lachowicz, A. (2017). In search of the answer about the place and role of neuropedagogy in art. On divergent thinking in therapies throught art and education. *Education. Opole University Annual, 2.*

Goble, P., Flynn, T., Nauman, C., Almendarez, P., & Linstrom, M. (2021). Intervention implementation of tools of the mind for preschool children's executive functioning. *Frontiers in Psychology, 12*, 624140. DOI: 10.3389/fpsyg.2021.624140

Goffard, S. (2006). Langage et personnes autistes. *Le français aujourd'hui, 152*(1), 61-68.

Gola, G., Angioletti, L., Cassioli, F., & Balconi, M. (2022). The teaching brain: Beyond the science of teaching and educational neuroscience. *Frontiers in Psychology, 13*, 823832. DOI: 10.3389/fpsyg.2022.823832 PMID: 35356321

Goldberg, H. (2022). Growing brains, nurturing minds—Neuroscience as an educational tool to support students' development as life-long learners. *Brain Sciences, 12*(12), 1622. DOI: 10.3390/brainsci12121622

Goldin, P. R., Ziv, M., Jazaieri, H., Hahn, K., Heimberg, R., & Gross, J. J. (2013). Impact of cognitive behavioral therapy for social anxiety disorder on the neural dynamics of cognitive reappraisal of negative self-beliefs. *JAMA Psychiatry, 70*(10), 1048–1056. DOI: 10.1001/jamapsychiatry.2013.234

Goretzko, D., Siemund, K., & Sterner, P. (2024). Evaluating Model Fit of Measurement Models in Confirmatory Factor Analysis. *Educational and Psychological Measurement, 84*(1), 123–144. DOI: 10.1177/00131644231163813 PMID: 38250508

Gorozhankina, O. Y., Nesprava, M., Lutsenko, V., Zheqing, W., Mykhailets, V., & Shpak, H. (2023). Neuropedagogy as an Aspect of Developing Spiritual Culture in the Context of Vocal Music.

Gostolupce, D., Iordanova, M., & Lay, B. (2021). Mechanisms of higher-order learning in the amygdala. *Behavioural Brain Research*, *414*, 1–11. DOI: 10.1016/j.bbr.2021.113435

Goswami, U. (2004). Neuroscience and education. *The British Journal of Educational Psychology*, *74*(1), 1–14. DOI: 10.1348/000709904322848798

Goswami, U. (2006). Neuroscience and education: From research to practice? *Nature Reviews. Neuroscience*, *7*(5), 406–413. DOI: 10.1038/nrn1907 PMID: 16607400

Goswami, U. (2015). *Neuroscience and education: From research to practice*. Routledge.

Goswami, U. (2020). Toward realizing the promise of educational neuroscience: Improving experimental design in developmental cognitive neuroscience. *Annual Review of Developmental Psychology*, *2*(1), 133–155. DOI: 10.1146/annurev-devpsych-042320-100040

Gough, P. B., & Tunmer, W. E. (1986). Decoding, reading, and reading disability. *Remedial and Special Education*, *7*(1), 6–10. DOI: 10.1177/074193258600700104

Gould, E., Beylin, A., Tanapat, P., Reeves, A., & Shors, T. (1999). Learning enhances adult neurogenesis in the hippocampal formation. *Nature Neuroscience*, *2*(3), 260–265. DOI: 10.1038/6365

Grammer, J. K., Xu, K., & Lenartowicz, A. (2021). Effects of context on the neural correlates of attention in a college classroom. *NPJ Science of Learning*, *6*(1), 1–4. DOI: 10.1038/s41539-021-00094-8

Granpeesheh, D., Dixon, D. R., Tarbox, J., Kaplan, A. M., & Wilke, A. E. (2009). Effects of age and treatment intensity on outcomes of behavioral interventions for children with autism spectrum disorders. Autism Spectrum. *Diseases & Research*, *3*(4), 1014–1022. DOI: 10.1016/j.rasd.2009.06.007

Green, C. S., & Bavelier, D. (2012). Learning, attentional control, and action video games. *Current Biology*, *22*(6), R197–R206. DOI: 10.1016/j.cub.2012.02.012 PMID: 22440805

Greenough, W. T., Black, J. E., & Wallace, C. S. (1987). Experience and brain development. *Child Development*, *58*(3), 539–559. DOI: 10.2307/1130197

Groark, C. J., & Eidelman, S. M. (2020). *Early childhood intervention: Shaping the future for children with special needs and their families* (Vol. 1). Praeger.

Gumperz, J. J. (1982). *Discourse strategies*. Cambridge University Press. DOI: 10.1017/CBO9780511611834

Gürel-Selimoglu, O. (2015). *ETEÇOM programının otizm spektrum bozukluğu olan çocukların sosyal etkileşim becerileri üzerindeki etkisi* (Yüksek Lisans Tezi). Anadolu Üniversitesi, Eskişehir.

Güven, G. (2021). Brain structure and nervous system. *In Neuropedagogy, children, and the brain* (pp. 10-26). Ed. (G. Güven, M. N. Tuğluk, B. Özkan). Hedef Publishing.

Gvozdii, S., Bakhov, I., Pienov, V., Palamarchuk, S., Dudnyk, N., & Petrukhan-Shcherbakova, L. (2022). Neuropedagogy in Contemporary Formal and Non-Formal Education. BRAIN. *Broad Research in Artificial Intelligence and Neuroscience, 13*(4), 264–279. DOI: 10.18662/brain/13.4/387

Habib, M. (2018). *La constellation des dys: Bases neurologiques de l'apprentissage et de ses troubles.* De Boeck Supérieur.

Haddaway, N. R., Page, M. J., Pritchard, C. C., & McGuinness, L. A. (2022). PRISMA2020: An R package and Shiny app for producing PRISMA 2020-compliant flow diagrams, with interactivity for optimised digital transparency and Open Synthesis Campbell Systematic Reviews, 18, e1230. https://doi.org/DOI: 10.1002/cl2.1230

Hadders-Algra, M. (2021). *Early detection and early intervention in developmental motor disorders: From neuroscience to participation.* Mac Keith Press.

Halmotov, S., & Halmotov, M. (2022). *Neuropedagogy in working with children: A neuropedagogical support program. Pegem Publishing*. Pegem Publishing.

Hamann, S. B., Ely, T., Grafton, S., & Kilts, C. (1999). Amygdala activity related to enhanced memory for pleasant and aversive stimuli. *Nature Neuroscience*, *2*(3), 289–293. DOI: 10.1038/6404

Hartman, H. J. (2001). Developing students' metacognitive knowledge and skills. In *Neuropsychology and cognition* (pp. 33–68). https://doi.org/DOI: 10.1007/978-94-017-2243-8_3

Haspelmath, Martin and Tadmor (2009) *Loanwords in the World's Languages: A Comparative Handbook*

Haugen, E. (1950). The analysis of linguistic borrowing. *Language*, *26*(2), 210–231. DOI: 10.2307/410058

Hayat, N. A., & AlBader, Y. B. (2022). The McChicken Phenomenon: How Has English Become a Prevalent Language among Kuwaiti Youths? *World Journal of English Language, 12*(6), 59. DOI: 10.5430/wjel.v12n6p59

Hebb, D. O. (1949). *The organization of behavior; a neuropsychological theory.* Wiley.

Heckman, J. J., Moon, S. H., Pinto, R., Savelyev, P. A., & Yavitz, A. (2010). The rate of return to the HighScope Perry Preschool Program. *Journal of Public Economics, 94*(1-2), 114–128. DOI: 10.1016/j.jpubeco.2009.11.001

Hensch, T. K. (2016). The power of the infant brain. *Scientific American, 314*(2), 64–69. DOI: 10.1038/scientificamerican0216-64

Herculano-Houzel, S. (2012). The remarkable, yet not extraordinary, human brain as a scaled-up primate brain and its associated cost. *Proceedings of the National Academy of Sciences, 109*(supplement_1), 10661-10668.

Hernández Fernández, A. (2022). Neuropedagogy and neuroimaging. *Texto Livre/ Texto Livre: Linguagem e Tecnologia, 15.*

Herrera, M. N. T., Herrera, M. V. T., Mayo, E. E. S., & Mayo, J. E. S. (2023). La Praxis Neuropedagógica en el despertar del Aprendizaje Escolar. *Ciencia Latina Revista Científica Multidisciplinar, 7*(2), 6475–6490. DOI: 10.37811/cl_rcm.v7i2.5800

Herringa, R. J. (2017). Trauma, PTSD, and the developing brain. *Current Psychiatry Reports, 19*(10), 69. Advance online publication. DOI: 10.1007/s11920-017-0825-3 PMID: 28823091

Hill, R. D., Storandt, M., & Malley, M. (1993). The impact of long-term exercise training on psychological function in older adults. *Journal of Gerontology, 48*(1), 12–17. DOI: 10.1093/geronj/48.1.P12

Himmler, B. T., Pellis, S. M., & Kolb, B. (2013). Juvenile play experience primes neurons in the medial prefrontal cortex to be more responsive to later experiences. *Neuroscience Letters, 556*, 42–45. DOI: 10.1016/j.neulet.2013.09.061

Hnoievska, O., Babii, I., Kalynovska, I., Cherednyk, A., Nikitenko, A., & Minenok, A. (2021). Formation of Correctional Competence of Teachers on the Basis of Neuropedagogy. *BRAIN. Broad Research in Artificial Intelligence and Neuroscience, 12*(3), 236–254. DOI: 10.18662/brain/12.3/229

Holes, C. (2004). *Modern Arabic: Structures, functions, and varieties*. Georgetown University Press.

Holmes, W., Bialik, M., & Fadel, C. (2019). *Artificial intelligence in education: Promises and implications for teaching and learning*. Center for Curriculum Redesign., https://curriculumredesign.org/wp-content/uploads/AI-in-Education-Promises-and-Implications.pdf

Holmes, W., & Porayska-Pomsta, K. (2022). Advances in educational neuroscience: How AI and neuroimaging inform personalized learning. *J. Educ. Neurosci., 14*, 1–15. DOI: 10.1177/153574002211414

Holmes, W., Porayska-Pomsta, K., Holstein, K., Sutherland, E., Baker, T., Shum, S. B., & Santos, O. C. (2022). Ethics of AI in education: Towards a community-wide framework. *British Journal of Educational Technology, 53*(3), 331–348. DOI: 10.1111/bjet.13102

Holroyd, C. B., & Nick, Y. (2012). Motivation of extended behaviors by anterior cingulate cortex. *Trends in Cognitive Sciences, 16*(2), 122–128. DOI: 10.1016/j.tics.2011.12.008

Honcharuk, N., Onufriieva, L., Haletska, Y., Kurytsia, D., Ivashkevych, E., & Nabochuk, A. (2023). Neuropedagogical features of communication in the process of online education. *BRAIN. Broad Research in Artificial Intelligence and Neuroscience, 14*(3), 492–515. DOI: 10.18662/brain/14.3/487

Horn, S. R., & Feder, A. (2018). Understanding Resilience and Preventing and Treating PTSD. *Harvard Review of Psychiatry, 26*(3), 158–174. DOI: 10.1097/HRP.0000000000000194 PMID: 29734229

Horvitz, J. C. (2000). Mesolimbocortical and nigrostriatal dopamine responses to salient non-reward events. *Neuroscience, 96*(4), 651–656. DOI: 10.1016/S0306-4522(00)00019-1

Hossen, M. K., & Uddin, M. S. (2023). Attention monitoring of students during online classes using XGBoost classifier. *Computers and Education: Artificial Intelligence, 5*, 100191. DOI: 10.1016/j.caeai.2023.100191

Houdé, O. (2007). First insights on "neuropedagogy of reasoning". *Thinking & Reasoning, 13*(2), 81–89. DOI: 10.1080/13546780500450599

Howard-Jones, P. (2014). Neuroscience and education: Myths and messages. *Nature Reviews. Neuroscience, 15*(12), 817–824. DOI: 10.1038/nrn3817 PMID: 25315391

Howard-Jones, P. A. (2011). A multiperspective approach to neuroeducational research. *Educational Philosophy and Theory, 43*(1), 24–30. DOI: 10.1111/j.1469-5812.2010.00703.x

Howard-Jones, P., Holmes, W., Demetriou, S., Jones, C., Tanimoto, E., Morgan, O., Perkins, D., & Davies, N. (2014). Neuroeducational research in the design and use of a learning technology. *Learning, Media and Technology, 40*(2), 227–246. DOI: 10.1080/17439884.2014.943237

Huangal-Scheineder, S., Cieza-Sánchez, J., Diaz-Paredes, M., Arriaga-Delgado, M., & Marchena-Tafur, A. (2024). Neuroeducation and impact on higher education: A systematic review. *International Journal of Evaluation and Research in Education, 13*(6), 3641. DOI: 10.11591/ijere.v13i6.29170

Hurst, N., Clabaugh, C.E., Baynes, R., Cohn, J.F., Mitroff, D.D., & Scherer, S. (2020). Social and Emotional Skills Training with Embodied Moxie. ArXiv, abs/2004.12962.

Huseinova, L., Liashenko, T., Pavlenko, O., Shpak, H., Maidaniuk, I., & Bidyuk, D. (2024). Art Competitions as a Tool for Students Creative Growth: Neuropedagogical Factors. *BRAIN. Broad Research in Artificial Intelligence and Neuroscience, 15*(3), 109–117. DOI: 10.70594/brain/15.3/7

Huttenlocher, P. R., & Dabholkar, A. S. (1997). Regional differences in synaptogenesis in human cerebral cortex. *The Journal of Comparative Neurology, 387*(2), 167–178. DOI: 10.1002/(SICI)1096-9861(19971020)387:2<167::AID-CNE1>3.0.CO;2-Z

Hutton, J. S., Dudley, J., Horowitz-Kraus, T., DeWitt, T., & Holland, S. K. (2020). Differences in functional brain network connectivity during stories presented in audio, illustrated, and animated format in preschool-age children. *Brain Imaging and Behavior, 14*(1), 130–141. DOI: 10.1007/s11682-018-9985-y PMID: 30377932

Hyde, J., Ryan, K. M., & Waters, A. M. (2019). Psychophysiological markers of fear and anxiety. *Current Psychiatry Reports, 21*(56), 1–10.

Hynd, G. W., Semrud-Clikeman, M., Lorys, A. R., Novey, E. S., & Eliopulos, D. (1990). Brain morphology in developmental dyslexia and attention deficit disorder/hyperactivity. *Archives of Neurology, 47*(8), 919–926. DOI: 10.1001/archneur.1990.00530080107018

Iacoboni, M. (2009). Imitation, empathy, and mirror neurons. *Annual Review of Psychology, 60*(1), 653–670. DOI: 10.1146/annurev.psych.60.110707.163604

Ibrahim, M. H. (1982). Arabic–English bilingualism: A code-switching and borrowing study. *Anthropological Linguistics, 24*(1), 55–68.

Ilic, P., Casebourne, I., & Wegerif, R. (2021). *Artificial intelligence in education: The intersection of technology and pedagogy*. Routledge.

Immordino-Yang, M. H., & Damasio, A. (2007). We feel, therefore we learn: The relevance of affective and social neuroscience to education. *Mind, Brain and Education : the Official Journal of the International Mind, Brain, and Education Society, 1*(1), 3–10. DOI: 10.1111/j.1751-228X.2007.00004.x

Indriani, L., & Bram, B. (2023, May). Lexical borrowing of social media terms in *liputan6.com* website. *Journal of Language.*, *5*(1), 11–22. DOI: 10.30743/jol.v5i1.6836

Jansen, K., & Kiefer, S. M. (2020). Understanding brain development: Investing in young adolescents' cognitive and social-emotional development. *Middle School Journal*, *51*(1), 18–25. DOI: 10.1080/00940771.2020.1787749

Jensen, E. (2005). *Teaching with the brain in mind.* Association for Supervision and Curriculum Development. https://www.google.co.in/books/edition/Teaching_with_the_Brain_in_Mind/KP5QBAAAQBAJ?hl=en&gbpv=1

Jensen, E. (2005). *Teaching with the brain in mind.* ASCD.

Jensen, E. (2008). *Brain-based learning: The new paradigm of teaching.* Corwin Press.

Jensen, E., & McConchie, L. (2020). *Brain-based learning: Teaching the way students learn.* SAGE Publications Ltd.

Ji, C., & Chen, Y. (2022). A Tentative Study on Translation Tactics of Culture-loaded Words Based on Domestication and Lexical borrowing: A Case Analysis of The Last Emperor Film. *Modern Languages, Literatures, and Linguistics, 1*(01).

Jirout, J. J., Ruzek, E., Vitiello, V. E., Whittaker, J., & Pianta, R. C. (2023). The association between and development of school enjoyment and general knowledge. *Child Development*, *94*(2). Advance online publication. DOI: 10.1111/cdev.13878 PMID: 36445041

Johnson, J. E., Rahn, N. L., & Bricker, D. (2015). *An activity-based approach to early intervention.* Brookes Publishing.

Jolles, J., & Jolles, D. D. (2021). On neuroeducation: Why and how to improve neuroscientific literacy in educational professionals. *Frontiers in Psychology*, *12*, 752151. Advance online publication. DOI: 10.3389/fpsyg.2021.752151

Jongsma, A. E.Jr, & Winkelstern, J. A. (2016). *The early childhood education intervention treatment planner.* Wiley.

Jovanovic, D., & Matejevic, M. (2014). Relationship between rewards and intrinsic motivation for learning. *Procedia: Social and Behavioral Sciences*, *149*, 256–260. DOI: 10.1016/j.sbspro.2014.08.287

Kagin, S. L., & Lusebrink, V. B. (1978). The expressive therapies continuum. *Art Psychotherapy*, *5*(4), 171–180. DOI: 10.1016/0090-9092(78)90031-5

Kalawski, J. P. (2020). The Alba Method and the Science of Emotions. *Integrative Psychological & Behavioral Science, 54*(4), 903–919. Advance online publication. DOI: 10.1007/s12124-020-09525-4 PMID: 32212066

Kandel, E. R., Schwartz, J. H., Jessell, T. M., Siegelbaum, S. A., & Hudspeth, A. J. (2013). *Principles of neural science* (5th ed.). McGraw-Hill Education.

Kane, M. J., & Engle, R. W. (2002). The role of prefrontal cortex in workingmemory capacity, executive attention, and general fluid intelligence: An individual-differences perspective. *Psychonomic Bulletin & Review, 9*(4), 637–671. DOI: 10.3758/BF03196323

Kang, S. H. K. (2016). Spaced repetition promotes efficient and effective learning. *Policy Insights from the Behavioral and Brain Sciences, 3*(1), 12–19. DOI: 10.1177/2372732215624708

Kania, B. F., Wrońska, D., & Zięba, D. (2017). Introduction to neural plasticity mechanism. *Journal of Behavioral and Brain Science, 7*(2), 41–49. DOI: 10.4236/jbbs.2017.72005

Kaplinskiy, V., Voloshyn, S., Stakhiv, L., Oleksyuk, O., Ruskulis, L., & Haidaienko, I. (2022). Educational Needs of Society: Neuropedagogy as One of the Main Aspects of Motivation in Learning within Formal and Non-Formal Education. *BRAIN. Broad Research in Artificial Intelligence and Neuroscience, 13*(3), 225–235. DOI: 10.18662/brain/13.3/364

Kaplinskyi, V., Stoliarenko, O., Stoliarenko, O., Berezyuk, O., Chumak, M., & Hatezh, N. (2024). Developing Future Teachers' Creativity as a Crucial Element of Systemic Work in the Neuropedagogical Environment. *Revista romaneasca pentru educatie multidimensionala, 16*(3), 375-385.

Kaptan, Z., & Üzüm, G. (2016). Erişkin hipokampal nörogenezin öğrenme ve hafıza fonksiyonlarındaki rolü. *Türk Nöroloji Dergisi = Turkish Journal of Neurology, 22*, 149–155. DOI: 10.4274/tnd.68889

Karamat, K. (2024). The Integration Between Neuropedagogy and Creativity in Higher Education. *American Journal of Technology and Applied Sciences, 20*, 67–71.

Karaolis, O. (2023). Not Just a Toy: Puppets for Autistic Teenagers. *Youth, 3*(4), 1174–1182. DOI: 10.3390/youth3040074

Karasievych, S., Halaidiuk, M., Kovalchuk, A., Oliinyk, M., Vykhrushch, V., Marionda, I., & Maksymchuk, I. (2021). Training future physical education teachers for physical and sports activities: Neuropedagogical approach. *BRAIN. Broad Research in Artificial Intelligence and Neuroscience*, *12*(4), 543–564. DOI: 10.18662/brain/12.4/264

Kasala, E. R., Bodduluru, N., Maneti, Y., & Thipparaboina, R. (2014). Effect of meditation on neurophysiological changes in stress mediated depression. *Complementary Therapies in Clinical Practice*, *20*(1), 74–80. DOI: 10.1016/j.ctcp.2013.10.001

Kasari, C., Kaiser, A., Goods, K., Nietfeld, J., Mathy, P., Landa, R., Murphy, S., & Almirall, D. (2014). Communication interventions for minimally verbal children with autism: A sequential randomized multiple assignment trial. *Journal of the American Academy of Child and Adolescent Psychiatry*, *53*(6), 635–646. DOI: 10.1016/j.jaac.2014.01.019 PMID: 24839882

Kelley, A. E., & Berridge, K. (2002). The neuroscience of natural rewards: Relevance to addictive drugs. *The Journal of Neuroscience : The Official Journal of the Society for Neuroscience*, *22*(9), 3306–3311. DOI: 10.1523/JNEUROSCI.22-09-03306.2002

Kempermann, G., & Gage, F. (2002). Genetic determinants of adult hippocampal neurogenesis correlate with acquisition, but not probe trial performance, in the water maze task. *The European Journal of Neuroscience*, *16*(1), 129–136. DOI: 10.1046/j.1460-9568.2002.02042.x

Kempermann, G., Kuhn, H., & Gage, F. (1998). Experience-induced neurogenesis in the senescent dentate gyrus. *The Journal of Neuroscience : The Official Journal of the Society for Neuroscience*, *18*(9), 3206–3212. DOI: 10.1523/JNEUROSCI.18-09-03206.1998

Kendeou, P., van den Broek, P., Helder, A., & Karlsson, J. (2014). A cognitive view of reading comprehension: Implications for reading difficulties. *Learning Disabilities Research & Practice*, *29*(1), 10–16. DOI: 10.1111/ldrp.12025

Kenwood, M. M., Kalin, N. H., & Barbas, H. (2022). The prefrontal cortex, pathological anxiety, and anxiety disorders. *Neuropsychopharmacology : Official Publication of the American College of Neuropsychopharmacology*, *47*(1), 260–275. DOI: 10.1038/s41386-021-01109-z

Kernas, A., Kotlomanitova, G., Kozyr, M., Myronenko, N., Sokolovska, S., & Stepanchenko, N. (2024). Professionalization of pedagogical activity of future teachers, formation of communicative competence as an aspect of neuropedagogy. *BRAIN. Broad Research in Artificial Intelligence and Neuroscience*, *15*(1), 77–88. DOI: 10.18662/brain/15.1/537

Kichuk, Y., Gurevych, R., Bohush, O., Zasypkina, L., Shvets, O., & Bevz, O. (2024). The Role of Pedagogical Reflexology in Fostering Teacher's Professional Reflection in Neuropedagogy. *BRAIN. Broad Research in Artificial Intelligence and Neuroscience*, *15*(4), 104–119. DOI: 10.70594/brain/15.4/8

Ki, J. J., Kelly, S., & Parra, L. (2016). Attention strongly modulates reliability of neural responses to naturalistic narrative stimuli. *The Journal of Neuroscience : The Official Journal of the Society for Neuroscience*, *36*(10), 3092–3101. DOI: 10.1523/JNEUROSCI.2942-15.2016

Kim, M. J., Gee, D., Loucks, R., Davis, F., & Whalen, P. (2011). Anxiety dissociates dorsal and ventral medial prefrontal cortex functional connectivity with the amygdala at rest. *Cerebral Cortex (New York, N.Y.)*, *21*(7), 1667–1673. DOI: 10.1093/cercor/bhq237

Kirov, S. A., Goddard, C., & Harris, K. (2004). Age-dependence in the homeostatic upregulation of hippocampal dendritic spine number during blocked synaptic transmission. *Neuropharmacology*, *47*(5), 640–648. DOI: 10.1016/j.neuropharm.2004.07.039

Kirschbaum, C., Wolf, O., May, M., Wippich, W., & Hellhammer, D. (1996). Stress- and treatment-induced elevations of cortisol levels associated with impaired declarative memory in healthy adults. *Life Sciences*, *58*(17), 1475–1483. DOI: 10.1016/0024-3205(96)00118-X

Knight, R. T., Hillyard, S. A., Woods, D. L., & Neville, H. J. (1981). The effects of frontal cortex lesions on event-related potentials during auditory selective attention. *Electroencephalography and Clinical Neurophysiology*, *52*(6), 571–582. DOI: 10.1016/0013-4694(81)91431-0

Knudsen, E. I. (2004). Sensitive periods in the development of the brain and behavior. *Journal of Cognitive Neuroscience*, *16*(8), 1412–1425. DOI: 10.1162/0898929042304796

Koegel, L. K., Singh, A. K., & Koegel, R. L. (2010). Improving academic motivation in children with autism. *Journal of Autism and Developmental Disorders*, *40*(9), 1057–1066. DOI: 10.1007/s10803-010-0962-6 PMID: 20221791

Koegel, R. L., & Koegel, L. K. (2006). *Pivotal response treatments for autism: Communication, social, and academic development*. Brookes Publishing., DOI: 10.1037/11485-000

Kohn, A. (1993). *Punished by rewards: The trouble with gold stars, incentive plans, A's, praise, and other bribes*. Mifflin and Company.

Köksal, N. (2024). *Brain-Based Learning*. Ed. Ö. Demirel. *New Directions in Education. Directions in education* (pp. 113-123). Pegem Publishing.

Kolb, B., & Gibb, R. (2011). Brain plasticity and behaviour in the developing brain. *Journal of the Canadian Academy of Child and Adolescent Psychiatry = Journal de l'Académie Canadienne de Psychiatrie de l'Enfant et de l'Adolescent, 20*(4), 265.

Kosola, S., Mundy, L. K., Sawyer, S. M., Canterford, L., van der Windt, D. A., Dunn, K. M., & Patton, G. C. (2017). Pain and learning in primary school. *Pain, 158*(9), 1825–1830. DOI: 10.1097/j.pain.0000000000000984 PMID: 28738407

Kostidakis, T. (2021). Dramatherapy and Greek Traditional Shadow Puppetry. In Hougham, R., & Jones, B. (Eds.), *Dramatherapy* (1st ed., pp. 99–113). Routledge., DOI: 10.4324/9781003042792-9

Koukourikos, K., Tsaloglidou, A., Tzeha, L., Iliadis, C., Frantzana, A., Katsimbeli, A., & Kourkouta, L. (2021). An Overview of Play Therapy. *Materia Socio-Medica, 33*(4), 293–297. DOI: 10.5455/msm.2021.33.293-297 PMID: 35210953

Koval, V., Prytulyk, N., Sharan, O., Streletska, N., Dudnyk, N., & Koltok, L. (2025). Neuropedagogical Technologies for Training Future Primary School Teachers. *BRAIN. Broad Research in Artificial Intelligence and Neuroscience, 16*(1 Sup1), 27-40.

Krull, K. R., Hardy, K. K., Kahalley, L. S., Schuitema, I., & Kesler, S. R. (2018). Neurocognitive Outcomes and Interventions in Long-Term Survivors of Childhood Cancer. *Journal of Clinical Oncology*, *36*(21), 2181–2189. DOI: 10.1200/JCO.2017.76.4696 PMID: 29874137

Kunduracı, H. Ö., & Aksoy, A. (2025). The Effects of" Mother Education Program" on Mothers' Parenting Knowledge, Parenting Self-Efficacy and Their Children's Development. *Education in Science*, *50*(221), 1–31.

Kuo, M.-F., Paulus, W., & Nitsche, M. (2006). Sex differences in cortical neuroplasticity in humans. *Neuroreport*, *17*(16), 1703–1707. DOI: 10.1097/01.wnr.0000239955.68319.c2

Kuznietsov, Y., & Kostiukevych, O. (2024). The influence of the integration of neuropedagogy, trend-watching, gamification, robotics, and immersive technologies on the development of pedagogical skills. *Scientia et societus, 1*(3), 92-103.

Kuznietsov, Y. (2024). *Innovative models of vocational education: A symbiosis of artificial intelligence, neuropedagogy, and the competency-based approach.* ПРОФЕСІЙНА ОСВІТА.

LaBar, K. S., & Cabeza, R. (2006). Cognitive neuroscience of emotional memory. *Nature Reviews. Neuroscience, 7*(1), 54–64. DOI: 10.1038/nrn1825

LaBerge, D. (2001). Attention, consciousness, and electrical wave activity within the cortical column. *International Journal of Psychophysiology, 43*(1), 5–24. DOI: 10.1016/S0167-8760(01)00176-3

LaBerge, D. (2002). Attentional control: Brief and prolonged. *Psychological Research, 66*(4), 220–233. DOI: 10.1007/s00426-002-0097-2

Lakhmotova, Y., Sadovets, O., Orlovska, O., Martynyuk, O., Myroshnychenko, V., & Lebedieva, L. (2024). Distance Learning of a Foreign Language in the Context of Neuropedagogical Factors. *BRAIN. Broad Research in Artificial Intelligence and Neuroscience, 15*(1), 105–121. DOI: 10.18662/brain/15.1/539

Lakoff, G., & Johnson, M. (2008). *Metaphors we live by*. University of Chicago Press.

Langer, A., Marshall, P. J., & Levy-Tzedek, S. (2023). Ethical considerations in child-robot interactions. *Neuroscience and Biobehavioral Reviews, 151*, 105230. DOI: 10.1016/j.neubiorev.2023.105230 PMID: 37169271

Lang, P. J. (1968). *Fear reduction and fear behavior: Problems in treating a construct. J. Schlien içinde, Research in Psychotherapy*. American Psychiatric Press.

Leaf, J. B., Leaf, R., McEachin, J., Taubman, M., Ala'i-Rosales, S., Ross, R. K., Smith, T., & Weiss, M. J. (2016). Applied behavior analysis is a science and, therefore, progressive. *Journal of Autism and Developmental Disorders, 46*(2), 720–731. DOI: 10.1007/s10803-015-2591-6 PMID: 26373767

Ledesma, R. D., Valero-Mora, P., & Macbeth, G. (2015). The Scree Test and the Number of Factors: A Dynamic Graphics Approach. *The Spanish Journal of Psychology, 18*, E11. DOI: 10.1017/sjp.2015.13 PMID: 26055575

LeDoux, J. E. (2015). Feelings: What are they & how does the brain make them? *Daedalus, 144*(1), 96–111. DOI: 10.1162/DAED_a_00319

Lehman, R. (2006). The role of emotion in creating instructor and learner presence in the distance education experience. *Journal of Cognitive Affective Learning, 2*(2), 12–26.

Lenska, S., Naumovska, N., Rudakova, N., Naumovska, O., Marchii-Dmytrash, T., & Sova, A. (2022). Neuropedagogical and Psychological Aspects of Play. *BRAIN. Broad Research in Artificial Intelligence and Neuroscience, 13*(4), 104–121. DOI: 10.18662/brain/13.4/378

Lester, S., & Russell, W. (2008). *Play for a change: Play, policy and practice – A review of contemporary perspectives*. Play England.

Leventon, J. S., Stevens, J., & Bauer, P. (2014). Development in the neurophysiology of emotion processing and memory in school-age children. *Developmental Cognitive Neuroscience, 10*, 21–33. DOI: 10.1016/j.dcn.2014.07.007

Li, L., Gow, A. D. I., & Zhou, J. (2020). The role of positive emotions in education: A neuroscience perspective. *Mind, Brain and Education : the Official Journal of the International Mind, Brain, and Education Society, 14*(3), 220–234. DOI: 10.1111/mbe.12244

Lillard, A. S., Lerner, M. D., Hopkins, E. J., Dore, R. A., Smith, E. D., & Palmquist, C. M. (2013). The impact of pretend play on children's development: A review of the evidence. *Psychological Bulletin, 139*(1), 1–34. DOI: 10.1037/a0029321

Lilley, R. (2011). The ABCs of Autism: Aspects of Maternal Pedagogy in Australia. *Social Analysis: The International Journal of Social and Cultural Practice, 55*(1), 134–159. https://www.jstor.org/stable/23182182

Lindau, M., Almkvist, O., & Mohammed, A. (2016). Effects of stress on learning and memory. G. Fink (Dü.) içinde, *Stress: Concepts, cognition, emotion, and behavior* [). Academic Press.]. *Cilt, 1*, 153–160.

Lindsay, E. K., Chin, B., Greco, C. M., Young, S., Brown, K. W., Wright, A. G. C., Smyth, J. M., Burkett, D., & Creswell, J. D. (2018). How mindfulness training promotes positive emotions: Dismantling acceptance skills training in two randomized controlled trials. *Journal of Personality and Social Psychology, 115*(6), 944–973. DOI: 10.1037/pspa0000134

Lin, M.-L., & Faldowski, R. A. (2023). The relationship of parent support and child emotional regulation to school readiness. *International Journal of Environmental Research and Public Health, 20*(6), 4867. DOI: 10.3390/ijerph20064867 PMID: 36981776

Liratni, M., & Blanchet, C. (2019). *Introduction. Enseigner les habiletés sociales aux enfants avec autisme: avec la méthode G.A.C.S (Groupe d'Apprentissage à la Communication et à la Socialisation)*. Dunod., https://shs.cairn.info/enseigner-les-habiletes-sociales-aux-enfants--9782100794966-page-17?lang=fr DOI: 10.3917/dunod.lirat.2019.01

Lisman, J., Yasuda, R., & Raghavachari, S. (2012). Mechanisms of CaMKII action in long-term potentiation. *Nature Reviews. Neuroscience, 13*(3), 169–182. DOI: 10.1038/nrn3192

Liu, S., Li, N., Zhang, X., Wang, L., & Liu, D. (2024). Effects of working memory and visual search skill on Chinese reading comprehension: Examining the simple view of reading. *Reading and Writing*, *38*(2), 329–351. DOI: 10.1007/s11145-024-10515-w

Llana, T., Fernandez-Baizan, C., Mendez-Lopez, M., Fidalgo, C., & Mendez, M. (2022). Functional near-infrared spectroscopy in the neuropsychological assessment of spatial memory: A systematic review. *Acta Psychologica, 224*, 103525. https://doi.org/, Y., Shi, L., & Musib, A.F. (2025) Effects of music training on executive functions in preschool children aged 3–6 years: systematic review and meta-analysis. *Front. Psychol.* 15:1522962. https://doi.org/DOI: 10.1016/j.actpsy.2022.103525Lu

Lohvynenko, T., Drozd, L., Marieieva, T., Hryntsiv, M., Prymakova, V., & Hrynyk, I. (2023). Neuropedagogical Principles as a Factor of Inclusive Education in the Context of Managerial Activity: European Experience. *BRAIN. Broad Research in Artificial Intelligence and Neuroscience*, *14*(4), 212–227. DOI: 10.18662/brain/14.4/501

López-Escribano, C., Escudero, A., & Pérez-López, R. (2021). An exploratory study about patterns of parental home literacy activities during the COVID-19 confinement among Spanish families. *Early Education and Development*, *32*(6), 812–829. DOI: 10.1080/10409289.2021.1916184

López-Resa, P., & Moraleda-Sepúlveda, E. (2023). Working memory capacity and text comprehension performance in children with dyslexia and dyscalculia: A pilot study. *Frontiers in Psychology*, *14*, 1191304. Advance online publication. DOI: 10.3389/fpsyg.2023.1191304

Lovaas, O. I. (1987). Behavioral treatment and normal educational and intellectual functioning in young children with autism. *Journal of Consulting and Clinical Psychology*, *55*(1), 3–9. DOI: 10.1037/0022-006X.55.1.3 PMID: 3571656

Luckin, R., Holmes, W., Griffiths, M., & Forcier, L. B. (2016). *Intelligence unleashed: An argument for AI in education*. Pearson Education.

Lupien, S. J., Fiocco, A., Wan, N., Maheu, F., Lord, C., Schramek, T., & Tu, M. (2005). Stress hormones and human memory function across the lifespan. *Psychoneuroendocrinology*, *30*(3), 225–242. DOI: 10.1016/j.psyneuen.2004.08.003

Lupien, S.J., & McEwen, B. (1997). The acute effects of corticosteroids on cognition: Integration of animal and human model studies. *Brain Research. Brain Research Reviews*, *24*(1), 1–27. DOI: 10.1016/S0165-0173(97)00004-0

Lupu, C., & Jurchescu, D. (2020). Neuropedagogia. Metoda de cunoa tere i cercetare a creierului de către copii. *Journal for Neurology & Psychiatry of Child & Adolescent in Romania, 26*(2).

Lyndina, Y., Martynyuk, Z., Tovstohan, V., Babichenko, A., Mytsyk, H., & Samoilenko, I. (2023). Psychological and pedagogical technologies in working with children with special educational needs: Neuropedagogical aspect. *BRAIN. Broad Research in Artificial Intelligence and Neuroscience, 14*(1), 302–318. DOI: 10.18662/brain/14.1/421

Ma, C.-L., Ma, X.-T., Wang, J.-J., Liu, H., Chen, Y.-F., & Yang, Y. (2017). Physical exercise induces hippocampal neurogenesis and prevents cognitive decline. *Behavioural Brain Research, 317*, 332–339. DOI: 10.1016/j.bbr.2016.09.067

Mácajová, M. (2013). Neuropedagogy and brain compatible learning--ideas for education in the 21st century. *Technologia Vzdelavania, 21*(3).

Macari, S., Chen, X., Brunissen, L., Yhang, E., Brennan-Wydra, E., Vernetti, A., Volkmar, F., Chang, J., & Chawarska, K. (2021). Puppets facilitate attention to social cues in children with ASD. *Autism research: official journal of the International Society for Autism Research, 14*(9), 1975-1985. DOI: 10.1002/aur.2552

MacArthur, C. A. (2009). Reflections on research on writing and technology for struggling writers. *Learning Disabilities Research & Practice, 24*(2), 93–103. DOI: 10.1111/j.1540-5826.2009.00283.x

Macias, L. D. C., Montoya, L. M. S., & Hernández, R. G. (2024). La neuropedagogía y sus herramientas educativas para mejorar la enseñanza en la educación técnica profesional en el área de contabilidad. *RECIMUNDO, 8*(1), 385–399. DOI: 10.26820/recimundo/8.(1).ene.2024.385-399

Madanipour, P., Garvis, S., Cohrssen, C., & Pendergast, D. (2025, January). Early childhood teachers' understanding of executive functions and strategies employed to facilitate them. [). Frontiers Media SA.]. *Frontiers in Education, 9*, 1488410. DOI: 10.3389/feduc.2024.1488410

Madi, B. (2014). *How does learning occur in the brain?* Efil Publishing.

Maguire, E. A., Frackowiak, R., & Frith, C. (1997). Recalling routes around london: Activation of the right hippocampus in taxi drivers. *The Journal of Neuroscience : The Official Journal of the Society for Neuroscience, 17*(18), 7103–7110. DOI: 10.1523/JNEUROSCI.17-18-07103.1997

Maguire, E. A., Spiers, H., Good, C., Hartley, T., Frackowiak, R., & Burgess, N. (2003). Navigation expertise and the human hippocampus: A structural brain imaging analysis. *Hippocampus, 13*(2), 250–259. DOI: 10.1002/hipo.10087

Mahoney, G., Nam, S., & Perales, F. (2014). The role of parents in early intervention: Implications for social–emotional development of children with disabilities. *Journal of Intellectual Disability Research, 58*(4), 333–345. DOI: 10.1111/jir.12095

Maidaniuk, I., Kavun, V., Tverdokhlib, N., Biryukova, L., Doroshenko, T., & Mashtaler, I. (2023). A Creative Approach to Preparing Inclusive Music Lessons: The Role of Neuropedagogy in Inclusive Music Education. *BRAIN. Broad Research in Artificial Intelligence and Neuroscience, 14*(4), 242–253. DOI: 10.18662/brain/14.4/503

Maino, D. M. (2009). Neuroplasticity: Teaching an old brain new tricks. *Revista Optometra.*

Mäki-Marttunen, V., Pickard, N., Solbakk, A.-K., Ogawa, K., Knight, R., & Hartikainen, K. (2014). Low attentional engagement makes attention network activity susceptible to emotional interference. *Neuroreport, 25*(13), 1038–1043. DOI: 10.1097/WNR.0000000000000223

Makrygianni, M. K., Gena, A., Katoudi, S., & Galanis, P. (2018). Effectiveness of Applied Behavior Analysis Interventions for Children with Autism Spectrum Disorders: A Meta-Analysis. *Research in Autism Spectrum Disorders, 51*, 18–31. DOI: 10.1016/j.rasd.2018.03.006

Mamaniyazovna, X. S. (2025). Ethical viewpoint formation through effective neuropedagogical methods and technologies. *International Journal of Pedagogics, 5*(02), 211–215. DOI: 10.37547/ijp/Volume05Issue02-57

Mamaniyozovna, K. S. (2025). Neuropedagogical Technologies That Develop Analysis, Critical and Creative Thinking. *CURRENT RESEARCH JOURNAL OF PEDAGOGICS, 6*(02), 42–47. DOI: 10.37547/pedagogics-crjp-06-02-09

Manav, F. (2011). Kaygı kavramı. *Toplum Bilimleri Dergisi, 5*(9), 201–211.

Marchak, D., Shvarts-Serebro, I., & Blonder, R. (2021). Crafting molecular geometries: Implications of neuro-pedagogy for teaching chemical content. *Journal of Chemical Education, 98*(4), 1321–1327. DOI: 10.1021/acs.jchemed.0c00306

Marc, L., & Philippette, T. (2021). L'évolution du rôle des enseignants d'élèves dyslexiques suite à l'utilisation d'un outil numérique en classe. *The Journal of Special Education, 45*(2), 88–100. DOI: 10.1007/s12630-021-00389-2

Marievych, N., Oksana, K. R. U. S., Martyniv, L., Komarovska, O., & Kryzhanovska, T. (2023). Music and Game Activity of Elementary School Students as an Aspect of Neuropedagogy. *BRAIN. Broad Research in Artificial Intelligence and Neuroscience, 14*(1), 269–284. DOI: 10.18662/brain/14.1/419

Markiv, O., Zarivna, O., Khymai, N., Shalova, N., Shemet, V., Markiv, I., ... & Tymkiv, O. (2025). Mentoring as a Neuro-Pedagogical Tool of Motivation for Health Culture Formation Among the Students During Periods of War and Global Challenges. BRAIN. Broad Research in Artificial Intelligence and Neuroscience, 16(1 Sup1), 165-178.

Márquez, F. (2025). The Relationship between Working Memory and Reading Comprehension in Elementary School Children. *Pensamiento Americano, 18*(36), 1–12. DOI: 10.21803/penamer.18.36.873

Marrero, N. D. L. M. P. (2023). Dinámica de formación neurodidáctica de docentes desde la neuropedagogía: Neuro-didactic Dynamics Training Teachers from Neuropedagogy. *Papeles, 15*(29).

Marrero, P., & de las Mercedes, N. (2023). Dinámica de formación neurodidáctica de docentes desde la neuropedagogía. *Papeles: Revista de la Facultad de Educación Universidad Antonio Nariño, 15*(29).

Marshall, L. L., & Bolt-Lee, C. E. (2022). A neuroeducation and cognitive learning-based strategy to develop active learning pedagogies for accounting education. *The Accounting Educators' Journal, 32*. https://www.aejournal.com/ojs/index.php/aej/article/view/689

Marusak, H. A., Iadipaolo, A. S., Harper, F. W., Elrahal, F., Taub, J. W., Goldberg, E., & Rabinak, C. A. (2017). Neurodevelopmental consequences of pediatric cancer and its treatment: Applying an early adversity framework to understanding cognitive, behavioral, and emotional outcomes. *Neuropsychology Review, 28*(2), 123–175. DOI: 10.1007/s11065-017-9365-1 PMID: 29270773

Maryati, S. S., Purwanti, I., & Mubarika, M. P. (2020). The effect of brain-based learning on improving students' critical thinking ability and self-regulation. *Indonesian Journal of Integrated Science Education, 2*(2), 162–171. DOI: 10.29300/ijisedu.v2i2.3333

Masten, A. S., Lucke, C. M., Nelson, K. M., & Stallworthy, I. C. (2021). Resilience in development and psychopathology: Multisystem perspectives. *Annual Review of Clinical Psychology, 17*(1), 521–549. DOI: 10.1146/annurev-clinpsy-081219-120307 PMID: 33534615

Matveev, M. (2024). Digital neuropedagogy: harnessing cognitive science and technology for educational efficiency. *Journal of Teaching English for Specific and Academic Purposes*, 693-712.

McEwen, B. S. (2006). Protective and damaging effects of stress mediators: Central role of the brain. *Dialogues in Clinical Neuroscience*, *8*(4), 367–381. DOI: 10.31887/DCNS.2006.8.4/bmcewen

McFarland, D. J. (2017). How neuroscience can inform the study of individual differences in cognitive abilities. *Reviews in the Neurosciences*, *28*(4), 343–362. DOI: 10.1515/revneuro-2016-0073

McGaugh, J. L., McIntyre, C., & Power, A. (2002). Amygdala modulation of memory consolidation: Interaction with other brain systems. *Neurobiology of Learning and Memory*, *78*(3), 539–552. DOI: 10.1006/nlme.2002.4082

McLeod, S. (2025). Working memory model. *Simply Psychology*. https://www.simplypsychology.org/a-level-memory.html?nowprocket=1

Medvedieva, S. O., Stepanova, I. S., Nykyporets, S. S., & Ibrahimova, L. V. (2023). The application of a neuropedagogical approach while teaching English to students of higher educational establishments. *Перспективи та інновації науки.Nº 8: 13-24.*

Mefteh, K. C. (2024). *Active pedagogy and neuroeducation: In-depth reflections for innovative teaching*. IntechOpen eBooks. https://doi.org/DOI: 10.5772/intechopen.114368

Melnyk, O., Petryk, O., Lysohor, L., Pavlyk, O., Boiaryn, L., & Tykhonova, S. (2022). Current approaches to organizing the educational process in primary school: A neuroscientific approach. *BRAIN. Broad Research in Artificial Intelligence and Neuroscience. Vol. 13,Nº 1, Sup. 1: 01-21.*

Mercan, O., & Kabadayı, F. (2023). Psychometric properties of the BALCI Turkish version. *Psicologia: Reflexão e Crítica : Revista Semestral do Departamento de Psicologia da UFRGS*, *36*(1), 7. Advance online publication. DOI: 10.1186/s41155-023-00248-0 PMID: 36853435

Mercer, N. (2019). *Language and the joint creation of knowledge: The selected works of Neil Mercer*. Routledge. DOI: 10.4324/9780429400759

Mesulam, M. M. (1983). The functional anatomy and hemispheric specialization for directed attention: The role of the parietal lobe and its connectivity. *Trends in Neurosciences*, *6*, 384–387. DOI: 10.1016/0166-2236(83)90171-6

Miller, J. E., & List, J. M. (2023). "Detecting Lexical Borrowings from Dominant Languages in Multilingual Wordlists". *Proceedings of the 17th Conference of the European Chapter of the Association for Computational Linguistics*, pages 2599–2605 May 2-6, ©2023 Association for Computational Linguistics. DOI: 10.18653/v1/2023.eacl-main.190

Ministry of Culture and Tourism. (2025). *Karagöz*. https://www.ktb.gov.tr/EN-98575/karagoz.html

Mirescu, C., & Gould, E. (2016). Stress and adult neurogenesis. *Hippocampus*, *16*(3), 233–238. DOI: 10.1002/hipo.20155

Mogg, K., & Bradley, B. P. (1998). A cognitive-motivational analysis of anxiety. *Behaviour Research and Therapy*, *36*(9), 809–848. DOI: 10.1016/S0005-7967(98)00063-1

Mohammadi, Y., Bozorgkhou, H., Hadavi, S. M., Shojaei, M., Khodadadi, F. R., Najafi, S., Karimi, Z., & Sarvestani, M. M. (2023). The effectiveness of neurofeedback on the management of academic performance in students with academic failure: Experimental research. *Annals of Medicine and Surgery (London)*, *85*(6), 2677–2682. DOI: 10.1097/MS9.0000000000000823

Moosapoor, M. (2023). The Effectiveness of Puppet Play Therapy On Increasing Communication Skills Through Social Stories for Children with Autism in Rasht. *International Journal of Innovation in Management. Economics and Social Sciences*, *3*(1), 30–39. DOI: 10.52547/ijimes.3.1.30

Moreira, P. A., Inman, R. A., Hanel, P. H., Faria, S., Araújo, M., Pedras, S., & Cunha, D. (2021). Engagement and disengagement with sustainable development: Further conceptualization and evidence of validity for the Engagement/Disengagement in Sustainable Development Inventory (EDiSDI). *Journal of Environmental Psychology*, *79*, 101729. DOI: 10.1016/j.jenvp.2021.101729

Moreno, R., & Mayer, R. (2007). Interactive multimodal learning environments: Special issue on interactive learning environments: Contemporary issues and trends. *Educational Psychology Review*, *19*(3), 309–326. DOI: 10.1007/s10648-007-9047-2

Morett, L. M., Morett, L. M., Hawes, Z., & Dommett, E. J. (2021). Why educational neuroscience needs educational and school psychology to effectively translate neuroscience to educational practice. *Frontiers in Psychology*, *11*(618449), 1–7.

Morett, L.M., Morett, L.M., & Hawes, Z., & Dommett, E.J. (2021). Educational neuroscience needs educational and school psychology to translate neuroscience into educational practice effectively. *Frontiers in Psychology, 11*(618449), 1–7. PMID: 33519642

Morgan, C. T. (1977). *A Brief Introduction to Psychology*. McGraw-Hill, Inc.

Moritz-Gasser, S., & Duffau, H. (2013). The anatomo-functional connectivity of word repetition: Insights provided by awake brain tumor surgery. *Frontiers in Human Neuroscience*, *7*(405), 1–4. DOI: 10.3389/fnhum.2013.00405

Morocco, U. N. I. C. E. F. (2020). *Annual report on early childhood education*. UNICEF.

Morris, R. (1984). Developments of a water-maze procedure for studying spatial learning in the rat. *Journal of Neuroscience Methods*, *11*(1), 47–60. DOI: 10.1016/0165-0270(84)90007-4

Moser, J. S., Schroder, H. S., Heeter, C., Moran, T. P., & Lee, Y. (2011). Mind your errors. *Psychological Science*, *22*(12), 1484–1489. DOI: 10.1177/0956797611419520

Moss-Zobel, A. (2024, July). Neuropedagogy in Higher Education. In *ARPHA Conference Abstracts* (Vol. 7, p. e129736). Pensoft Publishers. DOI: 10.3897/aca.7.e129736

Moumne, S., Hall, N., Böke, B. N., Bastien, L., & Heath, N. (2021). Implicit theories of emotion, goals for emotion regulation, and cognitive responses to negative life events. *Psychological Reports*, *124*(4), 1588–1620. DOI: 10.1177/0033294120942110 PMID: 32674669

Mudryk, O., Ivakhnenko, A., Odynchenko, L., Dmytriieva, I., Ivanenko, A., & Shelever, O. (2022). Mental and Pedagogical Techniques in Teaching Children with Special Educational Needs: Neuropedagogical Aspect. *BRAIN. Broad Research in Artificial Intelligence and Neuroscience*, *13*(4), 292–305. DOI: 10.18662/brain/13.4/389

Mundy, P., & Newell, L. (2007). Attention, joint attention, and social cognition. *Current Directions in Psychological Science*, *16*(5), 269–274. DOI: 10.1111/j.1467-8721.2007.00518.x PMID: 19343102

Murniati, N., Susilo, H., & Listyorini, D. (2023). Retention achievement in brain-based whole learning is supported by students' scientific literacy and concept mastery. *Pegem Journal of Education and Instruction*, *13*(3), 294–303. DOI: 10.47750/pegegog.13.03.30

Murray, E. A. (2007). The amygdala, reward and emotion. *Trends in Cognitive Sciences, 11*(11), 489–497. DOI: 10.1016/j.tics.2007.08.013

Murray, L., Levickis, P., McFarland, L., Eadie, P., Lee-Pang, L., Quach, J., & Page, J. (2025). Supporting Young Children's Social–Emotional Wellbeing in Early Childhood Education and Care: Perspectives from the Sector. *Education Sciences, 15*(5), 569. DOI: 10.3390/educsci15050569

Mutanga, M. B. (2024). Students' perspectives and experiences in project-based learning: A qualitative study. *Trends in Higher Education, 3*(4), 903–911. DOI: 10.3390/higheredu3040052

Mystakidis, S., Christopoulos, A., Fragkaki, M., & Dimitropoulos, K. (2023). Online professional development on educational neuroscience in higher education based on design thinking. *Information (Basel), 14*(7), 382. DOI: 10.3390/info14070382

Mzeau, M. (2005). *Neuropsychologie de l'enfant: Troubles développementaux et acquis*. Éditions Masson.

Näätänena, R., Gaillard, W. K., & Mäntysalo, S. (1980). Brain Potential Correlates of Voluntary and Involuntary Attention. *Progress in Brain Research, 54*, 343–348. DOI: 10.1016/S0079-6123(08)61645-3

Naumenko, N., Kozlov, A., Palevych, S., Denysenko, A., Tverdokhlib, T., & Bashkir, O. (2024). Advancing the Career Development for Future Primary School Teachers in Ukraine: New Neuropedagogical Challenges. *Revista Romaneasca Pentru Educatie Multidimensionala, 16*(4), 29–51. DOI: 10.18662/rrem/16.4/906

Nefedchenko, V., Ostapenko, E., Bokhonko, Y., Gurevych, R., Shanaieva-Tsymbal, L., & Rud, O. (2023). Features of Information and Communication Technologies in the Educational Process: Neuroscience in Education.

Nelson, C. A.III. (2017). Hazards to early development: The biological embedding of early life adversity. *Neuron, 96*(2), 262–266. DOI: 10.1016/j.neuron.2017.09.027

Neo, T., Amphawan, A., Hew, S., Neo, M., Hamidani, K., & Chang, Y. (2022). Inculcating student problem-solving skills through self-directed learning in a smart learning environment. *EDULEARN ... Proceedings, 1*, 326–332. DOI: 10.21125/edulearn.2022.0100

Nesic, M., Kostic, J., Cicevic, S., & Nesic, V. (2011). Neurofizioloske osnove paznje - Neurophysiology of attention. *Godisnjak za Psihologiju, 8*(10), 7–25.

Netton, I. R. (Ed.). (1985). *Arabia and the Gulf: From traditional society to modern states*. Croom Helm.

Ng, B. (2018). The neuroscience of growth mindset and intrinsic motivation. *Brain Sciences*, *8*(2), 20. DOI: 10.3390/brainsci8020020

Nievas, F., & Montes, M. (2023). Adapting pedagogical strategies through interdisciplinary neuroeducation: Meeting individual learning needs. *J. Educ. Psychol.*, *115*, 304–317. DOI: 10.1037/edu0000586

Nievas, P. P., & Del Pilar Gallardo-Montes, C. (2023). The neuroeducation training of students in the degrees of early childhood and primary education: A content analysis of public universities in Andalusia. *Education Sciences*, *13*(10), 1006. DOI: 10.3390/educsci13101006

Nijhof, S. L., Vinkers, C. H., van Geelen, S. M., Duijff, S. N., Achterberg, E. J. M., van der Net, J., Veltkamp, R. C., Grootenhuis, M. A., van de Putte, E. M., Hillegers, M. H. J., van der Brug, A. W., Wierenga, C. J., Benders, M. J. N. L., Engels, R. C. M. E., Kors van der Ent, C., Vanderschuren, L. J. M. J., & Lesscher, H. M. B. (2018). Healthy play, better coping: The importance of play for the development of children in health and disease. *Neuroscience and Biobehavioral Reviews*, *95*, 421–429. Advance online publication. DOI: 10.1016/j.neubiorev.2018.09.024 PMID: 30273634

Nikulochkina, O., Teslenko, T., Kokhanko, O., Sevastiuk, M., Yankovska, I., & Teletska, L. (2022). Neuro-pedagogical aspects of forming the professional competence of elementary school teachers and their interaction with students. *Revista Romaneasca Pentru Educatie Multidimensionala, 14*(4 Sup. 1), 128-154.

Nilsson, M., Perfilieva, E., Johansson, U., Orwar, O., & Eriksson, P. S. (1999). Enriched environment increases neurogenesis in the adult rat dentate gyrus and improves spatial memory. *Journal of Neurobiology*, *39*(4), 569–578. DOI: 10.1002/(SICI)1097-4695(19990615)39:4<569::AID-NEU10>3.0.CO;2-F

Nokia, M. S., Lensu, S., Ahtiainen, J. P., Johansson, P. P., Koch, L. G., Britton, S. L., & Kainulainen, H. (2016). Physical exercise increases adult hippocampal neurogenesis in male rats provided it is aerobic and sustained. *The Journal of Physiology*, *594*(7), 1855–1873. DOI: 10.1113/JP271552

Nores, M., Belfield, C. R., Barnett, W. S., & Schweinhart, L. (2005). Updating the economic impacts of the High/Scope Perry Preschool program. *Educational Evaluation and Policy Analysis*, *27*(3), 245–261. DOI: 10.3102/01623737027003245

Noureen, G., Awan, R. N., & Fatima, H. (2017). Effect of brain-based learning on academic achievement of seventh graders in mathematics. *Journal of Elementary Education*, *27*(2), 85–97.

Nouwens, S., Groen, M. A., & Verhoeven, L. (2017). How working memory relates to children's reading comprehension: The importance of domain-specificity in storage and processing. *Reading and Writing*, *30*(1), 105–120. DOI: 10.1007/s11145-016-9665-5

Novia, B. O. N., & Rachmawati, Y. (2025). Analysis of Parenting in Shaping Character in Early Childhood: Analisis Pola Asuh Orang Tua dalam Membentuk Karakter pada Anak Usia Dini. *PAUDIA: Jurnal Penelitian dalam Bidang Pendidikan Anak Usia Dini*, 1-12.

Nurmakhanova, D. E., Rakhmetova, A. K., Kassymbekova, D. A., Meiirova, G., & Rakhimzhanova, G. M. (2021). Neuropedagogy for improving the educational process in universities.

Nykyporets, S. S., Melnyk, O. D., Hadaichuk, N. M., Derun, V. H., & Chopliak, V. V. (2023). Neuropedagogical approach enhancing foreign language acquisition in non-linguistic higher education institutions. *Актуальні питання у сучасній науці.Nº 5: 341–355.*

O'Brien, L., & Murray, R. (2007). Forest School and its impacts on young children: Case studies in Britain. *Urban Forestry & Urban Greening*, *6*(4), 249–265. DOI: 10.1016/j.ufug.2007.03.006

O'Connor, R. (2018). Reading fluency and students with reading disabilities: How fast is fast enough to promote reading comprehension? *Journal of Learning Disabilities*, *51*(2), 124–136. DOI: 10.1177/0022219417691835

O'Neill, G., & Short, A. (2023). Relevant, practical and connected to the real world: What higher education students say engages them in the curriculum. *Irish Educational Studies*, •••, 1–18. DOI: 10.1080/03323315.2023.2221663

Oakes, L. M. (2017). Plasticity may change inputs as well as processes, structures, and responses. *Cognitive Development*, *42*, 4–14. DOI: 10.1016/j.cogdev.2017.02.012 PMID: 28993717

Oakes, L. M., & Rakison, D. H. (2019). *Developmental cascades: Building the infant mind*. Oxford University Press. DOI: 10.1093/oso/9780195391893.001.0001

Oakhill, J., & Cain, K. (2007). The precursors of reading ability in young readers: Evidence from a longitudinal study. *Reading and Writing*, *20*(1), 1–28. DOI: 10.1007/s11145-006-9021-5

Öcal, E., Karademir, A., Saatçioğlu, Ö., & Yılmaz, H. B. (2021). A cultural and artistic approach to early childhood science education: Shadow play. *Educational Policy Analysis and Strategic Research*, *16*(3), 209–244. DOI: 10.29329/epasr.2021.373.12

Oggiano, M. (2022). Neurophysiology of emotions. In *T. Heinbockel (Dü.), Neurophysiology - networks, plasticity, pathophysiology and behavior*. Intechopen. DOI: 10.5772/intechopen.106043

Oh, Y., & Son, H. (2023) "Lexical borrowing in Korean: a diachronic approach based on a corpus analysis", in *the Journal Corpus Linguistics and Linguistic Theory*. De Gruyter Mouton August 24, 2023

Okur, M., & Aksoy, V. (2025). The effect of a working memory intervention package on the working memory performance of primary school students with specific learning disabilities. *Behavioral Sciences (Basel, Switzerland)*, *15*(3), 3–22. DOI: 10.3390/bs15030356

Oliveira, J. E. (2024). Neuropedagogia e neurodidática na identificação precoce de transtornos no desenvolvimento cognitivo de crianças e adolescentes. *RECIMA21-Revista Científica Multidisciplinar-ISSN 2675-6218, 5*(2), e524886-e524886.

Olofin, S. O., & Olojo, O. J. (2022). Effect of brain-based strategy on senior secondary school students' performance in mathematics in Ekiti State. *International Journal of Education, Learning and Development, 10*(2), 1–15. DOI: 10.37745/ijeld.13/vol10no2pp.1-15

Ormrod, J. E. (1990). *Human learning: Principles, theories, and educational applications*. Merrill Publishing Co.

Ozcan, B., Sperati, V., Giocondo, F., Schembri, M., & Baldassarre, G. (2022). Interactive soft toys to support social engagement through sensory-motor plays in early intervention of kids with special needs. In *Proceedings of the 21st Annual ACM Interaction Design and Children Conference (IDC '22)*. Association for Computing Machinery, New York, NY, USA, 625-628. DOI: 10.1145/3501712.3535274

Özkan, B. (2015). *Development of a scientific process skills scale for children aged 60-72 months and the effect of a brain-based learning science program on scientific process skills.* Master's thesis. Marmara University.

Özkan, B., & Önder, A. (2021). Brain-based learning in children. *Neuropedagogy in Children and the Brain* (pp. 148-155). Ed. (G. Güven, M. N. Tuğluk, B. Özkan). Hedef Publishing.

Ozonoff, S., & Cathcart, K. (1998). Effectiveness of a home program intervention for young children with autism. *Journal of Autism and Developmental Disorders, 28*(1), 25–32. DOI: 10.1023/A:1026006818310 PMID: 9546299

Paciarotti, C., & Bertozzi, G. (2023). The impact of cross-cutting pedagogical features based on neuroeducation advances: Project-based learning vs. traditional lecturing in engineering education. *Journal of Engineering Education, 37*(3), 17–32. DOI: 10.16920/jeet/2024/v37i3/24002

Packer, M. J., & Moreno-Dulcey, F. A. (2022). Theory of puppets?: A critique of the use of puppets as stimulus materials in psychological research with young children. *Cognitive Development, 61*, 1–9. DOI: 10.1016/j.cogdev.2021.101146

Panksepp, J. (2007). Can PLAY diminish ADHD and facilitate the construction of the social brain?. *Journal of the Canadian Academy of child and adolescent psychiatry, 16*(2), 57-66.

Papanastasiou, G. P., Drigas, A. S., & Skianis, C. (2017). Serious games in preschool and primary education: Benefits and impacts on curriculum course syllabus. *International Journal of Emerging Technologies in Learning, 12*(1), 44. Advance online publication. DOI: 10.3991/ijet.v12i01.6065

Pashler, H., McDaniel, M., Rohrer, D., & Bjork, R. (2008). Learning styles. *Psychological Science in the Public Interest, 9*(3), 105–119. DOI: 10.1111/j.1539-6053.2009.01038.x

Patel, K., Katz, C. N., Kalia, S. K., Popovic, M. R., & Valiante, T. A. (2021). Volitional control of individual neurons in the human brain. *Brain, 144*(12), 3651–3663. DOI: 10.1093/brain/awab370

Patten, K. E. (2008). Toward a neuropedagogy of emotion.

Patten, K. E. (2011). The somatic appraisal model of affect: Paradigm for educational neuroscience and neuropedagogy. *Educational Philosophy and Theory, 43*(1), 87–97. DOI: 10.1111/j.1469-5812.2010.00712.x

Pávová, A., & Valent, M. (2020). Neuropedagogical knowledge in further education and counselling for teachers. In *10th International Adult Education Conference. Univerzita Karlova Pedagogická Fakulta, Prague.*

Peerbots, Inc. (2025). *Social robots for everyone*. https://www.peerbots.org/

Pehlivan, İ. (1995). *Yönetimde stres kaynakları*. Pegem Yayınları.

Pekrun, R. (2014). Emotions and learning. *Educational Practices Series, 24*, 1–31.

Pekrun, R., Goetz, T., Perry, R. P., Kramer, K., Hochstadt, M., & Molfenter, S. (2004). Beyond test anxiety: Development and validation of the test emotions questionnaire (TEQ). *Anxiety, Stress, and Coping, 17*(3), 287–316. DOI: 10.1080/10615800412331303847

Pellis, S. M., & Pellis, V. C. (2007). Rough-and-tumble play and the development of the social brain. *Current Directions in Psychological Science*, *16*(2), 95–98. DOI: 10.1111/j.1467-8721.2007.00483.x

Peng, P., Barnes, M. A., Wang, C., Wang, W., Li, S., Swanson, H. L., Dardick, W., & Tao, S. (2018). A meta-analysis on the relation between reading and working memory. *Psychological Bulletin*, *144*(1), 48–76. DOI: 10.1037/bul0000124

Perfetti, C., & Stafura, J. (2014). Word knowledge in a theory of reading comprehension. *Scientific Studies of Reading*, *18*(1), 22–37. DOI: 10.1080/10888438.2013.827687

Pergantis, P., Bamicha, V., Doulou, A., Christou, A. I., Bardis, N., Skianis, C., & Drigas, A. (2025). Assistive and Emerging Technologies to Detect and Reduce Neurophysiological Stress and Anxiety in Children and Adolescents with Autism and Sensory Processing Disorders: A Systematic Review. *Technologies*, *13*(4), 144. DOI: 10.3390/technologies13040144

Pergher, V., Vanbilsen, N., & Van Hulle, M. (2021). The effect of mental fatigue and gender on working memory performance during repeated practice by young and older adults. *Neural Plasticity*, *2021*, 6612805. Advance online publication. DOI: 10.1155/2021/6612805

Pericas, C., Clotas, C., Espelt, A., López, M. J., Bosque-Prous, M., Juárez, O., & Bartroli, M. (2022). Effectiveness of school-based emotional education program: A cluster-randomized controlled trial. *Public Health*, *210*, 142–148. DOI: 10.1016/j.puhe.2022.06.013 PMID: 35970016

Perry, T., & Malaia, E. (2013). Working memory intervention: A reading comprehension approach. In *Proceedings of the International Association for Development of the Information Society (IADIS) International Conference on Cognition and Exploratory Learning in the Digital Age (CELDA)* (pp. 3–9). IADIS.

Perry, B. D. (2002). Childhood experience and the expression of genetic potential: What childhood neglect tells us about nature and nurture. *Brain and Mind*, *3*(1), 79–100. DOI: 10.1023/A:1016557824657

Pervushina, N. A. (2018). Neuropedagogy And Bioethics Symbolism: Place In Knowledge Management. *European Proceedings of Social and Behavioural Sciences*.

Pervushina, N. A. (2019). A semiotic diagnostics of study kits in the era of neuropedagogy. *ΠΡΑΞΗΜΑ. Problemy vizual'noy semiotiki–ΠΡΑΞΗΜΑ. Journal of Visual Semiotics*, *4*, 194–205.

Pessoa, L. (2008). On the relationship between emotion and cognition. *Nature Reviews. Neuroscience*, *9*(2), 148–158. DOI: 10.1038/nrn2317

Peters-Scheffer, N., Didden, R., Korzilius, H., & Sturmey, P. (2011). A meta-analytic review of the effectiveness of comprehensive ABA-based early intervention programs for children with autism spectrum disorders. *Research in Autism Spectrum Disorders*, *5*(1), 60–69. DOI: 10.1016/j.rasd.2010.03.011

Phelps, E. A. (2006). Emotion and cognition: Insights from studies of the human amygdala. *Annual Review of Psychology*, *57*(1), 27–53. DOI: 10.1146/annurev.psych.56.091103.070234

Piaget, J. (1972). Development and learning. *Reading in child behavior and development*, 38-46.

Piddubna, O., Maksymchuk, A., Lytvychenko, D., Revutska, O., Moskalenko, M., & Sopina, O. (2023). Implementing neuropedagogical innovation in schools: From theory to practice. *BRAIN. Broad Research in Artificial Intelligence and Neuroscience*, *14*(2), 37–58. DOI: 10.18662/brain/14.2/443

Pinto, C. (2022). Neuropedagogy for multicultural classrooms: The neuromethodology for inclusion. *MLS Inclusion and Society Journal*, *2*(2), 207–218. DOI: 10.56047/mlsisi.v2i2.1676

Pinzón Blanco, D. M., & Téllez Sánchez, F. J. (2016). Neuropedagogical Tools: An Alternative to Improving Problem Solution Skills in Mathematics.

Polat, B., & Kara, M. (2023). The effect of toys and playing on child development. *Kastamonu University Faculty of Health Sciences Journal*, *2*(1), 1–10.

Polat, Ö., Akay, D., & Aydın, E. (2021). Examination of the Ministry of National Education's 2013 preschool education program from the perspective of brain-based learning. Brain-based learning approach. *National Education Journal*, *50*(229), 419–444.

Poole, K. L., Santesso, D. L., Van Lieshout, R. J., & Schmidt, L. A. (2018). Trajectories of frontal brain activity and socio-emotional development in children. *Developmental Psychobiology*, *60*(4), 353–363. DOI: 10.1002/dev.21620 PMID: 29457644

Poplack, S., Sankoff, D., & Miller, C. (1988). The social correlates and linguistic processes of lexical borrowing and assimilation. *Linguistics*, *26*(1), 47–104. DOI: 10.1515/ling.1988.26.1.47

Popovic, D., Ruef, A., Dwyer, D. B., Antonucci, L. A., Eder, J., Sanfelici, R., Kambeitz-Ilankovic, L., Oztuerk, O. F., Dong, M. S., Paul, R., Paolini, M., Hedderich, D., Haidl, T., Kambeitz, J., Ruhrmann, S., Chisholm, K., Schultze-Lutter, F., & Falkai, P. (2020). Traces of trauma: A multivariate pattern analysis of childhood trauma, brain structure, and clinical phenotypes. *Biological Psychiatry*, *88*(11), 829–842. DOI: 10.1016/j.biopsych.2020.05.020 PMID: 32782139

Posner, M. I., & Rothbart, M. K. (2007). Research on attention networks as a model for the integration of psychological science. *Annual Review of Psychology*, *58*(1), 1–23. DOI: 10.1146/annurev.psych.58.110405.085516 PMID: 17029565

Povoroznyuk, R., Pocheniuk, I., Gaidash, A., Rybakova, K., Ostropalchenko, Y., & Saifutdinova, O. (2024). Neuropedagogical guidelines for translation studies: Perceiving the linguistic-cultural markers of the other (foreign) in translation. *Revista Romaneasca pentru Educatie Multidimensionala, 16*(4), 185-209.

Pradeep, K., Anbalagan, R. S., Thangavelu, A. P., Aswathy, S., Jisha, V. G., & Vaisakhi, V. S. (2024). Neuroeducation: Understanding neural dynamics in learning and teaching. *Frontiers in Education*, *9*, 1437418. Advance online publication. DOI: 10.3389/feduc.2024.1437418

Pretorius, L. (2025). An active learning intervention for in-service teachers: Self-determination theory, heutagogy, neuroeducation and the (altered) flipped classroom in practice. *Curriculum Perspectives*, *45*(2), 1–14. DOI: 10.1007/s41297-024-00299-y

Proctor, C. P., Silverman, R. D., Harring, J. R., Jones, R. L., & Hartranft, A. M. (2020). Teaching bilingual learners: Effects of a language-based reading intervention on academic language and reading comprehension in grades 4 and 5. *Reading Research Quarterly*, *55*(1), 95–122. DOI: 10.1002/rrq.258

Pugh, K. R., Mencl, W. E., Shaywitz, B. A., Shaywitz, S. E., Fulbright, R. K., Constable, R. T., Skudlarski, P., Marchione, K. E., Jenner, A. R., Fletcher, J. M., Liberman, A. M., Shankweiler, D. P., Katz, L., Lacadie, C., & Gore, J. C. (2000). The angular gyrus in developmental dyslexia: Task-specific differences in functional connectivity within posterior cortex. *Psychological Science*, *11*(1), 51–56. DOI: 10.1111/1467-9280.00214 PMID: 11228843

Puglisi, A., Caprì, T., Pignolo, L., Gismondo, S., Chilà, P., Minutoli, R., Marino, F., Failla, C., Arnao, A. A., Tartarisco, G., Cerasa, A., & Pioggia, G. (2022). Social Humanoid Robots for Children with Autism Spectrum Disorders: A Review of Modalities, Indications, and Pitfalls. *Children (Basel, Switzerland)*, *9*(7), 953. DOI: 10.3390/children9070953 PMID: 35883937

Pyle, A., & Danniels, E. (2017). A continuum of play-based learning: The role of the teacher in play-based pedagogy and the fear of hijacking play. *Early Education and Development, 28*(3), 274–289. DOI: 10.1080/10409289.2016.1220771

Ragozzino, M. E. (2007). The contribution of the medial prefrontal cortex, orbitofrontal cortex, and dorsomedial striatum to behavioral flexibility. *Annals of the New York Academy of Sciences, 1121*(1), 355–375. DOI: 10.1196/annals.1401.013

Rahmani, E., Mahvelati, A., Alizadeh, A., Mokhayeri, Y., Rahmani, M., Zarabi, H., & Hassanvandi, S. (2022). Is neurofeedback effective in children with ADHD? A systematic review and meta-analysis. *Neurocase, 28*(1), 84–95. DOI: 10.1080/13554794.2022.2027456

Räisänen, T., & Kankaanranta, A. (2024). The use of English as corporate language in global knowledge work over a 15-year business career. *European Journal of International Management, 23*(4), 677–700. DOI: 10.1504/EJIM.2024.139611

Rakhmetova, A. K., Meiirova, G., Balpanova, D. T., Baidullayeva, A. K., & Nurmakhanova, D. E. (2024). The Use of Elements of Neuropedagogy in the Creation of Virtual Simulators for In-Depth Study of Chemistry in Higher Education. *Journal of Technology and Science Education, 14*(2), 473–483. DOI: 10.3926/jotse.2532

Ramey, C. T., & Ramey, S. L. (2023). Early childhood education that promotes lifelong learning, health, and social well-being: The Abecedarian Project and its replications. *Medical Research Archives, 11*(11). Advance online publication. DOI: 10.18103/mra.v11i11.4590

Rana, R., & Mahmood, N. (2010). The relationship between test anxiety and academic achievement. *Bulletin of Education and research, 32*(2), 63-74.

Rapport, M. D., Kofler, M., Alderson, R., Timko, T.Jr, & DuPaul, G. (2009). Variability of attention processes in ADHD: Observations from the classroom. *Journal of Attention Disorders, 12*(6), 563–573. DOI: 10.1177/1087054708322990

Rasch, B., & Born, J. (2013). About sleep's role in memory. *Physiological Reviews, 93*(2), 681–766. DOI: 10.1152/physrev.00032.2012

Rashwan, H. K. A. (2024). *Bridging the Gap between Neuroscience and Education: What are Teachers' Perceptions of Applying "Neuropedagogy" to High School Classrooms?* (Master's thesis, The American University in Cairo (Egypt)).

Rasskazova, O., Anholenko, V., Pecherytsia, N., Hryhorenko, V. A., Tsybulina, I., Andreieva, M., & Yefimtseva, H. (2023). An Overview of the Principles of an Inclusive Approach in Education in Ukraine in the First Decade of the 21st Century as a Neuroscientific Factor. *BRAIN. Broad Research in Artificial Intelligence and Neuroscience*, *14*(4), 373–387. DOI: 10.18662/brain/14.4/511

Reichow, B., Hume, K., Barton, E. E., & Boyd, B. A. (2018). Early Intensive Behavioral Intervention (EIBI) for young children with autism spectrum disorder (ASD). *Cochrane Database of Systematic Reviews*, *5*(10), CD009260. Advance online publication. DOI: 10.1002/14651858.CD009260.pub3 PMID: 29742275

Revelle, W., & Condon, D. M. (2019). Reliability from α to ω: A tutorial. *Psychological Assessment*, *31*(12), 1395–1411. DOI: 10.1037/pas0000754 PMID: 31380696

Ribtsun, Y., Bielova, O., Korolenko, V., Bolotnykova, T., Govorun, O., & Myttseva, O. (2023). Personality development in the paradigm of current neuropedagogy. *BRAIN. Broad Research in Artificial Intelligence and Neuroscience*, *14*(4), 388–403. DOI: 10.18662/brain/14.4/512

Riccardi, M. (2023). How neuroscience and brain-based learning theory can enhance skill development of students in higher education. *Journal of Homeland Security Education*, *16*, 1–6.

Riggleman, S., Higgins, J., & Lohmann, M. J. (2025). Crafting Behavior Goal Cocktails: What's in Yours? Writing Behavioral Goals in Early Childhood. *Beyond Behavior*, *34*(1), 14–23. DOI: 10.1177/10742956241313104

Riggs, K. J., McTaggart, J., Simpson, A., & Freeman, R. P. J. (2006). Changes in the capacity of visual working memory in 5- to 10-year-olds. *Journal of Experimental Child Psychology*, *95*(1), 18–26. DOI: 10.1016/j.jecp.2006.03.009

Ritchey, M., Murty, V. P., & Dunsmoor, J. E. (2016). Adaptive memory systems for remembering the salient and the seemingly mundane. *Behavioral and Brain Sciences*, *39*, 1–75. DOI: 10.1017/S0140525X15001922 PMID: 28347387

Ritonga, A. R., Ahmad, L., Rosniati, H., & Dasrizal, D. (2025). Optimizing learning environments through the lens of neuroscience: A study on the role of emotion, motivation, and brain plasticity. *Jurnal Pendidikan Islam*, *6*(1), 12–19.

Rizzolatti, G., & Craighero, L. (2004). The mirror-neuron system. *Annual Review of Neuroscience*, *27*(1), 169–192. DOI: 10.1146/annurev.neuro.27.070203.144230 PMID: 15217330

Rizzolatti, G., & Sinigaglia, C. (2016). The mirror mechanism: A basic principle of brain function. *Nature Reviews. Neuroscience, 17*(12), 757–765. DOI: 10.1038/nrn.2016.135

Robinson, O. J., Vytal, K., Cornwell, B. R., & Grillon, C. (2013). The impact of anxiety upon cognition: Perspectives from human threat of shock studies. *Frontiers in Human Neuroscience, 7*. Advance online publication. DOI: 10.3389/fnhum.2013.00203

Rocher, C. Spedding, M., Munoz, C., & Jay, T. (2004). Acute stress-induced changes in hippocampal/prefrontal circuits in rats: Effects of antidepressants. *Cerebral Cortex, 14*(2), 224-229.

Roediger, H. L.III, & Butler, A. C. (2010). The critical role of retrieval practice in long-term retention. *Trends in Cognitive Sciences, 15*(1), 20–27. DOI: 10.1016/j.tics.2010.09.003

Roe, J., & Aspinall, P. (2011). The restorative benefits of walking in urban and rural settings in adults with good and poor mental health. *Health & Place, 17*(1), 103–113. DOI: 10.1016/j.healthplace.2010.09.003

Roozendaal, B. (2003). Systems mediating acute glucocorticoid effects on memory consolidation and retrieval. *Progress in Neuro-Psychopharmacology & Biological Psychiatry, 27*(8), 1213–1223. DOI: 10.1016/j.pnpbp.2003.09.015

Roozendaal, B., McEwen, B. S., & Chattarji, S. (2009). Stress, memory and the amygdala. *Nature Reviews. Neuroscience, 10*(6), 423–433. DOI: 10.1038/nrn2651

Rose, D. H., & Dalton, B. (2009). Learning to read in the digital age. *Mind, Brain and Education : the Official Journal of the International Mind, Brain, and Education Society, 3*(2), 74–83. DOI: 10.1111/j.1751-228X.2009.01057.x

Ross, P. M., Scanes, E., & Locke, W. (2023). Stress adaptation and resilience of academics in higher education. *Asia Pacific Education Review*. Advance online publication. DOI: 10.1007/s12564-023-09829-1

Ruba, A. L., & Pollak, S. D. (2020). The Development of Emotion Reasoning in Infancy and Early Childhood. *Annual Review of Developmental Psychology, 2*(1), 503–531. DOI: 10.1146/annurev-devpsych-060320-102556

Rueckert, L., & Grafman, J. (1996). Sustained attention deficits in patients with right frontal lesions. *Neuropsychologia, 34*(10), 953–963. DOI: 10.1016/0028-3932(96)00016-4

Russell, J. D., & Herringa, R. J. (2021). Editorial: The Preschool Emotional Brain. *Journal of the American Academy of Child and Adolescent Psychiatry*, *60*(1), 29–31. DOI: 10.1016/j.jaac.2020.08.012 PMID: 32890671

Russ, S. W. (2023). *Play in child development and psychotherapy: Toward empirically supported practice* (3rd ed.). Routledge.

Rusydiana, I. (2023). Enhancing Learning Outcomes Through Neuropedagogy-Based Quantum Teaching. *Journal of Education and Religious Studies*, *3*(03), 76–83.

Ryan, R. M., & Deci, E. (2000). Self-determination theory and the facilitation of intrinsic motivation, social development, and well-being. *The American Psychologist*, *55*(1), 68–78. DOI: 10.1037/0003-066X.55.1.68

Ryan, R. M., & Deci, E. L. (2009). Promoting self-determined school engagement: Motivation, learning and well-being. In Wentzel, K. R., & Wigfield, A. (Eds.), *Handbook of motivastion at school* (pp. 171–195). Routledge.

Sadreimova, G., & Zhumabayeva, A. (2023). Neuropedagogical approaches to early intervention for children with autism spectrum disorder. *Education and Pedagogy Journal*, *15*(4), 221–236.

Şahin, H., & Seven, S. (2020). *Erken çocuklukta kaygı. H. Uzun (Dü.) içinde, Recent advances in education and sport researches*. Gece Kitaplığı.

Saputra, I., Kurniawan, A., Yanita, M., Putri, E. Y., & Mahniza, M. (2024). The evolution of educational assessment: How artificial intelligence is shaping the trends and future of learning evaluation. *Indonesian Journal of Computer Science*, *13*(6). Advance online publication. DOI: 10.33022/ijcs.v13i6.4465

Sarason, I. G., & Stoops, R. (1978). Test anxiety and the passage of time. *Journal of Consulting and Clinical Psychology*, *46*(1), 102–109. DOI: 10.1037/0022-006X.46.1.102 PMID: 627645

Sarrasin, J. B., Nenciovici, L., Brault Foisy, L.-M., Allaire-Duquette, G., Riopel, M., & Masson, S. (2008). Effects of teaching the concept of neuroplasticity to induce a growth mindset on motivation, achievement, and brain activity: A meta-analysis. *Trends in Neuroscience and Education*, *12*, 22–31. DOI: 10.1016/j.tine.2018.07.003

Savage, R., Lavers, N., & Pillay, V. (2007). Working memory and reading difficulties: What we know and what we don't know about the relationship. *Educational Psychology Review*, *19*(2), 185–221. DOI: 10.1007/s10648-006-9024-1

Savchenko, O., Prystai, H., Hulych, M., Sobol, L., & Stupnytska, H. (2023). Neuropedagogy of Communication-Imitation. Opportunities for the Ukrainian English Teacher. *BRAIN. Broad Research in Artificial Intelligence and Neuroscience*, *14*(3), 164–181. DOI: 10.18662/brain/14.3/468

Schaaf, R. C., & Case-Smith, J. (2014). Sensory interventions for children with autism. *Journal of Comparative Effectiveness Research*, *3*(3), 225–227. DOI: 10.2217/cer.14.18 PMID: 24969147

Schertz, K. E., Meidenbauer, K., & Berman, M. (2021). Understanding the affective benefits of interacting with nature.In E. Brymer, M. Rogerson, & J. Barton, *Nature and health. Physical activity in nature* (s. 7-22). Routledge. DOI: 10.4324/9781003154419-2

Schlaggar, B. L. (2007). Are We Ready for a Neuropedagogy?.

Schloesser, R. J., Huang, J., Klein, P. S., & Manji, H. K. (2008). Cellular plasticity cascades in the pathophysiology and treatment of bipolar disorder. *Neuropsychopharmacology : Official Publication of the American College of Neuropsychopharmacology*, *33*(1), 110–133. DOI: 10.1038/sj.npp.1301575

Schnitzer, K. E. (2019). *Discovering the educational implications of neuropsychological research: Understanding the impact of neuroeducation instruction on fifth-grade students and their teachers* (Doctoral dissertation, San Diego State University). ProQuest Dissertations Publishing. https://www.proquest.com/openview/79fd118aa695afe8d9dcca55afdba70c/1?pq-origsite=gscholar&cbl=18750&diss=y

Schonert-Reichl, K. A., Oberle, E., Lawlor, M. S., Abbott, D., Thomson, K., Oberlander, T. F., & Diamond, A. (2015). Enhancing cognitive and social–emotional development through a simple-to-administer mindfulness-based school program for elementary school children: A randomized controlled trial. *Developmental Psychology*, *51*(1), 52–66. DOI: 10.1037/a0038454

Schreibman, L., Dawson, G., Stahmer, A. C., Landa, R., Rogers, S. J., McGee, G. G., & Halladay, A. (2015). Naturalistic developmental behavioral interventions: Empirically validated treatments for autism spectrum disorders. *Journal of Autism and Developmental Disorders*, *45*(8), 2411–2428. DOI: 10.1007/s10803-015-2407-8 PMID: 25737021

Schultz, W. (2016). Dopamine reward prediction-error signalling: A two-component response. *Nature Reviews. Neuroscience*, *17*(3), 183–195. DOI: 10.1038/nrn.2015.26

Schwabe, L., Joëls, M., Roozendaal, B., Wolf, O. T., & Oitzl, M. S. (2012). Stress effects on memory: An update and integration. *Neuroscience and Biobehavioral Reviews, 36*(7), 1740–1749. DOI: 10.1016/j.neubiorev.2011.07.002

Schwabe, L., & Wolf, O. T. (2010). Learning under stress impairs memory formation. *Neurobiology of Learning and Memory, 93*(2), 183–188. DOI: 10.1016/j.nlm.2009.09.009

Schwanz, K. A., Palm, L., & Brallier, S. (2007). Attention problems and hyperactivity as predictors of college grade point average. *Journal of Attention Disorders, 11*(3), 368–373. DOI: 10.1177/1087054707305155

Selye, H. (1956). *The stress of life*. McGraw-Hill.

Semelius Granevald, V. (2025). Exploring factors related to special needs educators' work-related well-being in preschool settings. *European Journal of Special Needs Education, 40*(4), 1–16. DOI: 10.1080/08856257.2024.2421111

Sen, A. (2022). Revisiting Brain-Based Learning: Strategies And Implications In The Higher Education Scenario. In *INTED2022 Proceedings* (pp. 10084-10090). IATED.

Seo, J. H., Aravindan, P., & Sungkajun, A. (2017). Toward Creative Engagement of Soft Haptic Toys with Children with Autism Spectrum Disorder. In Proceedings of the 2017 ACM SIGCHI Conference on Creativity and Cognition (C&C '17). Association for Computing Machinery, New York, NY, USA, 75-79. DOI: 10.1145/3059454.3059474

Seth, R. (2023). Children with cancer: Shared care and transition of care. *Indian Journal of Pediatrics, 90*(12), 1232–1236. DOI: 10.1007/s12098-023-04644-3 PMID: 37368222

Shabatat, K., & Al-Tarawneh, M. (2016). The impact of a teaching-learning program based on a brain-based learning program on the achievement of female students in 9th grade in chemistry. *Higher Education Studies, 6*(2), 162–173. DOI: 10.5539/hes.v6n2p162

Shalom, M., & Luria, E. (2022). Neuro-pedagogy Course-Breaching the Borders Between Neuroscience and Education. *World Studies in Education, 23*(2), 51–67. DOI: 10.7459/wse/22.2.04

Sharma, A. (2024). Effectiveness of brain-based learning strategy using blended mode of teaching elementary school science students. *Educational Administration: Theory and Practice, 30*(4), 7294–7296. DOI: 10.53555/kuey.v30i4.2556

Shaywitz, S. E., & Shaywitz, B. A. (2008). Paying attention to reading: The neurobiology of reading and dyslexia. *Development and Psychopathology, 20*(4), 1329–1349. DOI: 10.1017/S0954579408000631 PMID: 18838044

She, C., Liag, Q., Jiang, W., & Xing, Q. (2023). Learning adaptability facilitates self-regulated learning at school: The chain mediating roles of academic motivation and self-management. *Frontiers in Psychology, 14*, 1162072. Advance online publication. DOI: 10.3389/fpsyg.2023.1162072

Shekh-Abed, A. (2024). Metacognitive self-knowledge and cognitive skills in project-based learning of high school electronics students. *European Journal of Engineering Education*, •••, 1–16. DOI: 10.1080/03043797.2024.2374479

Shields, G. S., Sazma, M. A., McCullough, A. M., & Yonelinas, A. P. (2017). The effects of acute stress on episodic memory: A meta-analysis and integrative review. *Psychological Bulletin, 143*(6), 636–675. DOI: 10.1037/bul0000100

Shiwlani, A., Hasan, S. U., & Kumar, S. (2024). Artificial intelligence in neuroeducation: A systematic review of AI applications aligned with neuroscience principles for optimizing learning strategies. *Journal of Digital and Social Sciences.* https://doi.org/DOI: 10.47205/jdss.2024(5-IV)50

Shiwlani, A., Hasan, S. U., & Kumar, S. (2024). Artificial Intelligence in Neuroeducation: A Systematic Review of AI Applications Aligned with Neuroscience Principles for Optimizing Learning Strategies. *Journal of Development and Social Sciences, 5*(4), 578–593.

Shloul, T. A., Mazhar, T., Abbas, Q., Iqbal, M., Ghadi, Y. Y., Shahzad, T., Mallek, F., & Hamam, H. (2024). Role of activity-based learning and ChatGPT on students' performance in education. *Computers and Education Artificial Intelligence, 6*, 100219. DOI: 10.1016/j.caeai.2024.100219

Shokhrukh, A. (2024). The Dominance of English in The Global Technology Industry: Implications for Non-English-Speaking Countries. *Universal Journal of Social Sciences. Philosophy and Culture, 2*(11), 41–55.

Shonkoff, J. P., & Phillips, D. A. (Eds.). (2000). *From neurons to neighborhoods: The science of early childhood development.* National Academy Press.

Shulha, L., Hnizdilova, O., Matishak, M., Marchii-Dmytrash, T., Yaroslavtseva, M., & Chorna, H. (2021). Developing Creative Abilities in Preschoolers in Painting Classes via the Principles of Neuropedagogy and Psychology of Creativity in Ukraine. *Revista Romaneasca Pentru Educatie Multidimensionala, 13*(4), 614–632. DOI: 10.18662/rrem/13.4/501

Shultz, K. S., Whitney, D. J., & Zickar, M. J. (2020). Confirmatory Factor Analysis. *Measurement Theory in Action, II*, 302–316. DOI: 10.4324/9781003127536-19

Shvarts-Serebro, I., Ben-Yehudah, G., Elgavi-Hershler, O., Grobgeld, E., Katzof, A., Luzzatto, E., Shalom, M., & Zohar-Harel, T. (2024, June). Agents of change: Integration of neuropedagogy in pre-service teacher education. [). Frontiers Media SA.]. *Frontiers in Education, 9*, 1369394. DOI: 10.3389/feduc.2024.1369394

Sigman, M., Peña, M., Goldin, A. P., & Ribeiro, S. (2014). Neuroscience and education: Prime time to build the bridge. *Nature Neuroscience, 17*(4), 497–502. DOI: 10.1038/nn.3672

SILVA, D. F. D. (2021). A neuropedagogia no processo de ensino e aprendizagem: uma abordagem da neurociência aplicada à educação no ensino fundamental I.

Silva-López, R. B., Fallad, J., Reyes-Ortiz, J. A., Bravo, M., & Rodriguez, J. (2015, December). Techno neuro pedagogy system: An instructional design methodology for customized online courses (virtual customized environment learning). In *2015 International Conference on Computational Science and Computational Intelligence (CSCI)* (pp. 281-286). IEEE. DOI: 10.1109/CSCI.2015.166

Silva-López, R. B., Reyes-Ortiz, J. A., Bravo, M., Federal, D., Fallad, J., de la Costa Sur, C. U., & Rodriguez, J. (2015). Techno Neuro Pedagogy System: an instructional design methodology for customized online courses. In *International Conference on Computational Science and Computational Intelligence*.

Singer, D., Golinkoff, R. M., & Hirsh-Pasek, K. (2006). *Play= Learning: How play motivates and enhances children's cognitive and social-emotional growth*. Oxford University Press. DOI: 10.1093/acprof:oso/9780195304381.001.0001

Siricharoen, N. (2023). Creative brain training apps and games can help improve memory, cognitive abilities, and promote good mental health for the elderly. *EAI Endorsed Transactions on Context-Aware Systems and Applications, 9*(1). Advance online publication. DOI: 10.4108/eetcasa.v9i1.3524

Skinner, B. F. (1957). *Behavior verbal*. Appleton-Century -Crofts. DOI: 10.1037/11256-000

Slavikivna, B. O., Viktor, R., Oleksandrivna, V. O., Alina, D., Yurii, K., & Svitlana, B. (2023). Innovative Learning Technologies for Future Elementary School Teachers in the Context of Neuropedagogy.

Slot, P. L., Mulder, H., Verhagen, J., & Leseman, P. P. (2017). Preschoolers' cognitive and emotional self-regulation in pretend play: Relations with executive functions and quality of play. *Infant and Child Development, 26*(6), e2038. DOI: 10.1002/icd.2038

Smakman, M., Vogt, P., & Konijn, E. A. (2021). Moral considerations on social robots in education: A multi-stakeholder perspective. *Computers & Education, 174*, 104317. Advance online publication. DOI: 10.1016/j.compedu.2021.104317

Smart, J. R. (1985). In Netton, I. R. (Ed.), *Language development in the Gulf: Lexical interference of English in the Gulf dialects* (pp. 202–212).

Smith, L. B., Jayaraman, S., Clerkin, E., & Yu, C. (2018). The developing infant creates a curriculum for statistical learning. *Trends in Cognitive Sciences, 22*(4), 325–336. DOI: 10.1016/j.tics.2018.02.004

Smith, R., Snow, P., Serry, T., & Hammond, L. (2021). The role of background knowledge in reading comprehension: A critical review. *Reading Psychology, 42*(3), 214–240. DOI: 10.1080/02702711.2021.1888348

Smith, T., & Iadarola, S. (2015). Evidence update on autism spectrum disorders. *Journal of Clinical Child and Adolescent Psychology, 44*(6), 897–922. DOI: 10.1080/15374416.2015.1077448 PMID: 26430947

Smith, T., & Jones, R. M. (2022). Advances in ABA: Integrating neuroscience into practice. *Journal of Applied Behavior Analysis, 55*(2), 210–225.

Snow, C. (2002). *Reading for understanding: Toward an R&D program in reading comprehension*. Rand Corporation.

Soichuk, R., Khrypun, D., Sydoruk, I., Serheieva, V., Shevchenko, V., & Shevchenko, S. (2022). Problems of organization of education of children with special educational needs in the conditions of contemporary primary school (in the context of neuropedagogy). *BRAIN. Broad Research in Artificial Intelligence and Neuroscience, 13*(4), 383–397. DOI: 10.18662/brain/13.4/394

Solano Orellana, G. P. (2025). Exploring innovative neuropedagogical implications in english as a forign language teaching.

Solano, G., & Vega, M. (2024). Exploring Innovative Neuropedagogical Implications in English as a Foreign Language Teaching. *RUNAS. Journal of Education & Culture, 5*(10), 12.

Soleiman, P., Moradi, H., Mahmoudi, M., Teymouri, M., & Pouretemad, H. R. (2021). Teaching turn-taking skills to children with autism using a parrot-like robot. arXiv. Retrieved from https://arxiv.org/abs/2101.12273

Song, C., Shin, S., & Shin, K. (2024). Implementing the dynamic feedback-driven learning optimization framework: A machine learning approach to personalize educational pathways. *Applied Sciences (Basel, Switzerland)*, *14*(2), 916. DOI: 10.3390/app14020916

Sotres-Bayon, F., & Quirk, G. (2010). Prefrontal control of fear: More than just extinction. *Current Opinion in Neurobiology*, *20*(2), 231–234. DOI: 10.1016/j.conb.2010.02.005

Sousa, D. A. (2011). *How the brain learns*. Corwin Press. DOI: 10.4135/9781452219684

Sousa, D. A. (2011). Mind, brain, and education: The ımpact of educational neuroscience on the science of teaching. *LEARNing Landscapes*, *5*(1), 37–43. DOI: 10.36510/learnland.v5i1.529

Soyalp, T. (2022). *The effect of brain-based learning theory on the achievement and attitudes of 8th-grade students in science education. Master's thesis. Gazi University.* Master's thesis. Gazi University.

Soysal, A. Ş., Yalçın, K., & Can, H. (2008). Bilişsel psikoloji kapsamında yer alan dikkat teorileri. *New Symposium Journal, 46*(1), 35-41.

Sözer Çapan, A. (2014). *An investigation of the effect of an education program prepared according to the brain-based learning approach on the creativity skills of 5-year- old children.* Doctoral thesis. Marmara University.

Spinka, M., Newberry, R. C., & Bekoff, M. (2001). Mammalian play: Training for the unexpected. *The Quarterly Review of Biology*, *76*(2), 141–168. DOI: 10.1086/393866

Squire, L. R. (2004). Memory systems of the brain: A brief history and current perspective. *Neurobiology of Learning and Memory*, *82*(3), 171–177. DOI: 10.1016/j.nlm.2004.06.005

Squire, L. R., Genzel, L., Wixted, J. T., & Morris, R. G. (2015). Memory consolidation. *Cold Spring Harbor Perspectives in Biology*, *7*(8), a021766. DOI: 10.1101/cshperspect.a021766

Srisang, P., & Everatt, J. (2021). Lower and higher level comprehension skills of undergraduate EFL learners and their reading comprehension. *LEARN Journal: Language Education and Acquisition Research Network*, *14*(1), 427–454.

Stahmer, A. C., Rieth, S. R., Dickson, K. S., Feder, J., Burgeson, M., Searcy, K., & Brookman-Frazee, L. (2020). Project ImPACT for Toddlers: Pilot outcomes of a community adaptation of an intervention for autism risk. *Autism*, *24*(3), 617–632. DOI: 10.1177/1362361319878080 PMID: 31565955

Stang, K. (2022). *Brain-based learning methods and student achievement.* Master's thesis. Bethel University.

Stanton, J. D., Sebesta, A. J., & Dunlosky, J. (2021). Fostering metacognition to support student learning and performance. *CBE Life Sciences Education, 20*(2), fe3. DOI: 10.1187/cbe.20-12-0289

Starkman, M. N., Gebarski, S., Berent, S., & Schteingart, D. (1992). Hippocampal formation volume, memory dysfunction, and cortisol levels in patients with Cushing's syndrome. *Biological Psychiatry, 32*(9), 756–765. DOI: 10.1016/0006-3223(92)90079-F

Stassinopoulos, R. L. (2023). *Cultivating student engagement and enhancing teaching self-efficacy in higher education STEM: A neuroeducation framework* (Doctoral dissertation, Johns Hopkins University). Johns Hopkins Institutional Repository. http://jhir.library.jhu.edu/handle/1774.2/68866

Stein, J. (2023). Theories about developmental dyslexia. *Brain Sciences, 13*(2), 208. DOI: 10.3390/brainsci13020208 PMID: 36831750

Stein, M. B., Simmons, A. N., Feinstein, J. S., & Paulus, M. P. (2007). Increased amygdala and insula activation during emotion processing in anxiety-prone subjects. *The American Journal of Psychiatry, 164*(2), 318–327. DOI: 10.1176/ajp.2007.164.2.318

Steinmetz, K. R., Addis, D., & Kensinger, E. (2010). The effect of arousal on the emotional memory network depends on valence. *NeuroImage, 53*(1), 318–324. DOI: 10.1016/j.neuroimage.2010.06.015

Stein, Z., & Fischer, K. (2011). Directions for mind, brain, and education: Methods, models and morality. *Educational Philosophy and Theory, 43*(1), 56–66. DOI: 10.1111/j.1469-5812.2010.00708.x

Stepanyants, A., Hof, P., & Chklovskii, D. (2002). Geometry and structural plasticity of synaptic connectivity. *Neuron, 34*(2), 275–288. DOI: 10.1016/S0896-6273(02)00652-9

Sternberg, R. J. (1985). *Beyond IQ: A triarchic theory of human intelligence.* Cambridge University Press.

Stevens Smith, D. A. (2020). Brain-based teaching: Differentiation in teaching, learning, and motor skills. *Journal of Physical Education, Recreation & Dance, 91*(7), 34–42. DOI: 10.1080/07303084.2020.1781717

Stiles, J., & Jernigan, T. (2010). The basics of brain development. *Neuropsychology Review, 20*(4), 327–348. DOI: 10.1007/s11065-010-9148-4

Strickland, K. (2003). *Brain-compatible learning in a high school classroom.* Master's thesis, Royal Roads University, British Columbia. Thesis, Royal Roads University, British Columbia.

Stringer, S., & Tommerdahl, J. (2015). Building bridges between neuroscience, cognition and education with predictive modeling. *Mind, Brain and Education : the Official Journal of the International Mind, Brain, and Education Society, 9*(2), 121–126. DOI: 10.1111/mbe.12076

Stuijfzand, S., Creswell, C., Field, A. P., Pearcey, S., & Dodd, H. (2018). Research Review: Is anxiety associated with negative interpretations of ambiguity in children and adolescents? A systematic review and meta-analysis. *Journal of Child Psychology and Psychiatry, and Allied Disciplines, 59*(11), 1127–1142. DOI: 10.1111/jcpp.12822

Suleiman, Y. (2013). *Arabic in the fray: Language ideology and cultural politics.* Edinburgh University Press.

Sundberg, M. L. (2008). *VB-MAPP: Verbal Behavior Milestone Assessment and Placement Program.* AVB Press.

Sundberg, M. L. (2008). *Verbal Behavior Milestone Assessment and Placement Program (VB-MAPP): A language and social skills assessment program for children with autism or other developmental disabilities.* AVB Press.

Supriatna, N., Fauzi, W. I., & Holilah, M. (2019). Social Studies Comic: Application of Neuropedagogy Approach To Social Studies Text Book of Smp Kelas Vii. *International Journal Pedagogy of Social Studies, 4*(2).

Swanson, H. L., & Beebe-Frankenberger, M. (2004). The relationship between working memory and mathematical problem solving in children at risk and not at risk for serious math difficulties. *Journal of Educational Psychology, 96*(3), 471–491. DOI: 10.1037/0022-0663.96.3.471

Swanson, H. L., & O'Connor, R. (2009). The role of working memory and fluency practice on the reading comprehension of students who are dysfluent readers. *Journal of Learning Disabilities, 42*(6), 548–575. DOI: 10.1177/0022219409338742

Syabila, H., & Irvan, M. (2022). The Effect of Interactive Hand Puppet on Joint Attention Ability in Children with Autism. *Proceedings of the International Conference on Education 2022 (ICE 2022).* DOI: 10.2991/978-2-38476-020-6_10

Syrotkina, Z., Bankul, L., Bukhniieva, O., Boychev, I., Gunko, N., & Chekhunina, A. (2022). The Arts as a Means of Developing Emotional Intelligence in the Context of Neuropedagogy. *BRAIN. Broad Research in Artificial Intelligence and Neuroscience, 13*(4), 306–320. DOI: 10.18662/brain/13.4/390

Szécsi, T., Varga, L., & Mák, V. (2018). Current trends, dilemmas and future directions in neuropedagogy in the field of early childhood. *Képzés és Gyakorlat: Neveléstudományi folyóirat, 16*(3), 51-58.

Taber, K. S. (2018). The Use of Cronbach ' s Alpha When Developing and Reporting Research Instruments in Science Education. *Research in Science Education, 48*(6), 1273–1296. DOI: 10.1007/s11165-016-9602-2

Tabibnia, G. (2024). Neuroscience education as a tool for improving stress management and resilience. *Current Opinion in Behavioral Sciences, 59*, 101401. DOI: 10.1016/j.cobeha.2024.101401

Tafuri, G., Scala, G., Di Lorenzo, G., & Gravino, G. (2024). Theoretical Review on inclusive education for children with special educational needs: From the main teaching techniques to the innovative aspects of neuropedagogy. *Journal of Inclusive Methodology and Technology in Learning and Teaching, 4*(2).

Tamis-LeMonda, C. S., & Masek, L. R. (2023). Embodied and embedded learning: Child, caregiver, and context. *Current Directions in Psychological Science, 32*(5), 369–378. DOI: 10.1177/09637214231178731

Tamm, L., Menon, V., & Reiss, A. L. (2006). Parietal attentional system aberrations during target detection in adolescents with attention deficit hyperactivity disorder: Event-related fMRI evidence. *The American Journal of Psychiatry, 163*(6), 1033–1043. DOI: 10.1176/ajp.2006.163.6.1033

Tan, P. Z., Oppenheimer, C. W., Ladouceur, C. D., Butterfield, R. D., & Silk, J. S. (2020). A review of associations between parental emotion socialization behaviors and the neural substrates of emotional reactivity and regulation in youth. *Developmental Psychology, 56*(3), 516–527. DOI: 10.1037/dev0000893 PMID: 32077721

Tanrıdağ, O. (2018). *The development of the child's brain*. Üsküdar University Publications.

Tarasenko, H., Zhurat, Y., Lipshyts, L., Soter, M., Chumak, L., Valchuk-Orkusha, O., & Melnyk, I. (2020). Developing Professional Subjectivity in Future Primary School Teachers in the Context of a Neuropedagogical Approach.

Tariq, M., Tariq, A., & Sadiq, A. H. B. (2024). Exploring Domestication and Lexical borrowing in the Urdu Translation of Doctor Faustus. *Harf-o-Sukhan, 8*(1), 291–299.

Téllez, M. N. B., Sotomayor, C. R., & Tobar, A. P. (2018). La gestión de los procesos neuropedagógicos del aprendizaje y la necesidad de un docente conectado con la neuropedagogía. *Opuntia Brava, 10*(2), 310–321.

Temirbekova, A. (2025). Neuropedagogical foundations of linguistics: Programming theory and practice. *International Journal of Pedagogics*, *5*(03), 203–205. DOI: 10.37547/ijp/Volume05Issue03-58

Thiessen, E. J., Gibson, H. D., Regis, D., Pehrsson, S. J., Ashley, K. T., & Smit, M. A. (2020). The distinct metamorphic stages and structural styles of the 1.94–1.86 Ga Snowbird Orogen, Northwest Territories, Canada. *Journal of Metamorphic Geology*, *38*(9), 963–992. DOI: 10.1111/jmg.12556

Thomas, M. S. C. (2020). *Educational neuroscience: Development across the life span*. Routledge. DOI: 10.4324/9781003016830

Thomas, M. S., Ansari, D., & Knowland, V. C. (2019). Annual research review: Educational neuroscience: Progress and prospects. *Journal of Child Psychology and Psychiatry, and Allied Disciplines*, *60*(4), 477–492. DOI: 10.1111/jcpp.12973

Thomason, S. G., & Kaufman, T. (1988). *Language contact, creolization, and genetic linguistics*. University of California Press. DOI: 10.1525/9780520912793

Thompson, L., & Thompson, M. (1998). Neurofeedback combined with training in metacognitive strategies: Effectiveness in students with ADD. *Applied Psychophysiology and Biofeedback*, *23*(4), 243–263. DOI: 10.1023/A:1022213731956

Tian, M. (2023). Research on the Application of Domestication and Lexical borrowing in Literary Translation. *International Journal of Education and Humanities*, *9*(1), 87–92. DOI: 10.54097/ijeh.v9i1.9364

Tian, X., Abdul Samat, N., & Zainal, Z. (2023). Gender differences in Chinese EFL learners' comprehension when reading across mediums. *English Language Teaching*, *17*(3), 32–44. DOI: 10.5539/elt.v17n3p32

Tillery, R., Howard Sharp, K. M., Okado, Y., Long, A., & Phipps, S. (2015). Profiles of Resilience and Growth in Youth With Cancer and Healthy Comparisons. *Journal of Pediatric Psychology*, *41*(3), 290–297. DOI: 10.1093/jpepsy/jsv091 PMID: 26423321

Tincani, M. and Devis, K. (2011). Quantitative synthesis and analysis of the components of single-participant studies on the image exchange communication system. *Education specialized and specialized, 32* (6), 458-470. https://doi.org/DOI: 10.1177/0741932510362494

Tokuhama-Espinosa, T. (2011). *Mind, brain, and education science: A comprehensive guide to the new brain-based teaching*. W. W. Norton.

Tokuhama-Espinosa, T. (2021). *Bringing the neuroscience of learning to online teaching: an educator's handbook.* Teachers College Press.

Tooley, U. A., Bassett, D. S., & Mackey, A. P. (2021). Environmental influences on the pace of brain development. *Nature Reviews. Neuroscience, 22*(6), 372–384. DOI: 10.1038/s41583-021-00457-5

Torres Martín, C. (2024). Neurodidáctica y transferencia del conocimiento a través del aprendizaje activo por competencias.

Touhami, F. (2020). L'intégration des TIC dans la prise en charge globale des enfants ayant des troubles spécifiques des apprentissages: Cas de la dyslexie (Master's thesis). Université Hassan II, Casablanca.

Trembath, D., Waddington, H., Sulek, R., Varcin, K., Bent, C., Ashburner, J., Eapen, V., Goodall, E., Hudry, K., Silove, N., & Whitehouse, A. (2021). An evidence-based framework for determining the optimal amount of intervention for autistic children. *The Lancet. Child & Adolescent Health, 5*(12), 896–904. DOI: 10.1016/S2352-4642(21)00285-6 PMID: 34672993

Trimingham, M. (2010). 'Objects in transition: The puppet and the autistic child'. *Journal of Applied Arts & Health, 1*(3), 251–265. DOI: 10.1386/jaah.1.3.251_1

Tsymbal-Slatvinska, S., Maksymchuk, B., Saienko, V., Babii, I., Behas, L., Lemeshchuk, M., Chepka, O., Dychok, T., & Maksymchuk, I. (2022). Psycho-pedagogical experience of intellectual education in the views of Ukrainian and foreign pedagogues as the basis of modern neuropedagogy. *BRAIN. Broad Research in Artificial Intelligence and Neuroscience, 13*(4), 321–346. DOI: 10.18662/brain/13.4/391

Turhan, B., & Özbay, Y. (2016). Erken çocukluk eğitimi ve nöroplastisite. *Uluslararası Erken Çocukluk Eğitimi Çalışmaları Dergisi, 1*(2), 54–63.

Turner, V. (2004). *The Anthropology of Performance*. PAJ Publications.

Umilta, C. (1988b). The control operations of consciousness. A. Marcel, & E. Bisiach (Dü) içinde, *Consciousness in contemporary science* (s. 334-356). Clarendon Press/Oxford University Press.

Umilta, C. (1988a). *Orienting of Attention. F. Boller, & J. Grafman (Dü) içinde, Handbook of Neuropsychology*. Elsevier.

Umurzakova, A. U. (2024). Arabic Language in the Era of Globalization: Problems and Solutions. *O'zbekiston davlat jahon tillari universiteti konferensiyalari*, 126-129.

UNESCO. (2018). Shadow play. UNESCO Intangible Cultural Heritage. Retrieved from https://ich.unesco.org/en/USL/shadow-play-01368

UNESCO. (2020). *Global education monitoring report 2020: Inclusion and education: All means all.* UNESCO.

UNESCO. (2023a). *Guidance for generative AI in education and research.* UNESCO Publishing.

UNESCO. (2023b). *Advancing preschool education in Morocco: Goals of inclusion, quality, and sustainable governance.* UNESCO. https://www.unesco.org/en/early-childhood-education/advancing-preschool-education-morocco-goals-inclusion-quality-and-sustainable-governance

UNICEF. (2025). *Childhood in a digital world: Innocenti report 2025.* UNICEF Office of Research–Innocenti.

Ur Rehman, S., Malik, A., Jawad, M., & Khan, M. (2025). The Influence of Technology on Contemporary English Vocabulary: Neologisms and Digital Discourse. *Review of Applied Management and Social Sciences, 8*(1), 157–168. DOI: 10.47067/ramss.v8i1.445

Vagg, P. R., Spielberger, C. D., & O'Hearn, T. P.Jr. (1980). Is the state-trait anxiety inventory multidimensional? *Personality and Individual Differences, 1*(3), 207–214. DOI: 10.1016/0191-8869(80)90052-5

Van den Berg, C. L., Hol, T., Van Ree, J. M., Spruijt, B. M., Everts, H., & Koolhaas, J. M. (1999). Play is indispensable for an adequate development of coping with social challenges in the rat. *Developmental Psychobiology, 34*(2), 129–138. DOI: 10.1002/(SICI)1098-2302(199903)34:2<129::AID-DEV6>3.0.CO;2-L

Van Mierlo, B., & Beers, P. J. (2018). Understanding and governing learning in sustainability transitions: A review. *Environmental Innovation and Societal Transitions, 34*, 255–269. DOI: 10.1016/j.eist.2018.08.002

Vance, D. E., Roberson, A., McGuinness, T., & Fazeli, P. (2010). How neuroplasticity and cognitive. *Journal of Psychosocial Nursing and Mental Health Services, 48*(4), 23–30. DOI: 10.3928/02793695-20100302-01

Vanderschuren, L. J., & Trezza, V. (2013). What the laboratory rat has taught us about social play behavior: role in behavioral development and neural mechanisms. *The neurobiology of childhood*, 189-212.

Vaninsky, A. (2017). Educational neuroscience, educational psychology, and classroom pedagogy as a system. *American Journal of Educational Research, 5*(4), 384–391. DOI: 10.12691/education-5-4-6

Varga, L., & Szécsi, T. (2018). Neuropedagogy in Early Childhood in Hungary: Foundations and Micro-investigation. *Képzés És Gyakorlat: Training And Practice, 16*(3), 67–74. DOI: 10.17165/TP.2018.3.8

Vargas Angulo, L. E., Manuel SellanIcasa, V., Escobar Torres, A. F., & Ramos Fuentes, L. F. (2022). Neuropedagogía, sugerencias metodológicas para su aplicación en la enseñanza superior. *Roca: Revista Científico-Educacional de la Provincia de Granma, 18*(1).

Vasilieva, S. A., Reipolska, O. D., Podoliuk, S., Sadova, I., Danyliak, R., & Lozenko, A. (2023). The relationship between neuropedagogic approaches and the formation of skills of primary school students. *Revista Romaneasca Pentru Educatie Multidimensionala, 1*(15), 352–365. DOI: 10.18662/rrem/15.1/700

Vecchi, V. (2010). *Art and creativity in Reggio Emilia: Exploring the role and potential of ateliers in early childhood education*. Routledge. DOI: 10.4324/9780203854679

Vernucci, S., Canet Juric, L., Introzzi, I., & Richards, M. (2019). Working memory training in children: A review of basic methodological criteria. *Psychological Reports, 123*(3), 1–18. DOI: 10.1177/0033294119832978

Virués-Ortega, J.Virués -Ortega. (2010). Behavior analytic intervention applied to autism in early childhood: Meta-analysis, meta-regression, and dose-response meta-analysis of multiple outcomes. *Clinical Psychology Review, 30*(4), 387–399. DOI: 10.1016/j.cpr.2010.01.008 PMID: 20223569

Voineskos, A. N. (2020). Mapping effects of childhood trauma onto brain systems and behavior. *Biological Psychiatry, 88*(11), 810–811. DOI: 10.1016/j.biopsych.2020.08.009 PMID: 33153524

Volpicelli, F., & Miniaci, M. C. (2024). Dopaminergic pathways and their impact on learning and motivation in educational contexts. *Biomedicines, 15*, 210–230. DOI: 10.1038/nrn1406

Vorotyntseva, O., Pozniak, O., Voitenko, A., Lopatina, H., Huz, I., & Husieva, T. (2022). The Preparation of Specialists for the Realization of Individual Education Path of Children with Special Educational Needs: Neuropedagogical Aspects. *BRAIN. Broad Research in Artificial Intelligence and Neuroscience, 13*(2), 97–112. DOI: 10.18662/brain/13.2/334

Vygotsky, L. S. (1978). *Mind in society: The development of higher psychological processes*. Harvard University Press.

Vynogradova, O., Zdanevych, L., Sivak, N., Melnychuk, S., Polianovska, O., & Motoziuk, L. (2021). The system of modern social work with children with disabilities in the context of neuropedagogy: Traditions and Innovations. BRAIN. *Broad Research in Artificial Intelligence and Neuroscience, 12*(3), 287–302. DOI: 10.18662/brain/12.3/232

Wang, S., & Aamodt, S. (2012). Play, stress, and the learning brain. *Cerebrum*,12.

Wang, J., Yang, Y., Li, L., Yang, X., Guo, X., Yuan, X., Xie, T., Yang, K., & Zhuang, J. (2024). Comparative efficacy of physical activity types on executive functions in children and adolescents: A network meta-analysis of randomized controlled trials. *Journal of Science and Medicine in Sport, 27*(3), 187–196. DOI: 10.1016/j.jsams.2023.11.006 PMID: 38042755

Wang, Y., Zhu, Z., Chen, B., & Fang, F. (2018). Perceptual learning and recognition confusion reveal the underlying relationships among the six basic emotions. *Cognition and Emotion*, •••, 1–14. DOI: 10.1080/02699931.2018.1491831 PMID: 29962270

Watagodakumbura, C. (2014). *Programming the brain: Educational neuroscience perspective, pedagogical practices and study skills*. Xlibris Corporation.

Watagodakumbura, C. (2017). Principles of curriculum design and construction based on the concepts of educational neuroscience. *Journal of Education and Learning, 6*(3), 54–69. DOI: 10.5539/jel.v6n3p54

Whitebread, D., & Basilio, M. (2013). *Play, culture and creativity*. Cultures of Creativity. Billund, Denmark. *The LEGO Foundation, 76*, 82.

Whitebread, D., Basilio, M., Kuvalja, M., & Verma, M. (2012). *The importance of play*. Toy Industries of Europe.

Whole Child Neuro. (2024, July 15). *How play supports cognitive, emotional, and social development in children*. Whole Child Neuro. https://www.wholechildneuro.com/blog/how-play-supports-cognitive-emotional-and-social-development-in-children

Widhiyanti, S. (2023). Brain based learning approach in early childhood learning. In *ICECEM 2022: Proceedings of the 1st International Conference on Early Childhood Education in Multiperspective, ICECEM 2022, 26th November 2022, Purwokerto, Central Java, Indonesia* (p. 103). European Alliance for Innovation. DOI: 10.4108/eai.26-11-2022.2339366

Wieser, M. J., Pauli, P., & Mühlberger, A. (2009). Probing the attentional control theory in social anxiety: An emotional saccade task. *Cognitive, Affective & Behavioral Neuroscience, 9*(3), 314–322. DOI: 10.3758/CABN.9.3.314

Wijayanti, K. D., & Sulaksono, D. (2018). Character building for early childhood learners through the shadow puppet-based Javanese language manners. In *Proceedings of the Third International Conference of Arts, Language and Culture (ICALC 2018).* Atlantis Press.

Williamson, B., Pykett, J., & Kotouza, D. (2025). Learning brains: Educational neuroscience, neurotechnology and neuropedagogy. *Pedagogy, Culture & Society*, •••, 1–21. DOI: 10.1080/14681366.2025.2521458

Williams, P., Sheridan, S., Garvis, S., & Mellgren, E. (2018). Early childhood education and care in Sweden: The context of Swedish preschool. In *International Perspectives on Early Childhood Education and Care* (pp. 189–201). Routledge. DOI: 10.4324/9780203730553-17

Willis, J. (2008). Building a bridge from neuroscience to the classroom. *Phi Delta Kappan*, *89*(6), 424–427. DOI: 10.1177/003172170808900608

Winnicott, D. W. (1953). Transitional objects and transitional phenomena. *The International Journal of Psycho-Analysis*, *34*, 89–97. PMID: 13061115

Winnicott, D. W. (1971). *Playing and Reality.* Tavistock Publications.

Wolf, M. (2007). Proust and the squid: The story and science of the reading brain. *New York.*

Wong, C., Odom, S. L., Hume, K. A., Cox, A. W., Fettig, A., Kucharczyk, S., Brock, M. E., Plavnick, J. B., Fleury, V. P., & Schultz, T. R. (2015). Evidence-based practices for children, youth, and young adults with autism spectrum disorder: A comprehensive review. *Journal of Autism and Developmental Disorders*, *45*(7), 1951–1966. DOI: 10.1007/s10803-014-2351-z PMID: 25578338

Woollett, K., & Maguire, E. A. (2012). Exploring anterograde associative memory in London taxi drivers. *Neuroreport*, *23*(15), 885–888. DOI: 10.1097/WNR.0b013e328359317e

Wulan, S., & Jamaris, M. (2023). Increasing Children's Character Overt Behaviours by Neuro Pedagogy-Based Play. *Jurnal Pendidikan Usia Dini*, *17*(2), 363–377. DOI: 10.21009/JPUD.172.12

Wu, S. (2024). Artificial intelligence applications in early childhood developmental assessment: Opportunities and challenges. *Frontiers in Psychology*, *15*, 1348294. DOI: 10.3389/fpsyg.2024.1348294

Yánez, L. Y. C., Paredes, R. R. P., Guamarica, S. M. P., Naranjo, V. M. G., & Andrade, R. E. A. (2025). Abordando los retos de la educación del siglo XXI: perspectivas de la neuropedagogía para el aprendizaje y el desarrollo cognitivo integral.: Addressing the challenges of XXI st century education: perspectives of neuro pedagogy for comprehensive learning and cognitive development. *Revista Científica Multidisciplinar G-Nerando, 6*(1), ág-255.

Yeager, D. S., & Dweck, C. S. (2012). Mindsets that promote resilience: When students believe that personal characteristics can be developed. *Educational Psychologist, 47*(4), 302–314. DOI: 10.1080/00461520.2012.722805

Yepes Landinez, Y. A., Barón Peña, J. D., Campuzano Rojas, D., Barrera Sepulveda, C. Y., Cantor Herrera, A., González Giraldo, C. S., ... & Embus Alzate, V. (2024). Overview of Neuroeducation Basic Principles.

Yermakova, S., Ivanova, O., Horytska, O., Polishchuk, V., Polukhtovych, T., & Vivcharenko, T. (2023). Influence of the Neuro-Educational Environment on One's Socialization under Total Digitalization. *BRAIN. Broad Research in Artificial Intelligence and Neuroscience, 14*(4), 593–611.

Yonamine, M. (2022). Domestication and lexical borrowing in interlingual subtitling: A systematic review of contemporary research. *Translation & Interpreting: The International Journal of Translation and Interpreting Research, 14*(1), 198–213.

Yonelinas, A. P., & Ritchey, M. (2015). The slow forgetting of emotional episodic memories: An emotional binding account. *Trends in Cognitive Sciences, 19*(5), 259–267. DOI: 10.1016/j.tics.2015.02.009

Yousuf, Mustafa (2022). "The Phenomenon of Language Borrowing at the Arabic Language Academy" (in Arabic) *Sardiyāt* , vol 12, issue 44, pp 85-136.

Yuan, X. (2022). Evidence of the spacing effect and influences on perceptions of learning and science curricula. *Cureus*. Advance online publication. DOI: 10.7759/cureus.21201

Yu, C. (2019). (in Review). Endocrine consequences of childhood cancer therapy and transition considerations. *Pediatrics, 48*(8), e326–e332. DOI: 10.3928/19382359-20190729-02 PMID: 31426101

Yuce, A. E. (2023). Physical, social and emotional needs of developing children: Comparison of neuroscientific findings and Bertrand Russell's ideas. *Journal of Theory and Practice in Education, 19*(1), 123–139.

Yu, H., & Choatchamrat, S. (2024). Integrating Jiang Han Ping Yuan Shadow Puppetry into Education for Cultural Protection and Literacy Development. *International Journal of Education and Literacy Studies, 12*(1), 206–212. DOI: 10.7575/aiac.ijels.v.12n.1p.206

Yurdakul, Y., Ilhan Ildız, G., & Ayhan, A. B. (2022). The examination of the relationship between self-regulation skills and prosocial behaviors in preschool children. *Mehmet Akif Ersoy University Journal of Education Faculty*, (62), 354–376. doi:10.21764/maeuefd.1008817

Zadina, J. N. (2015). The emerging role of educational neuroscience in education reform. *Psicologia Educativa, 21*(2), 71–77. DOI: 10.1016/j.pse.2015.08.005

Zamarreño, P., Mateos, P. M., & Valentín, A. (2024). Working memory training improves episodic memory in older people: Transfer based on controlled retrieval processes. *Frontiers in Psychology, 15*, 1–11. DOI: 10.3389/fpsyg.2024.1314483

Zambrano, I. G. V., & Mieles, J. E. C. (2023). Neuropedagogical strategies for the attention of simple language delay in infants. *Revista San Gregorio, 1*, 56–71.

Zeidner, M. (1998). Test anxiety: The state of the art.

Zhang, J., Yin, Z., Chen, P., & Nichele, S. (2020). Emotion recognition using multimodal data and machine learning techniques: A tutorial and review. *Information Fusion, 59*, 103–126. DOI: 10.1016/j.inffus.2020.01.011

Zhang, Z., Sangsawang, T., Vipahasna, K., & Pigultong, M. (2024). A Mixed-Methods Data Approach Integrating Importance-Performance Analysis (IPA) and Kaiser-Meyer-Olkin (KMO) in Applied Talent Cultivation. *Journal of Applied Data Sciences, 5*(1), 256–267. https://doi.org/https://doi.org/10.47738/jads.v5i1.170. DOI: 10.47738/jads.v5i1.170

Zhang, Z., Su, H., Peng, Q., Yang, Q., & Cheng, X. (2011). Exam anxiety induces significant blood pressure and heart rate increase in college students. *Clinical and Experimental Hypertension (New York, N.Y.), 33*(5), 281–286. DOI: 10.3109/10641963.2010.531850

Zhao, C., Deng, W., & Gage, F. (2008). Mechanisms and functional implications of adult neurogenesis. *Cell, 132*(4), 645–660. DOI: 10.1016/j.cell.2008.01.033

Zhao, S., Xiong, S. C., Pang, B., Tang, X., & He, P. (2025). Let AI read first: Enhancing reading abilities for individuals with dyslexia through artificial intelligence. *Journal of Artificial Intelligence in Education, 22*(4), 301–314. DOI: 10.1145/3706599.3720113

Zhurat, Y., Lipshyts, L., Soter, M., Chumak, L., Tarasenko, H., Valchuk-Orkusha, O., & Melnyk, I. (2021). Developing professional subjectivity in future primary school teachers in the context of a neuropedagogical approach. *BRAIN. Broad Research in Artificial Intelligence and Neuroscience, 11*(2Sup1), 64-81.

Zosh, J. M., Hopkins, E. J., Jensen, H., Liu, C., Neale, D., Pasek, K. H., ... & Whitebread, D. (2017). *Learning through play: A review of the evidence.*

Zull, J. E. (2002). *The art of changing the brain: Enriching the practice of teaching by exploring the biology of learning.* Stylus Publishing. https://moodle2.units.it/pluginfile.php/561006/mod_resource/content/1/el200409_zull.pdf

Zull, J. E. (2011). *From brain to mind: Using neuroscience to guide change in education.* Stylus Publishing. Tzirides, A. O. O., de Castro, V. C., Cope, B., & Kalantzis, M. (2025). Multimodality and transposition in collaborative language learning. In *Multimodal Literacy in English as an Additional Language in Higher Education* (pp. 67-86). Routledge.

About the Contributors

Driss Elomari is a prominent Moroccan scholar in pedagogical engineering and qualitative research. He earned his doctorate from Université Ibn Tofail and teaches at Université Sidi Mohamed Ben Abdellah in Fez. His research emphasizes knowledge engineering and the integration of digital tools in education, particularly augmented reality and online learning. Elomari is an active member of the Association de Technologie de l'Information pour l'Éducation et la Formation and has published extensively on collaborative skills and scientific knowledge construction. His contributions include designing professional development programs for educators and serving as a reviewer for notable journals. Elomari's innovative approach positions him as a leading figure in educational technology.

Nariman Aral, born in Turkey, has made significant strides in the field of child development, dedicating her career to understanding and improving the cognitive, emotional, and social development of children. She is currently a respected academic at Ankara University, where she is a key member of the faculty. Dr. Aral's journey in child development began early in her academic career. She has published numerous articles and studies on topics ranging from digital game addiction to media literacy in children, and the impacts of early childhood education. Her work often bridges theoretical pedagogy with practical applications, providing invaluable insights for educators and parents alike. One of her notable contributions is the examination of play behaviors in children with typical development compared to those with speech and language disorders. Her research has highlighted the crucial role of play in child development and has offered strategies for parents and educators to support children with developmental challenges. Dr. Aral's work extends beyond academia. She has been involved in various programs aimed at educating parents and caregivers on child development issues. Her commitment to enhancing the well-being of children is evident in her efforts to investigate the impacts of media literacy programs and early childhood education on young minds. Throughout her career, Dr. Aral has collaborated with other experts in the field, contributing to a broader understanding of child development across different cultural contexts. Her work has been published in numerous reputable journals, and she continues to be a leading voice in the field. Dr. Nariman Aral's dedication to child development and education has made a lasting impact on the field, inspiring many to follow in her footsteps. Her research and advocacy work continue to influence educational practices and policies, ensuring that children receive the support they need to thrive.

Bayram Deleş completed his undergraduate education at Eurasia University Faculty of Health Sciences, Department of Child Development. In 2020, he graduated from Üsküdar University Institute of Health Sciences, Department of Child Development. The same year, he started her doctorate education at Ankara University Institute of Health Sciences, Department of Child Development. He worked as a lecturer at Ardahan University Vocational School of Health Services, Department of Child Care and Youth Services in 2021. He was appointed as a lecturer at Erzincan Binali Yıldırım University Vocational School of Health Services, Department of Child Care and Youth Services, in 2022, and he is still working at the said university. The author has papers in congresses, articles in international and national journals, and chapter authorship in books. He is married and has two children

Mostafa Bouanani is Professor of Arabic linguistics, cognitive linguistics and didactic of languages at USMBA. He is the director of the International Institute for Research and Studies in Cognitive Sciences, deputy director of the Language Sciences, Literature, Arts, Communication and History Laboratory, director and editor-in-chief of the international peer-reviewed journal "Cognitive Research" and a member of the ALFA: ECM research team of the University of Quebec in Montreal, Canada. Founding director of the Cognitive Sciences Laboratory (2007-2017), Founding member of the International Transdisciplinary Research Group on Education (GRITE) and director of the research center "Languages, Communication and Arts" (2014-2017). His academic research focuses on phonetics, phonology and morphology. His research interests are in language teaching (Arabic and French), learning difficulties/disorders and cognitive linguistics (comprehension/ production of language, mental lexicon) and neuroeducation (methodologies/ strategies of teaching/ learning of languages, visual and auditory perception of language).

***

Ashraf Alam currently holds the position of Research Faculty at the Centre of Excellence in Public Policy, Sustainability and ESG Research, housed within the

Faculty of Law and Policy Studies at Alliance University, Bangalore. Renowned for his transdisciplinary acumen spanning education, technology, and policy studies, Dr. Alam has been distinguished as one of the World's Top 2% Scientists by Stanford University and Elsevier, an accolade that highlights the breadth and depth of his scholarly impact. His prolific academic output includes over fifty SCOPUS-indexed publications and more than one hundred conference presentations at esteemed national and international academic forums. His educational trajectory reflects both depth and versatility: a Ph.D. in Education from the Indian Institute of Technology (IIT) Kharagpur, an M.Ed. with a concentration in Mathematics Education, and a B.S. in Computer Science from the University of Delhi. He also holds postgraduate degrees in Public Administration (M.A.) and Mathematics (M.Sc.), supplemented by a suite of postgraduate diplomas in Higher Education, Guidance and Counselling, Educational Technology, Criminology and Police Administration, and Value Education. Dr. Alam is an active participant in global scholarly discourse. As Associate Editor of Frontiers in Education, he plays a pivotal role in curating and guiding intellectual contributions across the Educational, Pedagogical, and Learning Sciences. Concurrently, he serves as Founder and Director of Academic Chronicles Private Limited, where he orchestrates editorial board formation and develops strategic frameworks for peer-reviewed publishing in the Social, Behavioural, and Humanistic Sciences. His research has been disseminated through elite academic platforms, including Elsevier, Springer, Taylor & Francis, Wiley, Routledge, Sage, Emerald, and IEEE, and addresses a remarkably diverse array of topics such as pedagogical theories, educational administration, educational psychology, educational sociology, educational policy, technology-integrated learning, mathematics education, educational philosophy, educational technology, teacher education, and AI/ML in learning environments. Dr. Alam's scholarly rigor is further demonstrated by his success in qualifying multiple prestigious examinations including UGC-NET-JRF in both Education and Adult and Continuing Education, UGC- NET in Public Administration, and GATE in Humanities and Social Sciences. At the heart of Dr. Alam's intellectual ethos lies a steadfast belief in education as a catalytic and emancipatory force capable of engendering social justice, human flourishing, societal progress, and sustainable transformation. His recent explorations into 'Happiness Engineering' and holistic well- being in school ecosystems articulate a vision of education that transcends instrumentalist paradigms, prioritizing emotional intelligence, global consciousness, empathy, and psychosocial resilience among learners. His research agenda seeks to conceive educational praxis through the affordances of inclusive digital learning, gamified instructional design, and artificial intelligence (AIEd), thereby constructing robust, ethically grounded frameworks for 21st century education. At Alliance University, Dr. Alam remains committed to architecting pedagogical models that not only cultivate intellectual dexterity and cognitive excellence but also prepare learners for morally responsive leadership, intellectual nimbleness, and responsible global citizenship in an increasingly volatile, uncertain, complex, and ambiguous (VUCA) world.

Arzu Aydın, M.A., is a lecturer at the School of Foreign Languages, Karabük University, Türkiye. She earned her bachelor's degree in English Language Teaching from Akdeniz University and completed her master's degree in Curriculum and Instruction at Hacettepe University. She is currently a PhD candidate in Child Development and Education at Karabük University. She has been serving as a lecturer for 15 years. Her research interests include early childhood second language acquisition, children's literature, educational technologies, and the integration of artificial intelligence in early childhood education.

Flora Bakopoulou is a Professor of Pediatrics & Adolescent Medicine School of Medicine, National and Kapodistrian University of Athens

Abdellah Barebzi is a Moroccan researcher specializing in education and learning sciences, he has published several articles and books. He served as a university professor at the Higher School of Teachers (ENS) in Meknes, Moulay Ismail University, Morocco, and currently holds the position of head of the Department of Education Sciences and Educational Technology. Additionally, he is responsible for coordinating the Master's program in 'Education and Training Engineering,' along with other educational responsibilities at the Higher School of Teachers (ENS) in Meknes

Şehnaz Ceylan graduated from Gazi University, Faculty of Vocational Education, Department of Child Development and Preschool Education in 1999. She started to work as a research assistant at Gazi University, Faculty of Vocational Education, Department of Child Development and Preschool Education in 2000. Prof. Dr. Şehnaz Ceylan completed her master's degree in 2003 and PhD in 2009 at Gazi University Institute of Educational Sciences, Department of Child Development and Education. She started to work at Karabük University Safranbolu Vocational High School as an Assistant Professor in 2009. She became an Associate Professor at Karabük University, School of Health Sciences, and in 2019 he became a Full-Professor. Prof. Dr. Şehnaz Ceylan currently works as a faculty member and Head of the Child Development Department, Faculty of Health Sciences at Karabük University. She has several publications on child development, infancy development, early intervention, social skills, creative drama, child rights, baby library and family education.

Subharthi Das has completed a Master of Arts in Education from Kazi Nazrul University and has a strong interest in research, particularly in education, artificial intelligence, sustainability, and related fields. She has authored several book chapters published on both national and international platforms. She is currently pursuing a Bachelor of Education (B.Ed.) from Baba Saheb Ambedkar Education University.

Ender Durualp graduated from Istanbul University, Florence Nightingale School of Nursing in 1995. She received her expert of science degree (M.Sc.) in 1999 with her thesis entitled "The effects of giving catheter care education to Newborn Intensive Care Unit nurses on the type of agents and colonization in the umbilical catheter". She received a second expert of science degree (M.Sc.) from Ankara University, School of Home Economics, Department of Child Development and Education. Then, she received PhD from the same University and department with her thesis entitled "A Study on the Effects of Play-Based Social Skills Training on Social Adaptation and Skills of Six-year-old Preschool Children: Sample of Cankırı". She became associate professor in 2014. She was appointed to the professorship in 2022. She is working as academician of Ankara University, Faculty of Health Sciences, Department of Child Development. She has many national and international articles, books and papers in the field of child development.

Hamza Ghoura, is a PhD's student at the Doctoral Studies Center at the University of Sidi Mohamed Ben Abdellah, Fez - Morocco (USMBA), Laboratory of Language Sciences, Literature, Arts, Communication, History and Education (SLLACHE) at the Faculty of Literature and Humanities, Dhar El Mehraz, Fez, and is a member of the International Institute for Research and Studies in Cognitive Sciences (IRESCO). He holds a BA degree in Arabic language and literature - Specialization in linguistics - from Sidi Mohamed Ben Abdelah University in Fez, and a master's degree in Linguistics and Arabic Lexicography from the Doha Institute for Graduate Studies in Qatar.

Lügen Güneş adopted the principle of preserving the spirit of childhood. Her career path has been deeply influenced by her volunteer work with children battling cancer. She completed her non-thesis master's degree in 2017 and her thesis-based master's degree in 2020 in the Department of Child Development at Ankara University, Institute of Health Sciences. Since 2020, she has been pursuing her Ph.D. in the same department. Since 2019, she has served as a research assistant in the Department of Child Development at Ankara University, Faculty of Health Sciences. She worked as a volunteer teacher at LÖSEV Primary School for many years and held positions as a preschool teacher in various institutions. In recognition of her contributions, she was honored with the "Volunteer Academic of the Year" award by LÖSEV on December 5, 2023, within the scope of International Volunteer Day. She has completed the creative drama leadership training stages of the Contemporary Drama Association. As a children's book author, Güneş published her first illustrated storybook Pufpanya: The City of Lost Colors in 2023 with Parmak Çocuk Publishing, a subsidiary of Yağmur Publishing Group. Her second book, The Strongest Potion in the World: HOOOP Bittirus Iksirus, was published by Yağmur Çocuk Publishing in 2025. Believing that books are among the most meaningful tools for reaching children, Güneş continues to offer them stories from the magical world of imagination and color—seeking to touch their lives through her words.

Santu Karmakar has completed a Master of Arts in Education from Kazi Nazrul University and has a strong interest in research, particularly in education, artificial intelligence, sustainability, and related fields. He has authored several book chapters published on both national and international platforms, including notable publishers such as Springer Nature, Taylor & Francis, and IGI Global. He is currently pursuing a Bachelor of Education (B.Ed.) from Baba Saheb Ambedkar Education University.

Amine Khadraoui is a Moroccan researcher in the field of psychology and educational sciences. He is a visiting professor of "Docimology and Evaluation" at the Higher School of Teachers (ENS), Moulay Ismail University, Meknes, Morocco. He has published several collective books and studies on learning, attention, gamification, and educational technology. He was also the recipient of the National Reading Award in Morocco (2019). In addition, he serves as the Head of Office at the National Social Security Fund (CNSS) in Morocco.

Mohamed Labrouzi is a doctoral researcher at the Doctoral Studies Center at Sidi Mohamed Ben Abdellah University, Fes – Morocco (USMBA), in the Laboratory of Language Sciences, Literature, Arts, Communication, History, and Education (SLLACHE) at the Faculty of Arts and Humanities, Dhar El-Mahraz, Fes. He is a researcher in cognitive and clinical psychology and a member of the International Institute for Studies and Research in Cognitive Sciences (IRESCO). He holds a Bachelor's degree in Psychology from Sidi Mohamed Ben Abdellah University in Fes, and a Master's degree in Clinical Psychology from the same university in Fes, Morocco

Houda Tahesse is a researcher at the Laboratory of Language Sciences, Literature, Arts, Communication, History, and Education (SLLACHE) at Sidi Mohamed Ben Abdellah University in Fez. Her research centers on the integration of digital technologies into pedagogical frameworks to enhance teaching and learning processes. She has developed solid expertise in the use of digital tools within educational contexts, aiming to create more inclusive, interactive, and stimulating learning environments. Her current research focuses on the design and enhancement of online and hybrid learning systems, as well as the creation of innovative educational resources

Yasemin Taşkıner Şereflioğlu is an experienced science teacher in Ankara. She completed her master's degree in science education. She has presented papers at conferences, published articles, and book chapters. Her goal is to develop students' scientific thinking skills and actively prepare them for national exams, science events, and competitions. Fostering a love of science, cultivating curiosity, and promoting lifelong are always among her priorities.

Ayşe Tuna is a lecturer at Trakya University, Turkey since 2005. She has authored papers in international conference proceedings, and has been actively serving as a reviewer for international conferences and journals. Her research interests are support services for the elderly and disabled, education of autistic and related communication handicapped children, human-robot interaction, human-computer interaction, and data management methodologies.

Index

A

B

C

D

E

I

K

L

M

N

P

R

S

T

V

W

www.ingramcontent.com/pod-product-compliance
Lightning Source LLC
LaVergne TN
LVHW062339300926
849161LV00007B/1753